INTENSIVE CARE IN NEPHROLOGY

INTENSIVE CARE IN NEPHROLOGY

Edited by

PATRICK T MURRAY

Associate Professor of Medicine

Anaesthesia and Critical Care, and Clinical Pharmacology

University of Chicago

Chicago, Illinois, USA

HUGH R BRADY

President

University College Dublin

Dublin, Ireland

JESSE B HALL

Professor and Section Chief

Section of Pulmonary and Critical Care Medicine

University of Chicago

Chicago, Illinois, USA

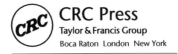

CRC Press
Taylor & Francis Group
Boca Raton London New York

CRC Press is an imprint of the
Taylor & Francis Group, an **informa** business

A TAYLOR & FRANCIS BOOK

First published 2006 by Taylor & Francis

Published 2019 by CRC Press
Taylor & Francis Group
6000 Broken Sound Parkway NW, Suite 300
Boca Raton, FL 33487-2742

© 2006 by Taylor & Francis Group, LLC
CRC Press is an imprint of Taylor & Francis Group, an Informa business

First issued in paperback 2019

No claim to original U.S. Government works

ISBN 13: 978-0-367-44644-4 (pbk)
ISBN 13: 978-1-84184-218-9 (hbk)

Visit the Taylor & Francis Web site at
http://www.taylorandfrancis.com

and the CRC Press Web site at
http://www.crcpress.com

A CIP record for this book is available from the British Library.

Library of Congress Cataloging-in-Publication Data
Data available on application

Composition by J&L Composition, Filey, North Yorkshire

Contents

CONTRIBUTORS

Robert C Albright Jr
Director of Dialysis
Division of Nephrology and Hypertension
Mayo Clinic College of Medicine
Rochester, MN
USA

Manar Alshahrouri
Section of Pulmonary and Critical Care Medicine
Rush University Medical Center
Chicago, IL
USA

John R Asplin
Nephrology
University of Chicago
Chicago, IL
USA

Robert A Balk
Section of Pulmonary and Critical Care Medicine
Rush University Medical Center
Chicago, IL
USA

Rinaldo Bellomo
Department of Intensive Care
Austin Hospital
Heidelberg, Victoria
Australia

Hugh R Brady
University College Dublin
Mater Misericordiae Hospital
Dublin
Ireland

William R Clark
Nephrology Division
Indiana University School of Medicine and
NxStage Medical, Inc.
Wishard Hospital
Indianapolis, IN
USA

Gilles Clermont
Department of Critical Care Medicine
University of Pittsburgh
Pittsburgh, PA
USA

Andrew Davenport
Centre for Nephrology
Royal Free Hospital
London
UK

John W Drover
Department of Surgery
Queen's University
Kingston, ON
Canada

William J Elliott
Department of Preventive Medicine
Rush University Medical Center
Chicago, IL
USA

Kevin W Finkel
Division of Renal Diseases and Hypertension
University of Texas MD Anderson Cancer Center
Houston, TX
USA

Marc Ghannoum
Division of Nephrology
Verdun Hospital
Montreal, QC
Canada

Tom A Golper
Vanderbilt University Medical Center
Professor of Medicine/Nephrology
Medical Director, Medical Specialities
Patient Care Center
Medical Center North
Nashville, TN
USA

Matthew D Griffin
Division of Nephrology and Hypertension
Mayo Clinic College of Medicine
Rochester, MN
USA

Kyle J Gunnerson
The Virginia Commonwealth University
Reanimation Engineering and Shock Center
(VCURES) Laboratory
Department of Anesthesiology, Division of Critical
Care
Department of Emergency Medicine
Virginia Commonwealth University Medical Center
Richmond, VA
USA

Jesse B Hall
Section of Nephrology
University of Chicago
Chicago, IL
USA

Daren K Heyland
Kingston General Hospital
Kingston, ON
Canada

Cheryl L Holmes
Critical Care Medicine
Kelowna General Hospital
Department of Medicine
University of British Columbia
Vancouver, BC
Canada

John Hotchkiss
CRISMA Laboratory
Department of Critical Care Medicine
University of Pittsburgh School of Medicine
Pittsburgh, PA
USA

Jose Iglesias
Clinical Associate Professor of Medicine
Department of Internal Medicine
Division of Nephrology
University of Medicine and Dentistry of
    New Jersey
School of Osteopathic Medicine
New Jersey, NJ
USA

Eduard A Iliescu
Department of Medicine
Queen's University
Kingston, ON
Canada

Munavvar Izhar
Department of Preventive Medicine
Rush University Medical Center
Chicago, IL
USA

John A Kellum
Critical Care and Medicine
University of Pittsburgh Medical Center
Pittsburgh, PA
USA

Niamh Kieran
Department of Medicine and Therapeutics
Mater Misericordiae University Hospital
Dublin
Ireland

Michael A Kraus
Nephrology Division
Indiana University School of Medicine
Indianapolis, IN
USA

Norbert Lameire
Renal Division
University Hospital Ghent
Ghent
Belgium

Martine Leblanc
Nephrology and Critical Care
Maisonneuve-Rosemont Hospital
Montreal, QC
Canada

Jerrold S Levine
Section of Nephrology
University of Illinois at Chicago
Chicago, IL
USA

Mark R Marshall
Nephrologist
Department of Renal Medicine
Middemore Hospital
Auckland
New Zealand

Gary R Matzke
Professor of Medicine and Pharmacy
Renal Division and Department of Pharmacy and
  Therapeutics
University of Pittsburgh
Pittsburgh, PA
USA

John McConville
Department of Medicine
University of Chicago
Chicago, IL
USA

Ravindra L Mehta
Clinical Nephrology and Dialysis Programs
Division of Nephrology
University of California at San Diego
  Medical Center
San Diego, CA
USA

Susan R Mendley
Departments of Pediatrics and Medicine
University of Maryland School of Medicine
Baltimore, MD
USA

Ayesa N Mian
Department of Pediatrics
University of Maryland School of Medicine
Baltimore, MD
USA

Patrick T Murray
Section of Nephrology
University of Chicago
Chicago, IL
USA

Neesh I Pannu
Divisions of Nephrology and Critical Care
University of Alberta
Edmonton, AB
Canada

Michael R Pinsky
Department of Critical Care Medicine
University of Pittsburgh School of Medicine
Pittsburgh, PA
USA

Rajiv Poduval
Southwest Kidney Institute
Phoenix, AZ
USA

Hamid Rabb
Division of Nephrology
Johns Hopkins University
Baltimore, MD
USA

Julie Raggio
Division of Nephrology and Hypertension
Georgetown University Medical Center
Washington, DC
USA

Miet Schetz
Department of Intensive Care Medicine
University Hospital Gasthuisberg
Leuven
Belgium

Gregory Schmidt
University of Chicago School of Medicine
Chicago, IL
USA

Andrew Shaw
Department of Critical Care
University of Texas MD Anderson Cancer Center
Houston, TX
USA

Joel Michels Topf
Section of Nephrology
Saint John Hospital
Detroit, MI
USA

Shigehiko Uchino
Departments of Intensive Care and Medicine
Austin & Repatriation Medical Centre
Melbourne
Australia

Jason G Umans
General Clinical Research Center
Georgetown University
Washington, DC
USA

Wim Van Biesen
Renal Division
University Hospital Ghent
Ghent
Belgium

Ramesh Venkataraman
CRISMA Laboratory
Department of Critical Care Medicine
University of Pittsburgh School of Medicine
Pittsburgh, PA
USA

Keith R Walley
UBC McDonald Research Laboratories
St Paul's Hospital
Vancouver, BC
Canada

Elaine Worcester
Section of Nephrology
University of Chicago
Chicago, IL
USA

Jack Work
Director
Interventional Nephrology
Department of Medicine
Emory University
Atlanta, GA
USA

Preface

Patrick T Murray, Hugh R Brady and Jesse B Hall

Renal dysfunction is extremely common in critically ill patients, in whom azotemia and abnormalities of fluid, electrolyte, or pH homeostasis are almost always present.[1,2] Whether managed by nephrologists, intensivists, or others caring for intensive care unit (ICU) patients, these problems present significant management challenges, requiring considerable expertise. The advent of ICUs, and, subsequently, the specialty of critical care medicine, has improved the management of critically ill patients. In some health systems, intensivists have largely assumed responsibility for management of renal, fluid, and electrolyte abnormalities in the ICU, including provision of renal replacement therapy with little or no nephrology input.[3] In other systems, nephrologists have primary or prominent consultative responsibility for the management of renal replacement therapy and other aspects of ICU nephrology.

Whoever is responsible, a common core of highly specialized knowledge is required to manage the range of disorders that could be considered ICU nephrology issues. This book is intended to be a resource for any practitioner responsible for the care of critically ill patients. It is organized in three sections, encompassing core topics in both critical care and nephrology, as well as specific related consultative topics. Section I provides up-to-date background information on the critically ill patient, including chapters on respiratory, circulatory, renal, and multiorgan failure. In Section II, core topics in ICU nephrology are discussed, including prevention and medical therapy of acute renal failure (ARF), and provision of a variety of renal replacement therapy (RRT) modalities. Finally, in Section III, a series of common ICU consultative nephrology topics is discussed.

This is an exciting time in critical care medicine. Our growing understanding of the pathogenesis of sepsis, shock, and organ dysfunction in ICU patients had led to the development of an increasing number of successful management strategies. The ARDSNet tidal volume study has determined a strategy for mechanical ventilation that decreases iatrogenic lung injury and improves outcome.[4] The same group is now investigating the optimal approach to management of fluid balance and hemodynamic monitoring in the critically ill. Improved use of sedation has also been demonstrated to improve outcome in patients with respiratory failure.[5] After years of failed trials of anti-inflammatory strategies and increased oxygen delivery to improve outcome in septic shock, we now have three positive trials in this population, utilizing anti-inflammatory (corticosteroids, activated protein C), anticoagulant (activated protein C), and hemodynamic therapies.[6–8] The management of early septic shock is improved by goal-directed therapy.[6] Corticosteroid therapy for adrenally insufficient patients with septic shock similarly improves survival.[7] Other approaches such as tighter glycemic control,[9] decreased use of harmful therapies such as inappropriate blood transfusion, and approaches to minimize nosocomial infection have also begun to improve outcome in ICU patients. Pivotal negative trials are also shaping the informed practice of critical care, such as the recent SAFE trial that showed no difference in outcome between crystalloid and colloid fluid resuscitation,[10] which has been an area of considerable controversy over the years. Coupled with advances in the management of acute coronary syndromes, we have many reasons to be optimistic that significant progress is being made in the understanding and management of critically ill patients.

Progress in the understanding, prevention, and management of human ARF has been less impressive than parallel advances in critical care in recent years. In nephrology, some long-cherished practices have been discarded following definitive studies, such as the negative ANZICS randomized controlled trial of low-dose dopamine for early ARF.[11,12] Other trials have provided the impetus for more aggressive RRT dosing in the ICU, with positive trials supporting the use of daily intermittent hemodialysis (IHD) or higher volumes of hemofiltration in this population.[13,14] Ongoing major trials will determine the answers to other major ICU nephrology questions:

- What is the preferred approach to fluid and hemodynamic management to prevent or treat ARF in critically ill patients?
- Should continuous renal replacement therapy (CRRT) or IHD be used for ARF, and at what doses?
- Is extracorporeal removal of inflammatory mediators a useful approach to the therapy of septic shock?

Many other topics must be addressed in this arena, however. ARF definitions and severity of illness scores that accurately predict ARF outcome in multiple populations (institutions, settings, etc.) are needed to improve the quality of diagnostic studies and clinical trials.[15,16] Real-time measures of renal perfusion and function (glomerular filtration rate or GFR) are not yet available.[2] Emerging biomarkers of renal injury may also help test and prove early interventions, in the same way that electrocardiographic findings and cardiac enzymes have facilitated progress in acute coronary syndromes. It remains a possibility that the discipline of genomics may yet reveal disease susceptibility genes for vascular disease or for acute renal failure specifically that predispose certain individuals to this complication. Identification of uremic mediators responsible for the adverse effects of ARF is clearly needed to guide the dosing of true acute 'renal replacement therapy'. Such information will do much to inform the design of studies to determine the optimal approach to avoidance, initiation, delivery, and withdrawal of RRT in ICU patients.

Multidisciplinary care with a team approach is the cornerstone of critical care medicine. It seems that the best approach to ICU care is to involve a variety of experts in consultation as needed with a trained intensivist and ICU team. Intensivists will never provide the full range of skills provided to care compre-hensively for every critically ill patient. Nephrologists are among those who we believe offer important skills to the ICU team. It is our hope that this book will provide important knowledge to nephrologists caring for ICU patients, and to intensivists who care for these problems, either alone or in a multidisciplinary group. We further hope that this school of thought will spur excellence and progress in the prevention and therapy of renal dysfunction in critically ill patients.

REFERENCES

1. Tang I, Murray PT. Prevention of perioperative ARF: What Works? Best Pract Res Clin Anesth 2004;18:91–111.
2. Murray PT, Le Gall JR, Dos Reis Miranda D et al. Physiologic end-points (efficacy) for acute renal failure studies. Curr Opin Crit Care 2002;8(6):519–25.
3. Murray PT, Hall JB. Renal replacement therapy for acute renal failure. Am J Respir Crit Care Med 2000;162:777–981.
4. ARDSNet. Ventilation with lower tidal volumes as compared with traditional tidal volumes for acute lung injury and the acute respiratory distress syndrome. N Engl J Med 2000;342:1301–8.
5. Kress JP, Pohlman AS, O'Connor MF, Hall JB. Daily interruption of sedative infusions in critically ill patients undergoing mechanical ventilation. N Engl J Med 2000;342:1471–7.
6. Rivers E, Nguyen B, Havstad S, et al. Early goal-directed therapy in the treatment of severe sepsis and septic shock. N Engl J Med 2001;345(19):1368–77.
7. Annane D, Sebille V, Charpentier C, et al. Effect of treatment with low doses of hydrocortisone and fludrocortisone on mortality in patients with septic shock. JAMA 2002;288:862–71.
8. Bernard GR, Vincent JL, Laterre PF, et al. Efficacy and safety of recombinant human activated protein C for severe sepsis. N Engl J Med 2001;344(10):699–709.
9. Van den Berghe G, Wouters P, Weekers F, et al. Intensive insulin therapy in the critically ill patients. N Engl J Med 2001;345(19):1359–67.
10. Finfer S, Bellomo R, Boyce N, et al. SAFE Study Investigators: a comparison of albumin and saline for fluid resuscitation in the intensive care unit. N Engl J Med 2004;350:2247–56.
11. Murray PT. Use of dopaminergic agents for renoprotection in the ICU. Yearbook of intensive care and emergency medicine. Berlin: Springer-Verlag; 2003:637–48.
12. ANZICS Clinical Trials Group. Low-dose dopamine in patients with early renal dysfunction: a placebo-controlled randomised trial. Lancet 2000;356:2139–43.
13. Schiffl H, Lang SM, Fischer R. Daily hemodialysis and the outcome of acute renal failure. N Engl J Med 2002;346:305–10.
14. Ronco C, Bellomo R, Homel P, et al. Effects of different doses in continuous veno-venous haemofiltration on outcomes of acute renal failure: a prospective randomized trial. Lancet 2000;356:26–30.
15. Kellum JA, Levin N, Bouman C, Lameire N. Developing a consensus classification system for acute renal failure. Curr Opin Crit Care 2002;8:509–14.
16. Halstenberg WK, Goormastic M, Paganini EP. Validity of four models for predicting outcome in critically ill acute renal failure patients. Clin Nephrol 1997;47(2):81–6.

I
Pathophysiologic principles

1

Shock

Cheryl L Holmes and Keith R Walley

INTRODUCTION

Shock is recognized at the bedside when hemodynamic instability leads to evidence of hypoperfusion of several organ systems. Accordingly, shock is a clinical diagnosis. Successful management of shock requires a primary survey directed at urgent initial resuscitation, which confirms or changes the working diagnosis, followed by a pause to ponder the broader differential diagnosis of the types of shock and the pathophysiology of shock, which leads to early definitive therapy of the underlying cause of shock. Shock has a hemodynamic component, which is the initial focus of resuscitation, but shock also has a systemic inflammatory component that leads to multiple system organ failure. Invasive hemodynamic monitoring should be goal-directed and discontinued as early as possible. Throughout this chapter, the importance of the tempo of resuscitation is emphasized.

SHOCK IS A CLINICAL DIAGNOSIS

Shock is present when there is evidence of multiple organ hypoperfusion. Clinical evidence of hypoperfusion includes tachycardia, tachypnea, low mean blood pressure, diaphoresis, mottled skin and extremities, altered mental status and decreased urine output (Box 1.1). An extremely low mean blood pressure will inevitably result in shock, as most organs require a head of pressure to maintain regional perfusion and function; therefore, shock is often recognized first when the blood pressure is low. An important caveat is that low blood pressure can present without shock and shock can be present despite elevated blood pressure. Therefore, shock must be recognized clinically by careful examination for evidence of multiple organ dysfunction.

Initial management of shock depends on the clinical hypothesis generation and testing at the bedside

A rapid clinical examination focused on determining the cause of shock is fundamental to successful resuscitation of the hypotensive patient. A simplified approach to the causes of shock allows the clinician to rapidly formulate a hypothesis and test that hypothesis by gauging the response to therapy.

While low blood pressure is not equivalent to shock, an extremely low blood pressure will result in shock, and a simplified 'Ohm's law' view suggests an initial approach to diagnosis of shock; i.e.

Mean arterial pressure (MAP) = Cardiac output (CO) × Venous resistance (VR)

Therefore, extremely low mean arterial pressure may be due to decreased cardiac output (which may be due to cardiac dysfunction or hypovolemia) or

---

Box 1.1 Defining features of shock

Low blood pressure
Rapid heart rate
High respiratory rate
Altered mentation
Low urine output
Metabolic acidosis

Table 1.1A   Rapid formulation of a working diagnosis of the etiology of shock.

	High cardiac output hypotension: vasodilatory shock	Low cardiac output hypotension: cardiogenic and hypovolemic shock
Is cardiac output reduced?	*No*	*Yes*
Pulse pressure	Wide	Narrow
Diastolic pressure	Very low	Low
Exremities, digits	Warm	Cool
Nailbed return	Rapid	Slow
Heart sounds	Crisp	Muffled
Temperature	Abnormally high or low	Normal
White blood cell count	Abnormally high or low	Normal
Site of infection	Present	Absent

Source: adapted from Walley and Wood[53] with permission.

Table 1.1B   Rapid formulation of a working diagnosis of the etiology of shock.

	Reduced pump function: cardiogenic shock	Reduced venous return: hypovolemic shock
Is the heart too full?	*Yes*	*No*
Symptoms, clinical context	Angina, abnormal ECG	Blood loss, volume depletion
Jugular venous pressure	High	Low
Gallop rhythm	Present	Absent
Respiratory examination	Crepitations	Normal
Chest radiograph	Large heart, pulmonary edema	Normal

Source: adapted from Walley and Wood[53] with permission.

decreased vascular resistance (Table 1.1). This approach suggests three useful questions.

The first question should be: 'Is there evidence of reduced cardiac output?' Evidence of reduced cardiac output is revealed at the bedside by cool extremities, peripheral and central cyanosis, poor peripheral pulses, sluggish nailbed return, muffled heart sounds, and a narrow pulse pressure. Reduced cardiac output occurs in hypovolemic shock and in cardiogenic shock.

The second question the clinician asks is: 'Is the heart too full?' A heart that is too full is manifest by elevated jugular venous pressure (JVP), peripheral edema, pulmonary edema and a large heart with extra heart sounds. Presence of these clinical signs strongly suggests cardiogenic shock, most often caused by ischemic heart disease, and they are

generally absent when low cardiac output results from decreased venous return (hypovolemia).

Hypovolemic shock is often suggested by the appropriate setting (trauma, childbirth, gastrointestinal bleeding), clinical manifestations of blood loss (hematemesis, tarry stools, abdominal distension) or dehydration (vomiting, diarrhea, thirst). Rapid differentiation between myocardial dysfunction and venous return is vitally important in management decisions (inotropic support and revascularization in cardiogenic shock and appropriate and rapid fluid infusions in hypovolemic shock) and requires that the bedside clinician possesses a basic understanding of factors that determine cardiac output.

Alternatively, the patient may present with evidence of a high cardiac output state despite evidence of multiple organ hypoperfusion such as low urine output and confusion, agitation or decreased level of consciousness. This patient will often have a wide pulse pressure, low diastolic pressure, warm extremities with good nailbed return and fever or hypothermia. These clinical findings strongly suggest a working diagnosis of vasodilatory shock of which septic shock is the paradigm. Appropriate therapy of septic shock includes fluid infusions, broad-spectrum antibiotic therapy, a search for reversible causes of sepsis, and vasopressor drug therapy.

The third question is: 'What doesn't fit?'. Often different etiologies of shock are combined at initial presentation so that the presentation is not classic. For example, if the initial clinical assessment suggests hypovolemic shock but aggressive fluid therapy fails to restore organ perfusion, the clinician must re-examine the patient and may need to re-address the hypothesis. Often, septic shock will initially present with clinical signs suggestive of hypovolemic shock but as the patient receives fluid, the pulse pressure widens, extremities become warm and pulses are bounding. Management must then be revised to ensure a successful outcome.

Alternatively, other specific etiologies of shock that fit within the broad categories defined by the first two questions (i.e. cardiogenic, hypovolemic, distributive) are identified. For example, obstructive shock due to pulmonary thromboembolism will present with (1) evidence of decreased cardiac output and (2) evidence that the heart is too full with distended jugular veins. However, examination of the chest does not suggest pulmonary edema, so that 'What doesn't fit?' requires re-examination of the broader differential diagnosis of this presentation of hypodynamic shock—leading to the caveat diagnosis of obstruction.

MANAGEMENT OF SHOCK

Successful management of shock depends on both the tempo of resuscitation and the administration of therapy appropriate to the cause of shock.

Urgent initial resuscitation should not be delayed

Urgent initial resuscitation aims to avoid later sequelae of organ system hypoperfusion by rapidly restoring an adequate circulation. Data from the thrombolysis in acute myocardial infarction trials demonstrate that time is tissue.[1,2] In fact, 'time is tissue' in all organ systems and all forms of shock. Prolonged ischemia results in a variety of cellular metabolic and ultrastructural changes that ultimately impair the patient's ability to recover even if blood pressure is eventually restored, a condition termed ischemia–reperfusion[3] (discussed later). The clinical manifestations include an intense inflammatory response, activation of the coagulation system, multiple organ dysfunction and death. Thus, all forms of shock eventually are manifest as an exaggerated systemic inflammatory response if hypoperfusion is prolonged.

Primary survey

The primary survey of a critically ill patient in shock should include:

- assessing and establishing an airway
- evaluating breathing and consideration of mechanical ventilator support;
- resuscitating the inadequate circulation.

The ultimate goal of the management of shock is to ensure adequate oxygen delivery to all tissues. The amount of oxygen delivered to the tissues (DO_2) is the product of cardiac output (CO), arterial oxygen saturation (SaO_2), and the oxygen-carrying capacity of the blood (= hemoglobin concentration $\times$ 1.36 ml O_2/g of hemoglobin [Hb]) plus a minor contribution from dissolved oxygen ($PaO_2 \times 0.003$ ml O_2/ml of blood).

$$DO_2 = CO \times (SaO_2 \times (Hb \times 1.36) + \text{Dissolved } O_2)$$

It follows that ensuring adequate oxygen delivery requires equal consideration of *cardiac output*, *arterial oxygenation*, and *oxygen-carrying capacity*.

Airway and breathing

Most patients in shock have one or more indications for airway intubation and mechanical ventilation that should be instituted early on, often before a blood gas is obtained. Significant hypoxemia is one indication for intubation and mechanical ventilation, as external masks may not reliably deliver an adequate fraction of inspired oxygen (FiO_2). Initially, a high FiO_2 should be administered until serial blood gas determinations allow a downward titration of oxygen therapy to less toxic levels. This is relevant in many patients, since pulmonary injury occurs early in shock due to the development of an intense inflammatory response. Acute respiratory distress syndrome (ARDS) is the name given to the lung injury that results from the impact of the systemic inflammatory response on the lung,[4] and is associated with hypoxemia.

Ventilatory failure should be recognized early in a patient who is clinically failing even before blood gases are obtained. It is important to recognize ventilatory failure clinically and not lose precious time in obtaining blood gases while the patient is rapidly deteriorating. Evidence of respiratory muscle fatigue includes labored breathing, inability to speak, tachypnea or an inappropriately low and falling respiratory rate, paradoxical abdominal respiratory motion, accessory muscle use, diaphoresis and cyanosis. Ventilatory failure should also be anticipated in patients who manifest a severe metabolic acidosis in association with shock, as they will eventually lose their ability to compensate for a variety of reasons, including respiratory muscle fatigue, mental obtundation and sedative drugs.

Airway intubation and mechanical ventilation along with sedation and paralysis will decrease oxygen demand of the respiratory muscles, allowing improved oxygen delivery to other hypoperfused tissue beds.[5] This is important during shock as respiratory muscles consume a disproportionate share of the whole body oxygen delivery, particularly for patients who are tachypneic due to acidosis, sepsis, pain or hypoxemia. Thus, multiple organ hypoperfusion (the definition of shock) is itself an indication for intubation and mechanical ventilation in order to redistribute blood flow from respiratory muscles to vital organs.

Thus, the indications for airway intubation and mechanical ventilation can be anticipated and are often clinically apparent in the absence of further diagnostic tests and procedures. Furthermore, in shock, airway intubation and mechanical ventilation should precede other complicated procedures, such as central venous catheterization, or complicated tests that require transportation of the patient.

Circulation: volume therapy is the cornerstone of initial management of shock

Based on the initial assessment of the patient in shock, the clinician formulates a working diagnosis. If the heart is not too full, the indicated intervention is a volume challenge. The rate and composition of the volume expanders is determined by the working diagnosis. Hemorrhagic

shock requires immediate hemostasis and rapid infusions of warmed blood substitutes (red cells, plasma, platelets, albumin). Hypovolemic shock due to dehydration requires rapid boluses of crystalloid—usually 1000 ml each. Cardiogenic shock without evidence of fluid overload requires smaller volume challenges—usually 250 ml of crystalloid. In vasodilatory shock, surprising large volumes of crystalloid are required, often 6–10 L. Many clinicians switch to colloid boluses (either albumin or pentastarch) in order to reduce the inevitable tissue edema that accompanies the capillary leak associated with this state, although evidence for the clinical benefit of this approach is controversial.

Regardless of the diagnosis or the fluid therapy chosen, the adequacy of volume expansion should be observed by titrating to an easily observable clinical endpoint: either benefit (increased blood pressure, decreased heart rate, increased pulse pressure, increased urine output) or harm (pulmonary edema, evidence of right heart dysfunction). Absence of either response indicates that the volume challenge was inadequate and ensuing volume challenges should continue along with rapid clinical reassessment of the response.

Since 'time is tissue', volume resuscitation should be rapid. The effects of 1 L saline infusion over 10 min can be readily identified and interpreted—leading to further similar infusions if necessary. In contrast, infusion of 1 L of normal saline over 1 hour does not reverse hypovolemic shock at an adequate pace and, in view of the many concurrent interventions and redistribution of saline to the entire extracellular compartment, is often difficult to assess.

Circulation: vasoactive therapy should be simplified and goal-directed

Too often, 'blanket' vasoactive therapy is applied early in shock without regard to the clinical diagnosis or the volume status of the patient. This strategy confounds the determination of an adequate circulating volume as well as the etiology of shock. Accordingly, we encourage early, rapid, aggressive volume resuscitation followed by vasoactive therapy if still required.

The choice of vasoactive therapy is surprisingly simple. The clinician must determine whether there is evidence of low cardiac output with high cardiac filling pressures that requires inotropic support or whether hypotension is accompanied by a high cardiac output state that requires pressor support. Adequate cardiac output is more important than blood pressure because adequate tissue oxygen delivery is the underlying goal. Adequate distribution of flow, however, depends on an adequate pressure head. At pressures below an autoregulatory limit, normal flow distribution mechanisms are lost, so that significant organ system hypoperfusion may persist in the face of elevated cardiac output owing to maldistribution of flow. This is the problem in vasodilatory (or septic) shock.

Generally, beta-adrenergic agonists are chosen for support of cardiac output and alpha-adrenergic agonists are chosen when maintainence of perfusion pressure is needed to maintain flow distribution to the tissues (Fig. 1.1). Commonly used alpha agonists are phenylephrine and norepinephrine. Norepinephrine will raise mean arterial pressure at the expense of cardiac output and therefore is only used when cardiac output is adequate or

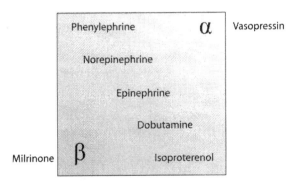

Figure 1.1 Approach to vasoactive therapy. This simplified approach to vasoactive therapy emphasizes differentiation between alpha-adrenergic agonists (α), which primarily have a pressor effect (pressure), and beta-adrenergic agonists (β), which primarily have an inotropic effect (flow). Phenylephrine is a pure alpha agonist that causes vasoconstriction. Norepinephrine is primarily alpha, but has some beta properties as well. Epinephrine is a powerful vasoconstrictor and positive inotropic agonist and is used in severe shock and impending cardiac arrest. Dobutamine has positive inotropic and vasodilating properties and is useful to enhance cardiac output in a well volume-resuscitated patient. Isoproterenol is a pure beta agonist and is used for its positive chronotropic properties in complete heart block. When alpha receptors are down-regulated and the patient no longer responds to alpha-adrenergic pressor agonists, vasopressin is an alternative as it has a pressor effect via the V1 receptor.[26] When the beta receptor is down-regulated and the patient no longer responds to beta agonists, a phosphodiesterase inhibitor such as milrinone is an alternative as it increases contractility by directly increasing cyclic AMP.

increased. Dobutamine is a common choice of a beta-adrenergic agonist. Dobutamine will increase cardiac output but will vasodilate the vasculature and blood pressure will drop unless venous return is augmented. If this occurs, a volume bolus is usually needed to restore blood pressure.

When beta-adrenergic receptor down-regulation occurs and dobutamine is no longer effective, an alternative choice is a phosphodiesterase inhibitor such as milrinone or amrinone. These agonists bypass the beta-adrenergic receptor and act to directly increase cyclic AMP levels and increase cardiac contractility. Likewise, when the patient is refractory to high-dose infusions of alpha-adrenergic agonists, vasopressin is an alternative agent. Vasopressin has several mechanisms of action in refractory vasodilatory shock. Vasopressin acts directly on vascular smooth muscle receptors to cause vasoconstriction, potentiates alpha agonists and blocks K_{ATP} channels, restoring vascular tone.[6] Epinephrine is used in severe shock and during acute resuscitation as it has both alpha- and beta-adrenergic effects. Prolonged use leads to flow inequalities and tissue ischemia[7] and therefore most clinicians step down therapy quickly.

Dopamine is an old friend to many clinicians. At low doses (<2 µg/kg/min) dopamine acts primarily on dopaminergic receptors augmenting renal and splanchnic blood flow. Up to doses of 5 µg/kg/min, beta-adrenergic effects are seen augmenting cardiac output. At higher doses, dopamine acts as an alpha-adrenergic agonist, maintaining blood pressure.[8] These effects have made dopamine a popular choice in the treatment of shock; however, several caveats exist. There is a very poor correlation between plasma dopamine level and infusion rate in hemodynamically stable critically ill adults.[9] This correlation actually worsened when only those patients on a 'renal dose' of 2–5 µg/kg/min were considered. Therefore, the concept of a selective renovascular low-dose dopamine infusion is invalid in critically ill patients. There is no evidence that low-dose dopamine improves renal function or prevents renal dysfunction in critical illness.[10] Additionally, there is compelling evidence that dopamine is harmful to the gastrointestinal,[11,12] endocrine,[13,14] immunologic[15] and respiratory systems[16] in critical illness. We prefer to use agonists with a more predictable hemodynamic response than dopamine, although there is currently no evidence that any pressor agent is preferable to any other.[17]

HEMODYNAMIC MONITORING SHOULD BE GOAL-DIRECTED AND DISCONTINUED WHEN STABILITY IS ACHIEVED

Hemodynamic monitoring of the critically ill using the pulmonary artery catheter is controversial.[18] An evidence-based meta-analysis by Heyland and colleagues showed that the attainment of supranormal hemodynamic goals did not significantly reduce mortality in critically ill patients.[19] Recently, Kern and Shoemaker reviewed 21 randomized controlled studies that described hemodynamic goals in acute, critically ill patients to evaluate the various influences that contributed to outcome.[20] They were able to identify seven studies in which the mortality in the control group was at least 20% and therapy was used before the onset of organ failure. In these studies, goal-directed therapy based on invasive hemodynamic monitoring to achieve supranormal goals was associated with a 23% absolute risk reduction in mortality ($p < 0.05$). There was no difference in mortality associated with goal-directed hemodynamic monitoring in less sick patients or in patients in whom organ failure had already occurred. They concluded, based on the studies, that increased cardiac index (CI) and oxygen delivery with a pulmonary arterial occlusion pressure <18 mmHg should be considered goals of therapy. When implemented early and aggressively, this reduces mortality in critically ill patients. Goal-directed therapy to achieve optimal goals is ineffective in the late stages after onset of organ failure because no amount of extra oxygen will restore irreversible oxygen debt, or reverse cellular death.

Rivers and colleagues conducted a randomized controlled trial of 263 patients with severe sepsis or septic shock, studying the application of early goal-directed therapy using a central venous catheter.[21] Patients randomized to early goal-directed therapy were managed for the first 6 hours in the emergency department. All patients were intubated, ventilated, and sedated as necessary. In the early goal-directed therapy group, crystalloid or colloid was infused to achieve a central venous pressure (CVP) of 8–12 mmHg and vasoactive agents were infused to achieve an MAP of at least 65 mmHg. Central venous oxygen saturation ($S_{CV}O_2$) was measured through the central venous catheter and used as a surrogate of cardiac output. A low $S_{CV}O_2$ correlates with low cardiac output and high $S_{CV}O_2$ correlates with high cardiac output.[22] If the $S_{CV}O_2$ was <70%, red cells were transfused until the hematocrit was >30%. If the $S_{CV}O_2$ remained low, inotropic agonists (dobutamine) were infused to achieve an $S_{CV}O_2$ of at least 70%. During the initial 6 hours of therapy, the patients assigned to early goal-directed therapy received significantly more fluid than those assigned to standard therapy ($p < 0.001$), more red cell transfusions ($p < 0.001$) and more inotropic support ($p < 0.001$), whereas similar proportions in the two groups received vasopressors and mechanical ventilation. Hospital mortality was significantly higher in the standard therapy group vs the treatment group (46.5% vs 30.5%, $p = 0.009$) as was 28-day mortality (49.2% vs 33.3%, $p = 0.01$) and 60-day mortality (56.9% vs 44.3%, $p = 0.03$).

The meta-analysis by Kern and Shoemaker demonstrates that goal-directed hemodynamic monitoring using a pulmonary artery (PA) catheter to achieve supranormal oxygen delivery is effective in critically ill patients when used before the onset of organ failure. The study by Rivers and colleagues highlights two important principles: to be effective, resuscitation must be initiated early and goal-directed. We do not favor one approach (use of a PA catheter and measurement of cardiac index and oxygen delivery) over the other (use of a central venous catheter and measurement of $S_{CV}O_2$ to guide therapy). The application of hemodynamic monitoring will depend on user familiarity, skill level, and resources. The actual goals of therapy should be individualized. What is most important in using hemodynamic monitoring to optimize therapy is that the goals should be clearly defined, whether they are physiological (urine output, skin perfusion, etc.) or measured (central venous pressure, oxygen saturation, cardiac index, etc.). As important, hemodynamic monitoring should be promptly discontinued when the information obtained no longer guides therapy.

DEFINITIVE THERAPY OF UNDERLYING CAUSES OF SHOCK IS IMPORTANT

Early in the resuscitation, the clinician should consider definitive therapy for the underlying cause of shock. Hemorrhagic shock requires prompt attempts at hemostasis and early surgical intervention. The mortality of cardiogenic shock has decreased in the past decade due to institution of an early and aggressive revascularization approach.[23,24] Shock due to massive pulmonary embolism is an indication for immediate thrombolysis.[25] Septic shock dictates early broad-spectrum antibiotic treatment, debridement of devitalized tissue and drainage of abscesses. Again, the requirement for definitive therapy in shock underscores the need to formulate a working hypothesis or diagnosis early on in the evaluation of the shock patient.

THE COMMON CAUSES OF SHOCK ARE HYPOVOLEMIC, CARDIOGENIC, AND VASODILATORY SHOCK

A number of classifications of shock are possible; here we discuss an approach that follows from the initial clinical examination (Table 1.2). Shock can result from inadequate circulating volume (hypovolemic shock), inadequate pump function (cardiogenic shock) or excessive vasodilation with inadequate venous return (vasodilatory shock). Rare forms of shock and overlapping etiologies of shock can confuse the diagnosis, and we will discuss an approach that follows when the clinical picture reveals findings that 'don't fit'.

Hypovolemic shock

Hypovolemic shock is the most common cause of shock caused by decreased venous return. Intravascular volume is decreased so that the venous capacitance system is not filled, leading to decreased driving pressure back to the heart. Cardiac output is reduced, leading to hypotension with a narrow pulse pressure, muffled heart sounds and thready pulses. Endogenous catecholamine levels are high as a compensatory mechanism that attempts to constrict the venous capacitance vessels and raise the pressure, driving blood back to the heart. This high catecholamine state leads to many of the clinical manifestations of hypovolemic shock: mottled, cool skin; tachypnea; tachycardia; and poor capillary refill.

Many causes of shock, that are related to hypovolemia and include trauma and burns also cause an intense inflammatory response that leads to capillary leak and third spacing of fluid, further aggravating decreased venous return. Other causes of shock that are caused by decreased venous return, thus resembling hypovolemic shock, include severe neurologic dysfunction, abdominal compartment syndrome, and drug ingestion by decreasing venous tone. The secondary survey with careful physical examination and search for toxidromes is therefore indicated and helpful.

Cardiogenic shock

Cardiogenic shock, like hypovolemic shock, demonstrates evidence of low cardiac output, yet differs due to evidence of a heart that is too full (high right-sided pressures) and evidence of pulmonary edema if left ventricular dysfunction is also present. Acute cardiac ischemia is the most common form of cardiogenic shock and confirmatory evidence should be sought early: electrocardiogram (ECG), and cardiac enzyme levels. It is important to realize, however, that other etiologies of cardiogenic shock include conditions such as acute valvular dysfunction, cardiac tamponade and pulmonary embolism. Once again, the secondary survey will reveal cardiac murmers and evidence of right-sided failure (high CVP) in the absence of left-sided failure (pulmonary congestion), respectively. Urgent confirmatory tests such as echocardiography, helical computed tomography (CT) scanning and/or cardiac catheterization may be indicated.

Table 1.2 What does not fit?		
Overlapping etiologies	**High right atrial pressure hypotension**	**Non-responsive hypovolemia**
Septic cardiogenic	High right-sided pressure, clear lungs:	Adrenal insufficiency
Septic hypovolemic	Pulmonary embolus	Anaphylaxis
Cardiogenic hypovolemic	Right ventricular infarction	Neurogenic shock
	Cardiac tamponade	

Source: adapted from Walley and Wood[53] with permission.

Table 1.3   Causes of shock.

Low cardiac output hypertension		High cardiac output hypotension
Cardiogenic shock	**Hypovolemic shock**	**Vasodilatory shock**
Left ventricular failure	**Reduced mean systemic pressure**	*Sepsis*
Systolic dysfunction	**Intravascular hypovolemia**	*Anaphylaxis*
Myocardial infarction ischemia	*Hemorrhage*	*Neurogenic shock*
Cardiomyopathy	Gastrointestinal	*Acute hepatic failure*
Depressant drugs	Trauma	*Ischemia-repefusion injury*
Beta-blocker overdose	Aortic dissection	(Prolonged shock of any cause)
Calcium channel blockers	Other internal sources	Hemorrhagic shock
Myocardia contusion	*Renal losses*	Post cardiac arrest
Metabolic derangements:	Diuresis – Osmotic, drug-induced	Cardiogenic shock
acidosis, hypophosphatemia,	Diabetes: insipidus, mellitus	Cardiopulmonary bypass
hypocalcemia	*Gastrointestinal losses*	
Diastolic dysfunction	Vomiting	**Probable vasodilatory shock**
Ischemia and global hypoxemia	Diarrhea	*Adrenal insufficiency*
Ventricular hypertrophy	Gastric suctioning	*Poisonings (hemoglobin and mitochondrial)*
Restrictive cardiomyopathy	Surgical stomas	Carbon monoxide
Greatly Increased Afterload	*Extravascular redistribution*	Metformin
Aortic stenosis/coarctation	Burns	Cyanide
Hypertrophic cardiomyopathy	Sepsis	Iron intoxication
Malignant hypertension	Trauma	
Valve and structural abnormality	Post-operative	**High cardiac output shock**
Mitral stenosis		Arteriovenous shunts
Endocarditis	**Increased resistance to venous return**	Dialysis
Severe mitral/aortic regurgitation	*Cardiac tamponade*	Paget's disease
Atrial myxoma/thrombus	Pericardial fluid collection	*Endocrine*
Papillary muscle rupture	Blood	Thyroid storm
Ruptured septum or free wall	Renal failure	Phaeochromocytoma
Right Ventricular Failure	Pericarditis with effusion	
Decreased contractility	Constrictive pericarditis	
Right ventricular infarction/ischemia	*High intrathoracic pressure*	
Greatly increased afterload	Tension pneumothorax	
Pulmonary embolism/hypertension	Massive pleural effusion	
Mechanical ventilation/high PEEP	Mechanical ventilation/PEEP	
Valvular and structural disease	*High intra-abdominal pressure*	
Obstruction; atrial myxoma,thrombus	Ascites	
Arrythmias	Abdominal trauma/surgery	

Source: adapted from Walley and Wood[53] with permission.

Vasodilatory shock

Vasodilatory (distributive) shock is often recognized initially as hypovolemic shock not responding to volume administration. Excessive vasodilation due to a number of factors[26] initially causes decreased venous return, which is evidenced clinically by hypotension with cool, mottled extremities, narrow pulse pressure and poor capillary refill. As volume is repleted, the syndrome is manifest as a high cardiac output state with a wide pulse pressure, crisp heart sounds, bounding pulses, warm extremities and rapid capillary refill. The usual cause of vasodilatory shock is sepsis due to infection but a number of other etiologies can cause the syndrome, including ischemia–reperfusion, anaphylaxis and some endocrine conditions.

Septic shock and sustained shock from any cause has an inflammatory component

Shock has a hemodynamic component that has been the focus of much of the previous discussion. Additionally, shock has an inflammatory component that is important to recognize because this component is much more important to clinical outcome. Shock is invariably accompanied by a degree of systemic inflammation, although the degree of inflammation varies greatly. A severe inflammatory response due to sepsis, pancreatitis, or burn injury can result in shock. Conversely, resuscitation of prolonged shock from any cause can result in an inflammatory response due to ischemia–reperfusion injury. Ischemia–reperfusion is a local and systemic inflammatory response characterized by production of toxic reactive oxygen species, complement activation, leukocyte–endothelial cell adhesion, transendothelial leukocyte migration, platelet–leukocyte aggregation, increased microvascular permeability, and decreased endothelium-dependent relaxation.[3]

Whereas the hemodynamic component of shock is often rapidly reversible, the systemic inflammatory component of shock is not, and is often the most important component of shock, leading to adverse outcomes including multiple system organ failure (MSOF). Mortality, in turn, is related to the number of organs failing.[27,28] The mortality from MSOF remains excessive and has not diminished over time.[29]

Overlapping etiologies can confuse the diagnosis

Septic shock can be accompanied by significant myocardial dysfunction,[30] which is associated with a high mortality. Conversely, cardiogenic shock can be complicated by aspiration pneumonitis that can cause an intense inflammatory response. These are examples of overlapping etiologies that can confuse the clinical diagnosis of shock. Invasive hemodynamic monitoring may be required to confirm the diagnosis and titrate therapy. The clinician must continually revise the working hypothesis based on new diagnostic information and response to therapy.

Nephrologists should be aware of unusual causes of shock

Abdominal compartment syndrome is an important cause of shock in patients with diverse conditions such as multiple trauma, pancreatitis, resuscitated ruptured abdominal aneurysm or ascites due to any cause.[31] Abdominal compartment syndrome is recognized clinically by the triad of a tense abdomen, increased ventilatory pressures, and decreased urine output. It is confirmed by measurement of bladder pressures. Bladder pressures over 35 cmH_2O mandate intervention: drainage of ascites or surgical decompression as indicated by the etiology.

A number of acute endocrinological conditions can present as shock. Acute adrenal insufficiency can present as shock in many settings, including trauma, hemorrhage,[32] childbirth (Sheehan's syndrome),[33] and adrenal insufficiency of sepsis.[34] Severe thyroid storm may lead to irreversible cardiovascular collapse, especially in the older patient who may have atypical features of thyrotoxicosis.[35] Pheochromocytoma is an explosive clinical syndrome characterized by severe hypertension associated with cardiac complications, hypotension, or even shock and sudden death. The key to diagnosing pheochromocytoma is to suspect it, then confirm it.[36]

Other unusual causes of shock include cellular poisonings such as cyanide, carbon monoxide and iron poisonings are suggested by the clinical setting and require specific therapy.

AN UNDERSTANDING OF THE PATHOPHYSIOLOGY OF CIRCULATORY DYSFUNCTION IS FUNDAMENTAL TO SUCCESSFUL MANAGEMENT OF SHOCK

Initial shock has a hemodynamic component; oxygen delivery to the tissues is severely impaired. Distinguishing types of shock is aided by understanding venous return curves, especially as they are coupled with cardiac function curves. Accordingly, we use these relationships to compare and contrast the cardiovascular mechanisms responsible for hypovolemic shock, cardiogenic shock and vasodilatory shock. We now discuss the hemodynamic factors that govern oxygen delivery.

Factors determining cardiac output

Cardiac output equals heart rate × stroke volume, so that a cursory analysis may conclude that cardiac output is determined by the heart: this is completely wrong. As heart rate increases from 50 to 150 beats/min, diastolic filling time and stroke volume decrease so that there is little or no change in cardiac output. Key exceptions are (1) right heart failure and (2) heart rates below 50 and above 150 (see below). Stroke volume is increased much more by increasing preload than by increasing ventricular contractility. The key exception is when ventricular contractility is markedly impaired (see below). Thus, heart rate × stroke volume may equal cardiac output, but this does not give any insight regarding the true determinants of cardiac output or what therapeutic options are available to increase cardiac output.

In animal experiments Guyton and colleagues[37] sought to determine the importance of the systemic vessels in controlling cardiac output. In control animals with a normally functioning heart, they found that an epinephrine (adrenaline) infusion approximately doubled cardiac output. They then replaced the heart with a pump that simply regulated its own flow in order to maintain right atrial pressure constant. Infusion of a similar amount of epinephrine in these animals without hearts resulted in a similar doubling of cardiac output. These data demonstrate that cardiac output is not determined by the heart but, rather, by factors governing venous return. A healthy heart has multiple mechanisms that allow it to respond to changes in venous return but the heart does not primarily determine cardiac output (which must equal venous return in the steady state).

Conversely, when cardiac function is greatly impaired, the heart cannot respond fully to changes in venous return. Thus, when the heart is the limiting factor in the cardiovascular circuit, heart function contributes substantially to regulation of cardiac output. The apparently competing views of heart vs veins as regulators of cardiac output can be unified by recognizing that regulation of cardiac output in health and disease depends on the interaction (intersection) of cardiac function with venous return.

Cardiac function curves

Cardiac function curves relate the input of the heart to the output (Fig. 1.2). As end-diastolic filling pressure increases, stroke volume of the heart increases. The cardiac function curve is shifted down and to the right by:

1. decreased ventricular contractility (because stroke volume is decreased by decreased ejection)
2. decreased diastolic compliance (because stroke volume is decreased by decreased diastolic filling)
3. increased afterload (which impedes systolic ejection and therefore decreases stroke volume).

The decrease in stroke volume due to decreased contractility, decreased diastolic compliance, and increased afterload can be understood by considering the ventricular pressure–volume loop that is followed during a cardiac cycle (Fig. 1.3).

The cardiac function curve derives from underlying ventricular pressure–volume characteristics and defines the relationship between input and output of the heart yet, by itself, does not define which specific cardiac output will occur. This depends on venous return.

Venous return curves

In most patients (other than those with overt heart failure) cardiac output is regulated by the venous circulation and not by the heart.[37] Venous return is driven by the difference between upstream pressure (mean systemic pressure) and downstream pressure (right atrial pressure) (Fig. 1.4). It follows that venous return at any right atrial pressure can be increased by increasing mean systemic pressure. Mean systemic pressure is, in turn, governed by the volume and compliance of the venous

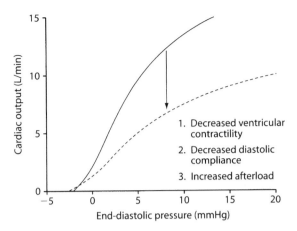

Figure 1.2 Starling function curves, or cardiac function curves, for the heart relate the input of the heart to output (dark solid line). Most frequently we use right atrial pressure (CVP) or left atrial pressure (approximated by pulmonary wedge pressure) as clinically measurable inputs to the heart. Cardiac output is a common measure of output of the heart. As the end-diastolic filling pressure of the heart increases, cardiac output also increases. The relationship is curvilinear. Decreased cardiac function is indicated by a shift down and to the right (dashed line), so cardiac output is lower at a given filling pressure (arrow). Decreased cardiac function may be due to decreased ventricular contractility. However, it is important to recognize that other factors, such as decreased ventricular compliance and increased afterload, have a profound influence on cardiac function curves. Understanding how these factors alter cardiac function requires consideration of ventricular pressure–volume relationships (Fig. 1.3). (Reproduced with permission of Holmes and Walley.[54])

compartment.[38] If the volume of the distensible venous compartment is increased, as in vasodilatory shock, mean systemic pressure increases. Alternatively, if the compliance of the venous compartment decreases by catecholamine infusion or increased sympathetic tone, pressure within the venous compartment increases without necessarily changing volume.

Intersection of cardiac function with venous return

Note that cardiac function curves and venous return curves can be plotted on the same set of axes (Fig. 1.5). In steady state, the amount of blood returning to the heart must equal the amount of blood leaving the heart, so that venous return must equal cardiac output. It follows that, at steady state, the intersection of these two relationships gives the value of the cardiac output and right

atrial pressure. Thus, cardiac output is determined by the interaction of factors governing venous return with factors determining cardiac function.

In health and in most critically ill patients, the cardiac function curve is already steep; therefore, increase in slope (inotrope administration, for example) has little impact on cardiac output, whereas small changes in the venous return curve (fluid administration, for example) can have very significant effects on cardiac output (Fig. 1.6). In patients with severe impairment of cardiac function, factors governing venous return have a lesser effect, since cardiac output is limited by the heart (Fig. 1.7).

Left ventricular dysfunction

Acute myocardial ischemia is the usual cause of left ventricular dysfunction. It can also be seen in critical illness from a variety of causes. In sepsis, ventricular function can be decreased due to both systolic and diastolic dysfunction.[39,40] In these patients, left ventricular ejection fraction is decreased. Sepsis is an 'afterload-reduced' state; therefore, ejection fraction should have been increased if contractility remained normal. In patients who survive, ejection fraction increases back to normal within 10 days.[39] In addition, survivors have dilated end-diastolic ventricles compared to nonsurvivors.[41] Dilation of end-diastolic ventricles is an appropriate and normal compensatory mechanism to maintain stroke volume in the face of the poorly ejecting, dilated end-systolic ventricle (Fig. 1.8).[42] Failure to increase end-diastolic volume limits stroke volume and therefore may contribute to mortality.

When myocardial function appears to be depressed, therapy focuses on correction of reversible causes of myocardial systolic and diastolic dysfunction such as hypoxia,[43] ischemia,[44] acidosis,[45,46] hypocalcemia,[47] hypophosphatemia, hypothermia, hyperthermia, and volume overload.[48] Bicarbonate infusion fails to improve myocardial dysfunction[49] and may, in fact, worsen it due to induction of hypocalcemia and worsening of intracellular acidosis. Thus, we do not recommend bicarbonate infusion for increased anion gap acidoses. Contributors to diastolic dysfunction due to increased intrathoracic pressure—positive pressure ventilation, positive end-expiratory pressure (PEEP), pleural effusion, distended abdomen, supine positioning of an obese patient—must be addressed. Meticulous attention to this level of detail often makes a substantial difference.

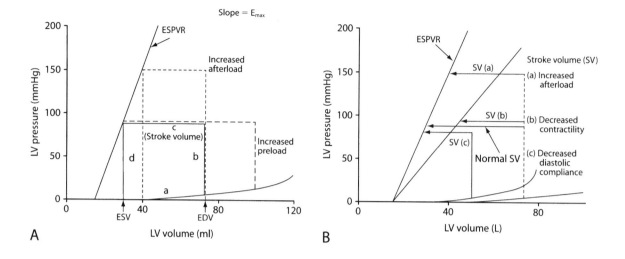

Figure 1.3 (A) Left ventricular pressure–volume relationships are illustrated. A single cardiac cycle pressure–volume loop is illustrated as a–d. During diastole the ventricle fills along a diastolic pressure–volume relationship (a) to end-diastolic volume (EDV). At the onset of systole left ventricular pressure rises with no change in volume (b). When left ventricular pressure exceeds aortic pressure, the aortic valve opens and the left ventricle ejects the stroke volume (c) to an end-systolic pressure–volume point. The ventricle then relaxes isovolumically (d). At increased pressure afterload the left ventricle is not able to eject as far (short interrupted lines). Conversely, at a lower afterload the left ventricle is able to eject further so that all end-systolic points lie along and define the end-systolic pressure–volume relationship (ESPVR). Increased preload (long interrupted lines) results in increased stroke volume from the larger EDV to an end-systolic volume (ESV) that lies on the same ESPVR. The slope of the ESPVR is E_{max}. An increase in contractility results in an increase in E_{max} so that the ventricle ejects to a smaller ESV at the same afterload. (B) Stroke volume (and hence cardiac output) is reduced from a normal stroke volume (longest arrow) by increased afterload (SV a, top arrow), by decreased contractility (SV b), and by decreased diastolic compliance (SV c). The cause of the decrease in stroke volume can be seen in each case by considering the illustrated left ventricular pressure–volume properties. (Reproduced with permission from Holmes and Walley.[54])

Administration of inotropic agonists such as dobutamine and milrinone can also be very helpful in improving cardiac output when systolic ventricular function is depressed (see Fig. 1.7). We rely on clinical evidence of improving organ system function (mentation, urine output), resolution of lactic acidosis, and improvement in mixed venous oxygen saturation to gauge response to therapy. Improving mixed venous oxygen saturation will often have a profound effect on arterial saturation. The main limitation to using dobutamine and milrinone is that patients who are inadequately volume resuscitated (i.e. venous return is limited by noncardiac factors) will become hypotensive due to the vasodilator effect of these agonists. If this happens, further volume resuscitation and judicious use of an additional vasoconstricting agent, such as norepinephrine, may allow beneficial use of dobutamine or milrinone to increase cardiac output. Balancing the competing goals of oxygenation vs cardiac output is often aided by the use of a PA catheter, so that response to therapy can be tested

by following the cardiac output, mixed venous oxygen saturation, and oxygen delivery.

Right ventricular dysfunction

In critically ill patients, pulmonary artery pressure may be elevated because of increased pulmonary vascular resistance caused by various pro-inflammatory mediators, hypoxia, acidosis, and by increased airway pressures due to positive pressure ventilation and PEEP. Increased pulmonary artery pressure is transmitted to the right ventricle, which dilates to maintain cardiac output. Fluid administration in right ventricular overload states may be detrimental.[50] A fluid challenge will produce a large increase in CVP. Within the constraints of the pericardium, a dilated right ventricle shifts the septum to the left and limits left ventricular filling, thereby decreasing left ventricular stroke volume and cardiac output. Right ventricular wall tension, which is the product of right ven-

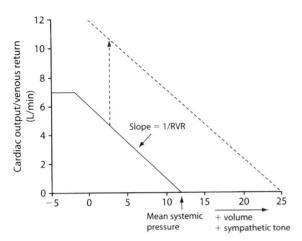

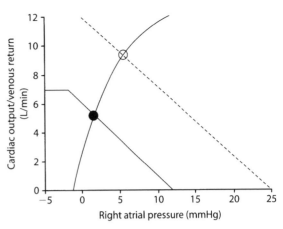

Figure **1.4** Right atrial pressure–venous return relationship. Venous return depends on the gradient between mean systemic pressure and right atrial pressure. Mean systemic pressure is a vascular compartment pressure that arises from venous blood volume distending the systemic veins. When right atrial pressure is so high that it equals mean systemic pressure (the intersection of the relationship with the x-axis), flow falls to zero. As right atrial pressure decreases, the pressure gradient driving venous return increases, so venous return increases. Flow is maximal when right atrial pressure is zero and cannot increase further because of collapsibility of the major veins. The inverse slope of this line is termed 'resistance to venous return' or RVR. An increase in venous volume or a decrease in compliance (induced by increased sympathetic tone, for example) increases mean systemic pressure (dashed line) so that at any given right atrial pressure venous return increases (vertical dashed arrow). (Reproduced with permission from Holmes and Walley.[54])

Figure **1.5** The cardiac function curve (solid curve) and the venous return curve (solid line) can be shown on the same axis. The intersection of the two relationships (●) defines the actual cardiac output and right atrial pressure. When venous return is increased (by volume expansion, which increases mean systemic pressure, dashed line), cardiac output increases substantially (○). In normal humans and most critically ill patients, factors that govern venous return are primarily responsible for changes in cardiac output, as illustrated here. (Reproduced with permission from Holmes and Walley.[54])

tricular radius and pressure, increases to the point where right ventricular ischemia may contribute to ventricular dysfunction. If this happens, right ventricular function may be improved by increasing mean aortic pressure, thus increasing coronary perfusion pressure, with vasoconstrictor agonists such as norepinephrine[51] and epinephrine.[52]

Therapeutically, increasing heart rate does not increase cardiac output unless right heart diastolic filling is limited by tamponade or right heart failure. In this setting, limited ventricular filling is completed early in diastole by high venous pressures. Prolonging diastole does not result in further diastolic filling or an increase in stroke volume. Since stroke volume is the limiting factor, increasing heart rate increases cardiac output proportionately. Increasing heart rate to 80 or even 100 beats/min, using a pacemaker or pharmacologic

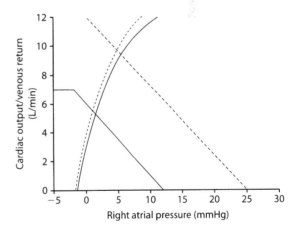

Figure **1.6** Healthy hearts already have a steep cardiac function curve (solid curve) so that a substantial increase in ventricular contractility cannot shift the cardiac function curve much (dashed curve). In this setting, the heart cannot contribute much to regulation of cardiac output. In contrast, a shift of the venous return curve due to an increase in mean systemic pressure (dashed line) results in a substantial increase in cardiac output. Thus, regulation of cardiac output is primarily accomplished by factors governing venous return when cardiac function is good. (Reproduced with permission from Holmes and Walley.[54])

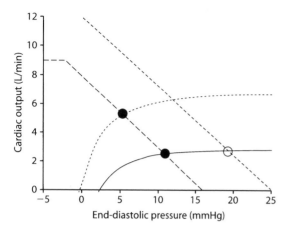

Figure 1.7 In contrast to Figure 1.6, when cardiac function is greatly decreased (solid curve), a shift of the venous return curve (solid line to dashed line by an increase in mean systemic pressure) does not increase cardiac output much (○). In this case, a shift up and to the left of the cardiac function curve (dashed curve) due to increased contractility, increased diastolic compliance, or decreased afterload, greatly increases cardiac output (●). Thus, when poor heart function limits cardiac output, the heart contributes substantially to regulation of cardiac output. (Reproduced with permission from Holmes and Walley.[54])

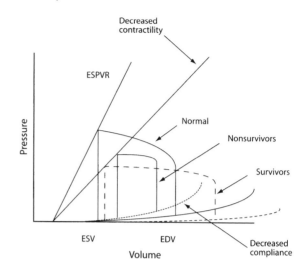

Figure 1.8 Theoretical ventricular pressure–volume relationships for normals, survivors, and nonsurvivors of septic shock. In both survivors and nonsurvivors, contractility is decreased by a decreased slope of the end-systolic pressure–volume relationship (ESPVR). Diastolic ventricles of survivors dilate as the normal compensatory response to decreased systolic contractility. Pathologic alterations of the myocardium prevent diastolic dilation in nonsurvivors so that stroke volume decreases due to both systole and diastole. ESV, end-systolic volume; EDV, end-diastolic volume. (Reproduced with permission from Holmes and Walley.[54])

agents, often beneficially increases cardiac output in right heart failure. The corollary is that when cardiac output is observed to be dependent on heart rate (when heart rate is in the range of 50–100 beats/min), right heart failure or limited diastolic filling (e.g. tamponade physiology) are probably present. At heart rates below 50 or above 150 beats/min, cardiac output does depend on heart rate (because diastolic filling is limiting), even in patients with relatively normal hearts.

The value to the clinician of understanding the pathophysiology of the circulation is to consider the heart as the problem in shock but also to recognize the importance of the peripheral circulation. If the heart is not the problem, attention must quickly turn to increasing venous return either by volume infusion, institution of vasoactive therapy or both. Understanding the pathophysiology of the circulation helps the bedside clinician to focus quickly on identifying and correcting the underlying problem.

SUMMARY

Shock is an emergency that requires continuous bedside evaluation, resuscitation, and re-evaluation. The initial bedside examination allows the clinician to determine whether the patient exhibits a clinical picture consistent with hypovolemic, cardiogenic, or vasodilatory shock. The primary survey dictates urgent initial resuscitation, usually consisting of intubation, ventilation, and volume support. Vasoactive therapy is started when the patient is well volume-resuscitated and consists of inotropic support for cardiogenic shock and pressor therapy for vasodilatory shock. The secondary survey is helpful in revealing the etiology of shock and necessary to institute early definitive therapy. Early shock has a hemodynamic component, which is often easily reversed. Septic shock and prolonged shock from any cause has an inflammatory component, which is not easily reversed and leads to MSOF and death. Success in treatment of shock depends on early recognition of shock and the tempo of resuscitation of the hemodynamic component of shock.

REFERENCES

1. Holmes DR Jr, Bates ER, Kleiman NS, et al. Contemporary reperfusion therapy for cardiogenic shock: the GUSTO-I trial experience. The GUSTO-I Investigators. Global utilization of streptokinase and tissue plasminogen activator for occluded coronary arteries. J Am Coll Cardiol 1995;26(3):668–74.
2. Califf RM. The rationale for thrombolytic therapy. Eur Heart J 1996;17(Suppl E):2–8.
3. Collard CD, Gelman S. Pathophysiology, clinical manifestations, and prevention of ischemia-reperfusion injury. Anesthesiology 2001;94(6):1133–8.
4. Kollef MH, Schuster DP. The acute respiratory distress syndrome. N Engl J Med 1995;332(1):27–37.
5. Hussain SN, Roussos C. Distribution of respiratory muscle and organ blood flow during endotoxic shock in dogs. J Appl Physiol 1985;59(6):1802–8.
6. Holmes CL, Patel BM, Russell JA, et al. Physiology of vasopressin relevant to management of septic shock. Chest 2001;120(3):989–1002.
7. Meier-Hellmann A, Reinhart K, Bredle DL, et al. Epinephrine impairs splanchnic perfusion in septic shock. Crit Care Med 1997;25(3):399–404.
8. D'Orio V, El Allaf D, Juchmes J, et al. The use of low-dose dopamine in intensive care medicine. Arch Int Physiol Biochim Biophys 1984;92:S11.
9. Juste RN, Moran L, Hooper J, et al. Dopamine clearance in critically ill patients. Intensive Care Med 1998;24(11):1217–20.
10. Bellomo R, Chapman M, Finfer S, et al. Low-dose dopamine in patients with early renal dysfunction: a placebo-controlled randomised trial. Australian and New Zealand Intensive Care Society (ANZICS) Clinical Trials Group. Lancet 2000;356(9248):2139–43.
11. Segal JM, Phang PT, Walley KR. Low-dose dopamine hastens onset of gut ischemia in a porcine model of hemorrhagic shock [see comments]. J Appl Physiol 1992;73(3):1159–64.
12. Dive A, Foret F, Jamart J, et al. Effect of dopamine on gastrointestinal motility during critical illness. Intensive Care Med 2000;26(7):901–7.
13. Van den Berghe G, de Zegher F, Lauwers P. Dopamine and the sick euthyroid syndrome in critical illness. Clin Endocrinol (Oxf) 1994;41(6):731–7.
14. Van den Berghe G, de Zegher F, Lauwers P, et al. Growth hormone secretion in critical illness: effect of dopamine. J Clin Endocrinol Metab 1994;79(4):1141–6.
15. McRitchie DI, Girotti MJ, Rotstein OD, et al. Impaired antibody production in blunt trauma. Possible role for T cell dysfunction. Arch Surg 1990;125(1):91–6.
16. Ward DS, Bellville JW. Effect of intravenous dopamine on hypercapnic ventilatory response in humans. J Appl Physiol 1983;55(5):1418–25.
17. Martin C, Viviand X, Leone M, et al. Effect of norepinephrine on the outcome of septic shock. Crit Care Med 2000;28(8):2758–65.
18. Connors AF Jr, Speroff T, Dawson NV, et al. The effectiveness of right heart catheterization in the initial care of critically ill patients. SUPPORT Investigators. JAMA 1996;276(11):889–97.
19. Heyland DK, Cook DJ, King D, et al. Maximizing oxygen delivery in critically ill patients: a methodologic appraisal of the evidence. Crit Care Med 1996;24(3):517–24.
20. Kern JW, Shoemaker WC. Meta-analysis of hemodynamic optimization in high-risk patients. Crit Care Med 2002;30(8):1686–92.
21. Rivers E, Nguyen B, Havstad S, et al. Early goal-directed therapy in the treatment of severe sepsis and septic shock. N Engl J Med 2001;345(19):1368–77.
22. Rivers EP, Ander DS, Powell D. Central venous oxygen saturation monitoring in the critically ill patient. Curr Opin Crit Care 2001;7(3):204–11.
23. Hollenberg SM, Kavinsky CJ, Parrillo JE. Cardiogenic shock. Ann Intern Med 1999;131(1):47–59.
24. Hochman JS, Sleeper LA, Godfrey E, et al. SHould we emergently revascularize Occluded Coronaries for cardiogenic shocK: an international randomized trial of emergency PTCA/CABG-trial design. The SHOCK Trial Study Group. Am Heart J 1999;137(2):313–21.
25. Wood KE. Major pulmonary embolism: review of a pathophysiologic approach to the golden hour of hemodynamically significant pulmonary embolism. Chest 2002;121(3):877–905.
26. Landry DW, Oliver JA. The pathogenesis of vasodilatory shock. N Engl J Med 2001;345(8):588–95.
27. Brun-Buisson C, Doyon F, Carlet J, et al. Incidence, risk factors, and outcome of severe sepsis and septic shock in adults. A multicenter prospective study in intensive care units. French ICU Group for Severe Sepsis. JAMA 1995;274(12):968–74.
28. Russell JA, Singer J, Bernard GR, et al. Changing pattern of organ dysfunction in early human sepsis is related to mortality. Crit Care Med 2000;28(10):3405–11.
29. Friedman G, Silva E, Vincent JL. Has the mortality of septic shock changed with time? Crit Care Med 1998;26(12):2078–86.
30. Kumar A, Haery C, Parillo JE. Myocardial dysfunction in septic shock. Crit Care Clin 2000;16(2):251–87.
31. Ivatury RR, Sugerman HJ, Peitzman AB. Abdominal compartment syndrome: recognition and management. Adv Surg 2001;35:251–69.
32. Claussen MS, Landercasper J, Cogbill TH. Acute adrenal insufficiency presenting as shock after trauma and surgery: three cases and review of the literature. J Trauma 1992;32(1):94–100.
33. Rusnak RA. Adrenal and pituitary emergencies. Emerg Med Clin North Am 1989;7(4):903–25.
34. Annane D, Sebille V, Troche G, et al. A 3–level prognostic classification in septic shock based on cortisol levels and cortisol response to corticotropin. JAMA 2000;283(8):1038–45.
35. Gavin LA. Thyroid crises. Med Clin North Am 1991;75(1):179–93.
36. Bravo EL. Pheochromocytoma. Cardiol Rev 2002;10(1):44–50.
37. Guyton AC, Lindsay AW, Abernathy B, et al. Mechanism of increased venous return and cardiac output caused by epinephrine. Am J Physiol 1958;192:126–30.
38. Goldberg HS, Rabson J. Control of cardiac output by systemic vessels. Circulatory adjustments to acute and chronic respiratory failure and the effect of therapeutic interventions. Am J Cardiol 1981;47(3):696–702.
39. Parker MM, Shelhamer JH, Bacharach SL, et al. Profound but reversible myocardial depression in patients with septic shock. Ann Intern Med 1984;100(4):483–90.
40. Russell JA, Ronco JJ, Lockhat D, et al. Oxygen delivery and consumption and ventricular preload are greater in survivors than in nonsurvivors of the adult respiratory distress syndrome. Am Rev Respir Dis 1990;141(3):659–65.

41. Parker MM, Shelhamer JH, Natanson C, et al. Serial cardiovascular variables in survivors and nonsurvivors of human septic shock: heart rate as an early predictor of prognosis. Crit Care Med 1987;15(10):923–9.

42. Parrillo JE, Parker MM, Natanson C, et al. Septic shock in humans. Advances in the understanding of pathogenesis, cardiovascular dysfunction, and therapy. Ann Intern Med 1990; 113(3):227–42.

43. Walley KR, Becker CJ, Hogan RA, et al. Progressive hypoxemia limits left ventricular oxygen consumption and contractility. Circ Res 1988;63(5):849–59.

44. Walley KR, Cooper DJ. Diastolic stiffness impairs left ventricular function during hypovolemic shock in pigs. Am J Physiol 1991;260(3 Pt 2):H702–12.

45. Teplinsky K, O'Toole M, Olman M, et al. Effect of lactic acidosis on canine hemodynamics and left ventricular function. Am J Physiol 1990;258(4 Pt 2):H1193–9.

46. Walley KR, Lewis TH, Wood LD. Acute respiratory acidosis decreases left ventricular contractility but increases cardiac output in dogs. Circ Res 1990;67(3):628–35.

47. Lang RM, Fellner SK, Neumann A, et al. Left ventricular contractility varies directly with blood ionized calcium. Ann Intern Med 1988;108(4):524–9.

48. Gaasch WH, Levine HJ, Quinones MA, et al. Left ventricular compliance: mechanisms and clinical implications. Am J Cardiol 1976;38(5):645–53.

49. Cooper DJ, Herbertson MJ, Werner HA, et al. Bicarbonate does not increase left ventricular contractility during L-lactic acidemia in pigs. Am Rev Respir Dis 1993;148(2):317–22.

50. Belenkie I, Dani R, Smith ER, et al. The importance of pericardial constraint in experimental pulmonary embolism and volume loading. Am Heart J 1992;123(3):733–42.

51. Martin C, Perrin G, Saux P, et al. Effects of norepinephrine on right ventricular function in septic shock patients. Intensive Care Med 1994;20(6):444–7.

52. Le Tulzo Y, Seguin P, Gacouin A, et al. Effects of epinephrine on right ventricular function in patients with severe septic shock and right ventricular failure: a preliminary descriptive study. Intensive Care Med 1997;23(6):664–70.

53. Walley KR, Wood LDH. Shock. In: Hall JB, Schmidt GA, Wood LDH, eds. Principles of critical care, 2nd edn. New York: McGraw-Hill; 1998:277–301.

54. Holmes CL, Walley KR. Cardiovascular management of ARDS. Semin Respi Criti Care Med 2001;22(3):307–15.

2

Respiratory failure

John McConville and Gregory Schmidt

CLASSIFICATION OF RESPIRATORY FAILURE

Respiratory failure (RF) is defined by the inability to provide adequate oxygen for consumption by the peripheral tissues and/or the inability to ventilate adequately. Four types or pathophysiologic mechanisms of RF are described (Table 2.1): Type I or acute hypoxemic RF is characterized by alveolar airspace flooding and resulting hypoxemia that does not correct easily with supplemental oxygen. Type II or ventilatory failure is characterized by relative alveolar hypoventilation. Hypoxemia may also be present in type II RF, but it is corrected easily with supplemental oxygen. Type III respiratory failure occurs in the perioperative period and is the end result of progressive atelectasis of dependent lung units. Type IV respiratory failure occurs in the setting of global hypoperfusion due to cardiogenic, hypovolemic, or septic shock. Inadequate cardiac output leads to progressive hypotension and increased work of breathing as the respiratory system attempts to compensate for the metabolic acidosis that often accompanies an underperfused state. In patients with shock, intubation and mechanical ventilation reduces the oxygen consumption of the respiratory muscles and prevents excessive 'steal' of the limited cardiac output by the respiratory system.

	Type I, acute hypoxemic		Type II, ventilatory	Type III, perioperative	Type IV, shock
Mechanism	$\dot{Q}s/\dot{Q}T$		$\dot{V}A$	Atelectasis	Hypoperfusion
Etiology	Airspace flooding		1. CNS drive	1. FRC	1. Cardiogenic
			2. N-M coupling	2. CV	2. Hypovolemic
			3. Work/dead-space		3. Septic
Clinical	Pulmonary edema		1. Overdose/CNS injury	1. Supine/obese,ascites/	1. Myocardial infarct,
Description	Cardiogenic		2. Myasthenia gravis,	peritonitis, upper	pulmonary hypertension
	ARDS		polyradiculitis/ALS,	abdominal incision,	2. Hemorrhage,
			botulism/curare	anesthesia	dehydration,
	Pneumonia		3. Asthma/COPD,	2. Age/smoking, fluid	tamponade
	Lung hemorrhage		pulmonary fibrosis,	overload, bronchospasm,	3. Endotoxemia,
			kyphoscoliosis	airway secretions	bacteremia

$\dot{Q}s/\dot{Q}T$: Shunt fraction, ARDS: Acute respiratory distress syndrome, $\dot{V}A$: Alveolar ventilation, CNS: Central nervous system, N-M coupling: Neuromuscular coupling, ALS: Amyotrophic lateral sclerosis, COPD: Chronic obstructive pulmonary disease, FRC: Functional residual capacity, CV: Closing volume.

Source: Principles of Critical Care reproduced from Schmidt et al[1].

THERAPY FOR RESPIRATORY FAILURE

Noninvasive ventilation

Noninvasive positive pressure ventilation (NIPPV) improves gas exchange and reduces the work of breathing for many patients with respiratory failure. There is also evidence that NIPPV is able to prevent intubation, reduce mortality and shorten intensive care unit (ICU) length of stay in patients with acute-on-chronic RF when compared with conventional mechanical ventilation.[1-7] Additional studies comparing NIPPV with 'conventional treatment' have proven its efficacy (decreased incidence of mechanical intubation and/or shorter hospital length of stay) in acute cardiogenic pulmonary edema, hypoxemic respiratory failure, and status asthmaticus.[8-10] Patients treated with NIPPV have a decreased need for sedation and paralysis, decreased incidence of nosocomial pneumonia, otitis, and sinusitis, and improved comfort as compared with patients requiring mechanical ventilation.[1-7]

It is often appropriate to attempt NIPPV in patients that formerly required endotracheal intubation. Once the decision to initiate NIPPV is made, it is important to explain the procedure to the patient as the ventilator and mask are being prepared. Before the mask is fixed tightly to the patient it is often beneficial to apply the mask to the patient's face by hand, with the ventilator connected, so that the patient can accommodate to the sensation of positive pressure ventilation and sense the relief of dyspnea it provides. A low level of pressure support of 5 cmH$_2$O and continuous positive airway pressure (CPAP) of 2 cmH$_2$O are good initial settings. These settings can be gradually increased until the respiratory rate decreases and the patient becomes more comfortable. A pressure support of 10 cmH$_2$O and CPAP of 5 cmH$_2$O will provide many patients with adequate ventilatory support. Waveforms can be helpful in determining whether significant autoPEEP (expiratory flow at end-expiration) is present and whether the patient's inspiratory effort is excessive.

NIPPV can be provided by conventional ICU ventilators or by bilevel pressure targeted ventilators. As decribed above, pressure support and CPAP are commonly used to provide NIPPV via conventional ventilators. In this setting, a PS/CPAP value of 10/5 provides 15 cmH$_2$O of inspiratory pressure and 5 cmH$_2$O of expiratory pressure. With bilevel ventilators, however, inspiratory and expiratory pressures are set separately. Thus, an inspiratory pressure of 10 cmH$_2$O and an expiratory pressure of 5 cmH$_2$O is not the same level of ventilatory assistance as PS/CPAP of 10/5 provided via a conventional ventilator. However, both modes of providing NIPPV can be adjusted to provide more or less ventilatory assistance. For example, increasing the CPAP via the conventional ventilator or increasing the expiratory pressure via the bilevel ventilator will reduce the work of breathing in a patient with airflow obstruction and significant autopeep. Although both conventional and bilevel ventilators are able to provide NIPPV, conventional ventilators are typically able to deliver higher levels of FiO$_2$ and also have waveform displays. For these reasons, conventional ventilators are used more frequently in our ICU when NIPPV is required.

The determination of NIPPV success or failure is a clinical judgment. Continuous pulse oximetry and an arterial blood gas determination are useful adjuvants, but clinical improvement, as determined by increased patient comfort and decreased work of breathing, are the endpoints used to determine NIPPV efficacy. If there is no visible improvement in the patient's respiratory status after 30 min of NIPPV, then intubation and mechanical ventilation should be considered. Sedatives and/or anxiolytics are often beneficial to patients receiving NIPPV, but they may increase the risk of aspiration, ventilatory failure, and respiratory arrest. The success of NIPPV depends on the coordinated efforts of nurses, respiratory therapists, and patients as well as physicians. Patients who are hemodynamically unstable, unable to protect their airway, or are in respiratory arrest should not have a trial of NIPPV and should be considered for intubation and mechanical ventilation immediately. While a large number of patients with RF are candidates for NIPPV, there are potential risks. These include skin necrosis, diminished control of a patient's ventilatory status compared with invasive ventilation, and possibly a small increased risk of aspiration of gastric contents. Also, patients requiring NIPPV should be thought of as being dependent on the ventilator (or bilevel ventilator) for respiratory assistance. Thus, initiating NIPPV has important implications for many other medical decisions. For example, sending a patient on NIPPV for a CT scan requires consideration of whether or not the patient can tolerate periods of time off assisted ventilation. Despite these potential complications, the risks of NIPPV are much less than mechanical ventilation and NIPPV has become the standard of care for many patients who develop respiratory failure.

Mechanical ventilation

Pressure, flow and volume waveforms from two patients on assist control ventilation are depicted in Figure 2.1. The second breath in each tracing has an end-inspiratory "pause" inserted. During this pause time there is no gas-flow along the airway, thus allowing equalization of pressures between the airway opening and the alveolus. The plateau airway pressure, measured during the period of no gas-flow, represents an estimation of alveolar airway pressure at a given tidal volume *if the patient is passive and is not making any respiratory efforts*. The peak to plateau pressure gradient is an important variable that should be monitored for all patients on volume-cycled ventilation. An elevated peak to plateau gradient (>15 cmH$_2$O) indicates increased airway resistance, typically seen in patients with obstructive lung disease (asthma, COPD) or secretions in the endotracheal tube. The expiratory waveform on the flow-time tracing can also reveal evidence of airflow obstruction. At the end of a normal exhalation there is a period of no airflow prior to the initiation of another breath. Airflow at the end of a passive exhalation is the definition of autopeep and is evidence that airflow obstruction

exists. Successful treatment of airflow obstruction, with beta-agonists and/or suctioning of the endotracheal tube, results in a reduction of the peak to plateau pressure gradient as well as a reduction in autopeep. Patients with airflow obstruction typically have normal or even increased lung compliance, meaning for a given change in lung volume there is a comparatively small change in transpulmonary pressure (alveolar pressure – pleural pressure). On the other hand, patients with acute respiratory distress syndrome (ARDS) have decreased lung compliance, requiring a greater change in transpulmonary pressure for a given change in lung volume. In these patients the peak to plateau pressure gradient tends not to be elevated, but the plateau airway pressures are elevated for a given lung volume as compared to patients with normal lung compliance. Careful attention to the plateau airway pressure is critical in patients with ARDS as a recent study has shown that low tidal volume ventilation (6 ml/kg), or lower to keep plateau airway pressures < 30 cmH$_2$O, reduces mortality in ARDS patients as compared with higher tidal volume ventilation (12 ml/kg).[18] (See section on acute hypoxemic respiratory failure below.)

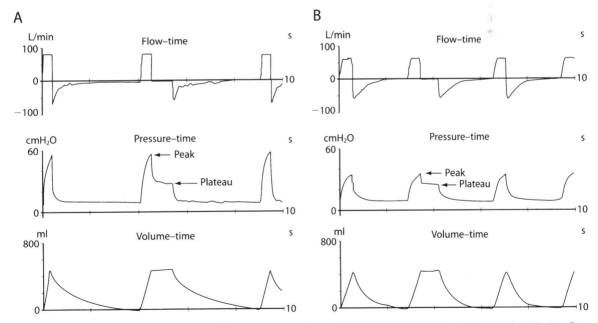

Figure 2.1 Tracings for flow–time, pressure–time, and volume–time curves from two patients on assist control ventilation. During the second breath in both examples an end-inspiratory pause time was inserted. Note that there is no flow during the pause and that the volume does not change during this period of no airflow. (A) Airflow obstruction is demonstrated by the increased peak to plateau gradient as well as a prolonged expiratory phase (>0.5 s). (B) This patient with ARDS has an elevated plateau airway pressure, despite low tidal volume ventilation, and a normal peak to plateau pressure gradient, consistent with reduced lung compliance.

Assist-control ventilation (ACV)

The set parameters of the assist-control mode are the inspiratory flow rate, frequency (f), and tidal volume (Vt). The ventilator delivers f equal breaths per minute, each of Vt volume. Vt and flow determine the inspiratory time (Ti), expiratory time (Te), and the inspiratory:expiratory (I:E) ratio. Plateau airway pressure (Pplat) is related to the Vt and the compliance of the respiratory system, while the difference between peak airway pressure (Ppeak) and Pplat includes contributions from flow and inspiratory resistance (Fig. 2.1). The patient has the ability to trigger extra breaths by exerting an inspiratory effort exceeding the preset trigger sensitivity, each at the set Vt and flow, and to thereby change Ti, Te, I:E ratio, and to potentially create or increase autoPEEP. Typically, each patient will display a preferred rate for a given Vt and will trigger all breaths when the controlled ventilator frequency is set a few breaths/min below the patient's rate; in this way, the control rate serves as an adequate support should the patient stop initiating breaths. When high inspiratory effort continues during the ventilator-delivered breath, the patient may trigger a second, superimposed ('stacked') breath (rarely a third as well). Patient effort can be increased (if the goal is to exercise the patient) by increasing the magnitude of the trigger or by lowering Vt (which increases the rate of assisting). Lowering f at the same Vt generally has no effect on work of breathing when the patient is initiating all breaths.

Synchronized intermittent mandatory ventilation (SIMV)

In the passive patient, SIMV cannot be distinguished from controlled ventilation in the ACV mode. Ventilation is determined by the mandatory f and Vt. However, if the patient is not truly passive, he may perform respiratory work during the mandatory breaths. More to the point of the SIMV mode, he can trigger additional breaths by lowering the airway opening pressure below the trigger threshold. If this triggering effort comes in a brief, defined interval before the next mandatory breath is due, the ventilator will deliver the mandatory breath ahead of schedule in order to synchronize with the patient's inspiratory effort. If a breath is initiated outside of the synchronization window, Vt, flow, and I:E are determined by patient effort and respiratory system mechanics, not by ventilator settings. The spontaneous breaths tend to be of small volume and are highly variable from breath to breath. The SIMV mode is often used to gradually augment the patient's work of breathing by lower-

ing the mandatory breath f (or Vt), driving the patient to breathe more rapidly in order to maintain adequate ventilation, but this approach appears to prolong 'weaning'.[11,12] Although this mode continues to be used widely, there is little rationale for it and SIMV is falling out of favor.

Pressure-control ventilation (PCV)

In the passive patient, ventilation is determined by f, the inspiratory pressure increment (Pinsp − PEEP), I:E ratio, and the time constant of the patient's respiratory system. In patients without severe obstruction (i.e. time constant not elevated) given a sufficiently long Ti, there is equilibration between the ventilator determined Pinsp and Palv, so that inspiratory flow ceases. In this situation, tidal volume is highly predictable, based on Pinsp (= Palv), and the compliance of the respiratory system (Crs). In the presence of severe obstruction or if Ti is too short to allow equilibration between ventilator and alveoli, Vt will fall below that predicted based on Pinsp and Crs (Fig. 2.2C).

The active patient can trigger additional breaths by reducing the airway opening pressure (Pao) below the triggering threshold, raising the I:E ratio. The inspiratory reduction in pleural pressure combines with the ventilator Pinsp to augment the transpulmonary pressure and the tidal volume. Because Ti is generally set by the physician, care must be taken to discern the patient's neural Ti (from the waveforms display) and adjust the ventilator accordingly, otherwise additional sedation might be necessary.

Pressure-support ventilation (PSV)

The patient must trigger the ventilator in order to activate this mode, so pressure support is not applied to passive patients. Ventilation is determined by Pinsp, patient-determined f, and patient effort. Once a breath is triggered, the ventilator attempts to maintain Pao at the physician-determined Pinsp, using whatever flow is necessary to achieve this. Eventually flow begins to fall due to cessation of the patient's inspiratory effort or to increasing elastic recoil of the respiratory system as Vt rises. The ventilator will maintain a constant Pinsp until inspiratory flow falls an arbitrary amount (e.g. to 20% of initial flow) or below an absolute flow rate. The patient's work of breathing can be increased by lowering Pinsp or making the trigger less sensitive, and can inadvertently increase if respiratory system mechanics change, despite no change in ventilator settings. Respiratory system mechanical parameters cannot be

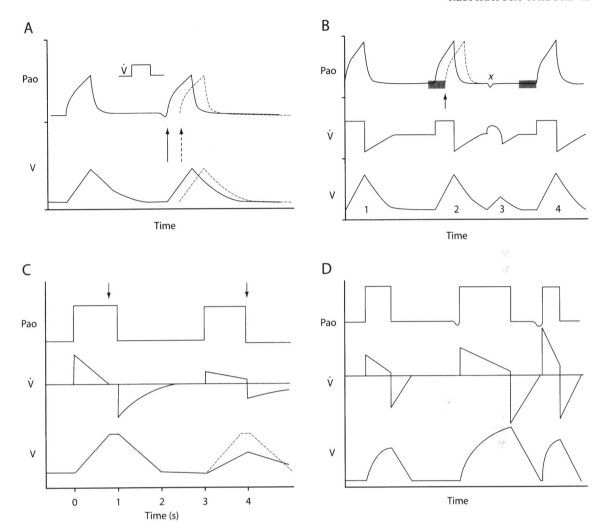

Figure 2.2 (A) Airway opening pressure (Pao) and lung volume (V) during ACV of a patient who is periodically triggering the ventilator. The second breath was set to be delivered at the time marked by the second arrow; instead, the patient lowers the Pao, triggering the ventilator at the time marked by the first arrow, thereby increasing the respiratory rate above the default value, decreasing the expiratory time (TE), and increasing the I:E ratio. (B) Airway opening pressure (Pao), flow (V), and lung volume (V) during SIMV. Breath 1 (a mandatory breath) is not triggered by the patient, who remains fully passive. V and V̇ are determined by the ventilator, while the Pao reflects the passive mechanical characteristics of the respiratory system. The shaded rectangle near the second breath denotes the interval during which the ventilator is programmed to synchronize with the patient's inspiratory effort, delivering the mandatory breath slightly ahead of schedule. At the end of this time interval (arrow), a mandatory breath would have been delivered (dotted tracing) if the patient had not triggered the ventilator. The synchronized breath (breath 2) has the same volume and flow as a mandatory breath. The Pao may not be the same as during a passive breath because of continued patient effort throughout inspiration. The third breath (3) is initiated before the synchronization interval at *x* and is therefore not assisted. Flow and tidal volume are totally determined by the patient's effort and mechanics. These breaths are typically shorter and smaller (as indicated) than the mandatory breaths. When the patient fails to trigger another breath within the next synchronization window, another mandatory breath (4) is delivered. (C) Pressure-control ventilation of a muscle-relaxed patient showing the effects of changed inspiratory resistance. The left-hand panel shows a pressure-control breath with normal resistance, during which Pinsp equilibrates with Palv before the inspiratory cycle is terminated (left arrow), flow ceases, and tidal volume can be predicted from the Pinsp and Cst (VT = Cst × Pinsp). In the right-hand panel, inspiratory resistance is elevated. Note that as the same Pinsp, inspiratory flow is reduced, the tidal volume is not reached until the inspiratory phase is terminated (right arrow), and the tidal volume (solid line) falls below that predicted by Cst and Pinsp (dotted line). Pao is airway opening pressure; V̇ is flow; V is volume. (D) Pressure-support ventilation. When a breath is

Continued.....

determined readily on this mode since the ventilator and patient contributions to Vt and flow are not represented by Pao; accordingly, these important measurements of Pplat, Ppeak−Pplat, and autoPEEP are measured during a brief, daily switch from pressure support to volume-preset ventilation. A potential advantage of PSV is improved patient comfort.

Mixed modes

Some ventilators allow combinations of modes, most commonly SIMV plus PSV. There is little reason to use such a hybrid mode, although some physicians use the SIMV as a means to add sighs to PSV, an option not otherwise generally available. Since SIMV plus PSV guarantees some backup minute ventilation (which PSV does not), this mode combination may have value in occasional patients at high risk for abrupt deterioration in central drive.

Waveforms

Assessing patient effort during mechanical ventilation has been greatly enhanced by the use of pressure, flow, and volume waveforms commonly found on most ventilators. When the goal of mechanical ventilation is full rest of the respiratory muscles, interpretation of waveforms can be helpful in establishing ventilator–patient synchrony. Typical waveforms for common modes of ventilation can be found in Figure 2.2.

Initial ventilator settings

Initial ventilator settings depend on the goals of ventilation (e.g. full respiratory muscle rest vs partial exercise), the patient's respiratory system mechanics, and minute ventilation needs. Although each critically ill patient presents myriad challenges, it is possible to identify five subsets of ventilated patients:

1. the patient with normal lung mechanics and gas exchange

2. the patient with severe airflow obstruction
3. the patient with acute-on-chronic respiratory failure
4. the patient with acute hypoxemic respiratory failure
5. the patient with restrictive lung or chest wall disease.

In all patients the initial FiO_2 (fraction of inspired oxygen) should usually be 0.5–1.0 to assure adequate oxygenation, although it can usually be lowered within minutes when guided by pulse oximetry and, in the appropriate setting, applying PEEP. In the first minutes following institution of mechanical ventilation, the physician should remain alert for several common problems. These include, most notably, airway malposition, aspiration, and hypotension. Positive-pressure ventilation may reduce venous return and so cardiac output, especially in patients with a low mean systemic pressure (e.g. hypovolemia, venodilating drugs, decreased sympathetic tone from sedating drugs, neuromuscular disease) or a very high ventilation-related pleural pressure (e.g. chest wall restriction, large amounts of PEEP, or obstruction causing autoPEEP). If hypotension occurs, intravascular volume should be rapidly expanded while steps are taken to lower the pleural pressure (smaller tidal volumes, less minute ventilation).

The patient with normal respiratory mechanics and gas exchange

Patients with normal lung mechanics and gas exchange can require mechanical ventilation:

1. because of loss of central drive to breathe (e.g. drug overdose or structural injury to the brainstem)
2. because of neuromuscular weakness (e.g. high cervical cord injury, acute idiopathic myelitis, myasthenia gravis)

---

triggered, Pao rises to the set level (Pinsp) with flow and Vt depending on the Pinsp, respiratory system mechanics, and patient effort. The first breath shown represents a patient who triggers the ventilator and then remains fully passive (a hypothetical circumstance used here for contrast with the usual patient efforts shown in the next two breaths). As long as there is no significant airflow obstruction, Vt nearly reaches the volume that would be predicted based on the compliance of the respiratory system (Vt = Crs × Pinsp). During the middle breath shown, the patient makes a moderate but prolonged inspiratory effort. The Pao remains at the set inspiratory level as long as patient effort maintains flow, and a much longer Ti and Vt result. In the final breath, a more powerful but briefer inspiratory effort is made, shortening the Ti but generating a larger Vt than during the passive breath. Pao is airway opening pressure; V̇ is flow; and V is volume.

Schmidt GA, Hall JB. Management of the ventilated patient. In: Hall JB, Schmidt GA, Wood LDH (eds). Principles of Critical Care (2nd edn). New York: McGraw-Hill; 1996:517–535.

3. as an adjunctive therapy in the treatment of shock
4. in order to achieve hyperventilation (e.g. in the treatment of elevated intracranial pressure following head trauma).

Following intubation, initial ventilator orders should be an FiO_2 of 0.5–1.0, tidal volume of 8–15 ml/kg, respiratory rate of 8–12 breaths/min, and inspiratory flow rate of 40–60 L/min. Alternatively, if the patient has sufficient drive and is not profoundly weak, PSV can be used. The level of pressure support is adjusted (usually to the range of 10–20 cmH_2O above PEEP) to bring the respiratory rate down into the low 20s, usually corresponding to tidal volumes of about 400 ml. If gas exchange is entirely normal, the FiO_2 can probably be lowered further, based upon pulse oximetry or arterial blood gas determinations.

Soon after the initiation of ventilation, airway pressure and flow waveforms should be inspected for evidence of patient–ventilator dyssynchrony or undesired patient effort. If the goal of ventilation is full rest, the patient's drive can often be suppressed by increasing the inspiratory flow rate, frequency, or tidal volume; of course, the latter two changes may induce respiratory alkalemia. If such adjustments do not diminish breathing effort, despite normal blood gases, to an undetectable level, sedation may be necessary. If this does not abolish inspiratory efforts and full rest is essential (as in shock), muscle paralysis should be considered. Measures to prevent atelectasis should include sighs (6–12/h at 1.5–2 times the Vt) or small amounts of PEEP (5–7.5 cmH_2O).

Patients with severe airflow obstruction

Severe obstruction is seen most commonly in patients with status asthmaticus, but also rarely in those with inhalation injury or central airway lesions, such as tumor or foreign body, that are not bypassed with the endotracheal tube. Many of these patients may benefit from NIPPV, but some will require invasive ventilation. These patients are usually extremely anxious and distressed. Deep sedation should be provided in such instances, supplemented in some patients by therapeutic paralysis, although the use of paralytic drugs occasionally causes long-lasting weakness. These interventions help to reduce oxygen consumption (and hence carbon dioxide production), to lower airway pressures, and to reduce the risk of self-extubation.

Because the gas exchange abnormalities of airflow obstruction are largely limited to ventilation–perfusion mismatch, an FiO_2 of 0.5 suffices in the vast majority of patients. Ventilation should be initiated using the ACV mode (or SIMV), the tidal volume should be small (5–7 ml/kg), and the respiratory rate 12–15 breaths/min. A peak flow of 60 L/min is recommended and higher flow rates do little to increase expiratory time. For example, if the Vt is 500 ml, the respiratory rate is 15 breaths/min, and the flow is 60 L/min, the expiratory time is 3.5 s. Raising flow (dramatically) to 120 L/min increases the expiratory time to only 3.75 s, a trivial improvement. In contrast, a small reduction in respiratory rate to 14 breaths/min increases the expiratory time to 3.8 s. This example serves to emphasize not only the relative lack of benefit of raising the flow rate but also the importance of minimizing minute ventilation when the goal is to reduce autoPEEP. Finally, if the patient is triggering the ventilator, some PEEP should be added to reduce the work of triggering.[13] Although this occasionally compounds the dynamic hyperinflation, potentially compromising cardiac output, usually autoPEEP increases little as long as PEEP is not set higher than about 85% of the autoPEEP.

The goals of ventilation are (1) to minimize alveolar overdistension (Pplat <30 cmH_2O) and (2) to minimize dynamic hyperinflation (autoPEEP below 10 cmH_2O or end-inspiratory lung volume <20 ml/kg), a strategy which largely prevents barotrauma.[14,15] Reducing minute ventilation to achieve these goals generally causes the PCO_2 to rise above 40 mmHg, often to 70 mmHg or higher. Although this requires sedation, such permissive hypercapnia is quite well-tolerated except in patients with increased intracranial pressure, and perhaps in those with ventricular dysfunction or critical pulmonary hypertension.[16]

Patients with acute-on-chronic respiratory failure

Acute-on-chronic respiratory failure (ACRF) is a term used to describe the exacerbations of chronic ventilatory failure, often requiring ICU admission, usually occurring in patients with chronic obstructive pulmonary disease (COPD). Unlike patients with status asthmaticus, patients in this population tend to have relatively smaller increases in inspiratory resistance, their expiratory flow limitation arising largely from loss of elastic recoil. The experience with NIPPV and its efficacy for patients with ACRF is well described.[1-6] NIPPV should always be considered as a treatment option in ACRF prior to mechanical ventilation. However, patients with ACRF will occasionally require mechanical ventilation and, in these patients, peak airway pressures on the ventilator tend not to be extraordinarily high, yet autoPEEP and its consequences are common. At the time of intubation, hypoperfusion is common, as manifested by tachycardia and relative hypotension, and typically responds to briefly ceasing ventilation combined with fluid loading.

Since the majority of these patients are ventilated after days to weeks of progressive deterioration, the goal is to rest the patient (and respiratory muscles) for 36–72 hours. Also, since the patient typically has an underlying compensated respiratory acidosis, excessive ventilation risks severe respiratory alkalosis and, over time, bicarbonate wasting by the kidney. For those who require intubation, the goals of rest and appropriate hypoventilation can usually be achieved with initial ventilator settings of a tidal volume of 5–7 ml/kg and a respiratory rate of 24–28 breaths/min, with either an ACV or an SIMV mode set on minimal sensitivity. Since gas exchange abnormalities are primarily those of ventilation–perfusion mismatch, supplemental oxygen in the range of an FiO_2 of 0.4 should achieve better than 90% saturation of arterial hemoglobin.

The majority of patients with COPD will appear exhausted at the time when mechanical support is instituted and will sleep with minimal sedation. To the extent that muscle fatigue has played a role in a patient's functional decline, rest and sleep are desirable. Two to three days of such rest presumably will restore biochemical and functional changes associated with muscle fatigue, but 24 hours is probably not sufficient. Small numbers of patients are difficult to rest on the ventilator, continuing to demonstrate a high work of breathing. Examination of airway pressure and flow waveforms can be very helpful in identifying this extra work, and in suggesting strategies for improving the ventilator settings. In many patients, this is the result of autoPEEP-induced triggering difficulty. Adding extrinsic PEEP to nearly counterbalance the autoPEEP dramatically improves the patient's comfort.

Patients with acute hypoxemic respiratory failure

Acute hypoxemic respiratory failure (AHRF) is caused by alveolar filling with blood, pus, or edema, and results in impaired lung mechanics and gas exchange. The gas exchange impairment results from intrapulmonary shunt, which is largely refractory to oxygen therapy. Acute respiratory distress syndrome (ARDS) constitutes a significant subset of patients with AHRF and is defined by

- the presence of bilateral infiltrates on chest radiograph
- pulmonary capillary wedge pressure ≤18 mmHg (if measured)
- PaO_2:FiO_2 ratio ≤200 (acute lung injury is considered to be present if the PaO_2:FiO_2 ratio is ≤300).

In ARDS, the significantly reduced FRC (functional residual capacity) due to alveolar flooding and collapse leaves many fewer alveoli to accept the tidal volume, making the lung appear stiff, and dramatically increasing the work of breathing. The ARDS lung should be viewed as a small lung, however, rather than a stiff lung. In line with this current conception of ARDS, it is now clearly established that excessive distension of the ARDS lung compounds lung injury and may induce systemic inflammation.[17,18] Ventilatory strategies have evolved markedly in the past decade, changing clinical practice and generating tremendous excitement.

The goals of ventilation are to reduce shunt, avoid toxic concentrations of oxygen, and choose ventilator settings which do not amplify lung damage. The initial FiO_2 should be 1.0 in view of the typically extreme hypoxemia. PEEP is indicated in patients with diffuse lung lesions, but may not be helpful in patients with focal infiltrates, such as lobar pneumonia. In patients with ARDS, PEEP should be instituted immediately, then rapidly adjusted to the least PEEP necessary to produce an arterial saturation of 90% on an FiO_2 no higher than 0.6 ('least PEEP approach'). An alternative approach is to set the PEEP at a value 2 cmH_2O higher than the lower inflection point of the inflation PV curve ('open-lung approach'), but this approach has not been validated, is rather complex, and is not recommended. Recruitment maneuvers have not been shown to be useful or necessary. The tidal volume should be 6 ml/kg of ideal body weight on ACV, higher tidal volumes being associated with higher mortality. Calculation of tidal volume must be based on ideal body weight, as use of daily weights may result in excessively large tidal volumes. Alternatively, PCV can be used, with an inspiratory pressure (PEEP plus the pressure increment) adjusted to drive tidal volumes of 6 ml/kg of ideal body weight. In either mode the respiratory rate should be set at 24–28 breaths/min as long as there is no autoPEEP. The combination of high levels of PEEP (especially when the open-lung approach is used) and low end-inspiratory pressures leaves only a small range for tidal ventilation. An occasional consequence is hypercapnia. This approach of preferring hypercapnia to alveolar overdistension is termed 'permissive hypercapnia'.

In May 2000 the Acute Respiratory Distress Syndrome Network (ARDS Network) published the results of a randomized, multicenter trial, which enrolled mechanically ventilated patients with acute lung injury (ALI) or ARDS.[19] Within 36 hours of intubation, patients were randomized to either of two mechanical ventilation strategies. The conventional group received tidal volumes of 12 ml/kg of predicted body weight (based on sex and height). If plateau airway pressures were greater than 50 cmH$_2$O with 12 ml/kg tidal volumes, then the tidal volume was decreased in a stepwise fashion with a goal of maintaining plateau airway pressures <50 cmH$_2$O but >45 cmH$_2$O. The low tidal volume group was ventilated with 6 ml/kg of predicted body weight. If ventilation with 6 ml/kg tidal volumes resulted in a Pplat of >30 cmH$_2$O then the tidal volume was decreased by 1 ml/kg in a stepwise fashion with a goal of maintaining plateau airway pressures of <30 but >25 cmH$_2$O. (A complete description of these methods can be found at www.ardsnet.org.) The trial was stopped after the enrollment of 861 patients, because mortality was lower (31.0% vs 39.8%, $p = 0.007$) and ventilator-free days within 28 days of randomization were greater (mean (±SD), 12 ± 11 vs 10 ± 11; $p = 0.007$) in the low tidal volume group.

It should be noted that measured weight exceeded predicted weight by 20% in this trial. Thus, it is essential to utilize the predicted body weight when calculating tidal volumes for mechanically ventilated patients (with ALI or ARDS) as use of measured weights will result in excessive tidal volumes that could exacerbate lung injury. (In the ARDSnet study, the predicted body weight of male patients = 50 + 0.91 (centimeters of height − 152.4); female patients = 45.5 + 0.91 (centimeters of height − 152.4).) Finally, patients ventilated with a low tidal volume strategy often require higher respiratory rates to maintain adequate minute ventilation (MV). Nevertheless, hypercapnia is often a consequence of this ventilation strategy.

The amount of PEEP used to maintain adequate oxygenation varies greatly in patients with ARDS. Typically, the FiO$_2$, inspiratory time, and PEEP are adjusted to keep oxygen saturation ≥88%. The 'least PEEP' approach advocates upward titration of PEEP until an acceptable level of oxygen saturation (≥88%) is achieved. In AHRF, 8–12 cmH$_2$O of PEEP is often required to achieve acceptable oxygen saturation, although it is not uncommon for 15–20 cmH$_2$O of PEEP to be required in severe ARDS.

The patient with restriction of the lungs or chest wall

Small tidal volumes (5–7 ml/kg) and rapid rates (18–24 breaths/min) are especially important in order to minimize the hemodynamic consequences of positive-pressure ventilation and to reduce the likelihood of barotrauma. The FiO$_2$ is usually determined by the degree of alveolar filling or collapse, if any. When the restrictive abnormality involves the chest wall (including the abdomen), the large ventilation-induced rise in pleural pressure has the potential to compromise cardiac output. This in turn will lower the mixed venous PO$_2$ and, in the setting of ventilation–perfusion mismatch (VQ mismatch) or shunt, the arterial partial pressure of oxygen (PaO$_2$) as well. If the physician responds to this falling PaO$_2$ by augmenting PEEP or increasing the minute ventilation, further circulatory compromise ensues. A potentially catastrophic cycle of worsening gas exchange, increasing ventilator settings, and progressive shock is commenced. This circumstance must be recognized, since the treatment is to reduce dead space (e.g. by lowering minute ventilation or correcting hypovolemia).

LIBERATION FROM MECHANICAL VENTILATION

When taking care of patients with respiratory failure, it is important to ask two questions each day: Does the patient still require mechanical ventilation? If so, why does the patient still require mechanical ventilation? These questions force the clinician to focus on the underlying causes of respiratory failure rather than focus on ventilator modes and settings. Initial ventilator settings are often chosen in an attempt to minimize the patient's work of breathing and maximize the ventilatory support. Once the underlying cause of respiratory failure has been identified and treated, the patient needs to resume spontaneous breathing prior to extubation. The term 'weaning' is often used to describe the process of moving from mechanical ventilation to spontaneous respiration without assistance. This implies a gradual process wherein the level of ventilator support is reduced to minimal levels prior to removal of the endotracheal tube. However, most patients are able to assume the work of breathing as soon as the underlying cause of respiratory failure has been treated. In fact, 76% of patients enrolled in two major trials investigating different liberation techniques had successful trials of spontaneous breathing prior to randomization into one of the 'weaning strategies'.[11,20] Because mechanical ventilation involves numerous risks, including pneumonia and pneumothorax, it is appropriate to initiate a spontaneous breathing trial (SBT) as soon as possible, with the goal of early extubation. The term 'liberation' from mechanical ventilation, as opposed to 'weaning', best describes this process and will be used throughout this chapter.

Once the underlying cause of respiratory failure has been treated, some assessment of the patient's ability to breathe spontaneously is required. Previously, weaning parameters such as negative inspired force (NIF), vital capacity, and maximum voluntary ventilation (MVV) were used to assess a patient's neuromuscular strength prior to initiating an SBT. Similarly, minute ventilation, respiratory compliance, and airways resistance were measured in an effort to determine the respiratory muscle load. While parameters suggesting poor respiratory muscle strength and excessive load may predict weaning failure, these measurements are not able to predict accurately which patients can breathe spontaneously and be extubated. In general, when patients are no longer in shock, have adequate oxygenation (PaO_2 >60 mmHg on FiO_2 ≤50% and PEEP ≤7.5 cmH_2O), and have a respiratory load that is not excessive (minute ventilation ≤20 L/min), an assessment of the patient's ability to breathe spontaneously can be made. Once these criteria are met, there is no need to measure daily 'weaning parameters' as *there is no substitute for a daily trial of spontaneous breathing.*

The index of rapid shallow breathing (RSBI or rate:volume ratio, RVR), has been studied in several large trials and has been shown to be an accurate predictor of who can breathe spontaneously.[23,24] This ratio measures the respiratory rate/the tidal volume (L) during a 1 min T-piece trial. A ratio of <105 breaths/min/L suggests that the patient is a candidate for liberation from the ventilator. Available evidence also suggests that CPAP of 5 cmH_2O or PSV of 5–8 cmH_2O are acceptable alternatives to an SBT utilizing a T-piece. In an effort to improve the predictive value of the ratio, many patients with an RVR of <105 during the initial 1 min trial have the SBT continued for 30–120 min. If the RVR remains <105 after the extended SBT, then the literature suggests that almost 90% of these patients can be successfully extubated, provided they have an adequate mental status or cough reflex. Patients who develop worsening gas exchange or have a RVR >125 breaths/min/L during a spontaneous breathing trial should be placed back on higher levels of ventilatory support and 'rested' until the following day. Therapy should be directed at decreasing the load on the respiratory system as well as improving the strength of the respiratory system prior to a repeat SBT the following day.

In patients who initially fail a trial of spontaneous breathing, performing a daily SBT results in earlier extubation than utilizing pressure support or intermittent mandatory ventilation (IMV)-directed weaning protocols.[20] Esteban and colleagues conducted a prospective, randomized, multicenter trial which enrolled 546 patients who had received mechanical ventilation for a mean of 7.6 ± 6.1 days. When the attending physician deemed these patients to be in stable condition and ready for weaning from the ventilator, they underwent a spontaneous breathing trial on a T-piece for up to 2 hours. Patients who did not develop a respiratory rate >35 breaths/min, O_2 saturation <90%, heart rate >140 beats/min, systolic blood pressure above 180 mmHg or below 90 mmHg, agitation, diaphoresis, or anxiety at the end of the trial were extubated. One hundred and thirty patients developed respiratory distress during the SBT and were subsequently randomized to one of four different 'weaning groups.' The groups were:

- IMV
- PSV
- two or more daily SBT with intermittent rest on ACV
- once-daily SBT with intermittent rest on ACV.

Standardized weaning protocols were used for each group and patients were extubated when they were able to breathe on minimal settings for 2 hours. Weaning was considered successful if rein-tubation was not required within 48 hours of extu-bation. The median duration of weaning was 5 days for the IMV group, 4 days for the PSV group, and 3 days for both of the SBT groups. There was no significant difference between either of the SBT groups. Thus, daily assessment of the patient's ability to breathe spontaneously, with full ventila-tory support for those who develop respiratory distress, results in earlier extubation than IMV or PSV protocols that call for a graded reduction in ventilatory support prior to extubation. However, not all studies examining methods for achieving liberation from mechanical ventilation have obtained similar results. Brochard[11] also studied patients who failed spontaneous breathing trials and randomly assigned 109 patients to T-piece trials, SIMV, or PS ventilation. The primary end point was liberation from mechanical ventilation at 21 days. The probability of remaining on mechani-cal ventilation 21 days after randomization was significantly lower for PS than for T-piece or SIMV (p <0.03). When all causes for liberation failure were considered, there were a lower number of failures on PS ventilation as compared with the T-piece and SIMV groups. This difference was statis-tically significant ($p = 0.05$) and became even more so (p <0.025) after excluding patients who had 'weaning' stopped for reasons not related to the 'weaning' process.

Additional studies by Ely et al have further demonstrated the importance of daily SBT in appropriate patients.[21] In their study, 300 mechan-ically ventilated patients were screened daily for their ability to undergo SBT using the following criteria:

- $PaO_2:FiO_2$ had to exceed 200
- PEEP could not exceed 5 cmH_2O
- there had to be adequate cough during suctioning
- the RVR could not exceed 105 breaths/min/L
- no infusions of vasopressor agents or sedatives.

Those patients in the intervention group who met all of the screening criteria had a daily SBT. When these patients successfully completed an SBT, the attending physician was notified. Patients in the control group had daily screenings for their ability to perform an SBT, but no other interventions. In both groups, the decision to discontinue mechani-cal ventilation was made by an attending physi-cian not involved in the study. The intervention group spent fewer days receiving mechanical ven-tilation (median of 4.5 days) as compared to the control group (median 6.0 days). Additionally, the intervention group had fewer complications (self-extubation, tracheostomy, and mechanical ventila-tion >21 days) and lower ICU costs than the control group. Again, patients are identified earlier and liberated from mechanical ventilation earlier if they are screened daily for their ability to undergo an SBT. Our practice is to initiate daily sponta-neous breathing trials for all patients who are hemodynamically stable, have acceptable oxy-genation (PaO_2 >60 on FiO_2 ≤50% and PEEP ≤7.5 cmH_2O) and have a minute ventilation <20 L/min (see Fig. 2). However, a recent study by Esteban et al looking at mechanical ventilation practices in North and South America, Spain and Portugal found great variability in how liberation from mechanical ventilation was achieved.[25] In this study PS ventilation (36%) was the most common modality used during 'weaning' trials.

Unfortunately, not everyone who is able to breathe spontaneously for 30–120 min is able to be extubated. Patients who develop upper air-way edema while receiving mechanical ventila-tion often do well on trials of spontaneous breathing, but require reintubation after develop-ing increased work of breathing after the endotra-cheal tube (ETT) has been removed. A 'cuff test' can help identify patients who have developed upper airway edema. Simply, deflate the balloon, occlude the ETT and have the patient take several breaths. Inability to move air around the ETT sug-gests upper airway edema and warrants an inspec-tion of the upper airway prior to removal of the ETT. Additionally, the ability to clear respiratory secretions and protect the airway is not measured during SBTs. After a successful SBT the patient's mental status and ability to clear secretions need to be judged prior to removal of the ETT.

Limiting the time patients spend on the ventila-tor is an important aspect of reducing ICU length of stay and ICU costs as well as reducing the com-plications associated with mechanical ventilation. A recent study by Kress et al indicates that how intubated patients are sedated in the ICU can affect the duration of mechanical ventilation.[22] In this randomized, controlled trial, 128 patients receiving mechanical ventilation and continuous infusions of sedative drugs were randomized to an interven-tion group, which had interruption of sedative infusions until they were able to follow instruc-tions, or a control group, in which the sedative drugs were infused at the discretion of the clini-cians in the ICU. Once patients were awake or

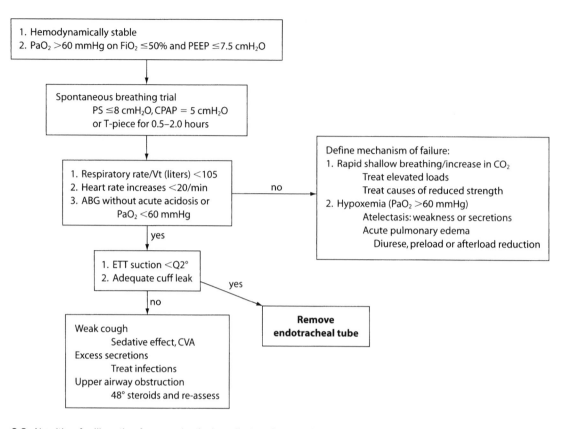

Figure 2.3 Algorithm for liberation from mechanical ventilation. See text for details. AGB = arterial blood gas; CVA = cerebral vascular accident; ETT = endotracheal tube; CPAP = continuous positive airway pressure; FiO_2 = fraction of inspired oxygen; PaO_2 = partial pressure of oxygen; PEEP = positive end-expiratory pressure.

became agitated in the intervention group, the sedative agents were restarted at half the original dose and titrated according to the need for sedation. The median duration of mechanical ventilation was 4.9 days in the intervention group and 7.3 days in the control group. Importantly, there was no increase in the rate of complications in the intervention group (self-extubation), and the type of sedatives used (midazolam or propofol) did not affect duration of mechanical ventilation. In this study, patients who had daily interruption of sedative agents were extubated earlier and spent less time in the ICU than patients who did not have daily cessation of sedative infusions.

REFERENCES

1. Wood LDH. The pathophysiology and differential diagnosis of acute respiratory failure. In: Hall JB, Schmidt GA, Wood LDH (eds). Principles of Critical Care (2nd edn). New York: McGraw-Hill; 1996:499–508.

2. Brochard L, Mancebo J, Wysocki M, et al. Noninvasive ventilation for acute exacerbations of chronic obstructive pulmonary disease. N Engl J Med 1995;333:817–22.

3. Kramer N, Meyer TJ, Meharg J, et al. Randomized, prospective trial of noninvasive positive pressure ventilation in acute respiratory failure. Am J Respir Crit Care Med 1995;151:1799–806.

4. Antonelli M, Conti G, Rocco M, et al. A comparison of noninvasive positive-pressure ventilation and conventional mechanical ventilation in patients with acute respiratory failure. N Engl J Med 1998;339:429–35.

5. Bott J, Carroll MP, Conway JH, et al. Randomized controlled trial of nasal ventilation in acute ventilatory failure due to chronic obstructive airways disease. Lancet 1993;341:1555–7.

6. Confalonieri M, Parigi P, Scartabellati A, et al. Noninvasive mechanical ventilation improves the immediate and long-term outcome of COPD patients with acute respiratory failure. Eur Respir J 1996;9:422–30.

7. Meduri GU, Abou-Shala N, Fox RC, et al. Noninvasive face mask mechanical ventilation in patients with acute hypercapnic respiratory failure. Chest 1991;100:445–54.

8. Bersten AD, Holt AW, Vedig AE, et al. Treatment of severe cardiogenic pulmonary edema with continuous positive airway pressure delivered by face mask. N Engl J Med 1991;325:1825–30.

9. Martin TJ, Hovis JD, Costantino JP, et al. A randomized, prospective evaluation of noninvasive ventilation for acute respiratory failure. Am J Respir Crit Care Med 2000;161:807–13.

10. Gehlbach B, Kress JP, Kahn J, et al. Correlates of prolonged hospitalization in inner-city ICU patients receiving noninvasive and invasive positive pressure ventilation for status asthmaticus. Chest 2002;122:1709–14.

11. Brochard L, Rauss A, Benito S, et al. Comparison of three methods of gradual withdrawal from ventilatory support during weaning from mechanical ventilation. Am J Respir Crit Care Med 1994;150:896–903.

12. Esteban A, Alía I, Gordo F, et al. Extubation outcome after spontaneous breathing trials with T-tube or pressure support ventilation. Am J Respir Crit Care Med 1997;156:459–65.

13. Ranieri VM, Giuliani R, Cinnella G, et al. Physiologic effects of positive end-expiratory pressure in patients with chronic obstructive pulmonary disease during acute ventilatory failure and controlled mechanical ventilation. Am Rev Respir Dis 1993;147:5–13.

14. Tuxen DV, Lane S. The effects of ventilatory pattern on hyperinflation, airway pressures, and circulation in mechanical ventilation of patients with severe air-flow obstruction. Am Rev Respir Dis 1987;136:872–9.

15. Tuxen DV, Williams TJ, Scheinkestel CD, et al. Use of a measurement of pulmonary hyperinflation to control the level of mechanical ventilation in patients with acute severe asthma. Am Rev Respir Dis 1992;146:1136–42.

16. Feihl F, Perret C. Permissive hypercapnia: how permissive should we be? Am J Respir Crit Care Med 1994;150:1722–37.

17. Ranieri VM, Suter PM, Tortoella C, et al. Effects of mechanical ventilation on inflammatory mediators in patients with acute respiratory distress syndrome: a randomized controlled trial. JAMA 1999;282:54–61.

18. Tremblay L, Valenza F, Ribeiro SP, et al. Injurious ventilatory strategies increase cytokines and c-fos m-RNA expression in an isolated rat lung model. J Clin Invest 1997;99:944–52.

19. The Acute Respiratory Distress Syndrome Network. Ventilation with lower tidal volumes as compared with traditional tidal volumes for acute lung injury and the acute respiratory distress syndrome. N Engl J Med 2000;342:1301–8.

20. Esteban A, Frutos F, Tobin MJ, et al. A comparison of four methods of weaning patients from mechanical ventilation. N Engl J Med 1995;332:345–50.

21. Ely EW, Baker AM, Dunagan DP, et al. Effect on the duration of mechanical ventilation of identifying patients capable of breathing spontaneously. N Engl J Med 1996;335:1864–9.

22. Kress JP, Pohlman AS, O'Connor MF, Hall JB. Daily interruption of sedative infusions in critically ill patients undergoing mechanical ventilation. N Engl J Med 2000;342:1471–7.

23. Yang ML, Tobin MJ. A prospective study of indexes predicting the outcome of trials of weaning from mechanical ventilation. N Engl J Med 1991;324:1445–50.

24. Jacob B, Chatila W, Manthous CA. The unassisted respiratory rate:tidal volume ratio accurately predicts weaning outcome in post-operative patients. Crit Care Med 1996;25:253–7.

25. Esteban A, Anzueto A, Alía I, et al. How is mechanical ventilation employed in the intensive care unit? Am J Respir Crit Care Med 2000;161:1450–8.

3

Multiple organ dysfunction/failure: pathophysiology and treatment

Manar Alshahrouri and Robert A Balk

INTRODUCTION

While critically ill patients of the past would have succumbed early in their course, improvements in management today permit many patients to develop evidence of multiple organ dysfunction syndrome (MODS) or multiple organ failure (MOF).[1-5] Multiple organ failure was first reported in 1969 and represented a consequence of the significant advances in the ability to provide early fluid resuscitation, ventilatory, and pharmacologic support for the critically ill patient.[3,6] Multiple organ system dysfunction has been reported in patients with all types of critical illness and/or extreme stresses of normal physiology.[7,8] It is evident that a patient's ultimate survival is dependent on factors other than the successful treatment of the initial disease process for which the patient was admitted. Multiple organ dysfunction/failure is now regarded as one of the most common causes of death in the noncoronary intensive care unit and is also a frequent cause of morbidity, prolonged hospitalization, and increased cost of care.[1]

DEFINITIONS OF MODS AND MOF

At this time a uniformly accepted definition for MODS or MOF is lacking, as is the exact definition of specific organ system dysfunction or failure.[6,9] In 1992 the American College of Chest Physicians and the Society of Critical Care Medicine put forward a consensus conference definition for MODS as the presence of altered organ function in an acutely ill patient such that homeostasis could not be maintained without intervention.[10] Although this concept is vague, it implies that there is a threshold of abnormality that requires some

intervention or the provision of organ replacement or supportive therapy. The consensus conference definition suggested that the dysfunction may be relative or absolute and recognized that there is a continuum of change from dysfunction to failure.[10] Unfortunately, this definition does not yield specific laboratory or functional criteria that serve as indicators of the dysfunction or mark the transition from a reversible dysfunction to an irreversible failure state. In addition, there is no uniformity in the provision of organ supportive or replacement therapy, so it is likely that not all patients with organ dysfunction/failure will be managed in a similar fashion.

It was also recognized that the initial injury might result from direct organ system involvement by an underlying disease or could be derived from hemodynamic alterations.[11] The initial multiple organ system dysfunction which accompanies the triggering insult has been termed primary MODS.[11] Secondary MODS refers to the later onset of organ dysfunction/failure that is frequently related to shock and the response to the initial insult or a series of insults. Many believe that multiple insults or 'hits' must be involved for the production of MODS/MOF.[6,11] These 'hits' probably involve the components of the host's response to insult, such as the systemic inflammatory response syndrome (SIRS), along with manifestations of the disease process and treatment-related effects.[6,11]

INCIDENCE AND EPIDEMIOLOGY

Given the lack of a uniformly agreed upon definition of MODS/MOF, it is not surprising that the actual incidence and prevalence is currently unknown.[6] Compounding the difficulty related to the lack of a uniform definition is the uncertainty related to the clinical impact of pre-existing organ dysfunction/failure on the morbidity and mortality associated with the insult. The most common clinical conditions and disorders associated with an increased risk for developing MODS/MOF are listed in Box 3.1[6,12] Sepsis and SIRS, shock, and prolonged periods of hypotension are among the most common clinical scenarios that predispose patients to the development of organ dysfunction.[6,12] Despite the lack of exact incidence data, MODS and MOF are currently recognized as the major causes of mortality in critically ill patients.[4,13–19]

PATHOGENESIS OF MODS/MOF

The pathogenesis of MODS/MOF is an extremely complex process that probably reflects the involvement and/or interaction of multiple potential pathways for the production of injury.[3,5,13,20–37] As previously stated, organ injury can occur early in the course of the insult or develop later as a consequence of the complex pathophysiologic responses that result from the systemic response to the initial injury (Box 3.2). Among the potential hypotheses to explain the development of MODS/MOF in the critically ill patient are circulating mediators, cellular elements, and/or

humoral factors, tissue bed ischemia with or without reperfusion, microcirculatory abnormalities, translocation of colonic bacteria and/or toxins from the gastrointestinal tract/lung, abnormal rheologic properties of the circulating red blood cells, programmed cell death (apoptosis), 'stunned organ function', and/or iatrogenic complications of therapy.[5,6,13,14,21,24–32,34,35,37]

The frequent association of MODS/MOF with critical illnesses such as sepsis, SIRS, acute respiratory distress syndrome (ARDS), trauma, and pancreatitis suggests that there may be similar pathophysiologic processes which result in the production of organ system injury.[14,23,25–27,38,39] Recent evidence has emphasized the complexity of the pathophysiologic processes and the interrelationship between inflammatory responses and coagulation pathways.[40] The inflammatory response itself is exceedingly complex and involves the balancing of a pro-inflammatory response with the appropriate anti-inflammatory response necessary to maintain homeostasis.[4] The proposed systemic inflammatory response (SIRS response) has been suggested to play a central role in the pathogenesis of the systemic manifestations and injury related to a wide variety of insults.[11,28,36,38,41–43] The patient's endogenous response to the activation of the SIRS pathway has been the rapid elaboration of a compensatory

---

Box 3.1 Major clinical risk factors for the development of MODS/MOF

Sepsis

Systemic inflammatory response syndrome (SIRS)

Shock and prolonged hypotension

Severe trauma

Chronic disease, including chronic renal disease and
   chronic liver disease

Pancreatitis

Ventilator-induced lung injury (VILI) to include
   volutrauma, barotrauma, atelectotrauma, biotrauma,
   systemic air embolism

Packed red blood cell transfusions during the initial 24
   hours of care

Coma

Excessive alcohol use

Elderly population

Box 3.2 Potential pathophysiologic mechanisms(s) involved in the production of MODS/MOF

Primary cellular injury

Inadequate tissue/organ perfusion
   Hypoperfusion
   Ischemia/reperfusion
   Microaggregation (platelets, leukocytes, red blood cells)
      and/or disseminated intravascular coagulation
      (DIC)

Diffuse endothelial cell injury

Circulating humoral factors (i.e. myocardial depressant
   substance)

Circulating immune/inflammatory mediators

Protein calorie malnutrition

Translocation of colonic bacteria and/or toxins

Defective red blood cells

Apoptosis

'Stunned or hibernating' organs

Adverse effect of directed treatment or medication

anti-inflammatory response syndrome (CARS), which represents the body's attempt to limit the damage from the SIRS response so that it is not counterproductive.[41] The resultant relationship or balance between the pro-inflammatory (SIRS) and anti-inflammatory (CARS) responses has been referred to as the mixed antagonistic response syndrome or MARS.[41] The components of the pro- and anti-inflammatory responses were readily identified in early experimental animal and clinical studies of injuries associated with the development of MODS/MOF. As such, the components of this inflammatory response represented attractive targets for the application of compounds that could neutralize, bind, or otherwise modify the given pathway or response.[44-48]

The delicate balance between pro- and anti-inflammatory response is oftentimes difficult to achieve. When there is a predominance or excessive pro-inflammatory reaction, organ dysfunction is likely to ensue.[41] On the other hand, when there is an overabundant anti-inflammatory response, the patient is at risk for opportunistic or secondary infections.[41] The development of secondary or nosocomial infections may then serve as an additional insult which can trigger a SIRS response and possibly serve as additional insults or 'hits' in the pathogenesis of MODS/MOF.[6]

Currently there is an ever-growing list of potential mediators, which includes humoral, cellular, and exogenous molecules or substances that may be instrumental in the host's response to injury (Box 3.3).[11,22,26,28,38,41,43,44,49-53] Humoral mediators include components of the complement system, products of arachidonic acid metabolism (both lipoxygenase and cyclooxygenase metabolites), tumor necrosis factor (TNF), interleukins 1–15 (IL-1 to IL-15), various growth factors, adhesion molecules, platelet activating factor (PAF), nitric oxide, procoagulants, fibronectin and opsonins, toxic oxygen free radicals, endorphins, vasoactive polypeptides and amines, bradykinin and other kinins, neuroendocrine factors, myocardial depressant factor, and coagulation factors along with their degradation products.

Various cells also participate in this process. Among the cellular inflammatory mediators are polymorphonuclear leukocytes (PMNLs), monocytes/macrophages, platelets, and endothelial cells. In addition, there may be exogenous mediators such as endotoxin, exotoxin and other toxins which may be involved in the production of specific organ or tissue injury.[6] The complexity of the response makes it likely that no single mediator or

component is the key to the production of the organ dysfunction/failure in all settings.[2,6,11,14,40] In the majority of clinical settings one may expect that there are multiple pathways and molecules involved in the production of organ system dysfunction/damage.[2,6,11,14,40] The complexity of this pathogenesis and the lack of a single pathway for the development of organ system dysfunction/failure makes early treatment extremely difficult. Much of the effort to date has been devoted toward improving organ-specific support therapies and developing effective strategies for prevention.[6] The development of MODS/MOF has a tremendous impact on patient outcome, resource utilization, and cost of care.[1,6,54]

Primary cellular injury may result from the direct effect of the underlying disease process or

---

Box 3.3 Potential mediators involved in the pathogenesis of MODS/MOF

Potential humoral mediators
Complement
Products of arachidonic acid metabolism:
 Lipoxygenase products
 Cyclooxygenase products
Tumor necrosis factor
Interleukins (1–15)
Growth factors
Adhesion molecules
Platelet activating factor
Procoagulants
Fibronectin and opsonins
Toxic oxygen free radicals
Endogenous opioids – Endorphins
Vasoactive polypeptides and amines
Bradykinin and other kinins
Neuroendocrine factors
Myocardial depressant factor
Coagulation factors and their degradation products

Cellular inflammatory mediators
Polymorphonuclear leukocytes
Monocytes/macrophages
Platelets
Endothelial cells

Exogenous mediators
Endotoxin
Exotoxin and other toxins

the direct toxicity from the systemically active components of the biological response to the initial insult.[11,25] This response may include activation of both pro- and anti-inflammatory pathways, activation of the complement and coagulation cascades, and the release of various enzymes and molecules.[4,11,14,26,28,38,40,41,52,55–60] Some investigators have speculated that a condition of inadequate tissue perfusion or the maldistribution of blood flow to critical tissue beds may exist in the setting of a number of critical illnesses.[14,24,27,50,61–66] This phenomenon, if present, would deprive the tissue bed of important nutrients, substrates, and oxygen, which are essential for proper function. Additionally, some investigators have hypothesized a maldistribution of tissue perfusion that could result from either decreased tissue oxygen delivery, decreased oxygen uptake by the cells or their mitochondria, impaired cellular metabolism, or a combination of these factors.[14,64–68] In some patients with sepsis and SIRS, there may be a decrease in cardiac output, decreased systemic perfusion pressure, or a selective alteration in the perfusion of an individual organ system, which may result in absolute or relative hypoperfusion or ischemia of the organ system.[48,63,66] The period of ischemia may be followed by reperfusion, which can compound the initial ischemic injury with an oxidative injury.[14] Organ and tissue bed ischemia may result from the microaggregation of microthrombi within the microcirculation.[6,11,14] The microcirculation has a diameter of 3–5 μm and this circulation can easily be obstructed by the microthrombi composed of platelets, PMNLs, red blood cells (RBCs), and fibrin, which may obstruct the small capillaries and impair the delivery of blood and substrate to the tissues.[11,20] Microcirculatory clots have been demonstrated in experimental models of acute lung injury and sepsis and may represent a subclinical form of disseminated intravascular coagulation (DIC).[6,11,14,62] In addition to the mechanical disruption of the microcirculation, some clinicians have speculated that even though adequate blood flow may reach the various tissue beds, there may be an inability of the mitochondria and/or cells to take up and/or utilize the delivered oxygen and substrate.[14,50,67] The ischemic or poorly perfused intestinal tract may have altered mucosal barrier function that can give rise to translocation of intestinal bacteria and/or toxins which may further the injury state (see below).[24,69] In summary, there are a number of mechanisms that may produce an ischemic/hypoxic injury to the tissues and result in the production of organ system dysfunction or failure.

Additionally, diffuse endothelial cell injury may result from elaborated mediators of the SIRS response, such as TNF and other pro-inflammatory cytokines.[14,25,26,38,42,43,52] This injury has been hypothesized as a mechanism for the development of acute lung injury and ARDS, which are frequently seen in the setting of sepsis and SIRS.[14] The vascular endothelial cell injury may produce a permeability defect that can compromise the integrity of the vascular endothelium and lead to pulmonary capillary leakage and edema.[14,25,38] This state has been termed 'malignant intravascular inflammation' and it may be a common manifestation of the SIRS response.[28]

When mechanical ventilatory support is provided with either excessive pressures or tidal volumes that result in alveolar overdistension, there is the potential to damage the capillary endothelial cells surrounding the alveolus, which can result in interstitial edema.[70] In addition, there have been reports of an accompanying increase in pro-inflammatory cytokines in the bronchoalveolar lavage fluid as well as the systemic circulation, which has been associated with the development of organ system dysfunction.[71] Alveolar overdistension may also damage the alveolar epithelial cells and has been linked to the potential for air embolization and/or translocation of airway bacteria.[72] Both of these processes can cause or potentiate a SIRS response and can lead to organ system injury.

A number of circulating humoral factors have been detected in critically ill patients and could be responsible for the development of organ system dysfunction.[14,53,73] One such substance has been termed myocardial depressant factor and is reported to be associated with the development of reversible biventricular failure in some patients with septic shock.[53,73] This reversible cardiomyopathy of sepsis is manifested by an increase in end-diastolic volume and a reduction in the ejection fraction, even though the stroke volume and the cardiac output may be adequately maintained or even increased.[73] Recent reports suggest that this process is probably the result of circulating TNF and IL-1. These pro-inflammatory cytokines stimulate the inducible form of nitric oxide synthase, leading to an increase in nitric oxide (NO), which can result in cardiac dilatation and decreased contractility.[53,74]

Critically ill patients are frequently hypercatabolic and may be particularly at risk for the development of protein calorie malnutrition.[13,75] The nutritional abnormalities may compromise immune function and the ability to mount an adequate inflammatory response against offending agents. A recent trial in patients with ARDS has demonstrated decreased organ dysfunction associated with the administration of an enteral diet containing eicosapentaenoic acid, γ-linolenic acid, and antioxidants.[76] Malnutrition and/or hypoperfusion of the gastrointestinal tract are both known causes of colonic bacteria and/or toxin translocation, at least in experimental animal models of injury.[13,21,75] Poor perfusion of the gastrointestinal tract, whether as a result of decreased cardiac output, hypotension, decreased splanchnic blood flow, or microthrombosis of the intestinal microcirculation, can result in abnormalities of the intestinal mucosal barrier function. These alterations can result in intestinal ischemia, which may be followed by reperfusion. The terminal ileum and cecum are vast storage areas for the colonizing Gram-negative bacteria and their associated endotoxin. With the alteration in the intestinal mucosal barrier function, the bacteria–endotoxin may enter the mesenteric lymph and/or systemic circulation, which can be a cause of a secondary infection or stimulus for the SIRS response.[14,21,24,29] This hypothesis has been supported by the observation of endotoxin in the peripheral blood samples of critically ill septic and SIRS patients.[44] Further support for this pathway of organ dysfunction is derived from the detection of endotoxemia in critically ill patients who lack clinical or microbiologic evidence of infection by Gram-negative bacteria.[44]

Recent reports have suggested that there are defective RBCs with altered shape or rheologic properties that may predispose to plugging or obstruction of the microvasculature, which can result in cellular or tissue ischemia.[14,52] In the presence of the activation of the coagulation system and endothelial abnormalities characteristic of the inflammatory state, these altered RBCs may further contribute to the perfusion abnormalities that may result in MODS/MOF. In addition, the transfusion of packed RBCs, which is a relatively common practice in the management of the critically ill patient, has been associated with an increased likelihood of organ dysfunction.[12] While the transfusion of packed RBCs may serve as a marker of disease severity, in-vitro studies have reported increased inflammatory cytokine production from PMNLs after exposure to the serum contained in packed cell transfusions that are older than 14 days.[77] The authors speculated that lysophosphatidylcholine and other possible serum compounds may be capable of inducing the inflammatory response from the primed cells.[77] This phenomenon was reduced when the packed cells were washed prior to application on the PMNLs. The practice of transfusing older packed RBCs may therefore have a possible role in the induction of organ system dysfunction by serving as an inflammatory trigger in keeping with the multiple-hit hypothesis.[37,77] Taylor and coworkers found that there was an increased risk for the development of nosocomial infections and increased mortality in critically ill patients who received packed RBC transfusions compared to those who were not transfused.[78]

A recent review of autopsy results from patients who died of sepsis reported a profound, progressive apoptosis-induced loss of cells of the adaptive immune system, which is directly opposite from what would have been intuitively expected.[35] This condition is marked by a depletion of lymphocytes. This review challenged the concept that immunosuppression is a compensatory response to the pro-inflammatory response to injury and suggests that immunosuppression is actually an important primary response to injury.[35] The authors cited the discordant histologic changes evident in autopsy studies performed shortly after death in patients dying of severe sepsis.[35] They noted a significant absence of severe histologic abnormalities in patients who manifested considerable biochemical and functional abnormalities of organ system function.[35] They postulated the presence of 'hibernating or stunned' organs as another explanation for organ system dysfunction.[35]

Finally, critically ill patients are at risk for the development of organ dysfunction that may be the consequence of the various interventions and therapies employed in the management of their illness.[6] A common example is renal dysfunction that may result from the administration of nephrotoxic agents such as intravenous contrast, aminoglycoside antibiotics, or amphotericin.[6,20] Many of the invasive diagnostic and therapeutic agents and procedures have the potential to produce undesirable adverse effects on a variety of organ systems.[6] Clinicians must constantly be aware of the potential adverse results of the therapeutic strategies and procedures used in the management of the critically ill patient and they should carefully weigh the potential risks against the expected benefits.

ASSESSMENT OF ORGAN FUNCTION

Severity of illness and organ dysfunction scores have been designed and used for the critically ill patient in the intensive care unit (ICU) to allow comparison of patients enrolled in clinical trials, to describe the population of patients cared for in the ICU, to monitor the effects of applied therapies, and in some circumstances to aid the intensivist in discussions concerning prognosis.[79–84] The main severity of illness scoring systems in clinical use include the acute physiology and chronic health evaluation (APACHE), simplified acute physiology score (SAPS), and the mortality probability model (MPM).[80] All of these scoring systems have had recent modifications. Teres and coworkers evaluated the Project Impact database to determine the percent of patients who had severe sepsis on admission to the ICU.[85] They reported that 11.3% (2434 patients) met the definition of severe sepsis on ICU admission and these patients had an increased severity of illness score, mortality rate, resource use, and ICU readmission rate compared to the nonseptic patients in the database.

In addition, there have also been specific organ dysfunction scoring systems, such as the multiple organ dysfunction score (MODS), sequential organ failure assessment (SOFA) score, and logistic organ dysfunction score (LODS).[80] As of this time, there has been no uniform acceptance of an assessment tool to determine abnormal organ function or prognosticate outcome for patients with suspected MODS. A majority of the tools employ an assessment of five to seven major organ systems, typically: respiratory, renal, hepatic, central nervous system, gastrointestinal system, hematological system, and the cardiovascular system. The MODS, SOFA, and LODS scores are used in the majority of current studies and reports to evaluate specific and global organ system function. The basic components of these scores are listed in Table 3.1. All of these scores have been demonstrated to track increased overall mortality and correlate with increased severity of illness.[86] Pettila and associates reported that the severity of the day 1 organ dysfunction score (MODS, SOFA, LODS) was predictive of outcome and tracked closely to the APACHE III score.[86] Previously, Knaus and coworkers reported that the presence of three or more organ dysfunctions for greater than or equal to 5 days was associated with 100% mortality rate in the 2719 patients they studied in their APACHE database.[79] Clearly, the more organs that are dysfunctional and the greater the duration of

Table 3.1   Comparison of three different organ dysfunction scoring systems.

Parameter	MODS	SOFA	LODS
Respiratory	PaO_2/FiO_2 ratio	PaO_2/FiO_2 ratio and need for ventilatory support	PaO_2/FiO_2 ratio and ventilation/CPAP status
Coagulation	Platelet count	Platelet count	White blood cell and platelet counts
Hepatic	Bilirubin concentration	Bilirubin concentration	Bilirubin concentration and prothrombin time
Cardiovascular	Heart rate × ratio of central venous pressure and mean arterial pressure (HR × [CVP/MAP])	Blood pressure and adrenergic support	Heart rate and systolic blood pressure
Central nervous system	Glasgow coma score	Glasgow coma score	Glasgow coma score
Renal	Creatinine concentration	Creatinine concentration or urine output	Urea and creatinine concentrations and urine output

MODS, multiple organ dysfunction score; SOFA, sequential organ failure assessment; LODS, logistic organ dysfunction score; PaO_2, arterial partial pressure of oxygen; FiO_2, fraction of inspired oxygen; CPAP, continuous positive airway pressure.
Source: modified from Vincent JL et al.[80]

dysfunction, the worse the outcome. More work is still necessary to refine our ability to determine a dysfunctional vs a failed organ system or, more importantly, differentiate between a reversibly injured and an irreversibly injured organ system.

TREATMENT/MANAGEMENT OF MODS/MOF

The current management of patients with MODS/MOF is predominantly supportive. Recent emphasis has been placed on the provision of early goal-oriented resuscitation of the critically ill patient and ventilatory support designed to minimize the risk for ventilator-induced lung injury (VILI).[66,70,71,87] Infection and sepsis are common predisposing conditions for the development of MODS/MOF and it is imperative to diligently investigate patients for the presence of active or inadequately treated infection.[6] It may be necessary to use sophisticated imaging techniques in addition to obtaining adequate culture specimens from the potential infective sites.[6] Clinical trials have demonstrated the importance of early administration of appropriate effective antibiotic therapy for improved survival in the management of patients with infections.[48] Adequate drainage and/or surgical debridement should also be utilized when necessary for effective management of closed space pus or infected tissues.[48]

The supportive measures for the patient with MODS/MOF include those basic management provisions that are essential for all critically ill patients. Pulmonary management is directed at supporting oxygenation and ventilation. The value of early intubation and mechanical ventilatory support to reduce the blood flow to the diaphragm and accessory muscles of respiration has been advocated by some clinicians, but there is a lack of supporting data from human studies.[6] The decision regarding early intubation and ventilatory support needs to be weighed against the potential complications associated with the procedure and the inability of the patient to protect his own airway. The use of lung protective ventilatory support strategies has been demonstrated to improve patient survival and is associated with decreased organ dysfunction.[70] The overdistension of alveoli can give rise to ventilator-associated lung injury and has also been associated with the elaboration of inflammatory molecules into the alveolus as well as the systemic circulation.[71] This has been termed biotrauma and, along with barotrauma (high airway pressure), volutrauma (large gas volumes), and atelectotrauma (alveolar collapse and re-expansion), is another component of the ventilator-induced injury that is associated with inappropriately high tidal volumes and/or lack of adequate positive end-expiratory pressure (PEEP).[88] Patients with acute lung injury (ALI) and ARDS who continue to manifest the physiologic, radiologic, and clinical abnormalities of injury after 7–10 days of supportive management are felt to have entered the fibroproliferative phase of injury.[89] Meduri and coworkers have demonstrated in a prospective, randomized, placebo-controlled, double-blind trial a significant improvement in survival associated with the administration of corticosteroids to this group of patients.[89] Along with the improvement in survival, there was a decrease in lung injury score and decreased organ dysfunction.[89]

Restoration and maintenance of hemodynamic stability is also an important aspect of management for the patient with organ system dysfunction.[6,87] The initial strategy should utilize fluid resuscitation to ensure that the circulating intravascular volume is appropriate.[6] There is controversy as to which type of fluid is preferable and a discussion of the pros and cons of crystalloid, colloid, blood products, and volume expanders is beyond the scope of this chapter. If hypotension persists after adequate volume resuscitation, vasoactive medications should be used to improve hemodynamic function and ensure adequate tissue oxygen delivery.[6,63,90,91]

The importance of early goal-directed hemodynamic resuscitation was recently emphasized by Rivers and colleagues.[66] The authors randomized critically ill SIRS patients with either hypotension or elevated lactates to standard resuscitation or to an early goal-oriented approach. The goal-directed approach targeted early administration of sufficient fluid (including blood products), vasopressors, and inotropes to achieve the following goals: central venous pressure 8–12 mmHg, mean arterial pressure >65 mmHg, urine output >0.5 ml/kg/h, and a central venous oxygen saturation ($ScVO_2$) >70%. In the situation where the $ScVO_2$ was <70%, therapy was directed to ensure the SaO_2 >93%, hematocrit >30%, and there was an adequate cardiac index and oxygen consumption. Patients randomized to the early goal-directed resuscitation strategy had a significantly reduced in-hospital (30.5% vs 46.5%, $p = 0.009$), 28-day, and 60-day mortality compared to patients who received conventional management. There was a significantly increased number of in-hospital deaths from sudden cardiovascular collapse in the conventional resuscitation group. This group also demonstrated a slight, but not significant increase in the percentage of patients with evidence of MODS (21.8% vs 16.2%, $p = 0.27$).[66]

There is general agreement regarding the importance of ensuring adequate tissue oxygen delivery. In the past, the definition of 'adequate' was a topic of debate and controversy.[54,92–95] The question of supply dependency of oxygen utilization in the setting of critical illness has been debated and may depend on individual patient factors and the methods used to assess oxygen consumption.[95] Studies performed predominantly in a surgical population demonstrated improved survival in those patients who were managed with strategies designed to increase tissue oxygen delivery.[94] Tissue oxygen delivery can be increased through the use of inotropic agents, which increase the cardiac output, or by increasing the hemoglobin with RBC transfusions to increase the oxygen-carrying capacity of the blood.[93,95] Potential undesirable effects associated with the use of inotropic and vasoactive agents include the development of arrhythmias and ischemia of selected organ beds.[93] The use of packed RBC transfusions to increase the oxygen-carrying capacity of blood needs to be counterbalanced by the potential risks, which include transmission of infectious agents, immune suppression, induction of a pro-inflammatory cytokine response from PMNLs, and microcirculatory dysfunction.[78,96] In blood that has been stored for longer than 15 days in citrate phosphate dextrose adenine 1 (CPDA-1), there may be a loss of normal RBC deformability with a potential for microcirculatory dysfunction. Many clinicians believe that the concept of oxygen supply dependence may actually reflect mathematical coupling, since this relationship was predominantly evident when both the oxygen delivery and the oxygen consumption were calculated using standard formulas.[95] Potential toxicity has been demonstrated in some patients who were subjected to strategies designed to greatly increase oxygen delivery by inotropic support of the cardiac output.[92] A large prospective randomized controlled trial failed to demonstrate improved survival using a therapeutic strategy designed to increase the tissue oxygen delivery to supranormal levels.[93]

In addition to ventilatory and hemodynamic support for the altered respiratory and circulatory dysfunction, respectively, other organ-specific support strategies are frequently utilized in the management of patients with MODS/MOF. Renal dysfunction can be supported by the provision of renal replacement therapy.[20,97,98] Hepatic support has recently been evaluated in selected centers using artificial and bioartificial support systems.[99] Abnormalities of the coagulation system can be addressed by replacing depleted coagulation factors with cryoprecipitate or fresh frozen plasma. Thrombocytopenia can be managed using platelet transfusions. A recent study evaluated erythropoietin as an alternative to packed RBC administration for the management of anemia in the critically ill patient.[96] While this treatment is not as immediate as packed RBC transfusions, it does appear to be a safe and cost-effective alternative.[96]

The importance of early enteral nutritional support to maintain the integrity of the intestinal mucosal barrier function and decrease the likelihood of bacterial toxin translocation has recently been emphasized.[24] Enteral nutrition also supports the integrity of the upper gastrointestinal tract and may prevent stress-related gastrointestinal bleeding. Other potential approaches to prevent stress-related gastrointestinal bleeding include the use of histamine type 2 blockers and cytoprotective agents. Patients at risk for the development of MODS/MOF are critically ill and are at risk for all of the potential complications and adverse events that are all too frequently encountered in this group of patients.[6] As such, strategies to prevent deep vein thrombosis and pulmonary emboli should be used unless there are specific contraindications.[6] The development of neuromuscular weakness has been recognized as a complication in the critically ill patient, particularly those with sepsis and MODS.[42] This condition is marked by axonal degeneration and is referred to as critical illness polyneuropathy and/or polymyopathy.[42] The pathophysiology of critical illness polyneuropathy probably results from the effects of pro-inflammatory mediators:[42] the axons may require 3–6 months to recover sufficiently. These disorders may explain prolonged ventilator dependency in some critically ill patients and may necessitate rehabilitation efforts, even after weaning or separation from ventilatory support, before the patient is able to return home and care for themselves.

PREVENTION OF MODS/MOF

In addition to the support management strategies for MODS, recent attention has been directed toward prevention in at-risk patients. Innovative clinical trials have evaluated a variety of strategies aimed at blocking, neutralizing, or removing the potential inflammatory mediators.[45–47,96,100,101] In addition, therapeutic success has been reported with the use of tight glucose control using supplemental doses of insulin, lung protective ventilatory support, and early goal-oriented hemodynamic resuscitation strategies.[54,63,66,70,90,93,102,103] Various antithrombotic agents, antioxidants, and nutritional support strategies have also been evaluated.[103–108] Unfortunately, up to this point in time, none of these approaches has been given approval for use based on demonstrated significant benefit in preventing or treating MODS/MOF in multicentered, prospective, randomized, controlled trials.

Trials of antiendotoxin therapy with the human and murine monoclonal antibodies against endotoxin demonstrated a decrease in development of multiple organ dysfunction.[100] The murine monoclonal antibody E-5 also demonstrated increased resolution of established organ dysfunction in the initial trials.[100] However, a subsequent confirmatory trial failed to find a statistical benefit to this form of treatment and neither form of antiendotoxin therapy has been approved for use in the management of patients with severe sepsis.[109] A large number of anti- and pro-inflammatory mediator trials have been conducted without the demonstration of significant improvement in outcome:[46,47] in fact, one trial of anti-TNF soluble receptor antibody was actually associated with increased mortality when higher levels of the monoclonal antibody were administered.[110] Additional approaches have evaluated the use of continuous venovenous hemofiltration, with or without adsorbent columns, as a means of removing circulating inflammatory mediators.[97] This technique also raises concern over the potential to remove the pro-inflammatory as well as the anti-inflammatory mediators. Further studies are ongoing in an attempt to define the role, if any, of antimediator therapy in the management of patients with MODS/MOF.

Strategies to limit additional 'hits' during the period of insult also have theoretical value as prevention for MODS/MOF. The time-consuming and expensive technique of selective digestive decontamination which couples topical and systemic antimicrobial therapy in an attempt to decrease the development of nosocomial infections has been shown to decrease the development of ventilator-associated pneumonia, but did not improve mortality.[111] Because of the great expense and time

commitment, coupled with a lack of significant improvement in survival, the true benefit of this technique remains to be established. Past reports have demonstrated decreased development of ARDS with the use of the thromboxane synthase inhibitor ketoconazole in surgical patients who were at increased risk for the development of MODS/MOF.[112] A subsequent multicentered, prospective, placebo-controlled clinical trial conducted by ARDSnet failed to demonstrate an improvement in the outcome of patients with ARDS and ALI.[113] Minimizing the administration of packed RBCs and blood products may also decrease the development of MODS.[37,77] A recent trial has demonstrated a relationship between the development of MODS and the transfusion of packed RBCs in critically ill patients.[17]

Therapeutic strategies directed at the activation of the coagulation system and disruption of the microcirculation from the generation of microthrombi have been addressed by the use of the endogenous anticoagulants antithrombin, protein C, and tissue factor pathway inhibitor.[105,106,114–118] The use of the serine protease AT III, antithrombin, replacement therapy was associated with a trend toward improved survival in a small trial of patients with septic shock and DIC.[115] A subsequent study of patients with sepsis and trauma demonstrated an improvement in the oxygenation index (PaO_2/FiO_2 ratio) in critically ill patients who were found to have less than 70% activity.[106] Eisele and colleagues reported on a meta-analysis of several studies of critically ill septic or post-trauma patients and reported that there was less organ dysfunction in the patients who had received antithrombin infusions compared to those treated with placebo.[105] Despite these promising early results, a recent multicenter, prospective, randomized, placebo-controlled clinical trial failed to demonstrate a significant survival benefit at 30, 60, or 90 days associated with antithrombin treatment of patients with severe sepsis and septic shock.[107] Similarly, a recent large multicenter trial of tissue factor pathway inhibitor vs placebo in septic patients failed to meet its targeted survival endpoint.[118]

Activated protein C – drotrecogin alpha (activated) – interrupts the coagulation cascade by inhibiting the action of factor Va and factor VIIIa.[117] In addition, activated protein C has been reported to have anti-inflammatory effects, as evidenced by a decrease in the IL-6 levels, and it can restore the fibrinolytic pathway by interfering with the generation of plasminogen activator inhibitor-1

(PAI-1).[117] All of these potential mechanisms of action could be beneficial in the septic cascade of events. A recent trial that evaluated the continuous 96-hour infusion of drotrecogin alpha (activated) vs placebo in patients with severe sepsis demonstrated a significant improvement in survival associated with the use of activated protein C.[117] A combination of anticoagulation and anti-inflammatory treatment would be expected to improve or prevent organ dysfunction by protecting or restoring the microcirculation. However, since activated protein C is an endogenous anticoagulant, there is a potential for increased bleeding complications. In subsequent analysis, the use of activated protein C was found to provide increased survival benefit in those patients who manifested the greatest baseline risk for mortality.[119] Vincent et al reported significant improvement in cardiovascular dysfunction with activated protein C therapy of severe sepsis.[120] Specifically, there was faster resolution of cardiovascular and respiratory dysfunction and a slower onset of hematologic dysfunction compared to placebo administration. Activated protein C treatment of severe sepsis was also found to be cost-effective and compared favorably with other lifesaving treatments.[121] The United States Food and Drug Administration (FDA) has recently approved the use of drotrecogin alpha (activated) for the treatment of adult patients with severe sepsis and a high risk for mortality as evidenced by an elevated APACHE II score or the presence of multiple organ dysfunction. There are cautions to restrict the use of this agent in patients with known hypersensitivity to it, the presence of increased risk for bleeding, or in those patients who have an epidural catheter in place. The cost per quality adjusted life year of activated protein C treatment of patients with severe sepsis and an APACHE II score >25 was US$27,400, while the mean cost per quality adjusted life year for the entire study population was $48,000.[121] The use of activated protein C in severe sepsis patients with an APACHE II score <25 was not found to be cost-effective.

In a study of postoperative patients, the majority of whom were being managed with mechanical ventilatory support, the use of continuous insulin infusions directed at maintaining the blood sugar between 90 and 110 mg/dl was associated with a significant improvement in outcome.[102] Not only was intensive care and hospital survival improved but also there was a fourfold decrease in the number of deaths associated with the development of organ failure associated with a septic source. In a subsequent analysis, the benefit of the tight glucose control was found to be related to the effects of glucose control and not from the administration of insulin.[122] These results suggest that paying attention to the basic metabolic needs of critically ill patients may be an important strategy to prevent the development of organ dysfunction and its attendant complications.[102,122]

PROGNOSIS

Multiple organ dysfunction/failure is a common occurrence in the critically ill patient and its presence is associated with a high risk for morbidity and mortality.[1-6] The development of MODS/MOF has been demonstrated to predict a high likelihood of death and is one of the two most common causes of death in the noncoronary intensive care unit.[1] Various trials have demonstrated that the mortality risk increases as the number of organ systems failing and the duration of the failure increase.[9,82] The ARDSnet database reported an increase in mortality rate, a longer time to wean from ventilatory support, and a longer stay in the ICU in elderly patients with ARDS compared to younger patients.[123] These results suggest that age may have a dramatic effect on outcome related to organ dysfunction.

A higher risk of mortality has been found in association with the dysfunction and/or failure of specific organ systems.[84,101,124-126] An increased mortality rate has been demonstrated with dysfunction/failure of the brain, liver, lung, and kidney.[84,101,124-126] Specific scoring systems have been used to quantify the level of organ dysfunction and have been primarily used in the evaluation of various investigational agents. The use of various organ dysfunction scores has been proposed as a prognostic index and has now been incorporated into many clinical trials as a means of quantifying the degree of organ dysfunction and the response to therapy. At the present time, we lack the ability to provide specific treatment for organ dysfunction/failure. Our current management of MODS/MOF relies on the treatment of the underlying, predisposing condition(s) and the provision of organ replacement or supportive therapy. The likelihood of recovery of organ function is quite variable and depends on multiple factors. Some clinicians view dysfunction as a more reversible form of injury in contrast to overt failure. It is also important to take into account those dysfunctions that were present prior to the injury, as their impact may be different from those dysfunctions/failures that were the result of the insult. Recent studies have emphasized that organ dysfunction in the setting of sepsis may reflect programmed cell death (apoptosis) and may be part of the normal physiologic response to the insult.[35] In addition, some clinicians have observed that altered organ function in various injury states may represent a form of 'stunned function' and, with the correction of the underlying injury or the passage of time, organ function will return to baseline.[35] Future efforts must also concentrate on strategies to prevent the development of organ dysfunction/failure.

SUMMARY

Multiple organ system dysfunction/failure is a common adverse sequel of critical illness and is one of the most common causes of death in the noncoronary ICU. The pathophysiology of the development of MODS is likely to be multifactoral and may take a number of different pathways. The frequency of specific organ system involvement is dependent on the definition used to describe the organ dysfunction. The presence of organ dysfunction/failure has great clinical impact on the underlying disease process and can prolong the hospital stay, increase the cost of care, and has been associated with an increase in mortality rate. At present, there is no recognized specific treatment for established organ failure; thus primary attention has been directed toward provision of organ support or replacement therapy and the prevention of subsequent organ dysfunction. Important components of the prevention strategy would include the provision of lung protective ventilatory support strategies, early goal-directed resuscitation, and control of hyperglycemia and other complications of critical illness, including nosocomial infection.

REFERENCES

1. Barie PS, Hydo LJ. Influence of multiple organ dysfunction syndrome on duration of critical illness and hospitalization. Arch Surg 1996;131:1318–24.
2. Beale R, Bihari DJ. Multiple organ failure: the pilgrim's progress. Crit Care Med 1993;21:S1–S3.
3. Carrico CJ, Meakins JL, Marshall JC, et al. Multiple-organ-failure syndrome. Arch Surg 1986;121:196–208.
4. Fry DE. Multiple system organ failure. Surg Clin North Am 1988;68:107–22.
5. Goris RJA, Boekhorst TPA, Nuytinck JKS, Gimbrere JSF. Multiple organ failure: generalized autodestructive inflammation. Arch Surg 1985;120:1109–115.
6. Balk RA. Pathogenesis and management of multiple organ dysfunction and failure in severe sepsis and septic shock. Crit Care Clin 2000;16:337–52.
7. Tilney NL, Bailey GL, Morgan AP. Sequential system failure after rupture of abdominal aortic aneurysms: an unsolved problem in postoperative care. Ann Surg 1973;178:117–22.
8. Eiseman B, Beart R, Norton L. Multiple organ failure. Surg Gynecol Obstet 1977;144:323–6.
9. Marshall JC. Criteria for the description of organ dysfunction in sepsis and SIRS. In: Fein AM, Abraham ED, Balk RA, et al, eds. Sepsis and multiorgan failure. Baltimore: Williams and Wilkins, 1997:286–96.
10. Members of the American College of Chest Physicians/Society of Critical Care Medicine Consensus Conference Committee. American College of Chest Physicians/Society of Critical Care Medicine Consensus Conference: definitions for sepsis and organ failure and guidelines for the use of innovative therapies in sepsis. Crit Care Med 1992;20:864–74.
11. Piper RD, Sibbald WJ. Multiple organ dysfunction syndrome: the relevance of persistent infection and inflammation. In: Fein AM, Abraham ED, Balk RA, et al, eds. Sepsis and multiorgan failure. Baltimore: Williams and Wilkins, 1997:189–208.
12. Tran DD, Cuesta MA, van Leeuwen PA, et al. Risk factors for multiple organ system failure and death in critically injured patients. Surgery 1993;114:21–30.
13. Barton R, Cerra FB. The hypermetabolism: multiple organ failure syndrome. Chest 1989;96:1153–60.
14. Dorinsky PM, Gadek JE. Mechanism of multiple nonpulmonary organ failure in ARDS. Chest 1989;96:885–92.
15. Montgomery AB, Stager MA, Carrico CJ, Hudson LD. Causes of mortality in patients with the adult respiratory distress syndrome. Am Rev Respir Dis 1985;132:485–9.
16. Regel G, Grotz M, Weltner T, Sturm JA, Tscherne H. Pattern of organ failure following severe trauma. World J Surg 1996;20:422–9.
17. Vincent JL, Baron JF, Reinhart K, et al, for the ABC Investigators. Anemia and blood transfusion in critically ill patients. JAMA 2002;288:1499–507.
18. Tran DD, Groeneveld J, van der Meulen J, et al. Age, chronic disease, sepsis, organ system failure, and mortality in a medical intensive care unit. Crit Care Med 1990;18:474–9.
19. Haire WD. Multiple organ dysfunction syndrome in hematopoietic stem cell transplantation. Crit Care Med 2002; 30:S257–62.
20. Corwin HL. Acute renal failure in sepsis and multiple organ failure. In: Fein AM, Abraham ED, Balk RA, et al, eds. Sepsis and multiorgan failure. Baltimore: Williams and Wilkins; 1997:5446–556.
21. Crouser ED, Dorinsky PM. Gastrointestinal tract dysfunction in critical illness: pathophysiology and interaction with acute lung injury in adult respiratory distress syndrome/multiple organ dysfunction syndrome. New Hor 1994;2:476–87.
22. Donnelly SC, Haslett C, Dransfield I, et al. Role of selectins in development of adult respiratory distress syndrome. Lancet 1994;344:215–19.
23. Ertel W, Friedl HP, Trentz O. Multiple organ dysfunction syndrome (MODS) following multiple organ failure in patients after severe blunt trauma. Crit Care Med 1994;23:474–80.
24. Fink MP, Aranow JS. Gut barrier dysfunction and sepsis. In: Fein AM, Abraham ED, Balk RA, et al, eds. Sepsis and multiorgan failure. Baltimore: Williams and Wilkins; 1997:383–407.
25. Hyers TM, Gee M, Andreadis NA. Cellular interactions in the multiple organ injury syndrome. Am Rev Respir Dis 1987;135:952–3.
26. Jansen MJJM, Hendriks T, Vogels MTE, van der Meer JWM, Goris RJA. Inflammatory cytokines in an experimental model for

the multiple organ dysfunction syndrome. Crit Care Med 1996;24:1196–202.

27. Michie HR. Metabolism of sepsis and multiple organ failure. World J Surg 1996;20:460–4.

28. Pinsky MR, Vincent JL, Deviere J, et al. Serum cytokine levels in human septic shock: relation to multiple-system organ failure and mortality. Chest 1993;103:565–75.

29. Swank GM, Deitch EA. Role of the gut in multiple organ failure: bacterial translocation and permeability changes. World J Surg 1996;20:411–17.

30. Power C, Fanning N, Redmond HP. Celllular apoptosis and organ injury in sepsis: a review. Shock 2002;18:197–211.

31. Papadoppoulos MC, Davies DC, Moss RF, Tighe D, Bennett ED. Pathophysiology of septic encephalopathy: a review. Crit Care Med 2000;28:3019–24.

32. Godin PJ, Buchman TG. Uncoupling of biological oscillators: a complementary hypothesis concerning the pathogenesis of multiple organ dysfunction syndrome. Crit Care Med 1996;24:1107–16.

33. Matuschak GM, Henry KA, Johanns CA, Lechner AJ. Liver–lung interactions following *Escherichia coli* bacteremic sepsis and secondary hepatic ischemia/reperfusion injury. Am J Respir Crit Care Med 2001;163:1002–9.

34. Doig CJ, Sutherland LR, Sandham JD, et al. Increased intestinal permeability is associated with the development of multiple organ dysfunction syndrome in critically ill ICU patients. Am J Respir Crit Care Med 1998;158:444–51.

35. Hotchkiss RS, Karl IE. The pathophysiology and treatment of sepsis. N Engl J Med 2003;348:138–50.

36. Pinsky MR, Matuschak GM. Multiple systems organ failure: failure of host defense homeostasis. Crit Care Clin 1989;5:199–220.

37. Aiboshi J, Moore EE, Ciesla DJ, Silliman CC. Blood transfusion and the two-insult model of post-injury multiple organ failure. Shock 2001;15:302–6.

38. Douzinas EE, Tsidemiadou PD, Pitardis MT, et al. The regional production of cytokines and lactate in sepsis-related multiple organ failure. Am J Respir Crit Care Med 1997;155:53–9.

39. Marshall JC, Christou NV, Horn R, Meakins JL. The microbiology of multiple organ failure. Arch Surg 1988;123:309–15.

40. Balk RA, Goyette RE. Multiple organ dysfunction syndrome in patients with severe sepsis: more than just inflammation. In: Balk RA, ed. International Congress and Symposium Series 249: advances in the diagnosis and management of the patient with severe sepsis. London: The Royal Society of Medicine Press, 2002:39–60.

41. Bone RC, Grodzin CJ, Balk RA. Sepsis: a new hypothesis for pathogenesis of the disease process. Chest 1997;112:235–43.

42. Bolton CF. Sepsis and the systemic inflammatory response syndrome: neuromuscular manifestations. Crit Care Med 1996;24:1408–16.

43. Schlag G, Redl H. Mediators of injury and inflammation. World J Surg 1996;20:406–10.

44. Casey LC, Balk RA, Bone RC. Plasma cytokine and endotoxin levels correlate with survival in patients with the sepsis syndrome. Ann Int Med 1993;119:771–8.

45. Fisher CJ Jr, Dhainaut JFA, Opal SM, et al. Recombinant human interleukin-1 receptor antagonist in the treatment of patients with sepsis syndrome. JAMA 1994;271:1836–43.

46. Zeni F, Freeman B, Natanson C. Anti-inflammatory therapies to treat sepsis and septic shock: a reassessment. Crit Care Med 1997;25:1095–100.

47. Eichacker PQ, Parent C, Kalil A, et al. Risk and the efficacy of anti-inflammatory agents: retrospective and confirmatory studies of sepsis. Am J Respir Crit Care Med 2002;166:1197–205.

48. Wheeler AP, Bernard GR. Treating patients with severe sepsis. N Engl J Med 1999;340:207–14.

49. Doughty L, Carcillo JA, Kaplan S, Janosky J. Plasma nitrite and nitrate concentrations and multiple organ failure in pediatric sepsis. Crit Care Med 1998;26:157–62.

50. Fink MP. Adequacy of gut oxygenation in endotoxemia and sepsis. Crit Care Med 1993;21:S4–8.

51. Francois B, Trimoreau F, Vignon P, et al. Thrombocytopenia in the sepsis syndrome: role of hemophagocytosis and macrophage colony-stimulating factor. Am J Med 1997;103:114–20.

52. Mallick AA, Ishizaka A, Stephens KE, et al. Multiple organ damage caused by tumor necrosis factor and prevented by prior neutrophil depletion. Chest 1989;95:1114–20.

53. Symeonides S, Balk RA. Nitric oxide in the pathogenesis of sepsis. Infect Dis Clin North Am 1999;13:449–63.

54. Boyd O, Grounds M, Bennett ED. A randomized clinical trial of the effect of deliberate perioperative increase of oxygen delivery on mortality in high-risk surgical patients. JAMA 1993;270:2699–707.

55. Baudo F, Caimi TM, de Cataldo F, et al. Antithrombin III (AT III) replacement therapy in patients with sepsis and/or post-surgical complications: a controlled, double-blind, randomized, multicenter study. Intens Care Med 1998;24:336–42.

56. Izumi M, McDonald MC, Sharpe MA, Chatterjee PK, Thiemermann C. Superoxide dismutase mimetics with catalase activity reduce the organ injury in hemorrhagic shock. Shock 2002;18:230–5.

57. Lorenz E, Mira JP, Frees KL, Schwartz DA. Relevance of mutations in the TLR4 receptor in patients with gram-negative septic shock. Arch Intern Med 2002;162:1028–32.

58. Tang GJ, Huang SL, Yien HW, et al. Tumor necrosis factor gene polymorphism and septic shock in surgical infection. Crit Care Med 2000;28:2733–6.

59. Mira JP, Cariou A, Grall F, et al. Association of TNF2, a TNF-α promoter polymorphism, with septic shock susceptibility and mortality. JAMA 1999;282:561–8.

60. Gerard C. Complement C5a in the sepsis sydrome – too much of a good thing? N Engl J Med 2003;348:167–9.

61. Fiddian-Green RG. Associations between intramucosal acidosis in the gut and organ failure. Crit Care Med 1993;21:S103–7.

62. Fourrier F, Chopin C, Goudemand J, et al. Septic shock, multiple organ failure, and disseminated intravascular coagulation. Chest 1992;101:816–23.

63. Landry DW, Oliver JA. The pathogenesis of vasodilatory shock. N Engl J Med 2001;345:588–95.

64. LeDoux D, Astiz ME, Carpati CM, Rackow EC. Effects of perfusion pressure on tissue perfusion in septic shock. Crit Care Med 2000;28:2729–32.

65. Taneja R, Marshall JC. Vasoactive agents and the gut: fueling the motor of multiple organ failure. Crit Care Med 2000;28:3107–8.

66. Rivers E, Nguyen B, Haystad S, et al. Early goal-directed therapy in the treatment of severe sepsis and septic shock. N Engl J Med 2001;345:1368–77.

67. Gutierrez G, Lund N, Bryan-Brown CW. Cellular oxygen utilization during multiple organ failure. Crit Care Clin 1989;5:271–88.

68. Mizock BA. Metabolic derangements in sepsis and septic shock. Crit Care Clin 2000;16:319–36.

69. Baue AE. The role of the gut in the development of multiple organ dysfunction in cardiothoracic patients. Ann Thorac Surg 1993;55:822–9.

70. Ventilation with lower tidal volumes as compared with traditional tidal volumes for acute lung injury and the acute respiratory distress syndrome. The Acute Respiratory Distress Syndrome Network. N Engl J Med 2000;342:1301–8.

71. Ranieri VM, Suter PM, Tortorella C, et al. Effect of mechanical ventilation on inflammatory mediators in patients with acute respiratory distress syndrome: a randomized controlled trial. JAMA 1999;282:54–61.

72. Cakar N, Akinci O, Tugrul S, et al. Recruitment maneuver: does it promote bacterial translocation? Crit Care Med 2002;30:2103–6.

73. Parker MM, McCarthy KE, Ognibene FP, Parrillo JE. Right ventricular dysfunction and dilatation, similar to left ventricular changes, characterize the cardiac depression of septic shock in humans. Chest 1990;97:126–31.

74. Heard SO, Perkins MW, Fink MP. Tumor necrosis factor causes myocardial depression in guinea pigs. Crit Care Med 1992;20:523–7.

75. Atkinson S, Sieffert E, Bihari D, on behalf of Guy's Hospital Intensive Care Group. A prospective, randomized, double-blind, clinical trial of enteral immunonutrition in the critically ill. Crit Care Med 1998;26:1164–72.

76. Gadek JE, DeMichele SJ, Karlstad MD, et al. Effect of enteral feeding with eicosapentaenoic acid, γ-linolenic acid, and antioxidants in patients with acute respiratory distress syndrome. Crit Care Med 1999;27:1409–20.

77. Zallen G, Moore EE, Ciesla DJ, et al. Stored red blood cells selectively activate human neutrophils to release IL-8 and secretory PLA2. Shock 2000;13:29–33.

78. Taylor RW, Manganaro L, O'Brien J, et al. Impact of allogenic packed red blood cell transfusion on nosocomial infection rates in the critically ill patient. Crit Care Med 2002;30:2249–54.

79. Knaus WA, Draper EA, Wagner DP, Zimmerman JE. Prognosis in acute organ-system failure. Ann Surg 1985;202:685–93.

80. Vincent JL, Ferreira F, Moreno R. Scoring systems for assessing organ dysfunction and survival. Crit Care Clin 2000;16:353–66.

81. Hebert PC, Drummond AJ, Singer J, et al. A simple multiple system organ failure scoring system predicts mortality of patients who have sepsis syndrome. Chest 1993;104:230–5.

82. Marshall JC, Cook DJ, Christou NV, et al. Multiple organ dysfunction score: a reliable descriptor of a complex clinical outcome. Crit Care Med 1995;23:1638–52.

83. Timsit JF, Fosse JP, Troche G, et al. for the OUTCOMEREA Study Group. Calibration and discrimination by daily Logistic Organ Dysfunction scoring comparatively with daily Sequential Organ Failure Assessment scoring for predicting hospital mortality in critically ill patients. Crit Care Med 2002;30:2003–13.

84. Bertleff MJOE, Bruining HA. How should multiple organ dysfunction syndrome be assessed? A review of the variations in current scoring systems. Eur J Surg 1997;163:405–9.

85. Teres D, Rapoport J, Lemeshow S, Kim S, Akhras K. Effects of severity of illness on resource use by survivors and nonsurvivors of severe sepsis at intensive care unit admission. Crit Care Med 2002;30:2413–19.

86. Pettila V, Pettila M, Sarna S, Voutilainen P, Takkunen O. Comparison of multiple organ dysfunction scores in the prediction of hospital mortality in the critically ill. Crit Care Med 2002;30:1705–11.

87. Delllinger RP. Cardiovascular management of septic shock. Crit Care Med 2003;31:946–55.

88. Dreyfuss D, Saumon G. Ventilator induced lung injury: lessons from experimental studies. Am J Respir Crit Care Med 1998;157:294–323.

89. Meduri GU, Headley AS, Golden E, et al. Effect of prolonged methylprednisolone therapy in unresolving acute respiratory distress syndrome: a randomized controlled trial. JAMA 1998;280:159–65.

90. Martin C, Viviand X, Leone M, Thirion X. Effect of norepinephrine on the outcome of septic shock. Crit Care Med 2000;28:2758–65.

91. de Backer D, Creteur J, Silva E, Vincent JL. Effects of dopamine, norepinephrine, and epinephrine on the splanchnic circulation in septic shock: Which is best? Crit Care Med 2003;31:1659–67.

92. Hayes MA, Yau EHS, Timmins AC, et al. Response of critically ill patients to treatment aimed at achieving supranormal oxygen delivery and consumption. Chest 1993; 103: 886–95.

93. Gattinoni L, Brazzi L, Pelosi P, et al. A trial of goal-oriented hemodynamic therapy in critically ill patients. N Engl J Med 1995;333:1025–32.

94. Shoemaker WC, Appel PL, Kram HB, et al. Prospective trial of supranormal values of survivors as therapeutic goals in high risk patients. Chest 1988;94:1176–86.

95. Russell JA, Phang PT. The oxygen delivery/consumption controversy. Am J Respir Crit Care Med 1994;149:533–7.

96. Corwin HL, Gettinger A, Pearl RG, et al, for the EPO Critical Care Trials Group. Efficacy of recombinant human erythropoietin in critically ill patients: a randomized controlled trial. JAMA 2002;288:2827–35.

97. Cole L, Bellomo R, Hart G, et al. A phase II randomized, controlled trial of continuous hemofiltration in sepsis. Crit Care Med 2002;30:100–6.

98. Metnitz PGH, Krenn CG, Steltzer H, et al. Effect of acute renal failure requiring renal replacement therapy on outcome in critically ill patients. Crit Care Med 2002;30:2051–8.

99. Kjacrard LL, Liu J, Als-Nielsen B, Gluud C. Artificial and bioartificial support systems for acute and acute-on-chronic liver failure. JAMA 2003;289:217–22.

100. Bone RC, Balk RA, Fein Am, et al. A second large controlled clinical study of E5, a monoclonal antibody to endotoxin: results of a prospective, multicenter, randomized, controlled trial. Crit Care Med 1995;23:994–1006.

101. Bone RC, Balk R, Slotman G, et al. Adult respiratory distress syndrome. Sequence and importance of development of multiple organ failure. The Prostaglandin E1 Study Group. Chest 1992;101:320–6.

102. Van Den Berghe G, Wouters P, Weelers lF, et al. Intensive insulin therapy in critically ill patients. N Engl J Med 2001;345:1359–67.

103. Kellum JA, Decker JM. Use of dopamine in acute renal failure: a meta-analysis. Crit Care Med 2001;29:1526–31.

104. Cerra FB, McPherson JP, Konstantinides FN, Konstantinides NN, Teasley KM. Enteral nutrition does not prevent multiple organ failure syndrome (MOFS) after sepsis. Surgery 1988;104:727–33.

105. Eisele B, Lamy M, Thijs LG, et al. Antithrombin III in patients with severe sepsis: a randomized, placebo-controlled, double-blind, multicenter trial plus a meta-analysis on all randomized, placebo-controlled, double-blind trials with antithrombin III in severe sepsis. Intens Care Med 1998;24:663–72.

106. Inthorn, D, Hoffman JN, Hartl WH, et al. Antithrombin III supplementation in severe sepsis: beneficial effects on organ dysfunction. Shock 1997;8:328–34.

107. Warren BL, Eid A, Singer P, et al. High-dose antithrombin III in severe sepsis: a randomized controlled trial. JAMA 2001;286:1869–78.

108. Molnar Z, Shearer E, Lowe D. N-acetylcysteine treatment to prevent the progression of multisystem organ failure: a prospective, randomized, placebo-controlled study. Crit Care Med 1999;27:1100–4.

109. Angus DC, Birmingham MC, Balk RA, et al. The third, and final, phase III trial of E-5 murine monoclonal anti-endotoxin antibody in gram-negative sepsis: results of a multicenter randomized controlled trial and implications for future sepsis trials. JAMA 2000;283:1723–30.

110. Fisher CJ Jr, Agosti JM, Opal SM, et al. Treatment of septic shock with the tumor necrosis factor receptor:Fc fusion protein. The Soluble TNF Receptor Sepsis Study Group. N Engl J Med 1996;334:1697–1702.

111. Heyland DK, Cook DJ, Jaeschke R, et al. Selective decontamination of the digestive tract. An overview. Chest 1994;105:1221–9.

112. Slotman GJ, Burchard KW, D'Arezzo A, Gann DS. Ketoconazole prevents acute respiratory failure in critically ill surgical patients. J Trauma 1988;28:648–54.

113. ARDS Network. Ketoconazole for early treatment of acute lung injury and acute respiratory distress syndrome: a randomized controlled trial. The Acute Respiratory Distress Syndrome Network. JAMA 2000;283:1995–2002.

114. Yan SB, Helterbrand JD, Hartman DL, Wright TJ, Bernard GR. Low levels of protein C are associated with poor outcome in severe sepsis. Chest 2001;120:915–22.

115. Fourrier F, Chopin C, Huart JJ, et al. Double-blind, placebo-controlled trial of antithrombin III concentrates in septic shock with disseminated intravascular coagulation. Chest 1993; 104:882–8.

116. Abraham E. Tissue factor inhibition and clinical trial results of tissue factor pathway inhibitor in sepsis. Crit Care Med 2000;28:S31–3.

117. Bernard GR, Vincent JL, Laterre PF, et al. Efficacy and safety of recombinant human activated protein C for severe sepsis. N Engl J Med 2001;344:699–709.

118. Chiron announces results of Phase III study of tifacogin in severe sepsis [press release]. Available at: http://biz.yahoo.com/prnews/011121/sfw016_1.html. Accessed December 12, 2001.

119. Ely EW, Laterre PF, Angus DC, et al, for the PROWESS Investigators. Drotrecogin alfa (activated) administration across clinically important subgroups of patients with severe sepsis. Crit Care Med 2003;31:12–19.

120. Vincent JL, Angus DC, Artigas A, et al, for the Recombinant Human Activated Protein C Worldwide Evaluation in Severe Sepsis (PROWESS) Study Group. Effects of drotrecogin alfa (activated) on organ dysfunction in the PROWESS trial. Crit Care Med 2003;31:834–40.

121. Angus DC, Linde-Zwirble WT, Clermont G, et al, for the PROWESS Investigators. Cost-effectiveness of drotrecogin alfa (activated) in the treatment of severe sepsis. Crit Care Med 2003;31:1–11.

122. Van den Berghe G, Wouters PJ, Bouillon R, et al. Outcome benefit of intensive insulin therapy in the critically ill: insulin dose versus glycemic control. Crit Care Med 2003;31:359–66.

123. Ely EW, Wheeler AP, Thompson BT, et al. Recovery rate and prognosis in older persons who develop acute lung injury and the acute respiratory distress syndrome. Ann Intern Med 2002;136:25–36.

124. Roumen RMH, Redl H, Schlag G, et al. Scoring systems and blood lactate concentrations in relation to the development of adult respiratory distress syndrome and multiple organ failure in severely traumatized patients. J Trauma 1993;35:349–55.

125. Schwartz DB, Bone RC, Balk RA, Szidon JP, Jacobs ER. Hepatic dysfunction in the adult respiratory distress syndrome. Chest 1989;95:871–5.

126. Sprung CL, Peduzzi PN, Shatney CH, et al. Impact of encephalopathy on mortality in the sepsis syndrome. The Veterans Administration Systemic Sepsis Cooperative Study Group. Crit Care Med 1990;18:801–6.

4

Renal effects of critical illness

Patrick T Murray and Michael R Pinsky

INTRODUCTION

Acute renal failure (ARF) is broadly defined as deterioration of renal function over days to weeks, a common occurrence in intensive care unit (ICU) patients; incidence and mortality estimates vary according to ARF definition and associated morbidities.[1-3] The mortality of ARF is 50–80% in ICU populations, and has not declined significantly since the initial marked benefit of acute dialysis therapy, despite numerous advances in renal replacement technologies and critical care over several decades.[4] Although multiple system organ failure (MSOF) and other comorbidities contribute to its high mortality rate, ARF independently increases morbidity and mortality.[5-8] The mechanisms by which ARF contributes to nonrenal organ dysfunction and death are incompletely understood. Emerging data suggest that isolated renal ischemia–reperfusion injury causes injury and dysfunction of distant organs in experimental ARF.[9-11] Apart from obviously lethal ARF sequelae such as severe hyperkalemia, the identities and precise effects of 'uremic' toxins have not been identified, particularly in ARF. Accordingly, it is likely that renal replacement therapy in its current form is only a partial solution to the multisystem problems caused by ARF.

Prevention or early diagnosis and amelioration of ARF are clearly the preferred approaches to diminishing the contribution of renal dysfunction to adverse outcomes in critically ill patients. Most ARF in ICU patients is caused by either prerenal azotemia (reversible renal insufficiency due to renal hypoperfusion) or acute tubular necrosis (ATN). ATN results from a variety of ischemic and nephrotoxic insults, often in additive or synergistic combination.[12] Multiple causes of renal hypoperfusion and injury are commonplace in the ICU, including systemic hypoperfusion (shock), the effects of mechanical ventilation,[13] renal vasoconstriction in patients with cirrhosis and sepsis,[14,15] increased intra-abdominal pressure,[16] and a variety of nephrotoxins (endogenous and exogenous). Because renal hypoperfusion plays a role in the pathogenesis of prerenal azotemia and ATN, and shock is common in critically ill patients who develop ARF, much attention is paid to optimization of renal perfusion, attempting to prevent or ameliorate ARF in the ICU. This chapter reviews the effects of critical illness on renal perfusion and function, and the impact of renal insufficiency on outcome in the ICU.

RENAL PERFUSION AND FUNCTION

The kidneys perform a variety of homeostatic functions, including regulation of fluid and electrolyte balance and tonicity, excretion of endogenous and exogenous wastes and toxins, and several endocrine functions such as the synthesis of erythropoietin (EPO) and renin and the activation of vitamin D. Much of the homeostatic and detoxification work of the kidneys is done through high-volume hemofiltration and selective filtrate reabsorption or modification. The best global index of renal function is the glomerular filtration rate (GFR), which is normally in the range of 100–125 ml/min. Of the 150–180 L filtered daily, only a small fraction ($\leq$1%, 1.5–1.8 L) typically appears as urine output (UOP). This is consistent with the concept that, beyond filtration, the major renal homeostatic function is the selective mass reabsorption of filtered fluid and electrolytes, apart from toxic nitrogenous wastes. Urine volume is determined by the requirement to excrete daily obligate solute load (electrolytes and nitrogenous wastes) in appropriately concentrated urine. Assuming maximal urine-concentrating ability (1400 mOsm/kg), the minimum daily urine output required to excrete the average daily solute load is 400 ml, below which positive solute balance and azotemia develop, thus the standard definition of oliguria (<400 ml/24 h). In terms of monitoring urine output, if urine is maximally concentrated (1.4 mOsm/ml), and excretion of 10 mOsm/kg/ day (700 mOsm/day in a 70-kg person) is required to avoid solute retention, this mandates urine output of 500 ml daily (21 ml/h or 0.3 ml/kg/h). Of course, if solute appearance increases (patient size, hypercatabolism, hyperalimentation) or maximal urinary concentrating ability is diminished (renal dysfunction, age), higher urine volumes are required to maintain adequate solute excretion. Since such conditions are more the rule than the exception, it seems more appropriate to expect solute retention at urine outputs below the more typical ICU monitoring target of 0.5–1.0 ml/kg/h (840–1680 ml/day). Of course, urine output targets must be sufficient to control fluid balance as well as solute excretion, so higher UOP values may be required for patients with large obligate fluid intakes. In a large study of 13 152 ICU patients, Le Gall and colleagues found that mortality increased with urine output below 750 ml/24 h, or above 10 L/day.[17] The cause–effect relationship between oliguria and adverse outcome, and the relative importance of solute retention vs fluid overload are unknown, but it seems clear that the higher minimum urine output target used in critically ill patients is justified. Of course, urine output must be assessed in context, relative to fluid intake, extrarenal fluid loss, diuretic use, systemic hemodynamic parameters, and overall fluid balance. Nonetheless, it is probably appropriate to use graded levels of oliguria, along with markers of GFR, to define the presence and severity of acute renal dysfunction. This approach underlies the recently proposed RIFLE criteria (risk, injury, failure, loss, end-stage) suggested for ARF definition by the ADQI group[3] (Fig. 4.1).

The kidneys normally receive 20–25% of cardiac output (CO), although their combined weight is less than 1% of total body weight, resulting in the highest tissue perfusion in the body. Basal renal oxygen consumption is 400 μmol/min/100 g of kidney, but this high value results in an arteriovenous oxygen content difference of only 1.7 vol%.[18] The vast majority of renal oxygen consumption is utilized to support tubular sodium reabsorption. As illustrated in Figure 4.2,[18] the kidneys are unique in having physiologic supply-dependent oxygen consumption. Decreasing renal oxygen delivery results in decreased oxygen consumption throughout a wide range,[19] because diminished GFR and sodium filtration requires proportionately less tubular oxygen consumption for reabsorptive work, and arteriovenous O_2 content difference is unchanged down to a renal blood

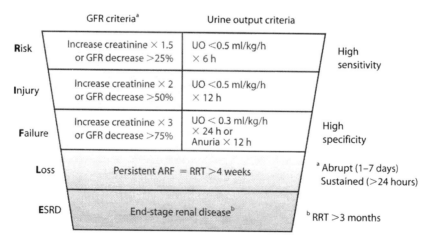

Figure 4.1 RIFLE classification system for acute renal failure. A new graded classification system has been proposed to 'stage' acute renal dysfunction, proposed by the Acute Dialysis Quality Initiative (ADQI) consensus group, incorporating levels of oliguria in addition to fractional serum creatinine elevation. The more severe of the GFR or UOP criteria is selected to determine ARF severity. [a] Serum creatinine increments must be abrupt (within 1–7 days) and sustained (>24 h). [b] Persistent ARF = 1–3 months of renal replacement therapy (RRT). ESRD = >3 months or more of RRT. (Reproduced with permission from Kellum et al.[3])

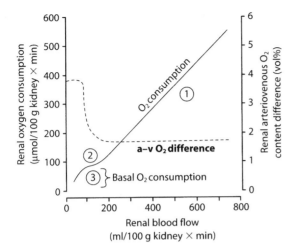

Figure 4.2 Renal oxygen consumption. Decreasing renal oxygen delivery results in decreased oxygen consumption throughout a wide range, because diminished glomerular filtration rate (GFR) and sodium filtration requires proportionately less tubular oxygen consumption for reabsorptive work. As renal blood flow is progressively decreased, renal oxygen consumption follows a *triphasic* pattern: Stage 1: renal oxygen consumption is decreased and arteriovenous (a–v) O₂ content difference is unchanged down to a renal blood flow of 150 ml/min/100 g of tissue. Stage 2: as renal blood flow and oxygen delivery decrease further below 150 ml/min/100 g, GFR ceases but the minimum threshold for supporting parenchymal oxygen consumption and viability is reached, oxygen extraction increases, and a–v content difference widens. Stage 3: Finally, as maximal oxygen extraction is exceeded (below a renal blood flow of 75 ml/min/100 g of kidney tissue), anaerobic metabolism, ATP depletion, and ischemic tubular injury ensue. (Reproduced with permission from Valtin H, Schafer JA: Renal function. Mechanisms preserving fluid and solute balance in health. Little, Brown and Company, Boston, 3rd edn, 1995. In: Chapter 6: Renal hemodynamics and oxygen consumption (figure 6–6, page 105); adapted from several papers.)

flow of 150 ml/min/100 g of tissue. This contrasts with other organs (notably myocardium, brain, and intestine) in which progressively increased O₂ extraction is required to maintain basal O₂ consumption and aerobic metabolism when delivery decreases. For example, the myocardium has the highest O₂ consumption in the body, associated with a much higher basal arteriovenous oxygen content difference of 11 vol%, so that decreased coronary flow rapidly leads to anaerobic metabolism.[18] In contrast, as renal blood flow and oxygen delivery decrease further below 150 ml/min/100 g, GFR ceases but the minimum threshold for supporting parenchymal oxygen consumption and

viability is reached, oxygen extraction increases, and arteriovenous O₂ content difference widens, events which normally occur much sooner during hypoperfusion of other organs. Finally, as maximal oxygen extraction is exceeded (below a renal blood flow of 75 ml/min/100 g of kidney tissue), anaerobic metabolism, ATP depletion, and ischemic tubular injury ensue. This phenomenon of physiologic supply dependence of renal oxygen consumption throughout a wide range of oxygen delivery underlies the distinct difference in renal tolerance of ischemic insults; renal artery crossclamp is better tolerated than insults of similar duration in the cerebral, coronary, or mesenteric circulations, but profound renal ischemia does cause ischemic injury.

Renal blood flow (RBF) is approximately 1.1 L/min (20–25% of CO), providing renal plasma flow (RPF) of 605 ml/min (assuming hematocrit of 45%).[20] There are three main determinants of RBF:

1. cardiac output (CO)
2. renal perfusion pressure (RPP)
3. renovascular resistance (RVR), which is primarily regulated by glomerular hemodynamic factors (afferent and efferent arteriolar tone).

$$RBF = RPP/RVR$$

RPP is the difference between renal arterial (inflow) and venous (outflow) pressures. Outflow pressure is negligible under normal circumstances, but may be increased by venous return impedance from extremely raised intrathoracic pressure (mechanical ventilation, discussed below) or intraabdominal pressure (see discussion of abdominal compartment syndrome in Ch. 5). Thus, RPP is proportional to mean arterial pressure (MAP) for practical purposes. The primary site of renovascular resistance is the afferent arteriole (Fig. 4.3). Afferent arteriolar resistance is modulated by several influences, both intrinsic (autoregulation) and extrinsic (neurogenic, paracrine, endocrine).[20,21] Autoregulation maintains RBF (and GFR) over a wide range of MAP levels by modulation of afferent arteriolar resistance. RBF increases by only 10% when MAP increases by 50% from 100 to 150 mmHg (Fig. 4.4).[20,22–26] This regulatory process is achieved by modulation of afferent arteriolar tone by two influences: a local myogenic reflex in the afferent arteriolar wall (increased stretch causes reflex vasoconstriction) and a process called *tubuloglomerular feedback* (TGF) (Figs 4.5 and 4.6).[21] The TGF mechanism functions as follows: the macula

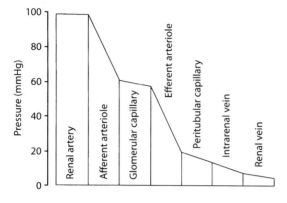

Figure 4.3 Renovascular resistance sites. The hydrostatic pressure profile in the canine renovascular tree is shown. The bulk of renovascular resistance occurs at the afferent and efferent arterioles. (Reproduced with permission from Valtin H, Schafer JA: Renal function. Mechanisms preserving fluid and solute balance in health. Little, Brown and Company, Boston, 3rd edn, 1995. In: Chapter 6: Renal hemodynamics and oxygen consumption (figure 6–1, page 97); adapted from another chapter.)

densa is a chloride-sensing nephron segment distal to the thick ascending limb of the loop of Henle (TALH); increased chloride delivery past the TALH results in afferent arteriolar vasoconstriction due to TGF, which normally serves to defend intravascular volume, by limiting GFR when salt excretion is excessive (see Fig. 4.6). Conversely, when renal perfusion, GFR, and tubular chloride concentration decrease, TGF and afferent tone are down-regulated. However, these mechanisms act to maintain RBF only in the range of 80–90 mmHg, and autoregulation fails precipitously at MAP lev-

els below 80 mmHg. RBF and GFR decrease linearly below 70–80 mmHg, and RBF ceases at a RPP of 30 mmHg (the critical closing pressure of the renal circulation; see Fig. 4.4).

Of course, GFR is not solely determined by renal plasma flow. The renal circulation is unique in featuring postcapillary (efferent) in addition to precapillary (afferent) arterioles. The efferent arteriole is the second major site in the renal circulation which determines renovascular resistance (see Fig. 4.3). The rate at which a portion of RPF traverses the filtration apparatus (GFR) is determined by the balance of hemodynamic (Starling) forces in the glomerular capillary (GC). Since the hydrostatic and oncotic pressures in Bowman's space are ordinarily negligible, the net filtration pressure (NFP) driving the GFR is the balance of intracapillary hydrostatic and oncotic pressures (Fig. 4.7). Early in the GC, hydrostatic pressure dominates and NFP and GFR are maximal. NFP progressively diminishes as hydrostatic pressure falls and oncotic pressure increases (by hemoconcentration), resulting in cessation of filtrate formation before blood enters the efferent arteriole (Fig. 4.8). The fraction of renal plasma flow which is filtered is called the *filtration fraction* (FF):

$$FF~(\%) = GFR~(ml/min)/RPF~(ml/min)$$

FF is normally approximately $\leq 20\%$ (GFR 125 ml/min $\div$ RPF 605 ml/min), determined by the balance of afferent and efferent arteriolar resistance (Fig. 4.9). Both afferent and efferent tone are increased by catecholamines, and back pressure from efferent resistance partly offsets decreased GC

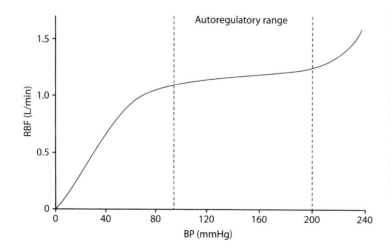

Figure 4.4 Autoregulation of renal blood flow (RBF). Autoregulation maintains RBF, and glomerular filtration rate (GFR), over a wide range of mean arterial pressure (MAP) levels by modulation of afferent arteriolar resistance. RBF increases by only 10% when MAP increases by 50% from 100 to 150 mmHg, but decreases precipitously when MAP falls below 70–80 mmHg. (Reproduced with permission from Vander AJ: Renal physiology, 5th Edn, McGraw-Hill, New York, 1995. In: Chapter 2: Renal blood flow and glomerular filtration (figure 2–4, page 34).)

A

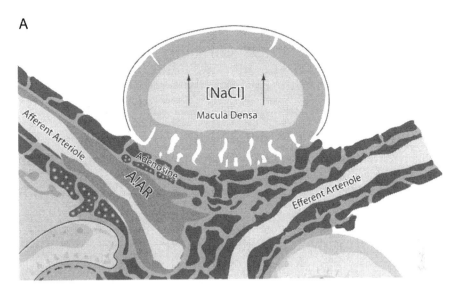

B

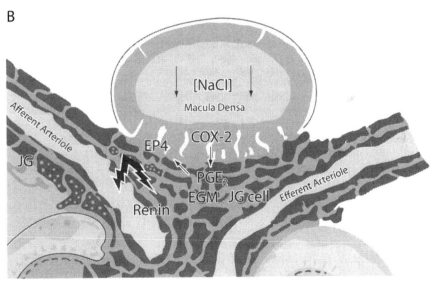

Figure 4.5 The juxtaglomerular apparatus (JGA) and tubuloglomerular feedback (TGF). The JGA consists of three components: (1) the granular cells (JG), which secrete renin; (2) the macula densa; and (3) the extraglomerular mesangial cells (EGM). (A) The effect of increasing salt (NaCl) delivery to the distal nephron (macula densa) increases levels of adenosine in the JGA interstitium, causing adenosine 1 receptor (A1AR)-mediated constriction of the afferent arteriolar smooth muscle cells. (B) The effect of decreasing salt delivery to the macula densa increases vasodilatory PGE_2 (made by cyclooxygenase-2, COX-2) in the JGA, along with renin release from granular cells (stimulated by PGE_2 receptor subtype EP4), resulting in vasodilation. (Reproduced with permission from Schnermann J.[21])

hydrostatic pressure due to catecholamine-induced afferent constriction, helping to augment FF and preserve GFR. In contrast, angiotensin II *preferentially* constricts the *efferent* arteriole, markedly increasing filtration fraction; this occurs because the efferent arteriole has only vasoconstrictor AT_1 recep-

tors, and lacks the AT_2 receptors which release vasodilatory nitric oxide (NO) and partly reverse angiotensin II-induced constriction in the afferent arteriole.[27] Various combinations of altered afferent and efferent arteriolar tone can change RBF and GFR, sometimes in opposite directions (see Fig. 4.9).

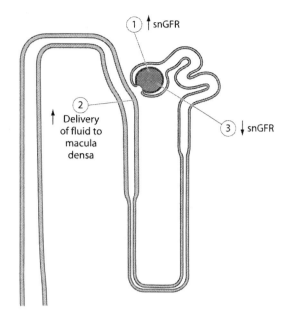

Figure 4.6 Single nephron GFR (snGFR) regulation by tubuloglomerular feedback (TGF). An increase in single nephron GFR (1) results in an increased rate of chloride delivery to the macula densa (2), activating TGF and afferent arteriolar vasoconstriction, resulting in decreased single nephron GFR (3). (Reproduced with permission from Valtin H, Schafer JA: Renal function. Mechanisms preserving fluid and solute balance in health. Little, Brown and Company, Boston, 3rd edn, 1995. In: Chapter 6: Renal hemodynamics and oxygen consumption (figure 6–5, page 103).)

It is important to understand the renal hemodynamic responses to shock. In response to hypotension, baroreceptor stimulation increases sympathetic outflow. Sympathetic outflow also indirectly activates the renin–angiotensin–aldosterone axis, through beta-adrenoceptor-stimulated renin release from the juxtaglomerular apparatus (JGA) in the afferent arteriolar wall (see Fig. 4.5). Renin release from the JGA is also stimulated locally by decreased afferent arteriolar stretch, and by autoregulation-dependent stimulation from the macula densa, sensing decreased distal salt delivery. Together, these influences augment filtration fraction, which tends to preserve GFR relative to decreased renal blood flow. In this setting, the combination of diminished RBF (inflow) and increased filtration fraction (outflow) results in concentration of unfilterable plasma proteins and increases glomerular capillary oncotic pressure; thus, NFP falls and glomerular filtration ceases earlier in the GC. The blood which traverses the efferent arteriole and peritubular capillaries

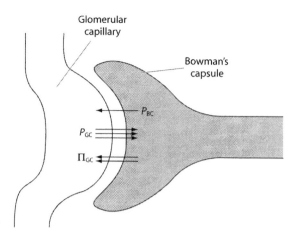

Figure 4.7 Net filtration pressure (NFP) and glomerular filtration rate (GFR). The NFP determining the GFR in the renal corpuscle is the glomerular capillary hydraulic pressure (P_{GC}) minus Bowman's capsule hydraulic pressure (P_{BC}) minus glomerular capillary oncotic pressure (Π_{GC}). (Reproduced with permission from Vander AJ: Renal physiology, 5th edn. McGraw-Hill, New York, 1995. In: Chapter 2: Renal blood flow and glomerular filtration (Figure 2–1, page 29).)

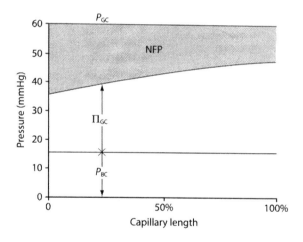

Figure 4.8 Net filtration pressure (NFP) forces along the glomerular capillary in humans. The forces involved in glomerular filtration change as renal blood flow moves from the afferent to the efferent end of the glomerular capillary. Although the glomerular capillary hydraulic pressure (P_{GC}) favoring filtration remains essentially unchanged (60 mmHg at the afferent end; 58 mmHg at the efferent end), and the hydraulic pressure in Bowman's capsule is unchanged (P_{BC}, 15 mmHg), oncotic pressure in the glomerular capillary (Π_{GC}) increases from 21 mmHg to 33 mmHg; thus NFP falls from 24 mmHg at the afferent end to 10 mmHg at the efferent end. (Reproduced with permission from Vander AJ: Renal physiology, 5th edn. McGraw-Hill, New York, 1995. In: Chapter 2: Renal blood flow and glomerular filtration (Figure 2-2, page 30). Data also from Table 2-1, page 29.).)

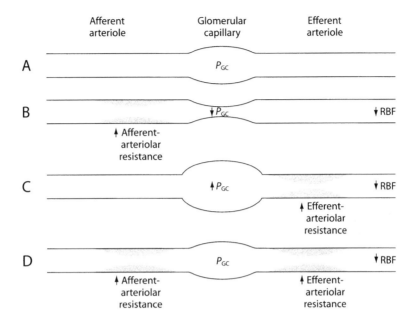

	Afferent arteriole	Glomerular capillary	Efferent arteriole

Figure 4.9 Effects of afferent- and efferent-arteriolar constriction on glomerular capillary hydraulic pressure (P_{GC}) and renal blood flow (RBF). RBF is altered *additively* by changes in total renal arteriolar (afferent and efferent) resistance, irrespective of site. Constriction of either the afferent (B) or efferent (C) arterioles decreases RBF, with additive effects of constricting both together (D). Glomerular capillary hydrostatic pressure (P_{GC}) and glomerular filtration rate (GFR) are *differentially* affected by increases in afferent tone (B, decreases P_{GC} and GFR) vs efferent tone (C, increases P_{GC} and GFR). Simultaneous constriction of afferent and afferent arterioles tends to decrease RBF, P_{GC}, and GFR, but efferent constriction helps maintain P_{GC} and GFR in this setting (D), by increasing filtration fraction. (Reproduced with permission from Vander AJ: Renal physiology, 5th edn. McGraw-Hill, New York, 1995. In: Chapter 2: Renal blood flow and glomerular filtration (Figure 2–3, page 32).)

has a higher oncotic pressure, increasing resorption of sodium and water in the proximal tubule, a phenomenon called *glomerulotubular balance* (Fig. 4.10). In the setting of systemic hypoperfusion, the pressor effects of catecholamines and angiotensin II also act to preserve systemic and renal perfusion pressure, and the same hormones promote sodium reabsorption throughout the nephron (angiotensin II both directly and via aldosterone). In addition, renal blood flow distribution is shifted from the superficial to the juxtamedullary nephrons, further facilitating salt retention (see below). In severe hypotension, nonosmotic vasopressin release has both pressor and fluid (water)-retaining effects.[28] Thus, the renal effects of the systemic pressor response to hypotension and hypoperfusion act to preserve GFR (by augmenting filtration fraction), and maximize salt and water retention to maintain intravascular volume. All of these systemic and renal responses are of course highly appropriate in response to a classic cause of shock and prerenal azotemia such as major hemorrhage, but increased systemic vascular resistance (SVR) and salt reten-

tion are maladaptive in congestive heart failure (CHF). The renal vasoconstrictor and salt-retaining effects of catecholamines and the renin–angiotensin–aldosterone axis are antagonized by activation of a variety of vasodilators (atrial natriuretic peptide (ANP), kinins, prostaglandins) and natriuretic substances (prostaglandins, ANP). Stimulation of afferent arteriolar release of vasodilator prostaglandins by catecholamines and angiotensin II partially offsets renal vasoconstriction in shock: thus, the adverse renal hemodynamic effects of nonsteroidal anti-inflammatory drugs (NSAIDs) in patients with systemic hypoperfusion and renal vasoconstriction. ANP is released in response to atrial stretch, and helps relieve the maladaptive salt retention and increased afterload caused by the other active hormonal systems in CHF.

There is a further level of sophistication in the design of the renal circulation which underlies the remarkable fluid-retaining capacity of the kidney. Solute and water retention are favored by the unique design of the intrarenal circulation. The

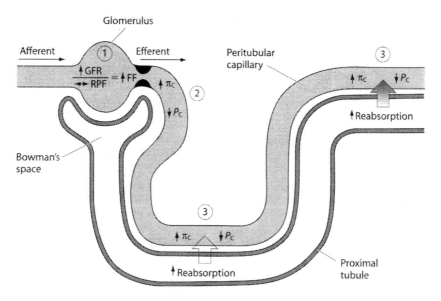

Figure 4.10 Glomerulotubular balance. Glomerulotubular balance is maintained by changes in filtration fraction (FF) and resulting Starling forces in the proximal tubulae and peritubular capillaries. If glomerular filtration rate (GFR) increases without a change in renal plasma flow (RPF) (Step 1) (e.g. afferent dilation with efferent constriction), then FF increases and more plasma water is filtered. This hemoconcentrates plasma proteins in the peritubular capillaries, raising plasma oncotic pressure (π_c), while hydrostatic pressure in the peritubular capillaries (P_c) is falling (due to efferent constriction) (Step 2). These changes in peritubular capillary Starling forces favor increased reabsorption of sodium and water in the proximal tubule (Step 3). Thus, although an unchanged *fraction* (approximately two-thirds) of the glomerular filtrate continues to be reabsorbed, the *amount* reabsorbed is greater, in proportion to the increase in GFR and FF. (Reproduced with permission from Valtin H, Schafer JA: Renal function. Mechanisms preserving fluid and solute balance in health. Little, Brown and Company, Boston, 3rd edn, 1995. In: Chapter 6: Renal hemodynamics and oxygen consumption (figure 7–10, page 141).

majority of nephrons are cortical (90%), but 10% are located deeper in the juxtamedullary region.[18,20,29] Juxtamedullary nephrons have a different efferent circulation than their superficial counterparts. Specifically, in cortical nephrons the efferent arteriole branches into a peritubular capillary network, which subsequently forms the renal venous system. In contrast, juxtamedullary efferent arterioles form long hairpin vessels called the vasa recta, which penetrate deep into the medulla and supply the thick ascending loops and distal proximal tubules of the deep nephrons (Fig. 4.11). The hairpin nature of the vasa recta is important to maintain the medullary solute concentration gradient, which permits maximal urinary concentration. However, the combination of major tubular oxygen consumption and countercurrent exchange of oxygen between vasa recta limbs makes the deep medulla a very hypoxic environment under normal circumstances.[30] Although renal oxygen consumption is driven largely by reabsorption of filtered sodium, as discussed above, the relationship between oxygen delivery and consumption

described above is not homogeneous throughout the kidneys. Although the kidneys are the most perfused organs in the body, this statement applies only to the cortex, not the medulla. The medulla receives only 6% of total renal blood flow (0.3 ml/min/g vs 5 ml/min/g to the cortex), and exists in a baseline hypoxic state (pO_2 10 mmHg vs 50 mmHg in cortex), despite containing two sites where a large proportion of tubular work and oxygen consumption occurs (the 'S_3' distal segment of the proximal tubule, and the TALH) (Fig. 4.12). It is not surprising that medullary hypoperfusion with predominant injury of the TALH and S3 segment is among the recognized models of ischemic ATN.[30]

RENAL EFFECTS OF SHOCK AND VASOACTIVE DRUGS

It is obvious that many cases of ARF in the ICU are caused by prerenal azotemia, which is decreased GFR resulting from diminished renal perfusion, often associated with shock. Prerenal azotemia is

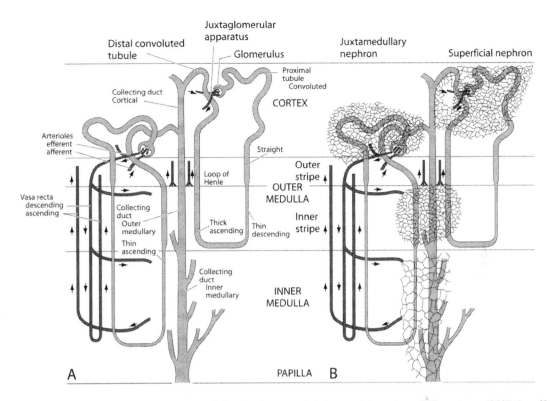

Figure 4.11 Superficial (cortical) and juxtamedullary nephrons and their vasculature. In cortical nephrons (90%) the efferent arteriole branches into a peritubular capillary network, which subsequently forms the renal venous system. Juxtamedullary nephrons (10%) have a different efferent circulation than their superficial counterparts. Juxtamedullary efferent arterioles form long hairpin vessels called the *vasa recta*, which penetrate deep into the medulla and supply the thick ascending loops and distal proximal tubules of the deep nephrons. (Reproduced with permission from Valtin H, Schafer JA: Renal function. Mechanisms preserving fluid and solute balance in health. Little, Brown and Company, Boston, 3rd edn, 1995. In: Chapter 1: Components of renal function (figure 1–2, page 5); adapted from Reference 29 and other sources.)

marked by decreased renal blood flow, renal vaso-constriction, increased filtration fraction, and avid salt and water reabsorption, through the mechanisms described above. In patients with prerenal azotemia, complete reversal of shock can normalize renal perfusion and function. Persistent systemic and/or renal hypoperfusion with unreversed prerenal azotemia may result in ischemic renal injury and ATN. It is unclear to what extent ATN is caused by ischemic injury in critically ill patients, an assumption which underlies most of the therapeutic approaches to the prevention or therapy of ARF over the past several decades. Systemic hypotension with shock is certainly a common precursor of ATN in humans, prerenal azotemia often precedes ATN, and decreased renal perfusion (renal vascular crossclamp, high-dose norepinephrine infusion) is a recognized model of renal injury in animals. Nonetheless, decreased

renal perfusion has not been documented to be of etiologic significance in the development of ATN in critically ill humans, apart from some clearcut insults such as surgical aortic crossclamp before ICU transfer. However, although other documented etiologic factors such as circulating nephrotoxins (drugs, pigments, cytokines), acidosis, and hypoxemia coexist in this population, it seems likely that ischemic (± reperfusion) injury plays an important role in the pathogenesis of much ATN in the ICU. Furthermore, since the vasoactive therapies which are used in the hemodynamic management of ICU patients may also alter renal blood flow, optimization of renal perfusion and function is a major endpoint in resuscitation. Taken together, available data suggest that optimization of renal perfusion is an important cornerstone of attempts to prevent and treat ARF in the ICU.

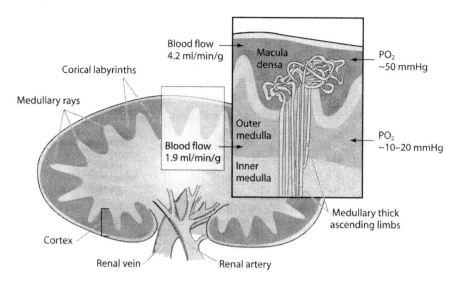

Figure 4.12 Medullary oxygen consumption. The renal cortex is highly perfused and well oxygenated, apart from medullary rays (supplied by medullary venous blood). Cortical blood flow is over double the medullary blood flow (per gram of tissue), and tissue pO_2 in the cortex is up to five-fold higher in the cortex. Poor medullary oxygenation is caused by a combination of O_2 consumption by the thick ascending loop of Henle, and countercurrent oxygen exchange in the vasa recta. (Reproduced with permission from Brezis and Rosen.[30]).

Although improving renal perfusion may reverse prerenal ARF (by definition), and diminish ischemic contributions to the pathogenesis of ATN, it is quite conceivable that in many cases ATN develops despite appropriate resuscitation and adequate renal perfusion. Zager and colleagues have shown in an endotoxemic rat model of septic ARF that paired combinations of insults (renal crossclamp, systemic endotoxin, aminoglycoside, temperature elevation) cause azotemia and renal pathologic findings of ATN, but these insults individually cause no renal dysfunction or injury.[12] We suspect that this synergistic injury model accurately reflects the pathogenesis of much ARF in the ICU. Other experimental data have shown that endotoxin, tumor necrosis factor, and numerous other inflammatory mediators are directly cytotoxic to renal endothelial and tubular cells.[14,31–33] Although ARF may be prevented or ameliorated by judicious use and monitoring of nephrotoxic drugs, and perhaps evolving cytoprotective and anti-inflammatory therapies, the major focus in ARF prophylaxis and therapy remains optimization of renal perfusion. The primary causes of renal hypoperfusion differ between the major types of shock, and therapies vary accordingly.

Renal effects of 'low-flow' shock (low CO states)

Decreased CO due to hypovolemia or cardiac dysfunction diminishes renal perfusion both directly and indirectly. Decreased CO not only directly lowers RBF (via inadequate CO, RPP, or both) but also activates a number of renal vasoconstrictor systems which increase RVR. Baroreceptor stimulation resulting from decreased CO activates neurohumoral responses (sympathetic nervous system, renin–angiotensin system, and vasopressin secretion) that have opposing effects on renal perfusion, tending to augment RPP but also cause renal vasoconstriction. Any intervention restoring CO and systemic perfusion therefore augments renal perfusion by reversing the aforementioned influences. Volume loading to prevent hypovolemia is probably the most effective preventive measure to avoid prerenal azotemia as well as ischemic and nephrotoxic ATN. As discussed elsewhere in this book, there are a variety of tools to guide fluid and vasoactive drug management in the ICU. It is important not to administer excessive fluid to avoid complications such as pulmonary edema, intra-abdominal hypertension, and poor wound healing with subcutaneous edema. It remains unresolved whether crystalloids or colloids are the preferred fluids to use to maintain adequate preload and renal function in hypovolemic shock.

The choice among available inotropes or vasodilators to improve renal function in patients with renal hypoperfusion secondary to CHF is similarly unclear. It is clear that the use of inotropes to achieve *supranormal* cardiac output and oxygen delivery does not improve renal function in critically ill patients,[34] and of course fails to improve or increase mortality.[34,35] Gattinoni and colleagues studied 762 ICU patients and found no difference in mortality or renal function (creatinine, urine output) with either supranormal CO/oxygen delivery or maintenance of mixed venous oxygen saturation (S_VO_2) $\geq$70% with dobutamine vs control management[34]. Hayes and colleagues found (in 100 ICU patients) that supranormal oxygen delivery (dobutamine) vs control resulted in increased mortality (54% vs 34%),[35] and this approach has fallen out of favor in the management of critically ill patients. However, as discussed in Chapters 1 and 5, there is a growing interest in *early* goal-directed therapy of septic shock, including the use of transfusion and inotropes to optimize oxygen delivery;[36] it is unknown if this approach will reduce the incidence of ARF.

The commonsense approach of using fluids and vasoactive drugs to achieve an adequate cardiac output, based on assessment of available hemodynamic and tissue perfusion markers (cardiac filling pressures, thermodilution or other cardiac output measurements, venous oxygen saturation), remains the primary approach to the prevention and reversal of ARF due to prerenal azotemia. However, restoration and maintenance of adequate intravascular volume and CO does not guarantee adequate renal perfusion. Renal blood flow is only optimized when CO is adequate *and* renal perfusion pressure is sufficient to distribute an appropriate proportion of systemic oxygen delivery to the kidneys. This requires a renal perfusion pressure above the lower autoregulatory threshold. It is particularly important to balance these factors when systemic vasodilators are used for afterload reduction to augment CO in CHF; excessive vasodilation may lower MAP and RPP below the renal autoregulatory threshold and negate some of the potential benefit of increased CO. Conversely, the use of vasopressors to support perfusion pressure in patients with vasodilatory shock may adversely affect tissue perfusion by creating excessive cardiac 'afterload' in the presence of significant myocardial dysfunction (pre-existing or acquired), in addition to any potential adverse effects on regional blood flow distribution (see below).

Renal effects of 'high-flow' (vasodilatory) shock

Although not generally regarded as a controversial critical care issue to the same degree as oxygen delivery strategies, the appropriate MAP and RPP target for titration of hemodynamic support is another area of clinical uncertainty. Importantly, the logic for defending renal perfusion pressure with vasoactive agents presumes both pressure-dependent renal flow and flow-dependent renal function. Standard recommendations have traditionally suggested that fluids and vasoactive drugs should be titrated to maintain an MAP $\geq$60 mmHg.[37,38] In the recent trial of goal-directed therapy in early septic shock, the target MAP range of 65–90 mmHg was (along with other parameters) associated with improved outcome, but renal function was not a reported endpoint in this study.[36] Although generally accepted as the target MAP in shock resuscitation and perioperative management, 60–65 mmHg is on the steep portion of the renal autoregulation curve (see Fig. 4.4), and is associated with a precipitous decrement in RBF and GFR from normal, in dogs and healthy human subjects.

The data demonstrating that 80 mmHg is the lower autoregulatory threshold in the renal circulation are primarily derived from animal studies.[22–26] Limited human data are consistent with prior experimental findings in animals, but definitive data from healthy humans are lacking.[39] Stone and Stahl demonstrated that hemorrhage in healthy humans, which decreased MAP from 80 to 67 mmHg, was associated with a 20% decrement of RBF and a 30% fall in GFR;[40] this study did not control for the contributory effects of decreased blood volume and CO on renal perfusion, however. It is certainly true that autoregulation extends predominantly over a high range of MAP (80–180 mmHg), impeding hypertensive renal injury, rather than truly protecting against decrements in RPP, RBF, and GFR. In patients with chronic hypertension, in whom the curve is right-shifted, this problem is probably exacerbated, but current recommendations for hemodynamic management do not account for this potential issue. In contrast, young healthy patients commonly have low normal baseline MAP and RPP values which are associated with shock and renal hypoperfusion in others. Apart from hypertension, other comorbidities, drugs, and other therapies may impair autoregulation. For example, experimental data suggest that angiotensin-converting enzyme (ACE) inhibitors and angiotensin receptor blockers may specifically impair autoregulation of GFR (but not renal blood flow) by blunting efferent arteriolar tone (Fig. 4.13).[25] In addition, it appears that RBF autoregulation is impaired by conditions such as sepsis and cardiopulmonary bypass (CPB).[41–45] Furthermore, if renal injury does result in ATN, experimental data suggest that autoregulation is lost, and that RBF becomes linearly pressure-dependent,[1,23,39] resulting in recurrent ARF with subsequent hypotension. Limited human biopsy data support the hypothesis that fresh ATN lesions develop with subsequent hypotension and hypoperfusion insults in humans with ATN.[46] Thus, maintenance of adequate MAP is important not only for prevention of renal injury/ATN but also its supportive management, in which maintenance of adequate RPP may become even more critical than in the presence of uncomplicated prerenal azotemia.

There are some precise experimental data examining the role of perfusion pressure in the pathogenesis of renal dysfunction in CPB patients. Animal studies support the concept that RBF during CPB is dependent on renal perfusion pressure,[41] suggesting loss of autoregulation, but pressor-induced increased MAP does not augment renal perfusion if pump flow is low.[42] Similarly, small studies in on-pump CABG (coronary artery bypass graft) patients suggest that increasing MAP by augmenting pump flow or adding a pressor in the presence of normal flow increases renal perfusion, but pressor use is ineffective for this purpose when pump flow is low.[43,44] There has not been a trial of higher vs lower renal perfusion pressure for the prevention of perioperative ARF in CABG patients at risk, and this was not examined as an endpoint in a trial which showed improved cardiovascular and neurologic outcomes.[45]

Uncertainty regarding the potential adverse renal effects of pressors is greatest in septic shock patients. In septic shock, recent consensus recommendations have suggested adoption of the MAP target from the early goal-directed therapy protocol ($\geq$65 mmHg) for initial resuscitation, with no specific guidance for later-phase pressor titration.[38] CO is normal or elevated in the majority of patients with fluid-resuscitated septic shock.

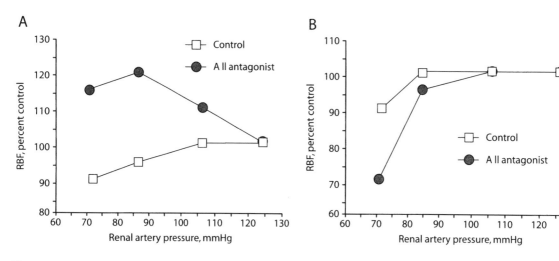

Figure 4.13 Angiotensin II and autoregulation of glomerular filtration rate (GFR). Reducing perfusion pressure is associated with preserved renal blood flow (RBF) (A) and GFR (B) in control dogs (open squares), until autoregulation falls below 105 mmHg (RBF) or 80 mmHg (GFR). RBF and GFR are expressed as a percentage of control values. In dogs receiving intrarenal infusion of angiotensin II antagonist (closed symbols), baseline RBF is higher (A), and RBF autoregulation is maintained. In contrast, autoregulation of GFR is impaired by intrarenal angiotensin II antagonist (B, closed circles), falling below 105 mmHg. (Reproduced with permission from Hall et al.[35] In Rose BD, Post TW: Clinical physiology of acid-base and electrolyte disorders, 5th edn. McGraw-Hill, New York, 2001. Chapter 2, page 41, figure 2–8.)

Prerenal azotemia in septic shock is caused by a wide-ranging variety of derangements, including hypovolemia (venodilation, capillary leak), vasoparesis causing refractory hypotension and decreased RPP, and relative myocardial depression (CO and stroke work are less than they should be, suggesting myocardial depression). In addition, occult renal vasoconstriction is a major cause of renal hypoperfusion in septic shock (see below).[14,46,47] Clinically, refractory arteriolar vasoparesis with pressor-resistant hypotension dominates management. In many patients, despite adequate preload and ventricular function, refractory hypotension develops with vasodilatory shock. The role of MAP/RPP in the pathogenesis of ARF in the ICU has not been explicitly evaluated in a prospective trial, and experimental data are limited. In experimental sepsis models, it is clear that administration of pressors to animals with inadequate fluid resuscitation is harmful, increasing the incidence of ARF and cardiovascular failure.[48] Treggiari and colleagues showed in volume-resuscitated endotoxemic pigs that administration of pressors to raise MAP from about 50 mmHg to about 60 mmHg resulted in increased cardiac output and renal blood flow. In this study, the use of higher doses to achieve MAP values of about 70 mmHg did not seem to improve renal perfusion, resulting in further increased cardiac output but also increased renovascular resistance and unchanged renal blood flow.[49] This is perhaps surprising in view of the fact that 60–70 mmHg is on the descending limb of the renal autoregulation curve, as discussed above (see Fig. 4.4).[22–26] In any case, it is unlikely that the threshold MAP to optimize renal perfusion is identical in animals and humans, so these experimental data are of limited relevance. More important is the concept that the use of alpha-adrenergic agonists in the presence of fluid-resuscitated, hyperdynamic, vasodilatory shock with refractory hypotension results in improved renal perfusion, rather than precipitating ARF. This was best shown in elegant studies by Bellomo and colleagues, who clearly demonstrated in canine endotoxemic shock that norepinephrine increased renal blood flow, not only increasing perfusion pressure but also lowering renovascular ohmic resistance and critical closing pressure.[50]

Clinical studies of patients in septic shock suggest that renal function and urine output improve once MAP is increased above 60 mmHg by the use of catecholamine vasopressor therapy. These studies are of poor quality (see recent extensive reviews),[51–52] however, and were hampered by the lack of a tool to measure blood flow in ICU patients. Of the available techniques to assess renal perfusion, p-aminohippuric acid (PAH) clearance is not a valid method to assess renal plasma flow, because tubular PAH extraction is impaired in critical illness, CPB, postrenal transplantation, and ATN.[53] In fact, it has never been documented whether or not renal autoregulation is intact in animal or human sepsis, and (if so) over what MAP/RPP range. Similarly, the choice of vasopressor is largely a matter of personal preference, without guidance from definitive prospective studies. Specific clinical scenarios and drug characteristics may lead to particular choices (e.g. norepinephrine for dopamine-refractory vasodilatory shock, phenylephrine for vasodilatory shock with arrhythmias on dopamine or norepinephrine). The hypothesis that higher perfusion pressures might prevent or reverse renal dysfunction in resuscitated patients with septic shock is untested by comparative clinical trials. There has only been one randomized trial comparing the effects of catecholamine pressor agents on renal function in septic shock; Martin and colleagues found that the use of norepinephrine was an effective pressor alone, and reversed shock refractory to high-dose dopamine, resulting in increased urine output, but GFR was not measured.[54] Several other descriptive studies have documented improving urine output in patients treated with norepinephrine,[55] but only a few also measured GFR, and none of these included comparison groups. Desjars and colleagues showed that initiation of norepinephrine in 22 of 25 septic shock patients increased MAP (54 to 80 mmHg), UOP (23 ml/h to 66 ml/h), and creatinine clearance (29 ml/min to 71 ml/min) after 24 hours of norepinephrine therapy.[56] Martin and colleagues similarly found that norepinephrine raised MAP in 24 patients refractory to fluids and dopamine and/or dobutamine, reversed oliguria in the majority (20/24), and was associated with increasing creatinine clearance.[57] Redl-Wenzel and colleagues studied 56 septic shock patients refractory to fluids and dopamine/dobutamine, and found that increased MAP (56 to 82 mmHg) was associated with increased creatinine clearance over 48 hours (75 ml/min baseline, 89 ml/min 24 hours, 102 ml/min 48 hours).[58] More recently, LeDoux and colleagues found that titration of norepinephrine to raise MAP from 65 mmHg to 85 mmHg in 10 patients resulted in significantly increased cardiac output, but no change in urine output (GFR was not measured).[59] Although recommendations for titration of catecholamine pressor therapy to

MAP targets of 60–70 mmHg have become routine, these are clearly not evidence-based guidelines.

Vasopressin is emerging as an alternative pressor for vasodilatory shock, and may have some advantages over catecholamines with respect to renal function. Vasopressin is a peptide hormone synthesized in the hypothalamus, stored in the posterior pituitary gland, and secreted in response to increased plasma osmolality, baroreflex activation (hypotension, hypovolemia), and other non-osmotic stimuli.[28,60–62] Vasopressin activates renal collecting duct V_2 receptors (increased tubular water reabsorption; 'ADH', antidiuretic hormone), and vascular V_1 receptors (vasoconstriction). Initial reports of successful use as a rescue agent in patients failing standard vasopressor therapy were followed by data showing that vasopressin *deficiency* (failure to adequately increase circulating vasopressin concentrations in response to hypotension), rather than altered vascular vasopressin responsiveness, was the underlying cause of this phenomenon.[63,64] Landry and colleagues have also demonstrated clinical utility of vasopressin for reversal of refractory vasodilation post-cardiac bypass, which is a clinical syndrome with many similarities to septic shock.[65–67] There is also an extensive literature suggesting advantages of vasopressin over epinephrine in cardiac arrest resuscitation.[68,69] Emerging data suggest that vasopressin deficiency plays a role in septic shock and in post-CPB hypotension. A small study suggested that prophylactic vasopressin administration reduces post-bypass hypotension and use of other vasoconstrictors.[70]

Data with regard to the effects of vasopressin on renal function in septic shock are promising.[28,71] These data suggest that vasopressin may augment GFR not only by raising MAP and RPP but also by increasing glomerular efferent arteriolar tone and filtration fraction, compensating for the counter-regulatory effect of septic afferent arteriolar vasoconstriction. Most compelling is in-vitro work that demonstrates an exclusive (preferential) *efferent arteriolar constriction* by vasopressin in renal glomerular microvessels.[72] This effect would tend in vivo to increase glomerular hydraulic pressure and GFR, and may explain the frequent observation that this agent *increases* UOP in septic shock, despite an anticipated ADH effect of water conservation/antidiuresis.[63,64,73] Preliminary data from a prospective, blinded study by Patel and colleagues suggest that vasopressin increases UOP and GFR compared with norepinephrine titrated to similar systemic endpoints.[73] Since other data showed

similar effects of adding vasopressin to norepinephrine or other pressors, we favor a direct glomerular hemodynamic effect of vasopressin as the explanation for improved UOP in human septic shock.[74–76] This is further supported by the recent work examining the effect of vasopressin on systemic and renal perfusion in septic animals.[77–79] Guzman and colleagues showed in a canine endotoxemia model that vasopressin increased renal blood flow towards baseline values, whereas norepinephrine titrated to similar systemic hemodynamic parameters did not.[77] In endotoxemic rats, vasopressin or L-canavanine (an inhibitor of inducible nitric oxide synthase) improved renal function, whereas norepinephrine titrated to similar MAP did not.[78] In septic sheep (cecal ligation and puncture), vasopressin therapy (alone or in combination with norepinephrine) improved urine output, renal histology, and survival compared to control or norepinephrine therapy.[79] Vasopressin seems to be a promising drug to improve renal function in vasodilatory shock, but in view of the potential for adverse effects on systemic and regional perfusion (notably skin necrosis and mesenteric ischemia), definitive outcome trials are required before recommending routine use in pressor-requiring vasodilatory shock. The 2000 subject VASST trial of vasopressin vs norepinephrine/placebo in septic shock is past 50% enrollment, and should provide the required data to determine safety and effectiveness (Dr Keith Walley pers comm).

Concerns for use in septic shock include potential for V_2-stimulated water intoxication/hyponatremia (not observed to date) and V_1-stimulated pulmonary arterial, coronary, cerebral, and mesenteric vasoconstriction. Pulmonary hypertension was not seen in any of the septic or other vasodilatory shock patients studied by Landry and colleagues or Tsuneyoshi and colleagues, and in the preliminary report by Patel and colleagues pulmonary artery pressures were lower in septic patients treated with vasopressin than norepinephrine.[73–76] Extrapolation from the cardiac arrest literature suggests that coronary and cerebral perfusion should not be compromised by vasopressin any more than by epinephrine or other catecholamines. As noted above, there is ongoing concern regarding potential effects of vasopressin on mesenteric perfusion. Although mesenteric ischemia was not specifically addressed by Tsuneyoshi et al's study, they did find that of their patients treated with vasopressin for septic shock, those that survived had decreased levels of lactate from baseline (a marker of more adequate systemic perfusion or improved liver function) compared to those that did not, and no correlation was found between vasopressin infusion and development of lactic acidosis.[74] More recent studies have not provided consistent conclusions regarding the effects of vasopressin therapy on splachnic perfusion in human septic shock, perhaps in part due to differences in perfusion measurement techniques and vasopressin dosing. Improved splachnic perfusion was found in human septic shock studies of terlipressin by Morelli and colleagues,[80] and of vasopressin by Dunser and colleagues.[81] Similarly, vasopressin therapy in ovine sepsis improved splanchnic perfusion and survival.[79] On the other hand, some studies in animals[82,83] and humans[84] suggest that vasopressin may cause splanchnic hypoperfusion in septic shock. Of course, these concerns must be balanced against the known systemic and regional adverse effects of conventional catecholamine vasopressors, which have been well-described to cause arrhythmias and regional tissue ischemia (by vasoconstriction and hypermetabolism) in human sepsis, particularly in the splanchnic circulation. Recent literature also highlights the known potential for pressor therapy (catecholamines, vasopressin, or both in combination) to cause or contribute to skin necrosis in vasodilatory shock.[85–87] In particular, peripheral intravenous administration increases the risk of skin necrosis;[85] accordingly, only central vein administration is recommended. Based upon available data, the use of vasopressin for vasopressor support in septic shock potentially represents the first major advance in this area since the introduction of catecholamine agents for this purpose. Results of the VASST trial are eagerly awaited. Meanwhile, the design of therapeutic regimens incorporating vasopressin should utilize every available tool to optimize systemic and regional perfusion and ensure full benefit is obtained from this innovation.

Taken together, the literature suggests that maintenance of adequate renal perfusion pressure is an important goal in optimizing renal blood flow, particularly in critically ill patients in whom autoregulation of RBF and GFR is probably impaired (sepsis, CPB, chronic hypertension, ACE inhibitors). Whether the benefit of any pressor in improving renal function is caused by increased global renal blood flow, alterations in renal blood flow distribution, or some other pressure-dependent mechanism is unclear, but it is agreed that patients with vasodilatory shock require

pressor therapy if hypotension is refractory to fluids and perhaps inotropic support. The literature does not provide a precise MAP target to achieve this goal, apart from specific circumstances such as aiming for 65 mmHg in protocol-driven resuscitation in early septic shock.[36,38] It appears that a minimum MAP target of 60–70 mmHg is appropriate for drug titration in patients with vasodilatory shock requiring pressors. However, some patients with myocardial dysfunction may require lower MAP targets (less afterload), whereas others (with prior hypertension in particular) may benefit from a higher renal perfusion pressure. Titration of therapy to individual response may require modifications of published protocols or guidelines.

Optimization of glomerular hemodynamics

Beyond provision of adequate CO and systemic oxygen delivery, and maintenance of optimal RPP, reversal of local renal vasoconstrictor influences is the third potential therapeutic component ensuring renal perfusion in shock. As discussed above, renal vasoconstriction occurs in shock, through multiple mechanisms. Even in septic shock and cirrhosis, two states marked by diminished SVR and hypotension, renal vasoconstriction occurs and is well documented to be the cause of hepatorenal syndrome. Specifically, in hepatorenal syndrome ARF occurs in cirrhotic patients with normal kidneys but profound renal vasoconstriction, which critically impairs renal perfusion and glomerular filtration; renal effects of chronic liver disease are further discussed in Chapter 5. Renal vasoconstriction is also thought to play a role in the pathogenesis of septic ARF, along with hypovolemia (septic venodilation, capillary leak) and impaired systemic oxygen delivery, leading to development of prerenal azotemia. Indeed, some evidence suggests that much septic ARF is in fact severe, unreversed prerenal azotemia, without apoptosis or necrosis on autopsy.[88] These data suggest that septic ARF can have a purely hemodynamic, vasoconstriction-mediated etiology, without apoptosis or necrosis, akin to hepatorenal syndrome. In combination, additive or synergistic nephrotoxic insults (inflammatory mediators, pigments, drugs, etc.) may then precipitate ATN when prerenal azotemia is not effectively prevented or reversed.

The relative importance of selective renal vasoconstriction and regional hypoperfusion vs systemic hypoperfusion or nephrotoxin exposure in causing ARF in critically ill patients has not been precisely defined. Theoretically, any agent which offsets renal vasoconstriction might decrease the incidence of prerenal azotemia and ATN in high-risk patients. It seems preferable to adopt a prophylactic strategy for prevention or reversal of vasoconstriction-induced prerenal azotemia, reversing an often clinically inapparent contributor to the pathogenesis of ATN, rather than attempting to intervene after frank renal injury has occurred. This concept, though theoretically attractive, remains unproven at this time. Increased renal vascular resistance may be reversed by use of generalized renal vasodilators, or by specific pharmacologic antagonists of known renal vasoconstrictor substances. Although the latter approach has been shown to increase renal perfusion and GFR in experimental ARF, with positive results using pharmacologic antagonists of endothelin, leukotrienes, thromboxane, and platelet-activating factor, definitive clinical studies have not been performed with any of these agents in critically ill humans. Of note, endothelin antagonism increased the rate of ARF in chronic renal insufficiency (CRI) patients receiving radiocontrast in a placebo-controlled study.[89] The former approach is best represented by the use of dopaminergic agonists and other vasodilators for renal vasodilation in high-risk patients, an approach which has proven unsuccessful in numerous clinical trials.[90–92]

Prolonged or severe prerenal azotemia may result in ATN, caused by ischemia alone or in combination with nephrotoxic insults. When ATN develops, decreased GFR results from a combination of renal vasoconstriction and parenchymal renal injury.[1] Several mechanisms probably account for the decrease in GFR in ATN, including the direct results of tubular injury (intratubular obstruction by necrotic tubular cell debris and 'backleak' of glomerular filtrate through damaged tubular epithelium) and a major functional element – renal afferent arteriole vasoconstriction via tubuloglomerular feedback (TGF). The effect of TGF is to decrease RBF and GFR in ATN as follows: afferent arteriole vasoconstriction is an adaptive response to the increased delivery of solutes to the macula densa in the distal tubule, preventing massive saline loss past injured proximal convoluted tubule and loop of Henle segments which have become incapable of reabsorptive work. If normal glomerular filtration of 150 L/day of isotonic saline has continued in the presence of impaired tubular sodium reabsorption, the adverse implications are obvious. The problem of inappropriate salt-wasting is exacerbated by the loss on cellular polarity in injured/apoptotic renal tubular cells,

which actively transfer sodium into the lumen. Indeed, the phenomenon whereby TGF-mediated afferent arteriolar constriction shuts down GFR in the presence of ATN has been termed 'acute renal success',[93] because hypovolemic death would be the alternative outcome.

Vascular contributions are important not only in the initiation of ATN and the subsequent vasoconstrictor-mediated decrement in GFR but also in extension and maintenance (see Chs 5 and 8). ATN also involves inflammatory mediators, reactive oxygen species formation, and leukocyte infiltration, all of which further damage the kidneys. Current strategies to prevent or treat ARF by increasing renal perfusion may be ineffective or even harmful in the presence of established ARF with ATN, because the phenomenon of physiologic supply-dependency of renal oxygen consumption dictates that increased RBF and GFR accordingly increase O_2 consumption. If renal vasodilators are to prove successful in ARF prevention and therapy, it is important that they favorably affect intrarenal blood flow distribution and the balance of regional O_2 delivery and consumption. Importantly, the potential for imbalance between oxygen supply and delivery in the medullary circulation suggests that the use of renal vasodilators is not without risk in ARF patients. Increased cortical blood flow favors glomerular filtration, but inadequate medullary blood flow may continue to deprive the S_3 and TALH segments (which must absorb this filtrate) of the necessary oxygen and nutrient supply to simultaneously perform reabsorptive work and remain viable. This may explain the failure of low-dose dopamine and a variety of other renal vasodilators to achieve benefit in ARF prophylaxis or therapy studies to date, despite the documented capacity to increase RBF.

It is possible that current resuscitation endpoints do not optimize renal perfusion, by failing to correct reversible septic myocardial depression, aiming for an inappropriately low renal perfusion pressure, and leaving renal vasoconstrictor influences unopposed, which results in the common occurrence of uncorrected prerenal azotemia. As mentioned above, uncorrected prerenal azotemia is the common substrate for synergistic renal injury and ATN,[12,94] and recurrent hypotension exacerbates renal injury in established ATN.[1,23] Therefore, although not guided by a comprehensive, evidence-based approach, the use of fluids and vasoactive drugs to optimize systemic and renal perfusion remains the mainstay of our efforts to prevent and reverse ARF in critically ill patients.

EFFECTS OF MECHANICAL VENTILATION ON RENAL FUNCTION

Positive pressure mechanical ventilation alters renal perfusion and function through a variety of mechanisms.[13] Elevation of intrathoracic pressure impedes venous return from the periphery, and may result in hypovolemic shock in patients with diminished effective arterial blood volume, particularly in the initial post-intubation period. Even in the absence of frank hypovolemia with hypotension, positive pressure ventilation alters a variety of neurohormonal systems. Positive pressure ventilation stimulates increased sympathetic outflow, activation of the renin–angiotensin–aldosterone axis, and nonosmotic vasopressin release, while suppressing ANP release. These effects lead to systemic and renal vasoconstriction, decreased renal blood flow and GFR, and fluid retention (salt and water) with oliguria. Increased pressure in the inferior vena cava and renal veins may also play a role in ventilator-induced renal dysfunction and fluid retention. Other data suggest that a shift of intrarenal perfusion from cortex to medulla is a contributor to the salt-retaining/oliguric effects of positive pressure ventilation,[95,96] but this has not been a consistent finding.[97]

Small studies have shown that fluid administration[98] and the use of vasoactive drugs, including dopamine ($5 \mu g/kg/min$) or fenoldopam (a pure vasodilator),[13,99,100] can ameliorate the renal hypoperfusion and decreased GFR associated with positive pressure ventilation and positive end-expiratory pressure (PEEP). However, hemodynamic and neurohormonal mechanisms may not be the major cause of ventilator-induced renal injury. A growing body of evidence suggests that the pro-inflammatory effects of positive pressure ventilation, particularly with (lung-) injurious ventilatory strategies, may be a source of acute renal injury.[101–104] Imai and colleagues elegantly demonstrated in a rabbit model of acute lung injury that an injurious ventilatory strategy led to increased acute renal failure, with pathologic evidence of renal tubular cell (and intestinal) apoptosis, and significant lung epithelial cell necrosis.[101] They further demonstrated that plasma from rabbits ventilated with injurious strategy induced increased apoptosis when incubated with cultured rabbit proximal renal tubular cells. In the ARDSNET Tidal Volume Trial, in addition to improved survival and ventilator-free days, the low tidal volume group had more days without circulatory, coagulation, and renal failure (renal: 20 ± 11 vs 18 ± 11 days, $p = 0.005$).[104] Similarly, Ranieri and colleagues showed that a 'lung-protective' mechanical ventilation strategy (lower tidal volume, higher PEEP) caused less systemic and intrapulmonary inflammation than standard management,[102] along with fewer patients with organ system failure, including markedly fewer with renal failure ($p < 0.04$) at 72 hours.[103] This topic is further discussed in Chapter 7. In summary, recent developments have shown us that a combination of appropriate hemodynamic support and lung-protective ventilatory strategies is the best current approach to minimize ventilator-induced renal dysfunction.

EFFECT OF RENAL INSUFFICIENCY ON FUNCTION OF OTHER ORGANS AND OUTCOME IN THE ICU

The mortality of ARF remains high, but it has often been said that modern ICU patients die 'with rather than of' ARF. The precise contribution of 'uremia' to their morbidity and mortality has been difficult to dissect, in part because severity of illness scores have perfomed poorly in prediciting ARF outcome. It is unclear how best to predict or stratify mortality in patients with ARF in the ICU, but there is sufficient evidence to doubt the predictive value of scores such as APACHE II and APACHE III, which seem to underestimate mortality in the presence of ARF.[105,106] Predictive scores designed specifically for ICU patients with renal failure, such as the Cleveland Clinic Score and the Liano Score, have better accuracy, but may not be applicable to other medical centers.[105,106] Renal failure-specific severity of illness scoring systems have been validated to predict prognosis in ICU ARF, accounting for both severity of renal failure and associated MSOF, but it is not known if these systems perform accurately outside of the institutions in which they were developed.[106,107]

It is becoming more apparent that increasing prevalence of septic ARF is the major impediment to improving ARF survival. For example, a recent prospective multicenter ICU study of ARF found that subjects with septic ARF had a far higher unadjusted mortality rate (74% vs 45%, $p < 0.001$) than those without sepsis.[108] Another prospective study of septic surgical ICU patients found that in-hospital mortality was 57% in those with ARF vs 28% without.[109] These findings are in agreement with the practical experience of every intensivist and nephrologist. Patients with hemodynamic instability are at greatest risk for developing ARF, are more difficult to provide renal replacement therapy for, and are most likely to die. Patients with septic shock, along with those with cardiogenic shock, remain our greatest management challenge, driving the current trends in ICU technology for RRT. Although MSOF and other comorbidities contribute to its high mortality rate, ARF independently increases morbidity and mortality. Studies in patients with radiocontrast nephropathy and ARF post-cardiac surgery have found that ARF independently increases mortality.[5,6] More recently, Metnitz and colleagues found that severe ARF requiring renal replacement therapy increased the risk of in-hospital death to a degree beyond that expected based on severity of illness scores.[7] Clermont and colleagues demonstrated that acute renal failure carries a higher odds ratio of death in critically ill patients than chronic renal failure with end-stage renal disease (ESRD), and this was unaccounted for by severity of illness scoring.[8] APACHE III scoring predicted outcome accurately in patients without renal failure, overestimated mortality in critically ill ESRD patients, but underpredicted mortality in those developing ARF after ICU admission. ARF patients had a higher mortality than ESRD patients even if they did not similarly require dialysis. Taken together, these and other studies have found that we lack a severity of illness scoring system which accurately predicts ARF outcome in ICU patients, and this is an impediment to appropriate stratification of multicenter, prospective trials in this population.

Many of the effects of ARF are difficult to identify and quantify independently. It is obvious that problems such as refractory hyperkalemia, pulmonary edema, or clearcut uremic manifestations such as pericarditis are related to ARF when they develop acutely in the appropriate setting. Other uremic manifestations may have several explanations (encephalopathy, acidosis), or may be occult causes of other complications (bleeding diathesis and gastrointestinal bleed, leukocyte dysfunction with immunosuppression, and nosocomial infection). In addition to the emergence of data which appear to confirm an independent role of ARF in increasing mortality in the ICU, it is also clinically obvious that ARF is a cause of significant morbidity and severely complicates ICU management. Many of these complications of renal dysfunction will be discussed in subsequent chapters of this book. Renal dysfunction (acute or chronic) impairs regulation of fluid and water balance, resulting in a tendency to develop volume overload and hyponatremia. A variety of other clinically apparent biochemical and acid–base disorders also develop in ARF patients, apart from accumulation of nitrogenous wastes, azotemia, and uremia. Other effects of renal dysfunction are more subtle. Elimination of many drugs, metabolites, and nephrotoxins is impaired in the presence of renal impairment. Nonrenal elimination (hepatic metabolism) of drugs may also be suppressed. The loss of proximal tubular function also prevents vitamin D hydroxylation at the 1α-position, contributing to hypocalcemia (along with hyperphosphatemia). Vitamin D may also play an immunoregulatory role. Similarly, renal tubules play a role in the removal of pro-inflammatory cytokines and the production of anti-inflammatory cytokines. As detailed in Chapter 7, renal ischemia–reperfusion injury may even cause acute lung injury.[10,11] Other data suggest that ARF causes injury to a variety of other distant organs.[9] Interstitial renal cells produce EPO, with deficiency causing anemia and perhaps contributing to multiple organ dysfunction (decreased oxygen delivery, EPO receptors on end-organs such as the brain), and EPO therapy may even improve outcome. Our attempts at renal replacement therapy probably fall far short of the goal of compensating for the loss of diverse renal functions. More sophisticated techniques may provide better acute RRT in the future; a bioartificial renal tubule assist device containing human proximal tubular cells is already entering phase II trials.[110–113] While our RRT options evolve, prevention (see Ch. 5) or amelioration (see Ch. 8) of ARF in the ICU is a major goal to improve outcome in critically ill patients.

REFERENCES

1. Tang I, Murray PT. Prevention of perioperative ARF: what works? Best Pract Res Clin Anesth 2004;18:91–111.
2. Murray PT, Hall JB. Renal replacement therapy for acute renal failure. Am J Respi Crit Care Med 2000;162:777–81.
3. Kellum JA, Levin N, Bouman C, Lameire N. Developing a consensus classification system for acute renal failure. Curr Opin Crit Care 2002;8:509–14.
4. Star RA. Treatment of acute renal failure. Kidney Int 1998;54:1817–31.
5. Levy EM, Viscoli CM, Horwitz RI. The effect of acute renal failure on mortality. A cohort analysis. JAMA 1996;275:1516–17.
6. Chertow GM, Levy EM, Hammermeister KE, et al. Independent association between acute renal failure and mortality following cardiac surgery. Am J Med 1998;104:343–8.
7. Metnitz PG, Krenn CG, Steltzer H, et al. Effect of acute renal failure requiring renal replacement therapy on outcome in critically ill patients. Crit Care Med 2002;30:2051–8.

8. Clermont G, Acker CG, Angus DC, et al. Renal failure in the ICU: comparison of the impact of acute renal failure and end-stage renal disease on ICU outcomes. Kidney Int 2002;62(4):886–96.
9. Kelly KJ. Distant effects of experimental renal ischemia/reperfusion injury. J Am Soc Nephrol 2003;14:1549–58.
10. Kramer AA, Postler G, Salhab KF, et al. Renal ischemia/reperfusion leads to macrophage-mediated increase in pulmonary vascular permeability. Kidney Int 1999;55:2362–7.
11. Rabb H, Wang Z, Nemoto T, et al. Acute renal failure leads to dysregulation of lung salt and water channels. Kidney Int 2003;63:600–6.
12. Zager RA. Endotoxemia, renal hypoperfusion, and fever: interactive risk factors for aminoglycoside and sepsis-induced acute renal failure. Am J Kidney Dis 1992;20:223–30.
13. Pannu N, Mehta RL. Mechanical ventilation and renal function: an area for concern? Am J Kidney Dis 2002;39(3):616–24.
14. Murray PT, Wylam ME, Umans JG. Nitric oxide and septic vascular dysfunction. Anesth Analg 2000;90:89–101.
15. Murray PT. Pathogenesis and management of septic shock. Semin Anesth Periop Med Pain 1999;18(3):192–203.
16. McNelis J, Marini CP, Simms HH. Abdominal compartment syndrome: clinical manifestations and predictive factors. Curr Opin Crit Care 2003;9(2):133–6.
17. Le Gall J-R, Klar J, Lemeshow S, et al. The Logistic Organ Dysfunction System. A new way to assess organ dysfunction in the intensive care unit. ICU Scoring Group. JAMA 1996;276:802–10.
18. Valtin H, Schafer JA, eds. Renal hemodynamics and oxygen consumption. In: Renal function, 3rd edn., Boston: Little, Brown, and Company; 1995:95–114.
19. Schlichtig R, Kramer DJ, Boston JR, Pinsky MR. Renal O₂ consumption during progressive hemorrhage. J Appl Physiol 1991;70:1957–62.
20. Vander AJ, ed. Renal blood flow and glomerular filtration. In: Renal physiology, 5th edn. New York: McGraw-Hill; 1995:24–50.
21. Schnermann J. The juxtaglomerular apparatus: from anatomical peculiarity to physiological relevance. J Am Soc Nephrol 2003;14:1681–94.
22. Shipley RE, Study RS. Changes in renal blood flow, extraction of inulin, glomerular filtration rate, tissue pressure and urine flow with acute alterations in renal artery pressure. Am J Physiol 1951;167:676–88.
23. Adams PL, Adams FF, Bell PD, Navar LG. Impaired renal blood flow autoregulation in ischemic acute renal failure. Kidney Int 1980;18:68–76.
24. Navar LG. Renal autoregulation: perspectives from whole kidney and single nephron studies. Am J Physiol 1977;233:F357.
25. Hall JE, Guyton AC, Jackson TE, et al. Control of glomerular filtration rate by renin–angiotensin system. Am J Physiol 1977;233:F366.
26. Schmid HE, Garrett RC, Spencer MP. Intrinsic hemodynamic adjustments to reduced renal pressure gradients. Circ Res 1964;14(Suppl):1170–7.
27. Siragy H. AT₁ and AT₂ receptors in the kidney: role in health and disease. Semin Nephrol 2004;24:93–100.
28. Holmes CL, Patel B, Russell JA, Walley KR. Physiology of vasopressin relevant to management of septic shock. Chest 2001;120:989–1002.
29. Kriz W, Bankir L. A standard nomenclature for structures of the kidney. Am J Physiol 1988;254 (Ren Fluid Electrolyte Physiol 23):F1–F8.
30. Brezis M, Rosen S. Hypoxia of the renal medulla – its implications for disease. N Engl J Med 1995;332:647–55.
31. Cunningham PN, Dyanov HM, Park P, et al. Acute renal failure in endotoxemia is caused by TNF acting directly on TNF receptor-1 in kidney. J Immunol 2002;168:5817–23.
32. Schnor N. Acute renal failure and the sepsis syndrome. Kidney Int 2002;61:764–76.
33. De Vriese AS. Prevention and treatment of acute renal failure in sepsis. J Am Soc Nephrol 2003;14:792–805.
34. Gattinoni L, Brazzi L, Pelosi P, et al. A trial of goal-oriented hemodynamic therapy in critically ill patients. N Engl J Med 1995;333:1025–32.
35. Hayes MA, Timmins AC, Yau E, et al. Elevation of systemic oxygen delivery in the treatment of critically ill patients. N Engl J Med 1994;330:1717–22.
36. Rivers E, Nguyen B, Havstad S, et al. Early goal-directed therapy in the treatment of severe sepsis and septic shock. New Engl J Med 2001;345(19):1368–77.
37. Task Force of the American College of Critical Care Medicine, Society of Critical Care Medicine. Practice parameters for hemodynamic support of sepsis in adult patients in sepsis. Crit Care Med 1999;27:639–60.
38. Dellinger RP, Carlet JM, Masur H, et al. Surviving Sepsis Campaign guidelines for management of severe sepsis and septic shock. Crit Care Med 2004;32:858–73.
39. Bersten AD, Holt AW. Vasoactive drugs and the importance of renal perfusion pressure. New Horizons 1995;3:650–61.
40. Stone AM, Stahl WM. Renal effects of hemorrhage in normal man. Ann Surg 1970;172:825–36.
41. Mackay JH, Feerick AE, Woodson LC, et al. Increasing organ blood flow during cardiopulmonary bypass in pigs: comparison of dopamine and perfusion pressure. Crit Care Med 1995;23:1090–8.
42. O'Dwyer C, Woodson LC, Conroy BP, et al. Regional perfusion abnormalities with phenylephrine during normothermic bypass. Ann Thorac Surg 1997;63:728–35.
43. Urzua J, Tronscoso S, Bugedo G, et al. Renal function and cardiopulmonary bypass: effect of perfusion pressure. J Cardiothorac Vasc Anesth 1992;6:299–303.
44. Andersson LG, Bratteby LE, Ekroth R, et al. Renal function during cardiopulmonary bypass: influence of pump flow and systemic blood pressure. Eur J Cardiothorac Surg 1994;8:597–602.
45. Gold JP, Charlson ME, Williams-Russo P, et al. Improvement of outcomes after coronary artery bypass: a randomized trial comparing intraoperative high versus low mean arterial pressure. J Thorac Cardiovasc Surg 1995;110:1302–14.
46. Badr KF. Sepsis-associated renal vasoconstriction: potential targets for future therapy. Am J Kidney Dis 1992;20:207–13.
47. Mitaka C, Hirata Y, Yokoyama K, et al. Improvement of renal dysfunction in dogs with endotoxemia by a nonselective endothelin receptor antagonist. Crit Care Med 1999;27(1):146–53.
48. Hinder F, Stubbe HD, Van Aken H, et al. Early multiple organ failure after recurrent endotoxemia in the presence of vasoconstrictor-masked hypovolemia. Crit Care Med 2003;31:903–9.
49. Treggiari MM, Romand J-A, Burgener D, Suter PM, Aneman A. Effects of increasing norepinephrine dosage on regional blood flow in a porcine model of endotoxin shock. Crit Care Med 2002;30:1334–9.
50. Bellomo R, Kellum JA, Wisniewski SR, Ondulik B, Pinsky MR. Effects of norepinephrine on the renal vasculature in normal and endotoxemic dogs. Am J Respir Crit Care Med 1999;159(4 Pt 1):1186–92.
51. Schetz M. Vasopressors and the kidney. Blood Purif 2002;20:243–51.
52. Lee RWC, Di Giantomasso D, May C, Bellomo R. Vasoactive drugs and the kidney. Best Pract Res Clin Anaesthesiol 2004;18:53–74.
53. Murray PT, Le Gall JR, Dos Reis Miranda D, Pinsky MR, Tetta C. Physiologic endpoints (efficacy) for acute renal failure studies. Curr Opin Crit Care 2002;8(6):519–25.

54. Martin C, Papazian L, Perrin G, et al. Norepinephrine or dopamine for the treatment of hyperdynamic septic shock? Chest 1993;103:1826–31.

55. Desjars P, Pinaud M, Potel G, et al. A reappraisal of norepinephrine therapy in human septic shock. Crit Care Med 1987;15:134–7.

56. Desjars P, Pinaud M, Bugnon D, et al. Norepinephrine therapy has no deleterious renal effects in human septic shock. Crit Care Med 1989;17:426–9.

57. Martin C, Eon B, Saux P, et al. Renal effects of norepinephrine used to treat septic shock patients. Crit Care Med 1990; 18(3):282–5.

58. Redl-Wenzl EM, Armbruster C, Edelmann G, et al. The effects of norepinephrine on hemodynamics and renal function in severe septic shock states. Intens Care Med 1993;19:151–4.

59. LeDoux D, Astiz ME, Carpati CM, Rackow EC. Effects of perfusion pressure on tissue perfusion in septic shock. Crit Care Med 2000;28:2729–32.

60. Schrier RW, Berl T, Anderson RJ. Osmotic and nonsomotic control of vasopressin release. Am J Physiol 1979;236(4):F321–32.

61. Cowley AW, Monos E, Guyton AC. Interaction of vasopressin and the baroreceptor reflex system in the regulation of arterial blood pressure in the dog. Circ Res 1974;XXXIV:505–14.

62. Leimbach WN, Schmid PG, Mark AL. Baroreflex control of plasma arginine vasopressin in humans. Am J Physiol 1984;247(4 Pt 2):H638–44.

63. Landry DW, Levin HR, Gallant EM, et al. Vasopressin pressor hypersensitivity in vasodilatory septic shock. Crit Care Med 1997;25:1279–82.

64. Landry DW, Levin HR, Gallant EM, et al. Vasopressin deficiency contributes to the vasodilation of septic shock. Circulation 1997;95:1122–5.

65. Argenziano M, Chen JM, Choudhri AF, et al. Management of vasodilatory shock after cardiac surgery: identification of presdisposing factors and use of a novel pressor agent. J Thorac Cardiovasc Surg 1998;116(6):973–80.

66. Mets B, Michler RE, Delphin ED, Oz MC, Landry DW. Refractory vasodilation after cardiopulmonary bypass for heart transplantation in recipients on combined amiodarone and angiotensin-converting enzyme inhibitor therapy: a role for vasopressin administration. J Cardiothorac Vasc Anesth 1998;12(3):326–9.

67. Argenziano M, Choudhri AF, Oz MC, et al. A prospective randomized trial of arginine vasopressin in the treatment of vasodilatory shock after left ventricular assist device placement. Circulation 1997;96(9 Suppl):II–286–90.

68. Lindner KH, Prengel AW, Brinkmann A, et al. Vasopressin administration in refractory cardiac arrest. Ann Intern Med 1996;124:1061–4.

69. Lindner KH, Prengel AW, Pfenninger EG, et al. Vasopressin improves vital organ blood flow during closed-chest cardiopulmonary resuscitation in pigs. Ann Intern Med 1995;91:215–21.

70. Morales DL, Garrido MJ, Madigan JD, et al. A double-blind randomized trial: prophylactic vasopressin reduces hypotension after cardiopulmonary bypass. Ann Thorac Surg 2003;75:926–30.

71. Schmid PG, Abboud FM, Wendling MG, et al. Regional vascular effects of vasopressin: plasma levels and circulatory responses. Am J Physiol 1974;227:998–1004.

72. Edwards RM, Trizna W, Kinter LB. Renal microvascular effects of vasopressin and vasopressin antagonists. Am J Physiol 1989; 256(RFE 25): F274–8.

73. Patel BM, Chittock DR, Russell JA, Walley KR. Beneficial effects of short-term vasopressin infusion during severe septic shock. Anesthesiology 2002;96(3):576–82.

74. Tsuneyoshi I, Yamada H, Kakihana Y, et al. Hemodynamic and metabolic effects of low-dose vasopressin infusions in vasodilatory septic shock. Crit Care Med 2001;29(3):487–93.

75. Malay MB, Ashton RC, Landry DW, Townsend RN. Low-dose vasopressin in the treatment of vasodilatory septic shock. J Trauma 1999;47(4):699.

76. Holmes CL, Walley KR, Chittock DR, Lehman T, Russell JA. The effects of vasopressin on hemodynamics and renal function in severe septic shock : a case series. Intens Care Med 2001; 27(8):1416–21.

77. Guzman JA, Rosado AE, Kruse JA. Vasopressin vs. norepinephrine in endotoxic shock: systemic, renal, and splanchnic hemodynamic and oxygen transport effects. J Appl Physiol 2003;95:803–9.

78. Levy B, Valee C, Lauzier F, et al. Comparative effects of vasopressin, norepinephrine, and L-canavanine, a selective inhibitor of inducible nitric oxide synthase, in endotoxic shock. Am J Physiol Heart Circ Physiol 2004;287:H209–15.

79. Sun Q, Dimopoulos G, Nguyen DN, et al. Low-dose vasopressin in the treatment of septic shock in sheep. Am J Respit Crit Care Med 2003;168(4):481–6.

80. Morelli A, Rocco M, Conti G, et al. Effects of terlipressin on systemic and regional haemodynamics in catecholamine-treated hyperkinetic septic shock. Intens Care Med 2004;30:597–604.

81. Dunser MW, Mayr AJ, Ulmer H, et al. Arginine vasopressin in advanced vasodilatory shock. A prospective, randomized, controlled study. Circulation 2003;107:2313–19.

82. Westphal M, Freise H, Kehrel BE, et al. Arginine vasopressin compromises gut mucosal microcirculation in septic rats. Crit Care Med 2004;32:194–200.

83. Martikainen TJ, Tenhunen JJ, Uusaro A, Ruokenen E. The effects of vasopressin on systemic and splanchnic hemodynamics and metabolism in endotoxin shock. Anesth Analg 2003;97:1756–63.

84. van Haren FM, Rozendaal FW, van der Hoeven JG, et al. The effect of vasopressin on gastric perfusion in catecholamine-dependent patients in septic shock. Chest 2003;124:2256–60.

85. Kahn JM, Kress JP, Hall JB. Skin necrosis after extravasation of low-dose vasopressin administered for septic shock. Crit Care Med 2002;30:1899–901.

86. Dunser MW, Mayr AJ, Tur A, et al. Ischemic skin lesions as a complication of continuous vasopressin infusion in catecholamine-resistant vasodilatory shock: incidence and risk factors. Crit Care Med 2003;31:1394–8.

87. Chen JL, O'Shea M. Extravasation injury associated with low-dose dopamine. Ann Pharmacother 1998;32:545–8.

88. Hotchkiss RS, Swanson PE, Freeman BD, et al. Apoptotic cell death in patients with sepsis, septic shock, and multiple organ dysfunction. Crit Care Med 1999;27:1230–51.

89. Wang A, Holcslaw T, Bashore TM, et al. Exacerbation of radiocontrast nephrotoxicity by endothelin receptor antagonism. Kidney Int 2000;57:1675–80.

90. ANZICS Clinical Trials Group. Low-dose dopamine in patients with early renal dysfunction: a placebo-controlled randomised trial. Lancet 2000;356:2139–43.

91. Kellum JA, Decker JM. Use of dopamine in acute renal failure: a meta-analysis. Crit Care Med 2001;29:1526–31.

92. Murray PT. Use of dopaminergic agents for renoprotection in the ICU. Yearbook of intensive care and emergency medicine. Berlin: Springer-Verlag; 2003:637–48.

93. Thurau K, Boylan JW. Acute renal success. The unexpected logic of oliguria in acute renal failure. Am J Med 1976;61(3):308–15.

94. Blantz RC. Pathophysiology of prerenal azotemia. Kidney Int 1998;53:512–23.

95. Hall SV, Johnson EE, Hedley White J. Renal hemodynamics and function with continuous positive-pressure ventilation in dogs. Anesthesiology 1974;41:452–61.

96. Moore ES, Glavez MB, Paton JB, et al. Effects of positive pressure ventilation on intrarenal blood flow in infant primates. Pediatr Res 1974;8:792–6.

97. Preibe HJ, Heimann JC, Hedley-White J. Mechanisms of renal dysfunction during positive end-expiratory pressure ventilation. J Appl Physiol 1981;50:643–9.

98. Ramamoorthy C, Rooney M, Dries DJ, et al. Aggressive hydration during continuous positive pressure ventilation restores atrial transmural pressure, plasma atrial natriuretic peptide concentrations, and renal function. Crit Care Med 1992;20:1014–19.

99. Poinsot O, Romand JA, Favre H, Suter PM. Fenoldopam improves renal hemodynamics impaired by positive pressure. Anesthesiology 1993;79:680–4.

100. Schuster HP, Suter PM, Hemmer M, et al. Fenoldopam improves renal dysfunction secondary to ventilation with PEEP. Intensivmedizin 1991;28:348–55.

101. Imai Y, Parodo J, Kajikawa O, et al. Injurious mechanical ventilation and end-organ epithelial cell apoptosis and organ dysfunction in an experimental model of acute respiratory distress syndrome. JAMA 2003;289:2104–12.

102. Ranieri VM, Suter P, Tortorella C, et al. Effect of mechanical ventilation on inflammatory mediators in patients with acute respiratory distress syndrome: a randomized controlled trial. JAMA 1999;282:54–61.

103. Ranieri VM, Suter PM, Slutsky AS. Mechanical ventilation as a mediator of multisystem organ failure in acute respiratory distress syndrome. JAMA 2000;284:43–4.

104. ARDSNet. Ventilation with lower tidal volumes as compared with traditional tidal volumes for acute lung injury and the acute respiratory distress syndrome. N Engl J Med 2000;342:1301–8.

105. Douma CE, Redekop WK, van der Meulen JH, et al. Predicting mortality in intensive care patients with acute renal failure treated with dialysis. J Am Soc Nephrol 1997;8(1):111–17.

106. Halstenberg WK, Goormastic M, Paganini EP. Validity of four models for predicting outcome in critically ill acute renal failure patients. Clin Nephrol 1997;47(2):81–6.

107. Liano F, Gallego A, Pascual J, et al. Prognosis of acute tubular necrosis: an extended prospectively contrasted study. Nephron 1993;63(1):21–31.

108. Neveu H, Kleinknecht D, Brivet F, Loirat P, Landais P. Prognostic factors in acute renal failure due to sepsis. Results of a prospective multicentre study. Nephrol Dial Transplant 1996;11(2):293–9.

109. Hoste EAJ, Lameire NH, Vanholder RC, et al. Acute renal failure in patients with sepsis in the surgical ICU: predictive factors, incidence, comorbidity, and outcome. J Am Soc Nephrol 2003;14:1022–30.

110. Humes HD, Fissell WH, Weitzel WF, et al. Metabolic replacement of kidney function in uremic animals with a bioartificial kidney containing human cells. Am J Kidney Dis 2002;39:1078–87.

111. Fissell WH, Lou L, Abrishami S, et al. Bioartificial kidney ameliorates gram negative bacteria-induced septic shock in uremic animals. J Am Soc Nephrol 2003;14:454–61.

112. Humes HD, Buffington DA, Lou L, et al. Cell therapy with a tissue-engineered kidney reduced the multiple organ consequences of septic shock. Crit Care Med 2003;31:2421–8.

113. Humes HD, Weitzel WF, Bartlett RH, et al. Renal cell therapy is associated with dynamic and individualized responses in patients with acute renal failure. Blood Purif 2003;21:64–71.

II
Renal failure in the intensive care unit

5

Prevention of acute renal failure in the intensive care unit

Kevin W Finkel, Patrick T Murray, and Andrew Shaw

INTRODUCTION

Acute renal failure (ARF) as a result of acute tubular necrosis (ATN) may develop in 10% of all patients admitted to the intensive care unit (ICU), and is associated with high morbidity and mortality rates.[1–3] Despite increased understanding of the pathophysiologic mechanisms operative in ATN, and the success of various treatments in reversing or ameliorating ATN in animal models, there are currently no proven therapies in human ARF, in which mortality rates remain in excess of 50%.[4]

Arguments offered to explain the discrepancy between laboratory and clinical studies include the lack of an appropriate model of human disease in the ICU, and the untimeliness of intervention in clinical trials.[5,6] The mechanisms of ARF in the ICU are complex, involving issues of renal hypoperfusion, nephrotoxic insults, and accompanying acute and chronic illness, often in the face of the systemic inflammatory response syndrome (SIRS) or sepsis. Additionally, the use of positive pressure ventilation and administration of vasopressor medications can have adverse effects on renal function.[7–9] The various animal models used to study ATN lack these complexities. Furthermore, ATN is an evolving process. Early on, renal ischemia and redistribution of renal blood flow play a prominent role.[10] Later, apoptosis and inflammation are key players.[11] Therefore, there is probably a limited time window for different therapeutic agents to provide benefit[12] (Fig. 5.1). In animal studies, the timing of a particular insult is known and therapy is applied without reliance on first detecting a fall in glomerular filtration rate (GFR). On the other hand, in clinical trials, because of the dependence on using changes in serum creatinine levels to detect a fall in GFR, there is an inherent delay in initiating potentially beneficial treatment. For vasoactive agents such as dopamine and atrial natriuretic peptide (ANP) to be effective it is possible they need to be given early in ARF, when renal ischemia is prominent. These agents may provide no benefit when given at a later stage of ATN. In the majority of studies on ARF in ICU patients, treatment is given late in its course.[13,14] The lack of efficacy of the various interventions could be the result of this delay, either because the mechanism of decreased GFR is no longer responsive to therapy or simply because too much functional renal mass has already been lost. Therefore, prevention of ATN remains a cornerstone in the treatment of the critically ill patient.

Prevention of ATN in patients in the ICU requires an understanding of certain key issues:

1. the pathophysiologic mechanism of a particular insult
2. risk factors for the development of ARF in the ICU
3. the contribution of acute and chronic organ dysfunction to renal failure
4. the effect of therapies such as vasopressors and positive pressure ventilation on renal function
5. the appropriate hemodynamic profile for a particular patient that optimizes renal blood flow (RBF).

Unfortunately, many of these factors are poorly understood or unknown.

GENERAL PRINCIPLES

In the ICU, patients are exposed to multiple potential renal insults. Frank ischemia or relative renal

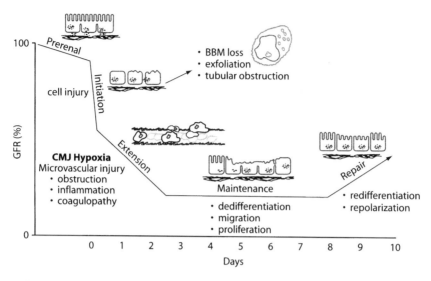

Figure 5.1 Relationship between the clinical phases and the cellular phases of ischemic acute renal failure (ARF), and the temporal impact on organ function as represented by the glomerular filtration rate (GFR). Prerenal azotemia exists when a reduction in renal blood flow causes a reduction in GFR. A variety of cellular and vascular adaptations maintain renal epithelial cell integrity during this phase. The initiation phase occurs when a further reduction in renal blood flow results in cellular injury, particularly the renal tubular epithelial cells, and a continued decline in GFR. Vascular and inflammatory processes that contribute to further cell injury and a further decline in GFR usher in the proposed extension phase. During the maintenance phase, GFR reaches a stable nadir as cellular repair processes are initiated in order to maintain and re-establish organ integrity. The recovery phase is marked by a return of normal cell and organ function that results in an improvement in GFR. (CMJ = corticomedullary junction, BBM = brush border membrane.) (Reproduced with permission from Sutton et al.[12])

hypoperfusion from capillary leak syndrome, hypoalbuminemia, and diuretics are frequently present in ICU patients. Potential exogenous insults to the kidneys, including myoglobin, radiocontrast media, aminoglycoside antibiotics, and amphotericin B preparations, often produce both ischemic and nephrotoxic damage. Distant organ dysfunction can contribute to the complexity by adversely affecting renal function, as occurs in hepatorenal syndrome and veno-occlusive disease of the liver (VOD). Therefore, it is difficult to devise a simple prevention strategy for all patients in the ICU (Fig. 5.2; Box 5.1).

Avoidance of potential nephrotoxins such as intravenous radiocontrast, aminoglycoside antibiotics, and antifungal agents is prudent, when possible. Although nonsteroidal anti-inflammatory drugs (NSAIDs), including cyclooxygenase-2 (COX-2) inhibitors, generally have a low nephrotoxic risk, the potential renal vasoconstrictive effect of these agents may be significant in selected patients, such as those with sepsis, heart failure, cirrhosis, nephrotic syndrome, volume depletion, and hypoalbuminemia. Single daily dosing of aminoglycoside antibiotics is associated with a lower risk of nephrotoxicity and equivalent antimicrobial efficacy compared to multiple dosing strategies.[15] Drug modifications such as nonionic radiocontrast and lipid-emulsified amphotericin B may also reduce the incidence of ATN.[16,17] Aggressive diuresis must be avoided when possible, particularly in conjunction with the use of angiotensin-converting enzyme (ACE) inhibitors or angiotensin receptor blockers, and must be accompanied by careful monitoring of fluid balance and renal function. Monitoring the serum levels of potentially nephrotoxic drugs such as aminoglycosides, cyclosporin A (CSA), tacrolimus, and vancomycin is recommended, although studies proving that therapeutic drug monitoring decreases the incidence of ATN are lacking. General measures that may decrease the incidence of ARF are listed in Box 5.1. The role of hemodynamic monitoring and support with fluids and vasoactive drugs in the prevention of ARF in the ICU is clearly important. The relationship between renal perfusion and function is discussed in depth in Chapter 4, but will be discussed in

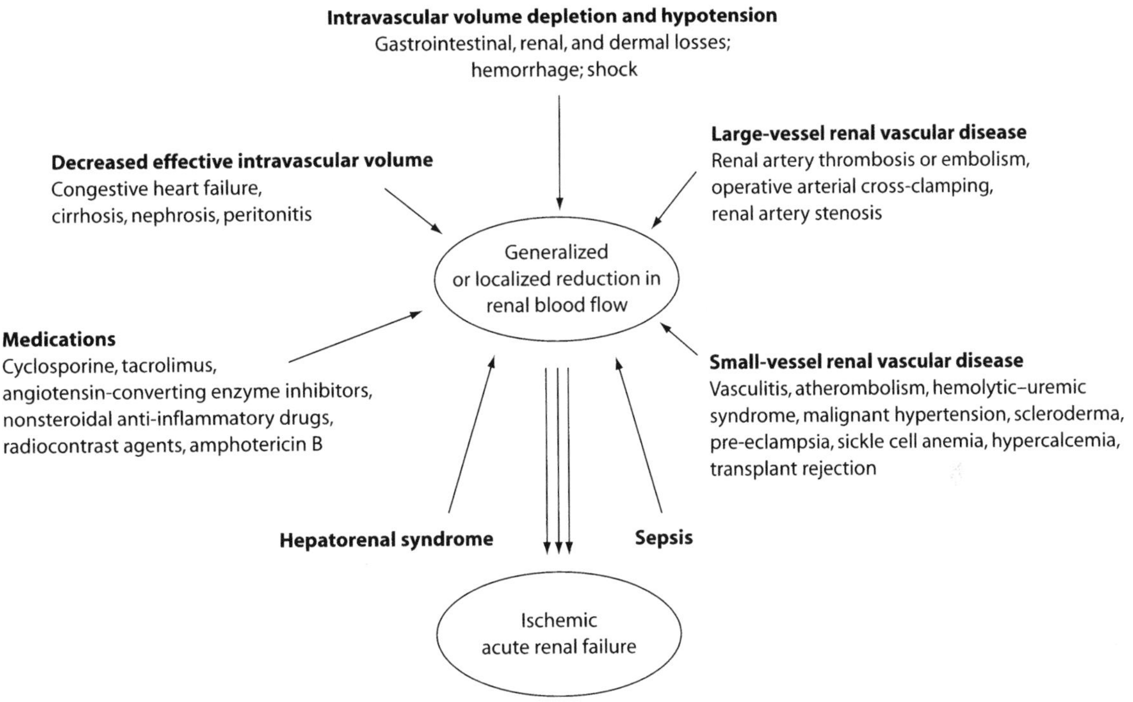

Figure 5.2 Conditions that lead to ischemic acute renal failure. A wide spectrum of clinical conditions can result in a generalized or localized reduction in renal blood flow, thus increasing the likelihood of ischemic acute renal failure. The most common condition leading to ischemic acute renal failure is severe and sustained prerenal azotemia. Kidney ischemia and acute renal failure are often the result of a combination of factors. (Reproduced with permission from Thadhani R, Pascual M, Bonventre JV. Acute renal failure. N Engl J Med 1996;334:1448–60.)

terms of ARF prophylaxis in this chapter, along with other approaches to avoid or ameliorate ARF in critically ill patients.

PREDICTION OF ACUTE RENAL FAILURE

For prevention of ARF to be an achievable goal, it is imperative that there is a means of accurately predicting the development of ARF. Although much research continues to center on predicting outcome in patients who experience ARF in the ICU, surprisingly little work has been done in the area of predicting who will develop ARF. To date, a reliable prediction model is not available. Studies using multiple linear or logistic regression analysis suggest that a combination of factors such as age, hypotension, hypoxia, the presence of two of four markers of SIRS, use of vasopressors, positive pressure ventilation, chronic renal failure, and sepsis have some prediction value, but none have the precision to allow application of true preventive

measures.[18–20] An analogous situation is found in attempting to predict mortality rates in ICU patients with ARF. Although scoring methods such as APACHE II and APACHE III are reasonably good at predicting overall mortality in ICU patients, they routinely underestimate the rate in the presence of ARF.[21,22] Predictive scores designed specifically for ICU patients with renal failure, such as the Cleveland Clinic Score and the Liano Score, have better accuracy, but may not be applicable to other medical centers.[22,23]

RENAL BLOOD FLOW

Providing adequate renal perfusion in the face of critical illness appears to be an appropriate goal. Often, patients in the ICU already have some component of prerenal failure that can progress to frank ischemic ATN if not corrected. However, what amount of perfusion is needed, where it should be distributed, and how to measure

---

Box 5.1   Strategies to decrease ARF in the ICU

Proven
Avoidance of nephrotoxins
Single daily dosing of aminoglycosides
Drug modifications:
  Liposomal amphotericin B
  Nonionic radiocontrast
Hydration:
  Radiocontrast
  Cisplatin
  Rhabdomyolysis
  Tumor lysis syndrome
Tight glycemic control in the critically ill

Possibly effective
Monitoring drug levels
Adequate renal perfusion
Low-dose fenoldopam
N-acetylcysteine (radiocontrast)
Alkalinization of the urine:
  Rhabdomyolysis
  Methotrexate
  Tumor lysis syndrome

Ineffective
Low-dose dopamine
Mannitol
Diuretics
Aminophylline
Atrial natriuretic peptide

---

adequacy are all unknown factors. A fall in renal perfusion is both a result and a response to injury. A decrease or a redistribution of blood flow away from a damaged tubule to prevent solute loss is an adaptive response to guard against hypovolemic shock.[24] When enough nephron loss occurs, nitrogenous waste accumulates and ARF ensues. As discussed in Chapter 4, indiscriminate increases in blood flow could have deleterious effects on the course of ATN by increasing solute loss, maintaining toxin exposure to injured tubules, or promoting reperfusion oxidant injury. In fact, although renal vasoconstriction in ATN could be viewed as a maladaptive response perpetuating ARF, this phenomenon should not be considered a purely inappropriate response like sodium retention in congestive heart failure (CHF). In CHF, although retention of sodium to improve cardiac preload is an adaptive response to perceived poor perfusion, it is detrimental to the patient and must be treated with diuretics. In contrast, increasing RBF with vasodilators in the presence of ATN may reverse a protective hemodynamic response of injured kidneys; this may be an inappropriate therapy for what has been termed 'acute renal success'.[24]

There are no reliable indicators of adequate RBF, except (presumably) normal renal function. Urine output correlates best with degree of renal injury (i.e. oliguric ATN has a worse prognosis, thought to reflect more severe renal injury). Except in the case of prerenal failure, where a volume infusion reverses the low flow state, urine output is an unreliable marker of renal perfusion. Most often, a predetermined mean arterial pressure (MAP) reading is considered proof of adequate renal perfusion. Vasopressor algorithms used in the ICU usually specify an arbitrary MAP goal for titration of the medications. However, the appropriate MAP for a critically ill patient with ARF is not defined. The three major determinants of renal blood flow are cardiac output, intravascular volume, and renal perfusion pressure.

Cardiac output

Increasing cardiac output by administration of intravenous fluid or cardiac inotropes should increase renal blood flow in low flow states such as cardiogenic shock and prerenal azotemia. In patients with ARF, decreased renal perfusion is the result of an imbalance between local renal vasoconstrictor and vasodilator influences. This imbalance causes both global renal hypoperfusion and shunting of blood flow away from the renal medulla. There is no evidence that increasing cardiac output to 'supranormal' levels counteracts this imbalance. Most studies in critically ill patients comparing normal to enhanced cardiac output measured by oxygen delivery or cardiac index have failed to show benefit on survival rates.[25] One recent study of aggressive hemodynamic management of 263 septic patients on arrival to the emergency center did demonstrate a survival benefit, but effects on renal function were not described, and its relevance to preventing ARF in established ICU patients is unknown.[26] Currently, there are no randomized controlled trials comparing different cardiac outputs and the subsequent development of ARF in high-risk individuals.

Intravascular fluid expansion

Both animal and human studies suggest that intravascular fluid expansion decreases the risk of ARF from radiocontrast agents and various nephrotoxic insults.[27,28] However, what role it plays in preventing ATN in patients in the ICU with multiple risk factors is purely speculative. Because ICU patients usually have capillary leak syndrome and impaired pulmonary function, indiscriminate fluid administration can have deleterious effects. Therefore, measuring volume status in ICU patients often requires invasive monitoring of right atrial pressure or pulmonary artery occlusion pressure. At this time, no data are available to indicate that a certain degree of intravascular filling is more protective of renal function than another.

The putative superiority of colloid over crystalloid fluids in the resuscitation of the critically ill patient has been a source of considerable controversy. Aggressive hydration with crystalloid solutions such as 0.9% sodium chloride can worsen interstitial edema and pulmonary function. Colloidal solutions such as various starches and human albumin might appear to be attractive alternatives, but there is little solid evidence of their superiority in clinical trials.[29,30] Systematic reviews of randomized controlled trials comparing crystalloids with colloids have yielded conflicting results. Some trials have found an increased mortality rate associated with the administration of human albumin and hydroxyethylstarch, whereas others have not.[31,32] Most recently, a large randomized, controlled prospective trial of albumin vs saline in almost 7000 critically ill patients found no benefit of one over the other.[33] Specifically, there was no demonstrable effect on mortality, renal function, or the frequency of renal replacement therapy. Of note, patients with cirrhosis were excluded from this trial, and limited data suggest that albumin is useful to prevent ARF in cirrhotic patients with spontaneous bacterial peritonitis (see below),[34] or undergoing large volume paracentesis. As discussed below, for prevention of radiocontrast nephropathy normal saline is superior to half-normal saline,[35] and an equimolar solution of sodium bicarbonate is superior to normal saline.[36] Otherwise, despite the importance of fluid therapy in the prevention of ARF, the nature of the optimum fluid resuscitation regimen remains a disputed topic. For the time being it appears that treatment of the underlying diagnosis, usually sepsis, and general supportive efforts are the mainstays of therapy.

Renal perfusion pressure

In the critically ill patient attention is usually focused on improving cardiac output and intravascular volume to maintain adequate perfusion to the heart and brain, the 'vital organs.' What is often unappreciated is that in the normal kidney loss of autoregulation of renal blood flow occurs at a MAP of 75–80 mmHg, and that the loss of autoregulation of GFR occurs at approximately 80–85 mmHg.[37,38] In the face of long-standing hypertension present in many ICU patients, autoregulation fails at even higher MAP levels. Therefore, ICU protocols that titrate vasopressors to an MAP of 65 or 70 mmHg can result in persistent renal ischemia (Fig. 5.3). There are no randomized controlled trials comparing MAP values and the development of ARF in ICU patients. However, the current treatment strategies may be inappropriate in some individuals.

PHARMACOLOGIC AGENTS

N-acetylcysteine (NAC, Mucomyst)

NAC is an antioxidant and causes renal vasodilation by generating increased levels of nitric oxide (NO). Based on these effects, NAC was used in several small human trials for the prevention of ARF from radiocontrast agents in high-risk individuals. The trials have shown that its administration results in a significantly smaller change from baseline of serum creatinine values compared to changes in the placebo group.[39,40] A recent meta-analysis of 8 randomized controlled trials supported the use of NAC to prevent radiocontrast nephropathy (RCN).[41] However, whether or not it prevents severe ARF and the need for dialysis has not been determined. Furthermore, emerging literature suggests that NAC causes a GFR-independent decrease in serum creatinine,[42] perhaps by inhibiting creatine phosphokinase-mediated generation of creatinine.[43] This may explain the puzzling but consistent decrease in serum creatinine below baseline levels observed in NAC-treated patients with chronic kidney disease undergoing RCN

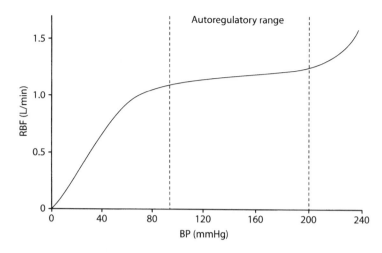

Figure 5.3 Autoregulation of renal blood flow (RBF). Autoregulation maintains RBF, and glomerular filtration rate (GFR) over a wide range of mean arterial pressure (MAP) levels by modulation of afferent arteriolar resistance. RBF increases by only 10% when MAP increases by 50% from 100 to 150 mmHg, but decreases precipitously when MAP falls below 70–80 mmHg. (Reproduced with permission from Vander AJ: Renal physiology, 5th edn. McGraw-Hill, New York, 1995. In: Chapter 2: Renal blood flow and glomerular filtration (Figure 2–4, page 34).)

prophylaxis, which was previously assumed to be an effect of volume expansion. It is thus conceivable that the putative renoprotective effect of NAC in contrast nephropathy is an artifact. NAC has also been administered intravenously to 100 critically ill patients in a randomized placebo-controlled trial to prevent progression of multiple organ dysfunction syndrome (MODS).[44] There was no significant difference between the groups in mortality rate, days of inotropic support, mechanical ventilation, ICU length of stay, or development of ARF.

At this point, it is probably harmless to provide NAC prior to radiocontrast administration in patients at risk for the development of ARF pending further research, provided that it is combined with appropriate volume expansion, and that the effect of NAC on serum creatinine is remembered while assessing post-dye renal function. However, there are no convincing data to support the routine administration of NAC in RCN or other clinical circumstances to prevent the development of ATN, and it may soon be proven ineffective for such purposes.

Low-dose dopamine

Low-dose dopamine administration (1–3 µg/kg/min) to normal individuals causes renal vasodilation and increased GFR, and acts as a proximal tubular diuretic. Due to these effects, numerous studies have used low-dose dopamine to either prevent or treat ATN in a variety of clinical settings. It has been given as prophylaxis for ARF

associated with radiocontrast administration, repair of aortic aneurysms, orthotopic liver transplantation, unilateral nephrectomy, renal transplantation, and chemotherapy with interferon.[45,46] Yet despite more than 20 years of clinical experience, prevention trials with low-dose dopamine have all been small, inadequately randomized, of limited statistical power, and with endpoints of questionable clinical significance. Furthermore, there is concern for the potential harmful effects of dopamine, even at low doses. It can trigger tachyarrhythmias and myocardial ischemia, decrease intestinal blood flow, cause hypothyroidism, and suppress T-cell function.[45–47] It has also been shown to increase the risk of RCN when given prophylactically to patients with diabetic nephropathy.[48]

Numerous trials using low-dose dopamine to treat established ATN have also been reported in the last several years and suggest its use is beneficial.[45,46,49] However, most studies were either uncontrolled case series or small randomized trials with limited statistical power. Kellum and Decker found no benefit of dopamine for prevention or therapy of ARF in an adequately powered meta-analysis.[50] More recently, a large randomized placebo-controlled trial in 328 critically ill patients, with early ARF sufficiently powered to detect a small benefit, reported no effect of low-dose dopamine on renal function, need for dialysis, ICU or hospital length of stay, or mortality.[51] These findings combined with the aforementioned potential deleterious effects of low-dose dopamine are strong arguments for abandoning its use entirely for the prevention and therapy of ARF.

Low-dose fenoldopam mesylate

Fenoldopam mesylate is a pure dopamine type-1 receptor agonist that has similar hemodynamic effects to dopamine in the kidney without α- and β-adrenergic stimulation. Limited trials suggested that administration of fenoldopam mesylate reduced the occurrence of ARF from radiocontrast agents and following aortic aneurysm repair.[52,53] However, a recently reported large randomized controlled trial of fenoldopam mesylate to prevent contrast nephropathy in 315 patients demonstrated that its administration had no beneficial effect on urine output, change in serum creatinine levels, incidence of ARF, or need for dialysis.[54] Promising data from a recent randomized, placebo-controlled pilot trial of low-dose fenoldopam mesylate in 155 ICU patients with early ATN showed that fenoldopam patients tended to have lower 21-day mortality rates and decreased need for dialysis, but the study was underpowered.[55] A larger study is required to determine if fenoldopam ameliorates the course of ATN.

Diuretics

Furosemide is a loop diuretic and vasodilator that may decrease oxygen consumption in the loop of Henle by inhibiting sodium transport, thus potentially lessening ischemic injury. By increasing urinary flow, it may also reduce intratubular obstruction and backleak of filtrate. Based on these properties, furosemide might be expected to prevent ARF (Fig. 5.4). However, there are little data to support its use. Furosemide was found to be ineffective or harmful when used to prevent ARF after cardiac surgery, and to increase the risk of ARF when given to prevent contrast nephropathy.[28,56]

Similarly, there is little evidence of benefit from diuretic therapy in established ARF. A single recent study in 100 patients with oliguric ARF after cardiac surgery suggested that a cocktail infusion of furosemide, mannitol, and dopamine improved renal function postcardiac surgery compared to intermittent loop diuretics alone.[57] In patients with established ATN, several studies have found no

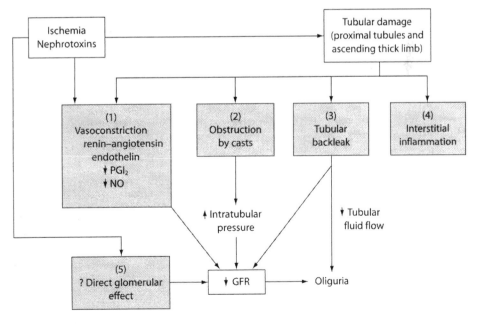

Figure 5.4 Pathophysiologic mechanisms of acute renal failure (ARF). Tubular damage by ischemia, nephrotoxins, or both, leads to decreased glomerular filtration rate (GFR) by a combination of mechanisms. (1) Renal vasoconstriction via activation of tubuloglomerular feedback, and decreased vasodilator substances (PGI$_2$, prostacyclin; NO, nitric oxide), is a prominent functional mechanism of decreased GFR in acute tubular necrosis (ATN). (2) Backpressure from tubular obstruction by casts directly decreases GFR. (3) Backleak of glomerular filtrate into peritubular capillaries decreases the efficiency of glomerular filtration, effectively decreasing GFR. (4) There is increasing evidence for a role of interstitial inflammation in the extension phase of ATN. (5) Direct glomerular effects (mesangial contraction, decreased filtration surface area) may also play a role in decreasing GFR in the presence of ATN.

benefit of loop diuretics:[58-62] their use did not accelerate renal recovery, decrease the need for dialysis, or reduce mortality. It was shown that the mortality rate of oliguric patients who responded to furosemide with a diuresis was lower than those who did not.[62,63] However, the clinical characteristics, severity of renal failure, and mortality rates were similar in patients with either spontaneous nonoliguric ARF or patients who became nonoliguric after furosemide. This implies that those patients able to respond to furosemide have less severe renal damage than nonresponders, rather than deriving any true therapeutic benefit from furosemide administration. Although administration of furosemide might facilitate improved fluid management if it induces a diuresis, a retrospective review of a recent trial in critically ill patients with ATN raised concerns of possible harm from loop diuretics in ARF. The authors found that diuretic use was associated with an increased risk of death and nonrecovery of renal function.[64] Most of the increased risk, however, was seen in those patients unresponsive to high doses of diuretics, implying they had more severe disease. Therefore, diuretics should be used with caution in critically ill patients, and iatrogenic hypovolemia and superimposed prerenal azotemia must be avoided. Diuretics should be withdrawn if there is no response, to avoid ototoxicity. In patients who experience an increase in urine output, hypotension must be avoided, since kidneys with ATN are susceptible to further damage from decreases in perfusion pressure. To maintain the diuresis, a continuous infusion of drug is probably preferable to intermittent bolus administration.[65] Although there are no large randomized controlled trials, the overall evidence suggests that continuous infusion of diuretics as opposed to bolus administration is more effective and associated with less toxicity and delayed development of diuretic resistance.

Mannitol is an osmotic diuretic that can decrease cell swelling, scavenge free radicals, and cause renal vasodilatation by inducing intrarenal prostaglandin production.[66] It may be beneficial when added to organ preservation solutions during renal transplantation and may protect against ARF caused by rhabdomyolysis if given extremely early.[66-68] Otherwise, mannitol has not been shown to be useful in the prevention of ARF. In fact, mannitol may aggravate ARF from radiocontrast agents.[28] Furthermore, mannitol may precipitate pulmonary edema if given to volume-overloaded patients who remain oliguric, can exacerbate the hyperosmolar state of azotemia,

and may even cause acute renal failure ('osmotic nephrosis').[69]

Atrial natriuretic peptide

Atrial natriuretic peptide causes vasodilation of the afferent arteriole and constriction of the efferent arteriole, resulting in an increased GFR. It also inhibits renal tubular sodium reabsorption. Most studies with ANP involved the treatment of established ATN. However, in two studies that administered ANP in renal transplant recipients to prevent primary renal dysfunction, no benefit was found.[70,71] As with mannitol and low-dose dopamine,[28,48] one study suggested that ANP prophylaxis might worsen renal function in diabetic patients receiving radiocontrast agents.[72]

Based on the positive results of small clinical studies using ANP to treat ATN, a randomized placebo-controlled trial of 504 critically ill patients with ARF was conducted.[13] Despite the large size of the trial, ANP administration had no effect on 21-day dialysis-free survival, mortality, or change in plasma creatinine concentration. Of note, the mean serum creatinine values at enrollment (about 4.4-5 mg/dl) in this study confirm that intervention in this trial was extremely late in the course of ATN. Although a subgroup analysis of the study suggested that ANP might be beneficial in those patients with oliguric renal failure, a subsequent trial in patients with oliguric renal failure failed to demonstrate any benefit of ANP.[73] Hypotension was significantly more common in ANP-treated patients in this study, and may have negated any potential benefit of renal vasodilation in these patients. Hence, there is no convincing evidence to support the use of ANP in the prevention or treatment of ARF. A new, promising, but underpowered (61 patients) positive study of ANP to treat ARF immediately following cardiac surgery showed a decreased rate of postoperative renal replacement therapy compared to placebo-treated patients;[74] a larger prospective trial in this setting appears warranted.

Insulin-like growth factor-1

Insulin-like growth factor-1 (IGF-1) increases renal blood flow and induces cell proliferation and differentiation. In addition, it reverses apoptosis. In animal models, it ameliorates renal injury associated with ischemia and may prevent injury following renal transplantation.[75,76] However, a recent small clinical trial found no benefit of IGF-1 therapy for delayed graft function in postcadaveric renal transplant in humans.[77]

IGF-1 has been given to a small group of patients in a single trial for prophylaxis of ARF following aortic aneurysm repair.[78] IGF-1 was started postoperatively in a randomized placebo-controlled fashion; it was well tolerated, and produced a modest increase in the creatinine clearance in the treated group compared to the placebo group, possibly by vasodilation rather than a 'trophic' effect. However, no patients developed ARF that necessitated dialysis. Hence, the role, if any, for IGF-1 in the prevention of ARF remains unknown.

Based on the positive effects of IGF-1 in animal models of ATN, a randomized placebo-controlled trial was conducted in 72 critically ill patients with established ARF.[14] The results showed there was no difference in the two groups in post-treatment GFR, need for dialysis, or mortality, although it should be noted that GFR at randomization was only 6.4–8.7 ml/min, and ATN was possibly too established for a successful intervention in this study population. In anuric patients, IGF-1 administration was associated with a slower rate of improvement in urine output and GFR. So, despite the ample evidence that IGF-1 accelerates renal recovery in animal models of ARF, there is no support for its use in humans.

Thyroxine

The administration of thyroid hormone following the initiation of ATN in a variety of ischemic and nephrotoxic animal models was found to be effective in promoting recovery of renal function.[79–82] Based on these results, thyroxine was administered to 59 patients with ARF in a randomized placebo-controlled trial.[83] Patients were well matched in baseline characteristics. Administration of thyroxine had no effect on any renal parameter. However, the trial was terminated early because of a significantly higher mortality rate in the patients who received thyroxine.

Intensive insulin therapy

Hyperglycemia associated with insulin resistance is common in critically ill patients, independent of a history of diabetes mellitus.[84] Studies involving nondiabetic patients have found that the plasma glucose level on admission is an independent predictor of prognosis after myocardial infarction or of the need for coronary artery bypass grafting.[85] Furthermore, the in-vitro responsiveness of leukocytes stimulated by inflammatory mediators is inversely correlated with glycemic control.[86] Based on these findings, a randomized controlled trial was conducted involving 1500 ICU patients who received either intensive or conventional glycemic control.[87] All patients were receiving mechanical ventilation, the majority postoperatively. The study was terminated early because the mortality rate in the intensive treatment group was significantly lower than in the conventional treatment arm. Moreover, the incidence of severe renal insufficiency (peak serum creatinine >2.5 mg/dl; 11.2% conventional, 7.7% intensive, $p = 0.04$) and need for renal replacement therapy (8.2% conventional, 4.8% intensive, $p = 0.007$) were significantly lower in the intensive glycemic control group. Whether these results can be readily extrapolated to patients in a nonsurgical ICU or to those with other types of critical illness is currently unknown. Similar trials in other groups of patients will be necessary to confirm the observed benefits.

Anti-TNF-α therapy

Tumor necrosis factor-α (TNF-α) is an inflammatory cytokine that plays a pivotal role in the host response to infection. In addition to systemic effects, TNF-α may have specific renal effects. In-vivo TNF-α infusion in animals or perfusion of the isolated rat kidney with TNF-α decreased GFR.[88] TNF-α caused leukocyte and fibrin accumulation in glomerular capillary lumens and induced apoptosis in glomerular endothelial cells.[89] A large number of studies in diverse animal models have shown that anti-TNF antibodies confer protection against the morbidity and mortality from both Gram-positive and Gram-negative sepsis, including the development of ARF.[90,91] Emerging animal data suggest that anti-TNF therapies may have the potential to prevent septic ARF, despite the failure of such therapies to improve mortality in sepsis syndrome. For example, Cunningham and colleagues found that renal susceptibility to renal injury in endotoxemic mice with or without TNF receptor knockouts was associated with TNF receptor expression in the kidneys rather than the hosts, as determined by performing renal transplants between knockouts and wild-type mice.[92] On the other hand, they recently found that *systemic* expression of Toll-like receptor-4 is also required for development of endotoxemic ARF.[93] Limited clinical data similarly suggest that TNF receptor expression may play a role in the susceptibility to ARF in patients with sepsis.[94]

Several large trials with neutralizing monoclonal anti-TNF-α antibodies or soluble TNF receptor fusion proteins have failed to consistently show significant survival benefits or a reduced incidence of ARF in patients with sepsis.[95–98] This apparent lack of efficacy may be related to the heterogeneity of the patient population. Age, immune status, and genetic predisposition may all alter the inflammatory reaction in critical illness and lead to different responses to anticytokine therapies. Therefore, despite the apparent success of anti-TNF therapies in animal models in decreasing both mortality and renal failure, the beneficial effects of these strategies in humans are marginal at best.

Inhibitors of coagulation

Disseminated intravascular coagulation is common in ICU patients and is associated with an adverse prognosis. It is characterized by a generalized activation of the coagulation cascade, resulting in the intravascular formation of fibrin clots and endothelial damage. Impaired tissue blood supply contributes to organ dysfunction, including ARF. Several agents that block coagulation at different levels have been evaluated as adjunctive therapy in sepsis.

Protein C is activated by the thrombin–thrombomodulin complex on endothelial cells and inhibits thrombin generation. Besides its effects on coagulation, activated protein C has direct anti-inflammatory properties, including impairment of leukocyte adhesion to the endothelium and inhibition of the production of inflammatory cytokines. In a randomized, multicenter trial conducted in 1690 patients with severe sepsis, recombinant human activated protein C significantly reduced mortality.[99] It was particularly effective in the most seriously ill patients, as assessed by the APACHE II score, the number of failing organs, and the presence of shock; effects on the incidence or course of ARF were not described in study publications.

Tissue factor forms a complex with factor VIIa and initiates thrombin generation. Tissue factor is inhibited by a natural anticoagulant, tissue factor pathway inhibitor (TFPI). A phase II trial comparing placebo and recombinant TFPI in 210 patients with severe sepsis showed a trend toward mortal-

ity reduction in the recombinant TFPI-treated group.[100] However, a recently completed pivotal phase III trial of TFPI in 1700 patients with sepsis or severe sepsis failed to show a survival benefit; ARF incidence in the groups was not reported.[101]

Antithrombin III blocks several proteases involved in coagulation and plasma levels are usually markedly reduced in patients with sepsis. In a double-blind, placebo-controlled multicenter trial of 2300 patients with severe sepsis and septic shock, high-dose antithrombin III had no effect on 28-day mortality and was associated with an increased risk of hemorrhage when co-administered with heparin.[102]

A complex interaction between the pro-inflammatory, coagulation, and fibrinolytic networks plays a pivotal role in organ damage in sepsis. Although several strategies to inhibit coagulation have been evaluated in sepsis, only the administration of activated protein C has proved successful, and its efficacy may depend on its combined effects on coagulation, fibrinolysis, and inflammation. Activated protein C is currently approved for the treatment of severe sepsis, although current trials are assessing its effectiveness in less-ill patients. Specific renoprotective effects have not been demonstrated in humans, but emerging data suggest that activated protein C may be broadly protective against ischemia–reperfusion injury in a variety of settings.[103]

Nitric oxide synthase inhibition

Nitric oxide (NO) is the metabolic product of L-arginine and is produced by three major NO synthase (NOS) isoforms: endothelial NOS (eNOS), neuronal NOS (nNOS), and inducible NOS (iNOS). Within the kidney, eNOS is constitutively expressed in endothelial cells and produces vascular relaxation and inhibition of leukocyte adhesion and platelet aggregation. Excessive generation of NO by iNOS has been implicated as an important mediator of the hemodynamic alterations in sepsis, particularly the vascular hyporesponsiveness and vasodilation.[104]

Animal studies using nonspecific inhibitors of NOS have yielded conflicting results, although use of specific iNOS inhibitors has been more encouraging. The ubiquitous nature and the pleiotropic effects of the NO system, as well as its complex alterations in sepsis and ARF, probably explain why NOS inhibition fails to show reproducible beneficial effects. NO release by the endothelial cells of the renal microcirculation is essential to counterbalance the vasoconstrictor influences and maintain RBF, to inhibit infiltration of leukocytes, and to prevent thrombosis. Several animal studies have shown that whereas nonselective NOS inhibition worsens septic ARF while raising blood pressure, iNOS-selective agents improve both systemic hemodynamics and renal function.[105]

The results of a phase II and a pivotal phase III trial of the nonspecific NO inhibitor L-NMMA were recently reported.[106,107] In the phase II trial of 315 patients with severe sepsis, compared to placebo, NO inhibition led to increased reversibility of shock.[106] However, in the phase III trial involving over 800 patients, the trial was stopped prematurely when interim analysis demonstrated increased mortality in the L-NMMA-treated group.[107] This discordant result may be due to differences in patient enrollment and hemodynamic management protocols, and the nonspecific nature of NOS inhibition. Future strategies that inhibit iNOS but amplify eNOS may prove beneficial.

Endothelin antagonism

Endothelin-1 (ET-1) is a peptide with potent vasoconstrictor effects on the renal microcirculation, thereby reducing RBF and GFR. Experimental studies with ET-receptor antagonists in animal models of ARF demonstrated improved renal function.[108] However, no studies with ET receptor antagonists have been performed in patients with sepsis. A nonselective ET antagonist increased the risk of contrast nephropathy in patients with chronic renal failure undergoing coronary angiography,[109] perhaps because ET_B receptors cause vasodilation and ET_A receptors cause vasoconstriction. This paradoxical finding may make it difficult to perform studies of ET antagonism in patients with ARF and sepsis, although results may be better with an ET_A receptor-selective agent.

Inhibitors of arachidonic acid metabolism

Metabolism of arachidonic acid by cyclooxygenase results in the generation of prostaglandins and thromboxanes, whereas lipoxygenase yields leukotrienes. Both prostaglandin E_2 and prostacyclin cause renal vasodilatation and natriuresis, whereas thromboxane A_2, leukotrienes, and prostaglandins F_2 and H_2 are potent renal vaso-

constrictors. Endotoxin and various inflammatory cytokines stimulate the synthesis of thromboxane A_2 and leukotrienes in the kidney and in inflammatory cells.[110]

In animal models of sepsis, cyclooxygenase inhibition with indomethacin, selective thromboxane inhibition, and leukotriene antagonism all had beneficial effects on renal function.[110–112] However, in 455 patients with sepsis, cyclooxygenase inhibition with intravenous ibuprofen reduced the synthesis of thromboxane and prostacyclin, but it had no effect on the development of shock or renal failure and did not improve survival.[113] In the absence of clinical studies with selective thromboxane or leukotriene inhibitors, no meaningful conclusions on their potential benefit can be drawn.

Inhibition of leukocyte adhesion

The recruitment of circulating leukocytes into a tissue is directed by specific adhesive interactions between the leukocyte and the vascular endothelium. Selectins mediate the initial contact between the leukocyte and the endothelium, and adherence and migration are mediated by interactions between integrins on the leukocyte and surface receptors on the endothelium such as intercellular adhesion molecule-1 (ICAM-1). Studies suggest that during sepsis and ischemia leukocytes infiltrate the kidneys, resulting in renal dysfunction, and provide a rationale for the inhibition of leukocyte recruitment in these settings.[114,115]

Treatment of experimental animals with anti-ICAM-1 antibodies or with antisense oligonucleotides for ICAM-1 prevents ischemic ATN and ameliorates the functional and histologic injury associated with experimental ischemic or septic ARF.[116,117] Several mechanisms may be operative in leukocyte-mediated renal injury. Leukocytes release reactive oxygen species and enzymes that may directly injure cells. The production of cytokines attracts additional inflammatory cells and up-regulates adhesion molecules, creating a cycle of injury. Release of vasoconstrictor arachidonic acid metabolites, as well as physical congestion of medullary capillaries, contributes to persistent hypoxia. However, no results from human trials with antibodies to leukocyte adhesion molecules are available. Inhibition of leukocyte recruitment is a potential promising approach in the treatment of septic ARF, but data in humans are required before relevant conclusions can be drawn.

SPECIFIC CLINICAL SCENARIOS

Radiocontrast agents

An acute rise in serum creatinine levels following administration of radiocontrast material is defined as contrast nephropathy. Clinical trials assessing the effectiveness of various prevention strategies have utilized different absolute changes in creatinine to define ARF, making comparisons between studies difficult and obscuring the actual benefit achieved. Preventing increases in serum creatinine values as small as 25% have been used to define successful intervention instead of relying on endpoints such as hospital length of stay, need for dialysis, or mortality rates. However, a retrospective review of 16 000 patients who received intravenous radiocontrast showed that patients with a 50% or more increase in serum creatinine had a 6-fold higher mortality rate compared to those who did not.[118] Hence, using modest changes in serum creatinine as a surrogate for more serious complications may be a reasonable approach. As shown in Box 5.2, numerous risk factors are known for the development of RCN, including chronic kidney disease (especially diabetic nephropathy), volume depletion, uncompensated CHF, and high contrast volume.

The pathogenesis of ARF from radiocontrast is complex and incompletely understood.[119–121] After intravenous injection, a brief period of renal vasodilation is followed by intensive vasoconstriction, in part mediated by endothelin and adenosine. Medullary blood flow is more profoundly affected than is cortical blood flow. Hence, concomitant administration of drugs that affect RBF particularly NSAIDs, may act synergistically with radiocontrast to produce ARF. This vasoactive mechanism probably explains the increased risk of contrast nephropathy observed in patients with CHF, volume depletion, and nephrotic syndrome, as well as the therapeutic benefit of saline loading. Direct tubular toxicity also contributes to ARF from radiocontrast. Proximal tubular cells exposed to contrast material demonstrate altered cellular metabolism and intracellular enzyme release, probably mediated by oxygen free radicals and reactive oxygen species.

Prevention strategies

Hydration. Intravenous administration of 0.45% saline has long been the standard of care therapy to reduce the incidence of contrast nephropathy in

---

Box 5.2   Risk factors for the development of radiocontrast nephropathy

Chronic renal insufficiency (particularly in diabetics)
Volume depletion
High contrast dose
Myeloma kidney
Nephrotic syndrome
Older age
Congestive heart failure
Nephrotic syndrome

---

high-risk patients undergoing coronary arteriography, although it has never been studied in a placebo-controlled trial. In a study of 78 patients with underlying renal dysfunction (mean baseline creatinine of 2.1 mg/dl), randomization to 0.45% saline was superior to 0.45% saline plus either mannitol or furosemide in preventing a 0.5 mg/dl increase in serum creatinine levels.[28] A variety of renal vasodilators (dopamine, fenoldopam, ANP) have proven ineffective in addition to saline. A more recent trial of comparable patients demonstrated that 0.9% saline was more beneficial than 0.45% saline in preventing contrast nephropathy.[35] Most recently, administration of an equimolar sodium bicarbonate solution was superior to normal saline for RCN prophylaxis, infused as 3 mEq/L/h for 1 hour precontrast, then 1 ml/kg/h for 6 hours.[36] It is interesting to note that experimental data from animals support the concept that urinary alkalinization ameliorates renal ischemia–reperfusion injury, but the mechanism is unexplained.

NAC. NAC is a free radical scavenger and, by generating nitric oxide, a renal vasodilator. By comparing changes in mean creatinine values for treatment groups or absolute changes in creatinine levels, several studies have demonstrated the effectiveness of Mucomyst (NAC) in preventing contrast nephropathy.[39,40] All studies to date have relied on these changes as surrogates for more meaningful endpoints such as need for dialysis and mortality rates. A recent meta-analysis of 8 randomized controlled trials involving 855 patients reported that the use of Mucomyst reduced the risk of radiocontrast by 59%.[41] However, emerging data suggest that NAC causes a decrement in serum creatinine (but not cystatin C) by a GFR-independent mechanism,[42] perhaps by inhibiting creatinine phosphokinase function.[43] Nevertheless, given the available data, oral administration of Mucomyst to patients at high risk of developing contrast nephropathy appears warranted.

Fenoldopam mesylate. Limited trials suggested that administration of fenoldopam mesylate reduced the occurrence of ARF from radiocontrast agents.[52,53] However, a large randomized placebo-controlled trial (the CONTRAST Trial) was published that refutes the evidence accumulated in the previous reports. In 315 patients at risk for contrast nephropathy undergoing coronary arteriography who were given a standardized hydration regimen, randomization to low-dose fenoldopam had no effect on urine output, change in serum creatinine levels up to 96 hours, or the need for dialysis.[54] This study is strong evidence against the indiscriminate administration of fenoldopam mesylate for prevention of contrast nephropathy.

Dialysis. Radiocontrast is a small molecule easily removed from the circulation by dialysis: therefore, there remains an interest in performing dialysis in high-risk individuals who receive radiocontrast to prevent the development of ARF. In two studies of postcontrast hemodialysis, the subsequent need for dialysis for ARF was unchanged or increased by prophylactic hemodialysis.[122,123]

A more recent randomized trial of hemofiltration started in high-risk patients before administration of radiocontrast demonstrated a benefit of therapy.[124] In this study, 114 consecutive patients with serum creatinine levels >2 mg/dl undergoing coronary interventions were randomly assigned to either hemofiltration in an ICU or isotonic saline hydration at a rate of 1 ml/kg/h in a step-down unit. Hemofiltration or hydration was initiated 4–8 hours before coronary intervention and continued for 18–24 hours after the procedure was completed. A 25% or more increase in baseline serum creatinine level, need for temporary dialysis, in-hospital mortality rate, and 1-year mortality rate were all significantly lower in the hemofiltration group compared to the hydration group. However, numerous concerns surround this study. Although arguments continue about the superiority of hemofiltration compared to hemodialysis in treating critically ill patients with ARF because of

better middle molecule removal with hemofiltration, there is no plausible explanation for its positive effects in removing a low-molecular-weight substance such as radiocontrast. Many of the control patients subsequently required dialysis for pulmonary edema, probably as a result of the hydration regimen used in these cardiac patients. Although such patients represent a therapeutic challenge, provocation of pulmonary edema with hydration does not prove the superiority of hemofiltration. It is also difficult to interpret the incidence of contrast nephropathy when one group has a fall in serum creatinine as a direct result of the intervention. It is interesting to speculate that bicarbonate administration in the hemofiltration group may have been another benefit of this therapy in RCN prophylaxis, in view of the subsequent data showing a protective effect of sodium bicarbonate.[36] It is also challenging to explain how limited hemofiltration would decrease the rate of acute myocardial infarction, ischemic stroke, and multiple organ failure, the most common causes of death in the hydration group. More to the point, treatment details of the placebo group were inadequately described. From the available data, it is unclear if the placebo group did worse because of the lack of hemofiltration or because ideal medical management was not provided. Given the cost and invasiveness of hemofiltration, further data will be required before it can be recommended as a preventive measure in contrast nephropathy.

In summary, volume expansion with saline or perhaps sodium bicarbonate remains the only proven method for RCN prophylaxis. Avoidance of iodinated radiocontrast agents in high-risk patients is preferred where possible, perhaps by using alternate imaging methods such as magnetic resonance angiography with gadolinium. When radiocontrast is required, the least nephrotoxic agent available is preferred. Currently, the iso-osmolar, dimeric, nonionic contrast medium, iodixanol is thought to be the least nephrotoxic agent available. In a study of 129 diabetics with chronic renal insufficiency, iodixanol caused significantly less RCN than the low-osmolar, nonionic, monomeric contrast medium, iohexol.[125] Although many positive studies suggest benefit, the value of NAC for RCN prevention is now uncertain. Finally, although a single positive study suggesting the use of prophylactic hemofiltration has added to the growing list of potentially effective preventive strategies, we do not regard this as a proven approach.

Aminoglycosides

Aminoglycosides cause ATN in approximately 10% of patients who are treated with them for more than 2–3 days. The serum creatinine typically rises 7–10 days after the drug is initiated. Aminoglycosides concentrate in the proximal tubular cells, causing cellular damage. Risk factors for aminoglycoside-induced ARF are advanced age, chronic kidney disease, volume depletion, liver disease, and prolonged use of the drug.

Aminoglycosides have concentration-dependent bactericidal activity as well as a 'post-antibiotic' effect on bacterial growth.[126] Therefore, single-daily dosing is as effective as multiple daily dosing in treating infections by Gram-negative bacteria. The rate of renal cortical uptake of aminoglycosides is saturable, so accumulation of drug is less when given in one large dose rather than in divided doses.[127] Therefore, single daily dosing of aminoglycosides should lower the incidence of nephrotoxicity. In a randomized controlled trial of 123 patients, single daily dosing of gentamicin was as effective in treating infection as multiple dosing, and significantly decreased the incidence of ARF. Two meta-analyses also support this conclusion.[15,128]

Amphotericin B

Amphotericin B and its liposomal derivatives are a common cause of ATN in the ICU, particularly in patients who have undergone bone marrow transplant. Eighty percent of patients who receive amphotericin B will develop some degree of renal impairment. The initial nephrotoxic injury from amphotericin B results from renal vasoconstriction of the preglomerular arterioles and predisposes the patient to an ischemic insult.[129,130] Direct tubular toxicity follows. The newer liposomal forms of amphotericin B lack the solubilizing agent deoxycholate that contributes to tubular toxicity. Although such agents have been shown to cause less nephrotoxicity, renal failure still develops in a significant proportion of patients.[131]

Effective strategies to prevent the nephrotoxicity of amphotericin B are not clearly defined due to the lack of rigorous clinical trials and the inherent complexities of patients who require amphotericin B. Several retrospective or uncontrolled prospective trials suggest that salt-loading reduces the risk of nephrotoxicity.[27,132] A small, randomized placebo-controlled trial of 20 patients confirmed

this finding.[133] Animal studies also suggest that administration of calcium channel blockers or aminophylline are protective, although no human trials have been reported.[134,135]

Cisplatin

Nephrotoxicity is the most common dose-limiting side effect of cisplatin administration. The primary site for clearance of cisplatin is the kidney. Cisplatin asserts its toxicity on the tubules, resulting in a tubular wasting syndrome that is often severe. The proximal tubule is most often affected but the distal nephron is also vulnerable. The direct tubular toxicity associated with cisplatin is exacerbated in a low-chloride environment. In the intracellular compartment, chloride molecules are replaced with water molecules in the *cis* position of cisplatin, forming hydroxyl radicals that injure the neutrophilic binding sites on DNA.[136,137] The decline in GFR associated with cisplatin toxicity usually occurs 7–14 days after the exposure. Doses of cisplatin >50 mg/m^2 are sufficient to cause renal insufficiency. The renal injury is typically reversible but repeated doses of cisplatin in excess of 100 mg/m^2 may cause irreversible renal damage.

Hydration and avoidance of concomitant nephrotoxins is the most effective way to prevent cisplatin-induced nephrotoxicity. Numerous trials proposing various hydration regimens have been reported, but it appears that 3 L of normal saline over 8–10 hours before and after cisplatin is sufficient to avoid most toxicity associated with conventional doses.[138,139] When cisplatin is given in very high doses (>100 mg/m^2), administration in 3% saline is also protective.[140] Amifostine has also been shown to reduce cisplatin nephrotoxicity.[141]

Calcineurin inhibitors

The calcineurin-inhibitors CSA and tacrolimus are widely used as immunosuppressants in solid organ and bone marrow transplantation. CSA and tacrolimus cause both ARF and chronic renal failure. The nephrotoxicity seen in the critically ill patient is the result of direct afferent arteriolar vasoconstriction, leading to a decrease in the glomerular filtration pressure and GFR. The vascular effect associated with CSA and tacrolimus is reversible with discontinuation of the drug. A dose reduction is sometimes enough to reverse the prerenal effect. Calcium channel blockers (CCBs) decrease ischemic damage and reverse CSA-induced renal vasoconstriction in animal models.[142] However, small clinical trials in humans have had conflicting results.[143,144] It has been suggested that the positive response to CCBs may be due to their ability to increase plasma levels of CSA, thereby decreasing acute rejection, as well as directly modifying T-cell function.[145]

Hemolytic uremic syndrome (HUS) is a rare complication of CSA and tacrolimus therapy. The mechanism of CSA- or tacrolimus-induced HUS is direct damage to the vascular endothelium in a dose-dependent fashion. With discontinuation of the drug, patients may have partial recovery.[146] The utility of therapeutic plasma exchange in the treatment of HUS induced by calcineurin inhibitors has not been well studied.

Myoglobin

The principal causes of pigment nephropathy are (1) rhabdomyolysis and (2) hemoglobinuria due to hemolysis. The majority of rhabdomyolysis cases are subclinical, with mild elevations in the creatine kinase, lactic dehydrogenase, or aspartate amino-transferase enzyme levels. In severe cases, ARF may ensue from myoglobinuria. Commonly encountered causes of rhabdomyolysis are listed in Box 5.3. Rhabdomyolysis has been thought to cause ATN through three mechanisms: renal vaso-constriction, intratubular cast formation, and heme-mediated proximal tubular injury. It is also known that oxidant stress is increased with the release of heme proteins. Free heme proteins are suspected of reducing the formation of nitric oxide and increasing endothelin levels, which results in vasoconstriction and the decline in GFR. Intratubular obstruction occurs with the inter-action of myoglobin and Tamm–Horsfall protein in an aciduric environment.[147]

To prevent and treat the ARF of rhabdomyolysis, aggressive hydration is effective. Alkalinization of the urine has also been advocated to increase the solubility of the heme proteins in the urine, with the goal of achieving a urine pH >6.5. Alkaliniza-tion may also reduce the production of reactive oxygen species, thus reducing the oxidant stress.[148] Caution must be exercised when administering bicarbonate, since the resulting alkalemia can worsen the hypocalcemia often present in patients with severe rhabdomyolysis and precipitate gener-alized seizures. Some of bicarbonate's salutary

---

Box 5.3 Causes of rhabdomyolysis

Direct injury
Crush injuries
Compression
Seizures
High-voltage electrical injury

Vascular insufficiency
Compartment syndrome
Shock

Metabolic disorders
Hypophosphatemia
Hypokalemia
Diabetic ketoacidosis
Hypothyroidism

Toxic injury
Alcohol
Amfetamines
Cocaine
Snake venom

Infections
Toxic shock syndrome
Influenza
Malaria
HIV infection

Myopathies
McArdle's disease
Phosphofructokinase (PFK) deficiency
Carnitine palmityl-transferase deficiency
Dermatomyositis
Polymyositis

---

effect stem from its serving as a nonreabsorbed solute which promotes an osmotic diuresis.[149] It is not known whether or not alkalinization of the urine is beneficial once a brisk diuresis is established with saline or diuretics.

Mannitol has also been advocated for the treat-ment of pigment nephropathy based on experi-mental models of myohemoglobinuric ARF. The protective effect has been attributed to its diuretic, renal vasodilatory, and hydroxyl scavenging prop-erties.[150,151] However, in a glycerol model of myo-globinuric ARF, mannitol's protective effect could be completely ascribed to a solute diuresis and increased heme excretion.[152] Also, although mannitol is a potent renal vasodilator, it may actually worsen cellular energetics during the induction of ARF. If administered immediately after renal ischemia, renal cortical ATP levels may abruptly decline by increasing the metabolic cost of sodium reabsorption by the loop of Henle.[151–153] Therefore, intravenous fluids or perhaps furosemide may be the preferable diuretic. If mannitol is used, it is essential to monitor serum osmolality to avoid a hyperosmolar state.

Because of its size, myoglobin removal by peritoneal dialysis or hemodialysis is poor, although a study by Amyot and colleagues suggests its clearance may be enhanced by continuous hemofiltration.[154] In addition, myoglobin levels fall exponentially with cessation of muscular release due to hepatic and splenic uptake.[155] It is also unclear whether or not myoglobin is a major contributor to the pathogenesis of rhabdomyolysis-induced ARF. Currently, there is no compelling evidence for the use of extracorporeal therapies in the treatment of myoglobinuric ARF.

Methotrexate

Methotrexate (MTX)-induced ARF is caused by the precipitation of the drug and its metabolites in the tubular lumen and is also a tubular cytotoxin.[137] High doses of MTX (>1 g/m^2) increase the risk of ARF. Once ARF develops, the excretion of MTX is reduced and the systemic toxicity of MTX is increased. Hydration and high urine output are essential to preventing MTX renal toxicity. Isotonic saline infusion and furosemide may be necessary to keep the urine output >100 ml/h. Alkalinization of the urine to a pH >6.5 is also recommended, to decrease tubular precipitation and increase renal MTX clearance. Once ARF has developed, it may be necessary to remove the drug with dialysis. Hemodialysis using high blood flow rates with a high-flux dialyzer is an effective method of removing methotrexate.[156] High-dose leucovorin therapy can reduce the systemic toxicity associated with MTX and ARF, and is routinely used when plasma levels are excessive 48 hours post-dose.[157,158]

Tumor lysis syndrome

Tumor lysis syndrome is often a dramatic presentation of ARF in patients with malignancy. It is characterized by the development of hyperphosphatemia, hypocalcemia, hyperuricemia, and hyperkalemia. Tumor lysis syndrome can occur spontaneously during the rapid growth phase of malignancies such as bulky lymphoblastomas and Burkitt's and non-Burkitt's lymphomas that have extremely rapid cell turnover rates.[159] More commonly, it is seen when cytotoxic chemotherapy induces lysis of malignant cells in patients with large tumor burdens. Tumor lysis syndrome has developed in patients with non-Hodgkin's lymphoma, acute lymphoblastic leukemia, chronic myelogenous leukemia in blast crises, small cell lung cancer, and metastatic breast cancer.[160] In most patients the ARF is reversible after aggressive supportive therapy including dialysis.

The pathophysiology of ARF associated with tumor lysis syndrome is related to two main factors: (1) pre-existing volume depletion prior to the onset of renal failure and (2) the precipitation of uric acid and calcium phosphate complexes in the renal tubules and tissue.[161] Patients may be volume-depleted from anorexia or nausea and vomiting associated with the malignancy, or from increased insensible losses from fever or tachypnea. Therefore, it is important to establish brisk flow of hypotonic urine to prevent or ameliorate ARF associated with tumor lysis syndrome.

Hyperuricemia is either present before treatment with chemotherapy or develops after therapy despite prophylaxis with allopurinol.[162] Uric acid is nearly completely ionized at physiologic pH, but becomes progressively insoluble in the acidic environment of the renal tubules. Precipitation of uric acid causes intratubular obstruction, leading to increased renal vascular resistance and decreased GFR.[163] Moreover, a granulomatous reaction to intraluminal uric acid crystals and necrosis of tubular epithelium can be found on biopsy specimens.

Hyperphosphatemia and hypocalcemia also occur in tumor lysis syndrome. In patients who do not develop hyperuricemia in tumor lysis syndrome, ARF has been attributed to metastatic intrarenal calcification or acute nephrocalcinosis.[164] Tumor lysis with release of inorganic phosphate causes acute hypocalcemia and metastatic calcification, resulting in ARF.

Therefore, ARF associated with tumor lysis syndrome is the result of the combination of volume depletion in the face of urinary precipitation of uric acid in the renal tubules and parenchyma, and acute nephrocalcinosis from severe hyperphosphatemia. Since patients at risk for tumor lysis often have intra-abdominal lymphoma, urinary tract obstruction can be a contributing factor in the development of ARF. Given the aforementioned pathogenetic factors for ARF, patients who are undergoing treatment with malignancies who are likely to experience rapid cell lysis should receive vigorous intravenous hydration to maintain good urinary flow and urinary dilution. In addition, because uric acid is very soluble at physiologic acid urine pH, sodium bicarbonate should be added to the intravenous fluid to achieve a urinary pH >6.5. Since metabolic alkalosis can aggravate hypocalcemia, caution should be exercised when using alkali in patients with low serum calcium levels. It is advisable to stop the infusion if the serum bicarbonate level is >30 mEq/L. Furthermore, it is conceivable that the use of urinary alkalinization to prevent uric acid nephropathy might actually precipitate or worsen calcium phosphate-induced ARF. Allopurinol is administered to inhibit uric acid formation. Through its metabolite oxypurinol, allopurinol inhibits xanthine oxidase and thereby blocks the conversion of hypoxanthine and xanthine to uric acid. During massive tumor lysis, uric acid excretion can still increase despite the administration of allopurinol, so that intravenous hydration is still necessary to prevent ARF. Since allopurinol and its metabolites are excreted in the urine, the dose should be reduced in the face of impaired renal function. Uricase has been recently approved for use in the United States. It converts uric acid to water-soluble allantoin, thereby decreasing serum uric acid levels and urinary uric acid excretion.[165] The use of uricase may obviate the need for urinary alkalinization, but good urine flow with hydration should be maintained given the probability of pre-existing volume depletion.

Dialysis for ARF associated with tumor lysis syndrome may be required for the traditional indications of fluid overload, hyperkalemia, hyperphosphatemia, or hyperuricemia unresponsive to medical management. There is some interest in using dialysis in patients at high risk of tumor lysis syndrome to prevent the development of renal failure. In a small trial involving five children, continuous hemofiltration was started prior to administration of chemotherapy and appeared to prevent renal failure in 80% of the patients.[166] However, given that continuous dialysis is complicated, expensive, and not without risk, its routine use as prophylaxis cannot be recommended.

Liver failure, bacterial peritonitis, and hepatorenal syndrome

Spontaneous bacterial peritonitis (SBP) is a common and severe disorder in patients with liver cirrhosis and ascites. In one-third of patients, renal impairment develops despite treatment of the infection with non-nephrotoxic antibiotics. Development of renal failure is the best predictor of hospital mortality in these patients and is thought to result from a decrease in the effective arterial blood volume caused by sepsis. In a randomized trial of 126 patients with SBP, administration of albumin plus antibiotics compared to antibiotics alone significantly decreased the incidence of renal impairment, in-hospital mortality, and 3-month mortality.[34] This study was not blinded, potentially introducing bias, and the quantity of albumin used was substantial, leading to significant cost. Also, there was no 'hydration' arm in the antibiotic-only group that would provide proof of the superiority of albumin over crystalloid solutions. However, these encouraging results will probably lead to further clinical investigations.

Hepatorenal syndrome (HRS) is a unique cause of renal vasoconstriction, with a decline in GFR in the face of normal renal histology that occurs in the setting of liver failure. The clinical picture associated with HRS is that of prerenal azotemia with oliguria and low FENa (urinary fractional excretion of sodium). In true HRS without confounding renal injuries, the renal failure will resolve with liver transplantation. The pathogenesis of HRS is incompletely understood. Systemic and splanchnic vascular resistance is decreased, leading to a decrease in the effective arterial blood volume and renal hypoperfusion. The compensatory hemodynamic response to systemic vasodilation includes an increase in the mediators of renal vasoconstriction, including increased renin–angiotensin–aldosterone activity, antidiuretic hormone (ADH) levels, sympathetic tone, and endothelin levels. The renal response is an increase in salt and water avidity, leading to worsening ascites and edema.[167,168] Liver transplant is the definitive therapy for HRS. However, patients who develop HRS prior to transplant have worse graft and patient survival.[169]

Newer pharmacologic therapy with vasopressin analogs (e.g. ornipressin and terlipressin), which are splanchnic vasoconstrictors, has shown some benefit.[170–172] Ornipressin and albumin was administered to a total of 16 patients with HRS for either 3 or 15 days (8 patients in each group). The 3-day regimen was associated with a normalization of the overactivity of renin–angiotensin and sympathetic nervous systems, ANP levels, and only a slight improvement in renal function. However, treatment for 15 days resulted in improved serum creatinine levels, renal plasma flow, and glomerular filtration rate. Similar results were seen in 9 patients who received intravenous terlipressin. However, a major complication associated with these medications is mesenteric ischemia. Oral midodrine (a selective α_1-adrenergic agonist) in combination with octreotide also showed benefit in renal function in a small series of patients.[173] Mucomyst given intravenously to 12 patients increased RBF without changing the hemodynamic derangements associated with HRS.[174] Several small studies have shown that transjugular intrahepatic portosystemic shunting (TIPS) has prolonged survival and improved renal function in patients with HRS.[175,176] Firm conclusions about efficacy of these therapies await the results of randomized controlled trials.

Renal transplantation

Acute renal failure remains a common complication of renal transplantation. It may occur at any time point in the life of the transplant, although it usually develops in the immediate postoperative period and is referred to as delayed graft function. The causes of delayed graft function are listed in Box 5.4, and include obstruction, volume depletion, and acute rejection, although the most common etiology remains ischemic ATN. Risk factors for ATN are advanced donor age, intraoperative or postoperative hypotension, prolonged warm or cold ischemia times, and initial high CSA dosage. Reperfusion injury as a result of direct endothelial trauma, oxygen free-radical generation, and neutrophil activation also contributes to the development of ATN.

Patients with delayed graft function have longer hospitalization rates and more complications, including a lower 5-year graft survival rate.[177] Therefore, prevention of ischemic ATN in the post-transplant setting may prolong renal survival. As in all patients at risk for the development of ischemic ATN, optimization of hemodynamic parameters in both recipient and donor is a key element and may require monitoring of central venous pressures; Carlier and colleagues showed that higher wedge pressures at the time of renal allograft revascularization were associated with

improved early graft function.[178] Some studies have suggested that intraoperative administration of mannitol decreases the incidence of ATN.[179] Decreasing warm and cold ischemia times should also decrease the occurrence of post-transplant delayed graft function. The use of the University of Wisconsin preservation solution during cold ischemia reduces the incidence of delayed graft function.[180] Renal vasodilators such as low-dose dopamine and fenoldopam, IGF-1, and ANP have not shown significant benefit in small clinical trials.[46,70] As previously discussed, although CCBs reverse CSA vasoconstriction and prevent ischemic injury in animal models, the benefit in clinical trials has been inconsistent. Current clinical trials aimed at lessening reperfusion injury by blocking adhesion molecule interactions are ongoing.[181,182]

Postoperative states

Many critically ill patients who undergo surgery will go on to develop ARF, and a large proportion of these will require renal replacement therapy.[183] In addition to the traditional risk factors for ARF present in any critically ill patient, the surgical patient may be exposed to the potentially harmful effects of cardiopulmonary bypass, hypothermic circulatory arrest, or aortic crossclamp.[184] The most common cause of ARF in the surgical setting is

---

Box 5.4 Causes of delayed graft function in renal transplant

Prerenal
Hypovolemia
Renal artery thrombosis

Renal
Ischemic ATN
Hyperacute rejection
Acute rejection
Acute calcineurin nephrotoxicity

Postrenal
Urinary tract obstruction
Lymphocele
Urinary leak
Ureteral necrosis

ischemic ATN that occurs in the face of critical illness and MODS. Often, there has been a preceding period of relative renal hypoperfusion from either true or effective volume depletion.

Risk assessment

In terms of risk assessment and characterization, there are no specific scoring systems that can predict accurately who will develop postoperative organ dysfunction.[185] The American Society of Anesthesiologists (ASA) scoring system is among the simplest and most reproducible general risk assessment tools.[186] It stratifies patients into high-, moderate-, or low-risk categories but does not specify the actual type of harm. Several studies have demonstrated that the presence of pre-existing renal disease, CHF, obstructive jaundice, diabetes mellitus, peripheral vascular disease, hypertension, and coronary artery disease are all risk factors for developing postoperative ARF.[187] This observation suggests that patient-related factors have a significant impact on the development of postoperative complications. In addition, overall risk can be thought of as having both genetic and environmental components. The environmental risk consists of the nature of the planned operation, its urgency, and the surgical skill of the personnel involved. The environmental risk further entails those unpredictable events such as catastrophic intraoperative hemorrhage and technical errors. Genetic risk is subtle and has only recently become recognized as important. The field of the genetics of complex-trait diseases is evolving, and the best tools for its analysis are still under debate. Currently, how genetic variability affects an individual's response to underlying illness, injury, treatment, and drug therapy is poorly defined. However, genetic variability probably has some effect on both the risk of developing a postoperative complication and on the response of the individual to its treatment.

Certain operations carry a higher risk for ARF because of the nature of the surgical procedure and the underlying medical condition of patients requiring the surgery. Patients undergoing surgery for either traumatic or thermal injuries are at high risk for ARF.[188] The ARF is usually multifactorial in nature, with ischemia, rhabdomyolysis, nephrotoxins, and sepsis all having a contributory role.

Cardiac surgery requiring cardiopulmonary bypass (CPB) may cause some degree of renal dysfunction in up to 50% of patients.[189,190] Cardiopulmonary bypass is a state of hypotension that triggers release of several renal vasoconstrictor agents, resulting in renal hypoperfusion. Although overt ARF may develop in less than 5% of patients with normal preoperative renal function, tubular enzymuria suggests that subclinical injury is much more common.[191] Preoperative left ventricular dysfunction and time on CPB increase the risk of ARF. The type of CPB (pulsatile or nonpulsatile) and bypass pressure do not appear to be significant factors in determining renal outcome.

Vascular surgery, particularly when cross-clamping the aorta is required, is associated with a higher incidence of postoperative ARF.[192] The best predictors of ARF are pre-existing renal insufficiency and hemodynamic instability during surgery.

Preoperative period

In general terms, the predisposition to a prerenal state can often be avoided by an overnight intravenous fluid infusion. Surgical patients are typically starved overnight, and administration of a bowel preparation routine can compound the volume depletion. Intravenous fluid administration is a simple means of preventing the development of a prerenal state from hypovolemia.

More specific therapies begun preoperatively to prevent postoperative ARF have not been proven effective. In part, because the incidence of postoperative ARF is low, large numbers of patients would need to be randomized in order to either demonstrate a positive effect, or to conclusively show such an effect does not exist. This problem has plagued ARF clinical research in general, and the surgical setting has been no exception. As previously detailed, various trials using low-dose dopamine, the diuretics furosemide and mannitol, growth factors, and ANP have failed to decrease the incidence of ARF. Small trials suggest that preoperative administration of fenoldopam mesylate and N-acetylcysteine may decrease the development of postoperative ARF,[193,194] but these require larger confirmatory effectiveness trials. However, to date, there are no large, randomized controlled clinical trials examining these agents in the operative setting.

Recently, studies have been published suggesting that for those patients with chronic renal impairment a period of elective renal replacement therapy may subsequently improve both renal and overall outcome. In a single study of 44 patients with chronic renal failure (mean serum creatinine level of 3.3 mg/dl) undergoing coronary artery bypass grafting (CABG) and CPB, randomization to prophylactic hemodialysis appeared to decrease mortality, hospital and ICU length of stay, and the incidence of postoperative ARF compared to standard care.[195] However, the study was small and details of medical therapy in the nondialysis arm (such as the use of ACE inhibitors, diuretics, and fluid balance) were not described. Furthermore, it is difficult to explain the benefits based on any sound physiologic principle. If frank fluid overload, which should have prompted therapeutic dialysis, was not present in these patients, then it is hard to explain how limited small solute clearance would decrease mortality or the incidence of postoperative ARF. In fact, there is good evidence that hemodialysis can prolong or perpetuate ARF by triggering ischemia or inflammation.[196,197] In an uncontrolled cohort study of patients on chronic hemodialysis, intensive dialysis prior to cardiothoracic surgery in 13 consecutive patients resulted in similar postoperative outcomes compared to patients with normal renal function.[198] Both of these studies probably demonstrate that in renal failure patients, aggressive management of fluid overload and electrolyte imbalances results in better postoperative outcomes. However, proof that dialysis is superior to medical management will depend on the results of large, randomized controlled clinical trials.

Intraoperative period
Most anesthetic agents cause dose-dependent venous and arterial vasodilatation, with an accompanying reduction in cardiac pre- and afterload. Hypotension may be exacerbated by neural impairment from spinal or epidural blockade. A mild reduction in blood pressure leads to less bleeding and is usually well tolerated, since anesthetic agents generally also reduce oxygen demand. Typically, crystalloid or colloid solutions are administered to expand the intravascular space in response to the mild drop in blood pressure that almost universally accompanies induction of anesthesia. A urine output of 1–2 ml/kg/h during surgery is considered evidence of adequate organ perfusion, although adequate urine output certainly does not preclude the presence of renal hypoperfusion and ischemia. Hemodynamic monitoring, including central venous pressure (CVP), cardiac index, systemic vascular resistance, and pulmonary artery occlusion pressure, is often used in critically ill patients. However, the ideal blood pressure, cardiac output, vascular tone, and intravascular volume for patients undergoing

major surgery are not known because of a lack of appropriate studies. No studies have proven that intensive hemodynamic monitoring improves outcome.[199,200] In fact, some studies actually suggest that the use of pulmonary artery catheters is associated with worse outcome.[201,202] For now, interventions that maximize the chance of good renal outcome include avoidance or treatment of hypoxemia, hypercarbia, hypotension, hyperglycemia, and anemia.

Postoperative period
Immediately after surgery, the emphasis on prevention of ARF shifts away from monitoring the minute-to-minute changes in hemodynamics to observation for bleeding, organ hypoperfusion, infection, and coagulation complications. Hypoxemia may arise from shunting through atelectatic areas of lung, or hypoventilation from narcotic analgesics or residual neuromuscular blockade. Impaired oxygen delivery can exacerbate any reduction in cardiac output, leading to decreased renal perfusion. Large fluid shifts may accompany major surgery and can manifest as severe anemia, electrolyte disturbances, acid–base abnormalities, or changes in cognition.

Later in the postoperative course, the greatest risk is posed by the development of severe sepsis syndrome, which can cause postoperative ARF from ischemic ATN. Sepsis induces vascular endothelial changes, organ and tissue ischemia, cellular apoptosis and necrosis, as well as coagulation abnormalities that exacerbate and accelerate the pathologic process.[203] To date, activated protein C has been the only agent administered to critically ill surgical patients that has significantly improved survival rates in the ICU.[99]

Abdominal compartment syndrome

Abdominal compartment syndrome (ACS) was first reported in 1876, in a paper describing the reduction in urine flow associated with elevated intra-abdominal pressure (IAP).[204] Acute increases in IAP are deleterious for both intra-abdominal and distant organ function, including the kidneys.[205] Acutely, the abdomen functions as a closed space; thus, any increase in the volume of its contents leads to a rise in compartmental pressure. Intra-abdominal hemodynamics are compromised when the IAP approaches and then exceeds 10 cmH$_2$O. ACS is present when the IAP reaches 20–25 cmH$_2$O, and unless decompressed, irreversible organ failure may result.[206] ACS is characterized by an acute rise in IAP, coupled with evidence of organ dysfunction, usually reduced urine output. The pathogenesis of this reduction in urine formation is complex and attributed to three major factors:

1. Compression of the great veins reduces venous return to the right heart, which manifests as relative hypovolemia and can become frank volume depletion if third spacing of fluid is extensive. Increased renal venous back pressure associated with high CVP may cause renal vein compression.
2. Direct pressure on the renal cortex can shunt blood away from the vulnerable corticomedullary junction by altering renal vascular resistance and induce an ischemic injury in this area.
3. Direct pressure on the ureters can lead to obstructive nephropathy, particularly if there is a predisposing condition such as extensive lymphadenopathy.

Regardless of the underlying cause, a reduction in urine output $\pm$ azotemia in the presence of a measured IAP over 15 cmH$_2$O is certainly cause for concern and should prompt intervention.

IAP can be measured in a number of ways, although the transvesical method is the most commonly used.[207] In this technique, 50–100 ml of sterile saline solution is instilled through the bladder catheter into the bladder and the drainage port then clamped distal to the sampling port. A conventional pressure monitoring line is then attached by hypodermic needle through the sampling port and the pressure measured directly, with the symphysis pubis taken as the zero reference point. This technique is straightforward, reliable, simple, and reproducible. An estimate of IAP can also be obtained by elevating the bladder catheter above the bed, since the pressure of urine in the bladder will then equilibrate with that in the tubing. This method represents a simple screening tool, and thus should be used in any patient who may be at risk of ACS.

The causes of an increased IAP are listed in Box 5.5. ACS should be managed with attention to preservation of underlying organ function, and is usually treated with urgent surgical decompression. Clearly, this is a highly complex situation and skilled surgical supervision is mandatory if the patient is ultimately to do well.

Multisystem trauma

Although the incidence of ARF following major trauma is generally low, it is associated with a high mortality rate.[208,209] Opinion has varied as to whether pre-existing medical conditions such as diabetes and hypertension are more important risk factors than the timeliness and type of resuscitation.[210]

Mechanical ventilation with high PEEP (positive end-expiratory pressure), hemoperitoneum, and rhabdomyolysis have been identified as the three conditions most strongly associated with ARF after major trauma.[211] Rhabdomyolysis may be caused by extensive skeletal muscle damage and worsened by subsequent infection, fever, drugs, and electrolyte abnormalities. The degree of elevation of serum creatine kinase is usually proportional to the extent of the muscle injury. Acute renal failure develops in rhabdomyolysis because of tubular obstruction, oxidant injury, and renal vasoconstriction, and thus preventive measures have been largely aimed at promoting tubular flow and restoring renal perfusion.[147] The single most important feature of ARF prevention is volume expansion. Alkalinization of the urine is usually recommended also, since this improves myoglobin washout, prevents lipid peroxidation, and minimizes renal vasoconstriction.[147] The use of mannitol is controversial. Although it has theoretic benefits such as reduced compartment pressure and cellular swelling, and mild antioxidant properties, it has not been shown to produce results superior to those of volume expansion alone.[212]

Box 5.5   Causes of increased intra-abdominal pressure

Peritoneal tissue edema (trauma, peritonitis)

Fluid overload in shock

Retroperitoneal hematoma

Surgical trauma

Reperfusion injury after bowel ischemia

Pancreatitis

Ileus or obstruction

Abdominal packing to control hemorrhage

Abdominal closure under tension

Severe ascites

SUMMARY

Acute renal failure as a result of ATN is a common development in critically ill medical and surgical patients that is associated with significant morbidity and mortality. Despite improvements in the understanding of the pathophysiologic mechanisms of ARF and the numerous agents effective in treating ARF in animal models, there are currently no effective treatments for ATN in human subjects. Therefore, prevention of ARF remains the best way to improve renal dysfunction-related outcome in the ICU. To date, most specific pharmacologic agents used to prevent ARF have been proven ineffective in clinical trials. Until further data are available, it seems that simple measures such as maintaining adequate renal perfusion, avoiding excessively aggressive diuresis and nephrotoxins, and monitoring levels of potentially nephrotoxic drugs are important goals in the care of the critically ill patient.

REFERENCES

1. Hou SH, Bushinsky DA, Wish JB, Cohen JJ, Harrington JT. Hospital–acquired renal insufficiency: a prospective study. Am J Med 1983;74:243–8.
2. Albright RC, Jr. Acute renal failure: a practical update. Mayo Clin Proc 2001;76:67–74.
3. Nash K, Hafeez A, Hou S. Hospital–acquired renal insufficiency. Am J Kidney Dis 2002;39:930–6.
4. Brivet FG, Kleinknecht DJ, Loirat P, Landais PJ. Acute renal failure in intensive care units—causes, outcome, and prognostic factors of hospital mortality; a prospective, multicenter study. French Study Group on Acute Renal Failure. Crit Care Med 1996;24:192–8.
5. Heyman SN, Lieberthal W, Rogiers P, Bonventre JV. Animal models of acute tubular necrosis. Curr Opin Crit Care 2002;8:526–34.
6. Rosen S, Heyman SN. Difficulties in understanding human 'acute tubular necrosis': limited data and flawed animal models. Kidney Int 2001;60:1220–4.
7. Annat G, Viale JP, Bui Xuan B, et al. Effect of PEEP ventilation on renal function, plasma renin, aldosterone, neurophysins and urinary ADH, and prostaglandins. Anesthesiology 1983;58:136–41.
8. Pannu N, Mehta RL. Mechanical ventilation and renal function: an area for concern? Am J Kidney Dis 2002;39:616–24.
9. Schetz M. Vasopressors and the kidney. Blood Purif 2002;20:243–51.
10. Heyman SN, Fuchs S, Brezis M. The role of medullary ischemia in acute renal failure. New Horiz 1995;3:597–607.
11. Kelly KJ, Molitoris BA. Acute renal failure in the new millennium: time to consider combination therapy. Semin Nephrol 2000;20:4–19.
12. Sutton TA, Fisher CJ, Molitoris BA. Microvascular endothelial injury and dysfunction during ischemic acute renal failure. Kidney Int 2002;62:1539–49.
13. Allgren RL, Marbury TC, Rahman SN, et al. Anaritide in acute tubular necrosis. Auriculin Anaritide Acute Renal Failure Study Group. N Engl J Med 1997;336:828–34.
14. Hirschberg R, Kopple J, Lipsett P, et al. Multicenter clinical trial of recombinant human insulin-like growth factor I in patients with acute renal failure. Kidney Int 1999;55:2423–32.
15. Hatala R, Dinh T, Cook DJ. Once-daily aminoglycoside dosing in immunocompetent adults: a meta-analysis. Ann Intern Med 1996;124:717–25.
16. Barrett BJ, Carlisle EJ. Metaanalysis of the relative nephrotoxicity of high- and low-osmolality iodinated contrast media. Radiology 1993;188:171–8.
17. Sorkine P, Nagar H, Weinbroum A, et al. Administration of amphotericin B in lipid emulsion decreases nephrotoxicity: results of a prospective, randomized, controlled study in critically ill patients. Crit Care Med 1996;24:1311–15.
18. Shusterman N, Strom BL, Murray TG, et al. Risk factors and outcome of hospital-acquired acute renal failure. Clinical epidemiologic study. Am J Med 1987;83:65–71.
19. de Mendonca A, Vincent JL, Suter PM, et al. Acute renal failure in the ICU: risk factors and outcome evaluated by the SOFA score. Intensive Care Med 2000;26:915–21.
20. Eriksen BO, Hoff KR, Solberg S. Prediction of acute renal failure after cardiac surgery: retrospective cross–validation of a clinical algorithm. Nephrol Dial Transplant 2003;18:77–81.
21. Douma CE, Redekop WK, van der Meulen JH, et al. Predicting mortality in intensive care patients with acute renal failure treated with dialysis. J Am Soc Nephrol 1997;8:111–17.
22. Halstenberg WK, Goormastic M, Paganini EP. Validity of four models for predicting outcome in critically ill acute renal failure patients. Clin Nephrol 1997;47:81–6.
23. Liano F, Gallego A, Pascual J, et al. Prognosis of acute tubular necrosis: an extended prospectively contrasted study. Nephron 1993;63:21–31.
24. Thurau K, Boylan JW. Acute renal success. The unexpected logic of oliguria in acute renal failure. Am J Med 1976;61:308–15.
25. Gattinoni L, Brazzi L, Pelosi P, et al. A trial of goal-oriented hemodynamic therapy in critically ill patients. SvO2 Collaborative Group. N Engl J Med 1995;333:1025–32.
26. Rivers E, Nguyen B, Havstad S, et al. Early goal-directed therapy in the treatment of severe sepsis and septic shock. N Engl J Med 2001;345:1368–77.
27. Stein RS, Albridge K, Lenox RK, Ray W, Flexner JM. Nephrotoxicity in leukemic patients receiving empirical amphotericin B and aminoglycosides. South Med J 1988;81:1095–9.
28. Solomon R, Werner C, Mann D, D'Elia J, Silva P. Effects of saline, mannitol, and furosemide to prevent acute decreases in renal function induced by radiocontrast agents. N Engl J Med 1994;331:1416–20.
29. Schierhout G, Roberts I. Fluid resuscitation with colloid or crystalloid solutions in critically ill patients: a systematic review of randomised trials. BMJ 1998;316:961–4.
30. Choi PT, Yip G, Quinonez LG, Cook DJ. Crystalloids vs. colloids in fluid resuscitation: a systematic review. Crit Care Med 1999;27:200–10.
31. Boldt J, Muller M, Mentges D, Papsdorf M, Hempelmann G. Volume therapy in the critically ill: is there a difference? Intensive Care Med 1998;24:28–36.
32. Schortgen F, Lacherade JC, Bruneel F, et al. Effects of hydroxyethylstarch and gelatin on renal function in severe sepsis: a multicentre randomised study. Lancet 2001;357:911–16.
33. Finfer S, Bellomo R, Boyce N, et al. A comparison of albumin and saline for fluid resuscitation in the intensive care unit. N Engl J Med 2004;350:2247–56.
34. Sort P, Navasa M, Arroyo V, et al. Effect of intravenous albumin on renal impairment and mortality in patients with cirrhosis and spontaneous bacterial peritonitis. N Engl J Med 1999;341:403–9.
35. Mueller C, Buerkle G, Buettner HJ, et al. Prevention of contrast media-associated nephropathy: randomized comparison of 2

hydration regimens in 1620 patients undergoing coronary angioplasty. Arch Intern Med 2002;162:329–36.

36. Merten GJ, Burgess WP, Gray LV, et al. Prevention of contrast-induced nephropathy with sodium bicarbonate: a randomized controlled trial. JAMA 2004;291:2328–34.

37. Shipley RE, Study RS. Changes in renal blood flow, extraction of inulin, gloerular filtration rate, tissue pressure, and urine flow with acute alterations in renal artery pressures. Am J Physiol 1951;167:676–88.

38. Bersten AD, Holt AW. Vasoactive drugs and the importance of renal perfusion pressure. New Horiz 1995;3:650–61.

39. Durham JD, Caputo C, Dokko J, et al. A randomized controlled trial of N-acetylcysteine to prevent contrast nephropathy in cardiac angiography. Kidney Int 2002;62:2202–7.

40. Kay J, Chow WH, Chan TM, et al. Acetylcysteine for prevention of acute deterioration of renal function following elective coronary angiography and intervention: a randomized controlled trial. JAMA 2003;289:553–8.

41. Alonso A, Lau J, Jaber BL, Weintraub A, Sarnak MJ. Prevention of radiocontrast nephropathy with N-acetylcysteine in patients with chronic kidney disease: a meta-analysis of randomized, controlled trials. Am J Kidney Dis 2004;43:1–9.

42. Hoffmann U, Fischereder M, Kruger B, Drobnik W, Kramer BK. The value of N-acetylcysteine in the prevention of radiocontrast agent–induced nephropathy seems questionable. J Am Soc Nephrol 2004;15:407–10.

43. Genet S, Kale RK, Baquer NZ. Effects of free radicals on cytosolic creatine kinase activities and protection by antioxidant enzymes and sulfhydryl compounds. Mol Cell Biochem 2000;210:23–8.

44. Molnar Z, Shearer E, Lowe D. N–Acetylcysteine treatment to prevent the progression of multisystem organ failure: a prospective, randomized, placebo-controlled study. Crit Care Med 1999; 27:1100–4.

45. Burton CJ, Tomson CR. Can the use of low–dose dopamine for treatment of acute renal failure be justified? Postgrad Med J 1999;75:269–74.

46. Denton MD, Chertow GM, Brady HR. 'Renal-dose' dopamine for the treatment of acute renal failure: scientific rationale, experimental studies and clinical trials. Kidney Int 1996; 50:4–14.

47. Segal JM, Phang PT, Walley KR. Low–dose dopamine hastens onset of gut ischemia in a porcine model of hemorrhagic shock. J Appl Physiol 1992;73:1159–64.

48. Weisberg LS, Kurnik PB, Kurnik BR. Risk of radiocontrast nephropathy in patients with and without diabetes mellitus. Kidney Int 1994;45:259–65.

49. Graziani G, Casati S, Cantaluppi A. Dopamine-furosemide therapy in acute renal failure. Proc EDTA 1982;19:319–24.

50. Kellum JA, M Decker J. Use of dopamine in acute renal failure: a meta-analysis. Crit Care Med 2001;29:1526–31.

51. Bellomo R, Chapman M, Finfer S, Hickling K, Myburgh J. Low-dose dopamine in patients with early renal dysfunction: a placebo-controlled randomised trial. Australian and New Zealand Intensive Care Society (ANZICS) Clinical Trials Group. Lancet 2000;356:2139–43.

52. Tumlin JA, Wang A, Murray PT, Mathur VS. Fenoldopam mesylate blocks reductions in renal plasma flow after radiocontrast dye infusion: a pilot trial in the prevention of contrast nephropathy. Am Heart J 2002;143:894–903.

53. Sheinbaum R, Ignacio C, Safi HJ, Estrera A. Contemporary strategies to preserve renal function during cardiac and vascular surgery. Rev Cardiovasc Med 2003;4 Suppl 1:S21–8.

54. Stone GW, McCullough PA, Tumlin JA, et al. Fenoldopam mesylate for the prevention of contrast–induced nephropathy: a randomized controlled trial. JAMA 2003;290:2284–91.

55. Tumlin JA, Finkel, K, Murray P, Shaw A. Dopamine 1 receptor agonists in early acute tubular necrosis: A prospective randomized double blind placebo-controlled trial of fenoldopam mesylate. J Am Soc Nephrol (abstract) 2003;14.

56. Lassnigg A, Donner E, Grubhofer G, et al. Lack of renoprotective effects of dopamine and furosemide during cardiac surgery. J Am Soc Nephrol 2000;11:97–104.

57. Sirivella S, Gielchinsky I, Parsonnet V. Mannitol, furosemide, and dopamine infusion in postoperative renal failure complicating cardiac surgery. Ann Thorac Surg 2000;69:501–6.

58. Cantarovich F, Galli C, Benedetti L, et al. High dose frusemide in established acute renal failure. Br Med J 1973;4:449–50.

59. Minuth AN, Terrell JB, Jr., Suki WN. Acute renal failure: a study of the course and prognosis of 104 patients and of the role of furosemide. Am J Med Sci 1976;271:317–24.

60. Kleinknecht D, Ganeval D, Gonzalez–Duque LA, Fermanian J. Furosemide in acute oliguric renal failure. A controlled trial. Nephron 1976;17:51–8.

61. Brown CB, Ogg CS, Cameron JS. High dose frusemide in acute renal failure: a controlled trial. Clin Nephrol 1981;15:90–6.

62. Shilliday IR, Quinn KJ, Allison ME. Loop diuretics in the management of acute renal failure: a prospective, double-blind, placebo-controlled, randomized study. Nephrol Dial Transplant 1997;12:2592–6.

63. Anderson RJ, Linas SL, Berns AS, et al. Nonoliguric acute renal failure. N Engl J Med 1977;296:1134–8.

64. Mehta RL, Pascual MT, Soroko S, Chertow GM. Diuretics, mortality, and nonrecovery of renal function in acute renal failure. JAMA 2002;288:2547–53.

65. Martin SJ, Danziger LH. Continuous infusion of loop diuretics in the critically ill: a review of the literature. Crit Care Med 1994;22:1323–9.

66. Schetz M. Should we use diuretics in acute renal failure? Best Pract Res Clin Anaesthesiol 2004;18:75–89.

67. Bonventre JV, Weinberg JM. Kidney preservation ex vivo for transplantation. Annu Rev Med 1992;43:523–53.

68. Better OS, Rubinstein I, Winaver JM, Knochel JP. Mannitol therapy revisited (1940–1997). Kidney Int 1997;52:886–94.

69. Visweswaran P, Massin EK, Dubose TD, Jr. Mannitol-induced acute renal failure. J Am Soc Nephrol 1997;8:1028–33.

70. Sands JM, Neylan JF, Olson RA, et al. Atrial natriuretic factor does not improve the outcome of cadaveric renal transplantation. J Am Soc Nephrol 1991;1:1081–6.

71. Ratcliffe PJ, Richardson AJ, Kirby JE, et al. Effect of intravenous infusion of atriopeptin 3 on immediate renal allograft function. Kidney Int 1991;39:164–8.

72. Kurnik BR, Allgren RL, Genter FC, et al. Prospective study of atrial natriuretic peptide for the prevention of radiocontrast–induced nephropathy. Am J Kidney Dis 1998;31:674–80.

73. Lewis J, Salem MM, Chertow GM, et al. Atrial natriuretic factor in oliguric acute renal failure. Anaritide Acute Renal Failure Study Group. Am J Kidney Dis 2000;36:767–74.

74. Sward K, Valsson F, Odencrants P, Samuelsson O, Ricksten SE. Recombinant human atrial natriuretic peptide in ischemic acute renal failure: a randomized placebo-controlled trial. Crit Care Med 2004;32:1310–15.

75. Petrinec D, Reilly JM, Sicard GA, et al. Insulin-like growth factor-I attenuates delayed graft function in a canine renal autotransplantation model. Surgery 1996;120:221–5;discussion 225–6.

76. Miller SB, Martin DR, Kissane J, Hammerman MR. Insulin-like growth factor I accelerates recovery from ischemic acute tubular necrosis in the rat. Proc Natl Acad Sci U S A 1992;89:11876–80.

77. Hladunewich MA, Corrigan G, Derby GC, et al. A randomized, placebo-controlled trial of IGF-1 for delayed graft function: a human model to study postischemic ARF. Kidney Int 2003;64:593–602.

78. Franklin SC, Moulton M, Sicard GA, Hammerman MR, Miller SB. Insulin-like growth factor I preserves renal function postoperatively. Am J Physiol 1997;272:F257–9.

79. Siegel NJ, Gaudio KM, Katz LA, et al. Beneficial effect of thyroxin on recovery from toxic acute renal failure. Kidney Int 1984;25:906–11.

80. Cronin RE, Brown DM, Simonsen R. Protection by thyroxine in nephrotoxic acute renal failure. Am J Physiol 1986;251:F408–16.

81. Cronin RE, Newman JA. Protective effect of thyroxine but not parathyroidectomy on gentamicin nephrotoxicity. Am J Physiol 1985;248:F332–9.

82. Sutter PM, Thulin G, Stromski M, et al. Beneficial effect of thyroxin in the treatment of ischemic acute renal failure. Pediatr Nephrol 1988;2:1–7.

83. Acker CG, Singh AR, Flick RP, et al. A trial of thyroxine in acute renal failure. Kidney Int 2000;57:293–8.

84. Shangraw RE, Jahoor F, Miyoshi H, et al. Differentiation between septic and postburn insulin resistance. Metabolism 1989;38:983–9.

85. Fietsam R, Jr., Bassett J, Glover JL. Complications of coronary artery surgery in diabetic patients. Am Surg 1991;57:551–7.

86. McManus LM, Bloodworth RC, Prihoda TJ, Blodgett JL, Pinckard RN. Agonist-dependent failure of neutrophil function in diabetes correlates with extent of hyperglycemia. J Leukoc Biol 2001;70:395–404.

87. van den Berghe G, Wouters P, Weekers F, et al. Intensive insulin therapy in the critically ill patients. N Engl J Med 2001;345:1359–67.

88. van der Veen AH, Seynhaeve AL, Breurs J, et al. In vivo isolated kidney perfusion with tumour necrosis factor alpha (TNF-alpha) in tumour-bearing rats. Br J Cancer 1999;79:433–9.

89. Bertani T, Abbate M, Zoja C, et al. Tumor necrosis factor induces glomerular damage in the rabbit. Am J Pathol 1989;134:419–30.

90. Fiedler VB, Loof I, Sander E, et al. Monoclonal antibody to tumor necrosis factor—alpha prevents lethal endotoxin sepsis in adult rhesus monkeys. J Lab Clin Med 1992;120:574–88.

91. Goldfarb RD, Parker TS, Levine DM, et al. Protein-free phospholipid emulsion treatment improved cardiopulmonary function and survival in porcine sepsis. Am J Physiol Regul Integr Comp Physiol 2003;284:R550–7.

92. Cunningham PN, Dyanov HM, Park P, et al. Acute renal failure in endotoxemia is caused by TNF acting directly on TNF receptor-1 in kidney. J Immunol 2002;168:5817–23.

93. Cunningham PN, Wang Y, Guo R, He G, Quigg RJ. Role of Toll-like receptor 4 in endotoxin-induced acute renal failure. J Immunol 2004;172:2629–35.

94. Iglesias J, Marik PE, Levine JS. Elevated serum levels of the type I and type II receptors for tumor necrosis factor-alpha as predictive factors for ARF in patients with septic shock. Am J Kidney Dis 2003;41:62–75.

95. Abraham E, Laterre PF, Garbino J, et al. Lenercept (p55 tumor necrosis factor receptor fusion protein) in severe sepsis and early septic shock: a randomized, double-blind, placebo-controlled, multicenter phase III trial with 1,342 patients. Crit Care Med 2001;29:503–10.

96. Albertson TE, Panacek EA, MacArthur RD, et al. Multicenter evaluation of a human monoclonal antibody to Enterobacteriaceae common antigen in patients with Gram-negative sepsis. Crit Care Med 2003;31:419–27.

97. Bunnell E, Lynn M, Habet K, et al. A lipid A analog, E5531, blocks the endotoxin response in human volunteers with experimental endotoxemia. Crit Care Med 2000;28:2713–20.

98. Reinhart K, Menges T, Gardlund B, et al. Randomized, placebo-controlled trial of the anti-tumor necrosis factor antibody fragment afelimomab in hyperinflammatory response during severe sepsis: The RAMSES Study. Crit Care Med 2001;29:765–9.

99. Bernard GR, Vincent JL, Laterre PF, et al. Efficacy and safety of recombinant human activated protein C for severe sepsis. N Engl J Med 2001;344:699–709.

100. Abraham E, Reinhart K, Svoboda P, et al. Assessment of the safety of recombinant tissue factor pathway inhibitor in patients with severe sepsis: a multicenter, randomized, placebo-controlled, single-blind, dose escalation study. Crit Care Med 2001;29:2081–9.

101. Abraham E, Reinhart K, Opal S, et al. Efficacy and safety of tifacogin (recombinant tissue factor pathway inhibitor) in severe sepsis: a randomized controlled trial. JAMA 2003;290:238–47.

102. Warren BL, Eid A, Singer P, et al. Caring for the critically ill patient. High-dose antithrombin III in severe sepsis: a randomized controlled trial. JAMA 2001;286:1869–78.

103. Levi M, Choi G, Schoots I, Schultz M, van der Poll T. Beyond sepsis: activated protein C and ischemia-reperfusion injury. Crit Care Med 2004;32:S309–12.

104. Landry DW, Oliver JA. The pathogenesis of vasodilatory shock. N Engl J Med 2001;345:588–95.

105. Murray PT, Wylam ME, Umans JG. Nitric oxide and septic vascular dysfunction. Anesth Analg 2000;90:89–101.

106. Bakker J, Grover R, McLuckie A, et al. Administration of the nitric oxide synthase inhibitor NG-methyl-L-arginine hydrochloride (546C88) by intravenous infusion for up to 72 hours can promote the resolution of shock in patients with severe sepsis: results of a randomized, double-blind, placebo-controlled multicenter study (study no. 144–002). Crit Care Med 2004;32:1–12.

107. Lopez A, Lorente JA, Steingrub J, et al. Multiple-center, randomized, placebo-controlled, double-blind study of the nitric oxide synthase inhibitor 546C88: effect on survival in patients with septic shock. Crit Care Med 2004;32:21–30.

108. Mitaka C, Hirata Y, Yokoyama K, et al. Improvement of renal dysfunction in dogs with endotoxemia by a nonselective endothelin receptor antagonist. Crit Care Med 1999;27:146–53.

109. Wang A, Holcslaw T, Bashore TM, et al. Exacerbation of radiocontrast nephrotoxicity by endothelin receptor antagonism. Kidney Int 2000;57:1675–80.

110. Klahr S. Role of arachidonic acid metabolites in acute renal failure and sepsis. Nephrol Dial Transplant 1994;9 Suppl 4:52–6.

111. Lugon JR, Boim MA, Ramos OL, Ajzen H, Schor N. Renal function and glomerular hemodynamics in male endotoxemic rats. Kidney Int 1989;36:570–5.

112. Badr KF, Kelley VE, Rennke HG, Brenner BM. Roles for thromboxane A2 and leukotrienes in endotoxin-induced acute renal failure. Kidney Int 1986;30:474–80.

113. Bernard GR, Wheeler AP, Russell JA, et al. The effects of ibuprofen on the physiology and survival of patients with sepsis. The Ibuprofen in Sepsis Study Group. N Engl J Med 1997;336:912–18.

114. Linas SL, Whittenburg D, Repine JE. Role of neutrophil derived oxidants and elastase in lipopolysaccharide-mediated renal injury. Kidney Int 1991;39:618–23.

115. Linas SL, Whittenburg D, Parsons PE, Repine JE. Mild renal ischemia activates primed neutrophils to cause acute renal failure. Kidney Int 1992;42:610–16.

116. Kelly KJ, Williams WW, Jr., Colvin RB, Bonventre JV. Antibody to intercellular adhesion molecule 1 protects the kidney against ischemic injury. Proc Natl Acad Sci U S A 1994;91:812–16.

117. Haller H, Dragun D, Miethke A, et al. Antisense oligonucleotides for ICAM-1 attenuate reperfusion injury and renal failure in the rat. Kidney Int 1996;50:473–80.

118. Levy EM, Viscoli CM, Horwitz RI. The effect of acute renal failure on mortality. A cohort analysis. JAMA 1996;275:1489–94.

119. Murphy SW, Barrett BJ, Parfrey PS. Contrast nephropathy. J Am Soc Nephrol 2000;11:177–82.

120. Solomon R. Contrast-medium-induced acute renal failure. Kidney Int 1998;53:230–42.

121. Bakris GL, Lass N, Gaber AO, Jones JD, Burnett JC, Jr. Radiocontrast medium-induced declines in renal function: a role for oxygen free radicals. Am J Physiol 1990;258:F115–20.

122. Huber W, Hennig M, Eckel F, Classen M. [Contrast medium-induced renal failure can not be prevented by hemodialysis]. Dtsch Med Wochenschr 2002;127:45–7.

123. Vogt B, Ferrari P, Schonholzer C, et al. Prophylactic hemodialysis after radiocontrast media in patients with renal insufficiency is potentially harmful. Am J Med 2001;111:692–8.

124. Marenzi G, Marana I, Lauri G, et al. The prevention of radiocontrast-agent-induced nephropathy by hemofiltration. N Engl J Med 2003;349:1333–40.

125. Aspelin P, Aubry P, Fransson SG, et al. Nephrotoxic effects in high-risk patients undergoing angiography. N Engl J Med 2003;348:491–9.

126. Vogelman B, Gudmundsson S, Leggett J, et al. Correlation of antimicrobial pharmacokinetic parameters with therapeutic efficacy in an animal model. J Infect Dis 1988;158:831–47.

127. Verpooten GA, Giuliano RA, Verbist L, Eestermans G, De Broe ME. Once-daily dosing decreases renal accumulation of gentamicin and netilmicin. Clin Pharmacol Ther 1989;45:22–7.

128. Barza M, Ioannidis JP, Cappelleri JC, Lau J. Single or multiple daily doses of aminoglycosides: a meta-analysis. BMJ 1996;312:338–45.

129. Sawaya BP, Briggs JP, Schnermann J. Amphotericin B nephrotoxicity: the adverse consequences of altered membrane properties. J Am Soc Nephrol 1995;6:154–64.

130. Sawaya BP, Weihprecht H, Campbell WR, et al. Direct vasoconstriction as a possible cause for amphotericin B-induced nephrotoxicity in rats. J Clin Invest 1991;87:2097–107.

131. Lopez–Berestein G, Bodey GP, Fainstein V, et al. Treatment of systemic fungal infections with liposomal amphotericin B. Arch Intern Med 1989;149:2533–6.

132. Arning M, Scharf RE. Prevention of amphotericin-B-induced nephrotoxicity by loading with sodium chloride: a report of 1291 days of treatment with amphotericin B without renal failure. Klin Wochenschr 1989;67:1020–8.

133. Llanos A, Cieza J, Bernardo J, et al. Effect of salt supplementation on amphotericin B nephrotoxicity. Kidney Int 1991;40:302–8.

134. Tolins JP, Raij L. Chronic amphotericin B nephrotoxicity in the rat: protective effect of calcium channel blockade. J Am Soc Nephrol 1991;2:98–102.

135. Gerkens JF, Heidemann HT, Jackson EK, Branch RA. Effect of aminophylline on amphotericin B nephrotoxicity in the dog. J Pharmacol Exp Ther 1983;224:609–13.

136. Leibbrandt ME, Wolfgang GH, Metz AL, Ozobia AA, Haskins JR. Critical subcellular targets of cisplatin and related platinum analogs in rat renal proximal tubule cells. Kidney Int 1995;48:761–70.

137. Ries F, Klastersky J. Nephrotoxicity induced by cancer chemotherapy with special emphasis on cisplatin toxicity. Am J Kidney Dis 1986;8:368–79.

138. Brock J, Alberts DS. Safe, rapid administration of cisplatin in the outpatient clinic. Cancer Treat Rep 1986;70:1409–14.

139. Finley RS, Fortner CL, Grove WR. Cisplatin nephrotoxicity: a summary of preventative interventions. Drug Intell Clin Pharm 1985;19:362–7.

140. Ozols RF, Corden BJ, Jacob J, et al. High–dose cisplatin in hypertonic saline. Ann Intern Med 1984;100:19–24.

141. Hensley ML, Schuchter LM, Lindley C, et al. American Society of Clinical Oncology clinical practice guidelines for the use of chemotherapy and radiotherapy protectants. J Clin Oncol 1999;17:3333–55.

142. Bia MJ, Tyler K. Evidence that calcium channel blockade prevents cyclosporine-induced exacerbation of renal ischemic injury. Transplantation 1991;51:293–5.

143. Ladefoged SD, Pedersen E, Hammer M, et al. Influence of diltiazem on renal function and rejection in renal allograft recipients receiving triple-drug immunosuppression: a randomized, double-blind, placebo-controlled study. Nephrol Dial Transplant 1994;9:543–7.

144. Neumayer HH, Wagner K. Prevention of delayed graft function in cadaver kidney transplants by diltiazem: outcome of two prospective, randomized clinical trials. J Cardiovasc Pharmacol 1987;10 Suppl 10:S170–7.

145. Lustig S, Shmueli D, Boner G, et al. Gallopamil reduces the posttransplantation acute tubular necrosis in kidneys from aged donors. Isr J Med Sci 1996;32:1249–51.

146. Medina PJ, Sipols JM, George JN. Drug-associated thrombotic thrombocytopenic purpura-hemolytic uremic syndrome. Curr Opin Hematol 2001;8:286–93.

147. Holt SG, Moore KP. Pathogenesis and treatment of renal dysfunction in rhabdomyolysis. Intensive Care Med 2001;27:803–11.

148. Moore KP, Holt SG, Patel RP, et al. A causative role for redox cycling of myoglobin and its inhibition by alkalinization in the pathogenesis and treatment of rhabdomyolysis-induced renal failure. J Biol Chem 1998;273:31731–7.

149. Zager RA. Studies of mechanisms and protective maneuvers in myoglobinuric acute renal injury. Lab Invest 1989;60:619–29.

150. Zager RA. Combined mannitol and deferoxamine therapy for myohemoglobinuric renal injury and oxidant tubular stress. Mechanistic and therapeutic implications. J Clin Invest 1992;90:711–19.

151. Zager RA, Mahan J, Merola AJ. Effects of mannitol on the postischemic kidney. Biochemical, functional, and morphologic assessments. Lab Invest 1985;53:433–42.

152. Zager RA, Foerder C, Bredl C. The influence of mannitol on myoglobinuric acute renal failure: functional, biochemical, and morphological assessments. J Am Soc Nephrol 1991;2:848–55.

153. Knox FG, Fleming JS, Rennie DW. Effects of osmotic diuresis on sodium reabsorption and oxygen consumption of kidney. Am J Physiol 1966;210:751–9.

154. Amyot SL, Leblanc M, Thibeault Y, Geadah D, Cardinal J. Myoglobin clearance and removal during continuous venovenous hemofiltration. Intensive Care Med 1999;25:1169–72.

155. Wakabayashi Y, Kikuno T, Ohwada T, Kikawada R. Rapid fall in blood myoglobin in massive rhabdomyolysis and acute renal failure. Intensive Care Med 1994;20:109–12.

156. Wall SM, Johansen MJ, Molony DA, et al. Effective clearance of methotrexate using high-flux hemodialysis membranes. Am J Kidney Dis 1996;28:846–54.

157. Ackland SP, Schilsky RL. High-dose methotrexate: a critical reappraisal. J Clin Oncol 1987;5:2017–31.

158. Kepka L, De Lassence A, Ribrag V, et al. Successful rescue in a patient with high dose methotrexate-induced nephrotoxicity and acute renal failure. Leuk Lymphoma 1998;29:205–9.

159. Cohen L BJ, Magrath I, Poplack D, Ziegler J. Acute tumor lysis syndrome. A review of 37 patients with Burkitt lymphoma. Am J Med 1980;68:486–91.

160. Silverman P, Distelhorst CW. Metabolic emergencies in clinical oncology. Semin Oncol 1989;16:504–15.

161. Arrambide K, Toto RD. Tumor lysis syndrome. Semin Nephrol 1993;13:273–80.

162. Kjellstrand CM CD, von Hartitzsch B, Buselmeier TJ. Hyperuricemic acute renal failure. Arch Intern Med 1974;133:349–59.

163. Conger J. Acute uric acid nephropathy. Semin Nephrol 1981;1:69–74.

164. Boles JM, Dutel JL, Briere J, et al. Acute renal failure caused by extreme hyperphosphatemia after chemotherapy of an acute lymphoblastic leukemia. Cancer 1984;53:2425–9.

165. Masera G, Jankovic M, Zurlo MG, et al. Urate-oxidase prophylaxis of uric acid-induced renal damage in childhood leukemia. J Pediatr 1982;100:152–5.

166. Saccente SL, Kohaut EC, Berkow RL. Prevention of tumor lysis syndrome using continuous veno-venous hemofiltration. Pediatr Nephrol 1995;9:569–73.

167. Kramer L, Horl WH. Hepatorenal syndrome. Semin Nephrol 2002;22:290–301.

168. Gines P, Guevara M. Good news for hepatorenal syndrome. Hepatology 2002;36:504–6.

169. Gonwa TA, Klintmalm GB, Levy M, et al. Impact of pretransplant renal function on survival after liver transplantation. Transplantation 1995;59:361–5.

170. Guevara M, Gines P, Fernandez-Esparrach G, et al. Reversibility of hepatorenal syndrome by prolonged administration of ornipressin and plasma volume expansion. Hepatology 1998;27:35–41.

171. Uriz J, Gines P, Cardenas A, et al. Terlipressin plus albumin infusion: an effective and safe therapy of hepatorenal syndrome. J Hepatol 2000;33:43–8.

172. Mulkay JP, Louis H, Donckier V, et al. Long-term terlipressin administration improves renal function in cirrhotic patients with type 1 hepatorenal syndrome: a pilot study. Acta Gastroenterol Belg 2001;64:15–19.

173. Angeli P, Volpin R, Gerunda G, et al. Reversal of type 1 hepatorenal syndrome with the administration of midodrine and octreotide. Hepatology 1999;29:1690–7.

174. Holt S, Goodier D, Marley R, et al. Improvement in renal function in hepatorenal syndrome with N-acetylcysteine. Lancet 1999;353:294–5.

175. Guevara M, Gines P, Bandi JC, et al. Transjugular intrahepatic portosystemic shunt in hepatorenal syndrome: effects on renal function and vasoactive systems. Hepatology 1998;28:416–22.

176. Brensing KA, Textor J, Perz J, et al. Long term outcome after transjugular intrahepatic portosystemic stent-shunt in nontransplant cirrhotics with hepatorenal syndrome: a phase II study. Gut 2000;47:288–95.

177. Koning OH, Ploeg RJ, van Bockel JH, et al. Risk factors for delayed graft function in cadaveric kidney transplantation: a prospective study of renal function and graft survival after preservation with University of Wisconsin solution in multi-organ donors. European Multicenter Study Group. Transplantation 1997;63:1620–8.

178. Carlier M, Squifflet JP, Pirson Y, Gribomont B, Alexandre GP. Maximal hydration during anesthesia increases pulmonary arterial pressures and improves early function of human renal transplants. Transplantation 1982;34:201–4.

179. van Valenberg PL, Hoitsma AJ, Tiggeler RG, et al. Mannitol as an indispensable constituent of an intraoperative hydration protocol for the prevention of acute renal failure after renal cadaveric transplantation. Transplantation 1987;44:784–8.

180. Ploeg RJ, van Bockel JH, Langendijk PT, et al. Effect of preservation solution on results of cadaveric kidney transplantation. The European Multicentre Study Group. Lancet 1992;340:129–37.

181. Salmela K, Wramner L, Ekberg H, et al. A randomized multicenter trial of the anti-ICAM-1 monoclonal antibody (enlimomab) for the prevention of acute rejection and delayed onset of graft function in cadaveric renal transplantation: a report of the European Anti-ICAM-1 Renal Transplant Study Group. Transplantation 1999;67:729–36.

182. Hourmant M, Bedrossian J, Durand D, et al. A randomized multicenter trial comparing leukocyte function-associated antigen-1 monoclonal antibody with rabbit antithymocyte glob-

ulin as induction treatment in first kidney transplantations. Transplantation 1996;62:1565–70.

183. Bellomo R, Goldsmith D, Russell S, Uchino S. Postoperative serious adverse events in a teaching hospital: a prospective study. Med J Aust 2002;176:216–18.

184. Weldon BC, Monk TG. The patient at risk for acute renal failure. Recognition, prevention, and preoperative optimization. Anesthesiol Clin North America 2000;18:705–17.

185. Shaw A, Boscoe MJ. Anaesthetic assessment and management of cardiac patients for non-cardiac surgery. Part I: Assessment [In Process Citation]. Int J Clin Pract 1999;53:281–6.

186. Meyer S. Grading of patients for surgical procedures. Anesthesiology 1941;2:281–5.

187. Carmichael P, Carmichael AR. Acute renal failure in the surgical setting. ANZ J Surg 2003;73:144–53.

188. Baxter C. Acute renal insufficiency complicating trauma surgery. In: Shires GT, ed. Principles of Trauma Care. New York: McGraw Hill, 1985:502.

189. Abel RM, Buckley MJ, Austen WG, et al. Etiology, incidence, and prognosis of renal failure following cardiac operations. Results of a prospective analysis of 500 consecutive patients. J Thorac Cardiovasc Surg 1976;71:323–33.

190. Mangano CM, Diamondstone LS, Ramsay JG, et al. Renal dysfunction after myocardial revascularization: risk factors, adverse outcomes, and hospital resource utilization. The Multicenter Study of Perioperative Ischemia Research Group. Ann Intern Med 1998;128:194–203.

191. Jorres A, Kordonouri O, Schiessler A, et al. Urinary excretion of thromboxane and markers for renal injury in patients undergoing cardiopulmonary bypass. Artif Organs 1994;18:565–9.

192. Myers BD, Miller DC, Mehigan JT, et al. Nature of the renal injury following total renal ischemia in man. J Clin Invest 1984;73:329–41.

193. Garwood S, Swamidoss CP, Davis EA, Samson L, Hines RL. A case series of low-dose fenoldopam in seventy cardiac surgical patients at increased risk of renal dysfunction. J Cardiothorac Vasc Anesth 2003;17:17–21.

194. Sekhon CS, Sekhon BK, Singh I, Orak JK, Singh AK. Attenuation of renal ischemia/reperfusion injury by a triple drug combination therapy. J Nephrol 2003;16:63–74.

195. Durmaz I, Yagdi T, Calkavur T, et al. Prophylactic dialysis in patients with renal dysfunction undergoing on-pump coronary artery bypass surgery. Ann Thorac Surg 2003;75:859–64.

196. Hakim RM, Wingard RL, Parker RA. Effect of the dialysis membrane in the treatment of patients with acute renal failure. N Engl J Med 1994;331:1338–42.

197. Schulman G, Fogo A, Gung A, Badr K, Hakim R. Complement activation retards resolution of acute ischemic renal failure in the rat. Kidney Int 1991;40:1069–74.

198. Okada H, Sugahara S, Nakamoto H, Omoto R, Suzuki H. Intensive perioperative dialysis can improve the hospital mortality of haemodialysis patients undergoing cardiac surgery. Nephrol Dial Transplant 1998;13:2713–14.

199. Sandham JD, Hull RD, Brant RF, et al. A randomized, controlled trial of the use of pulmonary-artery catheters in high-risk surgical patients. N Engl J Med 2003;348:5–14.

200. Richard C, Warszawski J, Anguel N, et al. Early use of the pulmonary artery catheter and outcomes in patients with shock and acute respiratory distress syndrome: a randomized controlled trial. JAMA 2003;290:2713–20.

201. Zion MM, Balkin J, Rosenmann D, et al. Use of pulmonary artery catheters in patients with acute myocardial infarction. Analysis of experience in 5,841 patients in the SPRINT Registry. SPRINT Study Group. Chest 1990;98:1331–5.

202. Connors AF, Jr., Speroff T, Dawson NV, et al. The effectiveness of right heart catheterization in the initial care of critically ill patients. SUPPORT Investigators. JAMA 1996;276:889–97.

203. Faust SN, Heyderman RS, Levin M. Coagulation in severe sepsis: a central role for thrombomodulin and activated protein C. Crit Care Med 2001;29:S62–7;discussion S67–8.

204. Wendt EC. Uber den Einflus des intra-abdominellen Druckes auf dies Absonderungsgeschwindigkeit des Hames. Arch Heilkunde 1876;17:527.

205. McNelis J, Marini CP, Simms HH. Abdominal compartment syndrome: clinical manifestations and predictive factors. Curr Opin Crit Care 2003;9:133–6.

206. Liolios A, Oropello JM, Benjamin E. Gastrointestinal complications in the intensive care unit. Clin Chest Med 1999;20:329–45, viii.

207. Iberti TJ, Kelly KM, Gentili DR, Hirsch S, Benjamin E. A simple technique to accurately determine intra-abdominal pressure. Crit Care Med 1987;15:1140–2.

208. Morris JA, Jr., Mucha P, Jr., Ross SE, et al. Acute posttraumatic renal failure: a multicenter perspective. J Trauma 1991;31:1584–90.

209. Regel G, Lobenhoffer P, Grotz M, et al. Treatment results of patients with multiple trauma: an analysis of 3406 cases treated between 1972 and 1991 at a German Level I Trauma Center. J Trauma 1995;38:70–8.

210. Tran DD, Cuesta MA, Oe PL. Acute renal failure in patients with severe civilian trauma. Nephrol Dial Transplant 1994;9 Suppl 4:121–5.

211. Vivino G, Antonelli M, Moro ML, et al. Risk factors for acute renal failure in trauma patients. Intensive Care Med 1998;24:808–14.

212. Homsi E, Barreiro MF, Orlando JM, Higa EM. Prophylaxis of acute renal failure in patients with rhabdomyolysis. Ren Fail 1997;19:283–8.

6

Diagnosis of acute renal failure

Julie Raggio and Jason G Umans

Acute renal failure (ARF) complicates the course of 7–23% of patients in the intensive care unit (ICU).[1-4] Early diagnosis and elucidation of its etiology guides successful treatment. This chapter will review definitions of ARF, clinical and laboratory evaluation, and the pathophysiology of ARF as they apply to the diagnosis of this disorder.

DEFINITIONS OF ARF IMPACTING ON ITS DIAGNOSIS

Critical evaluation of diagnostic strategies to detect and elucidate the causes of ARF has been limited by lack of consensus regarding its definition.[5] New and persisting anuria obviously connotes ARF. By contrast, decreased urinary volume may be an appropriate response to an ischemic or nephrotoxic insult. ARF has been defined operationally as a sudden decrease in renal function that results in anuria or the retention of nitrogenous wastes such as urea or creatinine.[6-9] However, there has been little agreement as to the magnitude of increase in these circulating filtration markers which would warrant designation as ARF.[5-7] Clearly, the sensitivity and specificity of diagnostic strategies would differ markedly were ARF to be defined as a 25% or 50% decrement in glomerular filtration rate (GFR) or as a fall in renal function to a GFR <10 ml/min. Likewise, authors differ as to the acuity implied in the diagnosis of 'acute' renal failure, with GFR decrements occurring over a period of hours to days to weeks.[5,7]

The serum creatinine concentration provides an inverse estimate of creatinine clearance, which itself is but an estimate of GFR. This estimation assumes both that creatinine production is constant and that creatinine is a flawless filtration marker; neither assumption is true. Skeletal myocytes release creatine, which is then dehydrated to creatinine. Creatine turnover is relatively constant in men with normal GFR, but has not been studied in women and may vary greatly in patients with myopathy, catabolic disorders, or in critical illness.[10] Due to the large creatine pool, small changes in fractional creatine turnover may lead to large changes in creatinine production. Intake of foods high in creatine or protein may also increase creatinine biosynthesis.[11]

Creatinine is filtered freely at the glomerulus without significant tubular reabsorption or metabolism. Proximal tubular cells, however, secrete creatinine, contributing more importantly to its clearance as GFR falls.[12] Patients with chronic renal insufficiency (CRI) eliminate more creatinine extrarenally, probably via the gut.[11] Changes in serum creatinine must thus be interpreted differently in patients with acute-on-chronic renal failure.

While changes in GFR lead to predictable, delayed, changes in serum creatinine, given basic assumptions regarding its production rate and volume of distribution,[13] this relationship may vary due to pathologic changes in total body water or tubular secretion.[12,14] At lower baseline creatinine levels, small (and clinically inapparent) increments of serum creatinine, even within a normal range, may reflect large changes in GFR.

More recently, cystatin C (CysC) has been proposed as an alternative serum GFR marker which may provide greater sensitivity than creatinine in the diagnosis of ARF. CysC is a 13 kDa protein produced in all nucleated cells at an apparently constant rate. Due to its small size and basic pH, it is freely filtered at the glomerulus and is not secreted. Filtered CysC is then reabsorbed by proximal tubular epithelial cells and fully catabolized, such that none returns to the circulation.[15] Thus, urinary excretion of CysC could provide an early marker of proximal tubular epithelial injury,[16] whereas its serum levels should correlate inversely with GFR.[17]

In contrast to creatinine, CysC levels appear similar in men and women, and in African-Americans and Caucasians.[18,19] Serum levels of CysC may detect renal dysfunction more sensitively than serum creatinine, particularly in patients with less muscle mass, such as the elderly and cirrhotics.[18–22] Likewise, CysC levels appear to rise earlier than those of creatinine in patients with ARF.[23,24] Currently, however, the usual immunonephelometric assays for CysC are poorly standardized, so that normal ranges vary considerably and differing norms may apply in patients with malignant disease, in those receiving glucocorticoids, and in those with renal allografts.[15,19,20] Nevertheless, larger studies should define the utility of this new filtration marker, which may soon aid in the earlier diagnosis of ARF.

PATHOPHYSIOLOGY AS IT IMPACTS DIAGNOSIS OF ACUTE RENAL FAILURE

ARF is often categorized as falling into one of three broad pathophysiologic categories:

- reversible 'prerenal' (PR) ARF due to renal hypoperfusion
- 'intrinsic' ARF due to nephron injury
- 'post renal' ARF due to urinary obstruction.

Of course, multiple etiologies may contribute to ARF in a given patient.

Prerenal etiologies

Prerenal ARF occurs when absolute or effective hypovolemia impairs renal perfusion. GFR is defended by coordinated afferent arteriolar dilation and efferent vasoconstriction; failure of these compensatory mechanisms, including interference with intrarenal effects of vasodilator prostanoids or angiotensin II, worsens the decrement in GFR.[25] The appropriate tubular response to volume depletion is increased reabsorption of water and solute, and thus urinary concentration. The definitive diagnosis of PR ARF depends on prompt recovery of GFR with restoration of effective volume.[26] Hospital-acquired PR ARF is often secondary to decreased effective volume rather than to measur-

able decrements in total body water or its compartments.[27]

Cyclosporine, nonsteroidal anti-inflammatory drugs (NSAIDs) including cyclooxygenase-2 inhibitors, radiographic contrast agents, and hypercalcemia may all increase afferent arteriole tone and therefore impair GFR in patients whose GFR depends on afferent vasodilation, such as those with physiologic activation of the renin–angiotensin system.[7] Likewise, ARF may be precipitated by administration of angiotensin-converting enzyme (ACE) inhibitors or angiotensin receptor blockers in any patient with decreased effective volume or impaired afferent arteriolar flow, e.g. patients with congestive heart failure (CHF), bilateral renal artery stenosis, cirrhosis, or the nephrotic syndrome.[6]

Intrinsic acute renal failure

Either extensive glomerular or tubular damage may lead to intrinsic ARF. Glomerular damage also typically leads to proteinuria and urinary sediment abnormalities, both aiding in its diagnosis. Similarly, diagnosis of tubular injury is aided by its resulting impairment of solute reclamation and urinary concentration.

Acute tubular necrosis (ATN) is the most common cause of intrinsic ARF in hospitalized patients.[28,29] Fifty percent of cases are due to ischemic injury.[9] Ischemia may lead to a continuum of disease, with PR ARF progressing to ATN, and then to irreversible cortical necrosis if the kidneys are not reperfused.[26] Nephrotoxins such as aminoglycosides and radiographic contrast agents may cause 25–35% of reported ATN cases.[9,28] The kidneys seem particularly susceptible to toxic damage, in part because they can concentrate toxins within the medullary interstitium and in tubular epithelial cells. If other potential insults occur concurrently, the risk of renal damage increases.

Postrenal acute renal failure

Obstruction of urine flow at any point from the tubules to the urethral outlet may result in postrenal ARF. It is crucial to rule out functional obstruction because urinary drainage may restore and preserve renal function. In most cases obstruction only leads to clinically apparent decrements in GFR when bilateral or when a patient has but one functional kidney, which is then obstructed.

Intratubular obstruction by crystalline or proteinaceous material increases pressure more proximally and opposes filtration. Drugs such as acyclovir, indinavir, or sulfonamides may precipitate, as can uric acid, calcium oxalate, or myeloma proteins. More distally, nephrolithiasis or retroperitoneal fibrosis may lead to ureteral obstruction. Prostatic hypertrophy or bladder dysfunction due to autonomic neuropathy may lead to lower tract obstruction. Likewise, lower tract obstruction may result from atropinic or α-adrenergic drug effects which either decrease detrusor function or increase bladder sphincter tonicity.

MAKING THE DIAGNOSIS OF ACUTE RENAL FAILURE

A careful history and physical examination, including review of laboratory tests, will reveal the most likely etiology of ARF in the majority of hospitalized patients.[30,31] Record review, urinalysis (UA), and possibly bladder catheterization or ultrasound (US) examination should be part of the initial assessment.[8] More detailed evaluation, including urinary diagnostic indices and specialized serum assays, are performed subsequently as indicated (Table 6.1).

History

Pre-existing conditions, such as CHF, cirrhosis, human immunodeficiency virus (HIV) infection, and malignancy, medications (including over-the-counter medications and herbs), and as full a review of systems as possible should be elicited. A history of voluminous diarrhea, CHF exacerbation, ingestion of ACE inhibitors or NSAIDs or the complaints of thirst or orthostatic dizziness might suggest PR causes, which account for 21–60% of inpatient ARF, and 17% of cases in the ICU.[1,8,29,32] Systemic symptoms such as rash, arthralgias, sinusitis, hemoptysis, or fever may suggest autoimmune disease, vasculitis, allergic interstitial nephritis (AIN, generally drug-induced) or a pulmonary–renal syndrome, responsible for >2% of ARF in the ICU.[29] Flank pain is consistent with catastrophic renal vein thrombosis,[25] nephrolithiasis, obstruction, or infarction. A recent history of hypotension, especially while under the influence of general anesthetic agents, or of exposure to nephrotoxic medications suggests ATN, which may account for 76% of ICU ARF.[29] Obstructive

symptoms or the use of medications with anticholinergic or α-adrenergic properties in uncatheterized patients suggests the possibility of postrenal ARF, responsible for 1–10% ARF in hospitalized patients and for 0.8–4% of cases in the ICU.[1–3,8,27,29,32–34]

Investigation should not halt at the identification of one potential insult, especially in patients with normal baseline renal function.[34] Risk factors significantly associated with ICU ARF include sepsis, nephrotoxins, hypotension, older age, prior chronic disease, and multiorgan failure.[1–3,29,32]

Careful charting of a hospitalized patient's daily fluid inputs and output, daily weight, exposure to medications and radiocontrast agents, fluctuation in blood pressure, and invasive interventions in relation to BUN and creatinine is invaluable. BUN and creatinine frequently rise 24–48 hours after contrast, peaking 3–5 days following exposure, and in most cases returning to normal values 7–10 days post insult. Renal dysfunction secondary to ATN may appear hours to days after ischemia or nephrotoxin exposure, usually lasts 1–2 weeks, but sometimes as long as 1–11 months. Aminoglycoside-induced ATN is usually not evident until 7–10 days of aminoglycoside treatment, but may present earlier in the setting of concomitant renal insults or of baseline impairment of renal function.[35] Atheroembolic complications may present 1 day to 7 weeks following arterial intervention.

Laboratory values or symptoms consistent with chronic kidney disease suggest acute-on-chronic renal failure, and an alternate differential diagnosis. Pre-existing symptoms such as anorexia, dysgeusia, and nausea suggest underlying uremia. Hyperphosphatemia, anemia, and hypocalcemia do not generally differentiate between acute and chronic renal dysfunction.[31] Carbamylated hemoglobin, reflecting chronic azotemia, may be elevated in patients with chronic kidney disease, but is not used clinically.[36,37]

Physical examination

The physical examination should focus on hemodynamics, assessment of volume status, and a search for signs of systemic disorders which could lead to renal injury. Hypotension and either hypothermia or fever might indicate sepsis or a systemic inflammatory response, associated with up to 70% of ARF cases in the ICU.[1–3] Severe hypertension may accompany ARF due to acute glomerulonephritis (GN), scleroderma, malignant

Table 6.1 Approach to the diagnosis of acute renal failure (ARF).

Initial evaluation in all patients	Further evaluation as clinically indicated	More specialized testing as appropriate
History: focus on PR insults such as diarrhea/NSAIDs; symptoms consistent with autoimmune disease, obstructive symptoms	Urine diagnostic indices (urinary Na, FeNa, FeUN, urinary Cl) most helpful in differentiating PR ARF from ATN	Doppler US or MR imaging of renal vasculature if vascular obstruction or thrombosis suspected
Record review: including fluid in's and out's, episodes of hypotension, exposure to nephrotoxic medications or contrast	Renal ultrasound: rule out obstruction unless another etiology highly likely, evaluate size and echogenicity	MAG3 furosemide renogram: may aid in evaluation of functional obstruction if US findings are equivocal
Physical: assessment of volume status, complete physical examination, complete metabolic panel and CBC	Consider fluid challenge if PR state suspected	Therapeutic trial: discontinuance of nephrotoxic medications or treatment of heart failure
Urinary bladder catheterization if oligoanuric	Consider invasive hemodynamic monitoring if volume status unclear	Biopsy: particulary if sediment reveals RBC casts/WBC casts c/w GN, new onset proteinuria >1 g/day, symptoms consistent with autoimmune disease or vasculitis, or evidence of thrombotic microangiopathy
Urinalysis: urine specific gravity, urine osmolality, urine protein, hematuria	Serum assays as indicated: ANA, anti-dsDNA, p-ANCA, c-ANCA, anti-GBM antibody, C3, C4, CH50, antistreptolysin O, creatine kinase, uric acid, serum protein electrophoresis, cryoglobulins	Arteriography may aid in diagnosis of polyarteritis nodosa
Sediment examination: RBCs, WBCs, hyaline, granular, tubular, RBC and WBC casts. Examination of fresh urine by physician seems key	Urine assays as indicated: prot:creat ratio, eosinophils by Hansel's stain, myoglobin, urine protein electrophoresis	CT may aid in identifying obstructive nephrolithiasis or in detecting obstruction in the setting of cystic disease. Antegrade or retrograde pyelogram aid in evaluation of obstruction

PR, prenatal; NSAIDs, nonsteroidal anti-inflammatory drugs; ATN, acute tubular necrosis; FeNa, fractional excretion of sodium; FeUN, fractional excretion of urea nitrogen; US, ultrasound; GN, glomerulonephritis; MR, magnetic resonance; RBC, red blood cells; WBC, white blood cells; CBC, complete blood count.

hypertension, or pre-eclampsia. Orthostatic vital signs should be assessed if at all possible, and weight compared to the patient's baseline.

Signs consistent with a PR state include skin tenting, dry mucous membranes, furrowed tongue, peripheral cyanosis, sunken eyes, and dry axillae. A postural increase in pulse (supine to standing) of at least 30 beats/min is 96% specific for clinically significant volume depletion, whereas systolic pressure may fall 20 mmHg upon standing in 10% of normal individuals and in up to 30% of patients over 65 years old.[38] The inability of a patient to stand because of severe lightheadedness is a relatively specific sign of hypovolemia.[38] Edema, ascites, elevated jugular venous pressure, and pulmonary rales suggest total body volume excess, but do not rule out effective hypovolemia.

Examination of the head and neck is key. Scleritis or uveitis suggest an autoimmune disease. Fundoscopy may reveal signs of malignant hypertension, endocarditis, or of underlying diabetic microvascular disease. New murmurs or extra heart sounds would focus further evaluation on acute cardiac disease. The abdominal examination should seek evidence of ascites, hepatosplenomegaly, vascular bruits, and of abdominal aortic aneurysm. Bladder palpation and percussion may reveal distension due to obstruction, while rectal examination may reveal a diffusely enlarged prostate, albeit urethral obstruction is usually due to median lobe hypertrophy. Decreased peripheral pulses may be consistent with peripheral arterial disease, though normal lower extremity pulses do not exclude atheroembolic ARF.[25] Otherwise unexplained altered mental status might lead one to suspect sepsis, thrombotic thrombocytopenic purpura (TTP), or systemic vasculitis. Examination of skin and nailbeds may provide evidence of chronic liver disease, atheroemboli, endocarditis, vasculitis, or drug allergy.

Bladder catheterization should be considered whenever the patient is anuric, oliguric, or has anuria alternating with polyuria.[8] If volume status remains unclear following physical examination, invasive hemodynamic monitoring with a pulmonary artery catheter may guide treatment. Diagnostic evaluation may include a trial of fluids: if urine output increases and creatinine falls, one has diagnosed PR ARF.

Basic laboratory tests

Serum levels of creatinine and blood urea nitrogen (BUN) provide initial estimates of renal function, but are subject to misinterpretation. Several medications may impair creatinine clearance without altering GFR. Pyrimethamine, probenecid, cimetidine, and trimethoprim may all do so by competing with creatinine at its site of proximal tubular secretion.[11,12,39,40] In these cases, the lack of a parallel increase in BUN should provide evidence that GFR may not have changed.

Serum urea nitrogen concentration is usually less useful in the estimation of GFR than is creatinine.[41] Urea is generated primarily via hepatic amino acid catabolism.[40] It is filtered freely at the glomerulus, but, in contrast to creatinine, 40–50% is reabsorbed, principally in the proximal tubule and medullary collecting duct. Gastrointestinal bleeding, corticosteroids, or any inflammatory or catabolic stimulus may increase urea synthesis, elevating BUN without decreasing renal function.

The normal serum BUN: creatinine ratio is about 8:1; a ratio greater than 20:1 suggests a prerenal state.[42] As urine flow falls, tubular reabsorption of urea is increased. An elevated BUN:creatinine ratio is not specific for PR ARF, however, as gastrointestinal bleeding and glucocorticoids may disproportionately elevate BUN. Conversely, a decreased BUN:creatinine ratio may accompany rhabdomyolysis, in which muscle breakdown increases creatinine selectively.[40] Hyperkalemia may raise suspicions of NSAID or ACE inhibitor ingestion, rhabdomyolysis, or tumor lysis syndrome.[30] Likewise, severe hypercalcemia may itself lead to ARF.

Microangiopathic hemolytic anemia can lead to ARF in a diverse set of clinical scenarios, including hemolytic uremic syndrome (HUS), TTP, malignant hypertension, scleroderma, pre-eclampsia, and following several drugs.[43,44] It should be ruled out if there is any evidence of thrombocytopenia or hemolysis. Peripheral eosinophilia should prompt consideration of AIN or atheroembolic disease.[45]

Urine volume

Minimal daily solute production is 400–600 milliOsmoles (mOsmol), requiring a minimum urine volume of 300–500 ml, assuming maximal urine concentration to about 1200 mOsmol/L. Oliguria is thus defined as 100–400 ml of urine/day and anuria as <100 ml/day, even though urinary concentrating ability is often lost in ARF.

Anuria suggests bilateral acute cortical necrosis, severe ATN, obstructive uropathy, overwhelming acute GN,[46] or bilateral renal artery or vein occlusion. Obstruction may result in anuria, polyuria, or in fluctuation between the two.[47]

Volume-depleted patients are often, but not always, oliguric. Nonoliguric PR failure may be seen if patients have diminished ability to concentrate urine secondary to an osmotic diuresis, central or nephrogenic diabetes insipidus, CRI, or malnutrition.[48] Marked oliguria typifies hepatorenal syndrome (HRS).[49]

Urinalysis

Urine specific gravity (SG) and osmolality provide measures of urinary concentration, which is impaired in the setting of tubular injury, as in ATN. A urine SG >1.020 or osmolality >500 mOsm/kg accompanying oliguria suggests PR ARF, whereas isosthenuria (SG of 1.010–1.012 or osmolality 300–350 mOsm/kg) is consistent with ATN or AIN.[42,50,51] These measures of urinary concentration are both sensitive to low-molecular-weight solutes and interfering substances such as contrast agents or glucose. CRI, hypokalemia, or loop diuretics may impair urinary concentration, resulting in a spuriously dilute urine despite hypovolemia. Conversely, acute GN or acute obstruction can each lead to concentrated urine in the absence of volume depletion.[52] By contrast, chronic obstruction usually results in isosthenuria.

Albuminuria or nonselective proteinuria connotes a defect in glomerular barrier function. Usual dipstick tests for proteinuria detect albumin selectively but vary in their sensitivity due to variation in urinary concentration. Dipstick tests are now available to assess ratios of urinary albumin to creatinine. Laboratory methods to detect all urinary proteins, e.g. sulfosalycilic acid, are required to detect immunoglobulin fragments, as in multiple myeloma. Proteinuria may be confirmed by assessment of the urine protein:creatinine ratio or total measurement in a timed urine specimen. Proteinuria is usually limited to <1 g/day in ATN.

Glomerular, vascular, interstitial, or lower urinary tract pathology may lead to hematuria. A UA positive for blood (heme) without hematuria suggests either hemoglobinuria or myoglobinuria; in the former, both plasma and urine are tinged pink.

Sediment analysis

Light microscopic examination of the urine sediment depends on a fresh, relatively concentrated urine and is often aided by staining of the sediment. Urinary cells and casts will disintegrate with time, perhaps contributing to the low diagnostic yield of routine urinalysis in the hospital laboratory.[53]

Nonglomerular bleeding results in relatively normal-appearing urinary erythrocytes, whereas dysmorphic red cells identify a glomerular source. AIN, papillary necrosis, and pyelonephritis may all lead to leukocyturia. Hyaline and granular casts may be seen in prerenal ARF, whereas broad casts (>3 white blood cells (WBCs) in diameter) suggest underlying CRI. Muddy brown tubular casts or free renal tubular epithelial cells are specific for ATN, but may be missed in 20–30% of ischemic ATN cases. GN, vasculitis, or, in some cases AIN, may all lead to red cell casts. Biopsy-proven GN without either urinary erythrocytes or red cell casts in a freshly voided specimen examined by a nephrologist is quite uncommon.[53] WBC casts can be associated with AIN, pyelonephritis, or with GN.

Uric acid crystals may be seen in any concentrated urine, but if numerous, uric acid nephropathy, tumor lysis syndrome, or other catabolic state should be considered. Oxalate crystals may accompany ethylene glycol intoxication. Sulfonamide, triamterene, or indinavir crystals suggest tubular obstruction by these agents.

Urine eosinophils are best visualized using Hansel's stain.[54] Eosinophiluria is associated with AIN, especially in a clinical presentation which includes an appropriately timed drug exposure, fever, and peripheral eosinophilia. However, eosinophiluria may also be observed in the setting of atheroembolic disease as well as in prostatitis, GN, or cystitis.[8,54]

Urine sodium concentration

The urine sodium concentration (urine [Na]) is typically low (<10–20 mEq/L) in HRS, PR ARF, and in GN. Urine [Na] >40 mEq/L is consistent with ATN or intrinsic renal disease, whereas a urine [Na] between 20 and 40 mEq/L is nonspecific.[42] As in the case of urinary concentration, urine [Na] may be <10 mEq/L in acute obstructive uropathy,[55] but high following chronic obstruction. Loop or thiazide diuretics may falsely elevate urine Na despite hypovolemia. Urine [Na] may also be elevated due to osmotic diuresis, salt-losing nephropathy, mineralocorticoid deficiency, or CRI. Conversely, a urine [Na] <10 mEq/L has been reported in cases of ATN due to myoglobinuria, hemoglobinuria, sepsis, cirrhosis, or radiocontrast agents, due apparently to renal vasoconstriction.[56–60] Patients with salt-avid states who develop ATN may continue to retain Na, suggesting nephron heterogeneity (obstructed or 'backleaking' tubules may not contribute to urine production, whereas less severely injured, salt-retaining tubules can produce urine with low sodium).[61]

FeNa

The fractional excretion of sodium (FeNa) describes the fraction of filtered Na that is excreted in the urine. It is used to compensate for variation in urine volume. FeNa is the amount of Na excreted (urine [Na] × urine flow) divided by the amount of Na filtered (plasma [Na] × GFR), which simplifies arithmetically to:

$$FeNa = \frac{U/P\ [Na]}{U/P\ [creat]} \times 100\%$$

FeNa may be more accurate than urine Na alone in discriminating between prerenal ARF and ATN. FeNa is generally low (<1%) in oliguric patients with prerenal states, where tubular reabsorption of sodium increases, and often >2% in ATN. Miller and colleagues prospectively evaluated 102 patients hospitalized with ARF and found an FeNa <1% in 94% of prerenal patients but in only 4% of ATN cases.[42] Patients who had received diuretics within 24 hours were excluded, as were patients with CRI, cirrhosis, adrenal insufficiency, and bicarbonaturia. However, as FeNa merely provides another measure of renal salt avidity, it is subject to the same diagnostic associations and pitfalls as is interpretation of urinary sodium concentration. It may be falsely elevated in patients with CRI, during an osmotic diuresis, or following either loop or thiazide diuretics. Filtered anions such as bicarbonate, beta lactams and ketoacids trap sodium in the tubular lumen, increasing its excretion; in these cases, urinary chloride concentration remains low (<15 mEq/L) and diagnostic of a PR state.[25,62,63]

FeUN

The fractional excretion of urea nitrogen (FeUN) has been proposed as a more sensitive and specific marker than FeNa of PR ARF, especially in patients who have received high doses of diuretics:

$$FeUN = \frac{U/P\ [UN]}{U/P\ [creat]} \times 100\%$$

The normal FeUN is 50–65%. Urea reabsorption is trivial in the thick ascending limb and distal convoluted tubule. Hypovolemia results in increased urea absorption, decreased urea clearance, and thus a lower FeUN.[64] Loop and thiazide diuretics, which act at the thick ascending limb and distal convoluted tubule, do not interfere directly with urea reabsorption and should not alter FeUN. However, proximal tubule diuretics and osmotic diuresis decrease proximal reabsorption of urea and may produce an inappropriately high FeUN.

Carvounis and coworkers prospectively evaluated 102 hospitalized patients referred for evaluation of ARF.[65] Patients were divided into three groups: 50 were deemed PR; 27 were deemed PR with diuretics given up to the day of consultation (details are not provided as to whether diuretics were given 1 or 23 hours prior to the urine sample); and 25 were diagnosed with ATN. Patients with AIN, GN, and obstructive nephropathy were excluded. FeNa was <1%, as expected, in 92% of group 1 patients, but in only 48% of the PR patients treated with diuretics. In contrast, 90% of the group 1 patients and 89% of those given diuretics had an FeUN <35%. The ATN patients evidenced a mean FeUN of 59%. An FeUN <35% had 85% sensitivity, 92% specificity, 99% positive predictive value, and 75% negative predictive value, for a PR state.[65]

Other urinary indices

Less commonly used urinary indices, such as the renal failure index (RFI), urine:plasma UN, urine:plasma creat, FeUricAcid, FeLi, and urine UA:creat, have been proposed to facilitate differentiation of PR ARF from ATN. The nonspecific RFI is essentially the FeNa, not indexed for serum Na; a value <1 is consistent with PR ARF, whereas a value >1 is consistent with ATN.[42] A urine to plasma urea nitrogen (urine:plasma UN) ratio >8[42] or >20[66] is consistent with a PR state, while ratios <3[42] or <10[66] suggest ATN. Urine to plasma creatinine ratios (urine:plasma creat) provide an alternative measure of urinary concentration, with ratios ≥40 suggesting PR ARF and ratios ≤20 consistent with intrinsic dysfunction.[65,67]

In tandem with FeNa and FeUN, the fractional excretion of uric acid (FeUricAcid) and of lithium (FeLi) decrease during volume contraction and rise during volume expansion. Uric acid is not reabsorbed beyond the proximal tubule, so that loop diuretics do not interfere with utility of FeUricAcid, though the sensitivity of this measure is limited.[68] In one study an FeLi value of <15% was 72% specific and 93% sensitive for PR ARF, and was not affected by loop or thiazide diuretics.[68] However, glucosuria, theophylline and proximally or distally acting diuretics may falsely elevate FeLi.

A study of five patients with acute uric acid nephropathy suggested that a urinary uric acid to creatinine concentration ratio (UA:creat) of >1 is consistent with this diagnosis.[69] Others, however, have found a urine UA:creat concentration ratio >1 in the absence of uric acid nephropathy, possibly related to increased catabolism.[70]

Markers to assess tubular injury

The physiologically based diagnostic strategies in current use and summarized above all focus on detecting decreased GFR and then determining, in oliguric patients, whether tubular function is well preserved, suggesting a physiologic response to renal hypoperfusion. These strategies will usually fail to detect ARF early following an insult, when intervention might be most beneficial, and are of but limited utility in patients with nonoliguric ATN. An alternative approach would be to detect markers of tubular injury, independent of resulting changes in renal function. A large, older literature suggested some utility in measuring tubular proteinuria, including markers such as β_2-microglobulin and urinary excretion of tubular brush border enzymes such as N-acetyl-β-D-glucosaminidase as markers of acute nephrotoxic injury.[71] More recently, the severity of tubular injury, as assessed by urinary excretion of CysC or α_1-microglobulin, has been suggested to correlate with clinical outcome in patients with nonoliguric ATN.[16]

An emerging literature has focused on measurement of the urinary kidney injury molecule 1 (Kim-1) as a selective and sensitive early marker of proximal tubular cell injury. Kim-1 is a type 1 transmembrane protein, with immunoglobulin and mucin domains, whose expression is markedly up-regulated in proximal tubular cells following experimental ischemia–reperfusion injury or nephrotoxin exposure in the rat.[72,73] Its ectodomain is shed from cells into urine and can be detected in patients with biopsy-proven ischemic ATN, though it seems of little utility in detection of other forms of ARF, including contrast nephropathy.[74] Whether other markers of tubular cell damage such as spermidine/spermine N-acetyltransferase or neutrophil gelatinase-associated lipocalin (NGAL), both of which allow early detection of ischemic tubular cell injury, will result in a clinically useful urinary diagnostic marker remains unknown.[75,76] Recent research has applied gene expression profiling and proteomic techniques to discover markers of nephrotoxicity. While clearly of benefit in assessing toxic mechanisms of environmental agents and pharmaceuticals, this strategy should lead to the identification of other candidate markers which may be of diagnostic utility in man.[76,77]

Imaging – ultrasound

The kidneys of most ARF patients should be imaged by US unless either ATN or PR causes are strongly suspected and obstruction seems very unlikely.[78] The major role for US is to detect obstruction, as hydronephrosis or collecting system dilation, in the setting of a suggestive history.[79] When clinical suspicion centers on lower urinary tract obstruction, catheterization to measure postvoiding residual urine volume may provide the same diagnostic insight as US. In one series of 192 patients with ARF, moderate-to-severe hydronephrosis was unrelated to obstruction in 11% of cases, whereas a false-negative rate of 0.5% was noted.[80] Normal pregnancy, cystic diseases, or brisk diuresis secondary to overhydration, medications, osmotic factors or nephrogenic diabetes insipidus can all lead to collecting system dilation in the absence of obstruction.[78,80–82] Conversely, US may fail to detect collecting system dilation early in the course of obstructive uropathy, or in volume-depleted patients with oliguria.[31,81,83–85] Maillet and coworkers noted that 4 of 80 patients with obstructive nephropathy failed to demonstrate US evidence of urinary tract dilation even, in one case, after 34 days of anuria.[85] Finally, dilation may be prevented if the ureters are encased, as by retroperitoneal fibrosis or by periureteral tumor.[83,84]

The kidneys of ARF patients are normal or slightly increased in size. Kidney size varies with body size, but a length of 10–12 cm is generally expected for adults of average height.[78] Large kidneys are occasionally seen in ATN and GN, whereas the kidneys in PR ARF are usually normal in size.[79,86] Asymmetric kidneys are suggestive of renal artery stenosis (RAS) or unilateral renal vein thrombosis; a >2 cm difference is abnormal.[78] Bilaterally, small kidneys suggest chronic renal disease.

In addition to assessing renal size and collecting system distension, US permits an assessment of echogenicity, reflecting increased interstitial fibrosis, density, and vascularity, and usually taken to reflect chronicity of underlying kidney disease. Normal renal cortex is less echogenic than liver after infancy.[78] However, the increased echogenicity common to CRI is observed occasionally in ARF and does not permit discrimination between various etiologies of renal failure.[78,79,86–88]

Ultrasound vascular evaluation

Estimates of renal vascular flow velocity by Doppler ultrasound may be useful in the diagnosis of RAS, renal vein or artery thrombosis, and renal infarction. Estimates of sensitivity of Doppler US for diagnosis of RAS range from 0 to 100%, and of specificity from 37 to 100%.[89] If RAS is strongly suspected, Doppler US may be insufficiently sensitive, warranting magnetic resonance angiography (MRA).[78] Elevated Doppler resistive indices provide a nonspecific measure of intrarenal vasoconstriction and have been observed in patients with ATN, AIN, HRS, rapidly progressive glomerulonephritis (RPGN), and HUS.[79,89]

Specific laboratory assays

Antinuclear antibodies, antibodies to double-stranded DNA, and serum complements should be measured if immune-mediated GN is suspected. Antineutrophil cytoplasmic antibodies can focus attention on vasculitis or pauci-immune GN. Antiglomerular basement membrane antibody titers can guide therapy in Goodpasture's syndrome. Complement levels are often low in rapidly progressive ARF due to systemic lupus erythematosus (SLE), severe postinfectious GN, and, occasionally, in atheroembolic disease. Antistreptolysin O titers may be elevated in 75% of patients with postinfectious GN following a streptococcal upper respiratory infection, though in only 40% following a streptococcal skin or soft tissue infection.[90]

Increased creatinine kinase or myoglobinuria point toward rhabdomyolysis. Peripheral eosinophilia is common in either AIN or atheroembolic disease. Serum and urine protein electrophoresis may be required to elucidate the etiology of ARF due to unsuspected multiple myeloma.

Imaging studies other than ultrasound

Evaluation of ARF rarely requires imaging other than US. Magnetic resonance imaging (MRI) or MRA may be used to diagnose renal vein thrombo-

sis and RAS.[78] Noninfused spiral computed tomography (CT) provides the gold standard for diagnosis of potentially obstructing kidney stones.[91] However, only retrograde pyelography and, in some cases, the response to ureteral stenting or percutaneous nephrostomy can definitively confirm or exclude the diagnosis of obstructive uropathy in difficult cases (e.g. extensive, encasing pelvic tumor).

Given their use of potentially nephrotoxic contrast, CT with contrast, angiography and pyelograms should be performed infrequently, and only when US, MR, or noncontrast CT results are equivocal. CT with contrast may be needed to evalute hydronephrosis in patients with renal cysts. Intravenous pyelogram (IVP) is highly sensitive and specific for hydronephrosis, and has been utilized to rule out obstruction if it is strongly suspected but not visualized on US.[83,85] Arteriography is used infrequently to evaluate the possibility of large- or medium-sized vessel vasculitis. Although Doppler ultrasound, MRI/MRA, and CT are used more frequently in evaluation of thromboembolic disease and acute cortical necrosis, renal venography provides the gold standard in diagnosing renal vein thrombosis.

Radionuclide scans using Tc 99m mercaptoacetyltriglycine (MAG3) can provide information on renal function and are commonly used to identify pathologic obstruction in the setting of ARF. However, both PR and intrarenal ARF can produce delayed intratubular excretion of radionuclide, limiting its diagnostic utility.

Renal biopsy

Indications for biopsy in the setting of ARF include diagnosis of suspected glomerular or microvascular disease, definitive diagnosis of AIN, or evaluation of patients with persisting undiagnosed ARF who might benefit from specific therapy.[92,93] Potential complications of renal biopsy include hematuria, leading to hypotension in 1–2% of cases, and to transfusion in 0.1–0.3% of cases. Percutaneous biopsy in the prone position has largely replaced open biopsy in critically ill intubated patients, and transjugular biopsy may provide an additional alternative in coagulopathic patients.[92,94]

CONCLUSION

In conclusion, a thorough history, physical examination, and record review are essential in making

Table 6.2 Typical laboratory assays and imaging seen in ATN, PR ARF, GN, HRS, AIN, and Post RF; for exceptions to these generalizations, please refer to text.

Assay	ATN	PR	GN	HRS	AIN	Post RF
BUN:creat	8:1	>20:1	8:1	8:1	8:1	8:1
Urine volume	Oliguric or nonoliguric	Oliguric	Nonoliguric, rarely anuric	Oliguric	Nonoliguric	Anuric, polyuric or alternation between two
Urine SG	1.010–1.012	>1.020	>1.020	>1.020	1.010	>1.020 acutely, <1.020 chronically
Urine osmolality (mOsm/kg)	<350	>500	>350	>350	<350	>400 acutely, 300 chronically
Sediment	Tubular cells, tubular casts, muddy brown granular casts	Bland; hyaline, granular casts	Dysmorphic RBCs, RBC casts, rare WBC casts	Bland; <50 RBCs/hpf, <500 mg protein/day	Eosinophils, WBCs, RBCs, WBC casts	Bland, occasional RBCs
Urinary Na	>40	<20	<20	<10	>40	<20 acutely, >40 chronically
FeNa	>2%	<1%	<1%	<1%	>2%	<1% acutely, >1% chronically
FeUN	>35%	<35%				
Urinary Cl	>15	<15				
Serum assays; symptoms	Nonspecific	Thirst, orthostatic symptoms	+ ANA, DS-DNA, ANCA, anti-GBM ab, ASO, C3, C4, CH50; rash, arthralgias, hemoptysis, sinus symptoms	Abnormal LFTs, serum Na <130; symptoms consistent with hepatic failure	Peripheral eosinphilia; fever, rash	Metabolic acidosis with high K and Cl if chronic
US	Normal or large-sized kidneys, at times with increased echogenicity	Normal in size, echogenicity	Sometimes enlarged with increased echogenicity	Increased resistive indices possible	Increased echogenicity possible	Dilated collecting system or hydronephrosis

ATN, acute tubular necrosis; PR, prerenal; GN, glomerulonephritis; HRS, hepatorenal syndrome; AIN, acute interstitial nephritis; BUN, blood urea nitrogen; RBC, red blood cells; WBC, white blood cells; Na, sodium; FeNa, fractional excretion of sodium; FeUN, fractional excretion of urea nitrogen, Cl, chloride; K, potassium; US, ultrasound.

the diagnosis of ARF. The multiple factors contributing to ARF in the ICU often prevent clear differentiation of ARF cases into prerenal, intrinsic, and postrenal ARF. Serum and urine assays as well as US may help in diagnosis (Table 6.2), but should be interpreted with caution. New approaches which focus on detecting renal parenchymal injury prior to evidence of severely decreased GFR will probably become key to early diagnosis and intervention for ARF occurring in the ICU setting.

REFERENCES

1. Brivet FG, Kleinknecht DJ, Loirat P, Landais PJ. Acute renal failure in intensive care units – causes, outcome, and prognostic factors of hospital mortality; A prospective, multicenter study. French Study Group on Acute Renal Failure. Crit Care Med 1996;24:192–8.
2. Groeneveld AB, Tran DD, van der Meulen J, Nauta JJ, Thijs LG. Acute renal failure in the medical intensive care unit: Predisposing, complicating factors and outcome. Nephron 1991;59:602–10.
3. Menashe PI, Ross SA, Gottlieb JE. Acquired renal insufficiency in critically ill patients. Crit Care Med 1988;16:1106–9.
4. Wilkins RG, Faragher EB. Acute renal failure in an intensive care unit: incidence, prediction and outcome. Anaesthesia 1983;38:628–34.
5. Bellomo R, Kellum JA, Ronco C. Defining acute renal failure: physiological principles. Intensive Care Med 2004;30:33–7.
6. Anderson RJ, Linas SL, Berns AS, et al. Nonoliguric acute renal failure. N Engl J Med 1977;296:1134–8.
7. Brady HR, Clarkson MR, Lieberthal W. Acute renal failure. In: Brenner BM, ed. The Kidney, 7th edn. Philadelphia: WB Saunders; 2004:1215–92.
8. Nolan CR, Anderson RJ. Hospital-acquired acute renal failure. J Am Soc Nephrol 1998;9:710–18.
9. Thadhani R, Pascual M, Bonventre JV. Acute renal failure. N Engl J Med 1996;334:1448–60.
10. Clark WR, Mueller BA, Kraus MA, Macias WL. Quantification of creatinine kinetic parameters in patients with acute renal failure. Kidney Int 1998;54:554–60.
11. Perrone RD, Madias NE, Levey AS. Serum creatinine as an index of renal function: new insights into old concepts. Clin Chem 1992;38:1933–53.
12. Shemesh O, Golbetz H, Kriss JP, Myers BD. Limitations of creatinine as a filtration marker in glomerulopathic patients. Kidney Int 1985;28:830–8.
13. Moran SM, Myers BD. Course of acute renal failure studied by a model of creatinine kinetics. Kidney Int 1985; 27:928–37.
14. Doolan PD, Alpen EL, Theil GB. A clinical appraisal of the plasma concentration and endogenous clearance of creatinine. Am J Med 1962;32:65–79.
15. Laterza OF, Price CP, Scott MG. Cystatin C: an improved estimator of glomerular filtration rate? Clin Chem 2002;48:699–707.
16. Herget-Rosenthal S, Poppen D, Husing J, et al. Prognostic value of tubular proteinuria and enzymuria in nonoliguric acute tubular necrosis. Clin Chem 2004;50:552–8.
17. Dharnidharka VR, Kwon C, Stevens G. Serum cystatin C is superior to serum creatinine as a marker of kidney function: A meta-analysis. Am J Kidney Dis 2002;40:221–6.
18. Newman DJ, Thakkar H, Edwards RG, et al. Serum cystatin C measured by automated immunoassay: a more sensitive marker of changes in GFR than serum creatinine. Kidney Int 1995;47:312–18.
19. Uhlmann EJ, Hock KG, Issitt C, et al. Reference intervals for plasma cystatin C in healthy volunteers and renal patients, as measured by the Dade Behring BN II system, and correlation with creatinine. Clin Chem 2001;47:2031–3.
20. Coll E, Botey A, Alvarez L, et al. Serum cystatin C as a new marker for noninvasive estimation of glomerular filtration rate and as a marker for early renal impairment. Am J Kidney Dis 2000;36:29–34.
21. Fliser D, Ritz E. Serum cystatin C concentration as a marker of renal dysfunction in the elderly. Am J Kidney Dis 2001;37:79–83.
22. Orlando R, Mussap M, Plebani M, et al. Diagnostic value of plasma cystatin C as a glomerular filtration marker in decompensated liver cirrhosis. Clin Chem 2002;48:850–8.
23. Rickli H, Benou K, Ammann P, et al. Time course of serial cystatin C levels in comparison with serum creatinine after application of radiocontrast media. Clin Nephrol 2004;61:98–102.
24. Delanaye P, Lambermont B, Chapelle JP, et al. Plasmatic cystatin C for the estimation of glomerular filtration rate in intensive care units. Intensive Care Med 2004;30:980–3.
25. Abuelo JG. Diagnosing vascular causes of acute renal failure. Ann Int Med 1995;123:601–14.
26. Brady HR, Singer GS. Acute renal failure. Lancet 1995;346:1533–40.
27. Hou SH, Bushinsky DA, Wish JB, Cohen JJ, Harrington JT. Hospital-acquired renal insufficiency: a prospective study. Am J Med 1983;74:243–8.
28. Anderson RJ, Schrier RW. Acute renal failure. In: Schrier RW, ed. Diseases of the Kidney and Urinary Tract, 7th edn. Philadelphia: Lippincott, Williams and Wilkins; 2001:Chapter 41.
29. Liano F, Junco E, Pascual J, Madero R, Verde E. The spectrum of acute renal failure in the intensive care unit compared with that seen in other settings. The Madrid Acute Renal Failure Study Group. Kidney Int 1998:53,(Suppl):S16–24.
30. Johnson DC, Anderson RJ. Acute renal failure, part 2: zeroing in on the diagnosis. J Crit Illness, 2002;17:301–5.
31. Faber MD, Kupin WL, Krishna GG, Narins RG. The differential diagnosis of acute renal failure. In: Lazarus JM, Brenner BM, eds. Acute Renal Failure, 3rd edn. New York: Churchill Livingstone; 1993:133–92.
32. Liano F, Pascual J. Epidemiology of acute renal failure: a prospective, multicenter community-based study. The Madrid Acute Renal Failure Study Group. Kidney Int 1996;50:811–18.
33. Davidman M, Olson P, Kohen J, Leither T, Kjellstrand C. Iatrogenic renal disease. Arch Int Med 1991;151:1809–12.
34. Rasmussen HH, Ibels LS. Acute renal failure: multivariate analysis of causes and risk factors. Am J Med 1982;73:211–18.
35. Humes HD. Aminoglycoside nephrotoxicity. Kidney Int 1988;13:900–11.
36. Han JS, Kim YS, Chin HJ, et al. Temporal changes and reversibility of carbamylated hemoglobin in renal failure. Am J Kidney Dis 1997;30:36–40.
37. Stim J, Shaykh M, Anwar F, et al. Factors determining hemoglobin carbamylation in renal failure. Kidney Int 1995;48:1605–10.
38. McGee S, Abernethy WB 3rd, Simel DL. The rational clinical examination: Is this patient hypovolemic? JAMA 1999;281:1022–9.
39. Opravil M, Keusch G, Luthy R. Pyrimethamine inhibits renal secretion of creatinine. Antimicrob Agents Chemother 1993;37:1056–60.
40. Jurado R, Mattix H. The decreased serum urea nitrogen-creatinine ratio. Arch Int Med 1998;158:2509–11.

41. Anderson RJ. Clinical and laboratory diagnosis of acute renal failure. In: Molitoris BA, Finn WF, eds. Acute Renal Failure: a companion to Brenner & Rector's The Kidney, 1st edn. Philadelphia: WB Saunders; 2001.

42. Miller TR, Anderson RJ, Linas SL, et al. Urinary diagnostic indices in acute renal failure: a prospective study. Ann Intern Med 1978;89:47–50.

43. Humphreys BD, Sharman JP, Henderson JM, et al. Gemcitabine-associated thrombotic microangiopathy. Cancer 2004;100:2664–70.

44. Pisoni R, Ruggenenti P, Remuzzi G. Drug-induced thrombotic microangiopathy: incidence, prevention and management. Drug Saf 2001;24:491–501.

45. Kasinath BS, Corwin HL, Bidani AK, et al. Eosinophilia in the diagnosis of atheroembolic renal disease. Am J Nephrol 1987;7:173–7.

46. Klahr S, Miller SB. Acute oliguria. N Engl J Med 1998;338:671–5.

47. Harrington JT, Cohen JJ. Acute oliguria. N Engl J Med 1975;292:89–91.

48. Miller PD, Krebs RA, Neal BJ, McIntyre DO. Polyuric prerenal failure. Arch Int Med 1980;140:907–9.

49. Gines P, Arroyo V. Hepatorenal syndrome. J Am Soc Nephrol 1999;10:1833–9.

50. Lins RL, Verpooten GA, De Clerck DS, De Broe ME. Urinary indices in acute interstitial nephritis. Clin Nephrol 1986;26:131–3.

51. Liano F, Gamez C, Pascual J, et al. Use of urinary parameters in the diagnosis of total acute renal artery occlusion. Nephron 1994;66:170–5.

52. Hilton PJ, Jones NF, Barraclough MA, Lloyd-Davies RW. Urinary osmolality in acute renal failure due to glomerulonephritis. Lancet 1969;2:655–6.

53. Goorno W, Ashworth CT, Carter NW. Acute glomerulonephritis with absence of abnormal urinary findings. Diagnosis by light and electron microscopy. Ann Int Med 1967;66:345–53.

54. Nolan CR 3rd, Anger MS, Kelleher SP. Eosinophiluria – a new method for detection and definition of the clinical spectrum. N Engl J Med 1986;315:1516–19.

55. Hoffman L, Suki WN. Obstructive uropathy mimicking volume depletion. JAMA 1976;236(18):2096–7.

56. Corwin HL, Schreiber MJ, Fang LS. Low fractional excretion of sodium: occurrence with hemoglobinuric- and myoglobinuric-induced acute renal failure. Arch Int Med 1984;144:981–2.

57. Steiner RW. Low fractional excretion of sodium in myoglobinuric renal failure. Arch Int Med 1982;142:1216–17.

58. Vaz AJ. Low fractional excretion of urinary sodium in acute renal failure due to sepsis. Arch Int Med 1983;143:738–9.

59. Diamond JR, Yoburn DC. Nonoliguric acute renal failure associated with a low fractional excretion of sodium. Ann Int Med 1982;96:597–600.

60. Fang LS, Sirota RA, Ebert TH, Lichtenstein NS. Low fractional excretion of sodium with contrast media-induced acute renal failure. Arch Int Med 1980;140:531–3.

61. Zarich S, Fang LS, Diamond JR. Fractional excretion of sodium: exceptions to its diagnostic value. Arch Int Med 1985;145:108–12.

62. Nanji AJ. Increased fractional excretion of sodium in prerenal azotemia: need for careful interpretation. Clin Chem 1981;27:1314–15.

63. Anderson RJ, Gabow PA, Gross PA. Urinary chloride concentration in acute renal failure. Miner Electrolyte Metab 1984;10:92–7.

64. Goldstein MH, Lenz PR, Levitt MF. Effect of urine flow rate on urea reabsorption in man: urea as a 'tubular marker'. J Appl Physiol 1969;26:594–9.

65. Carvounis CP, Nisar S, Guro-Razuman S. Significance of the fractional excretion of urea in the differential diagnosis of acute renal failure. Kidney Int 2002;62:2223–9.

66. Perlmutter M. Urine-serum urea nitrogen ratio: simple test of renal function in acute azotemia and oliguria. JAMA 1959;170:1533–7.

67. Albright RC. Acute renal failure: a practical update. Mayo Clin Proc 2001;76:67–74.

68. Steinhauslin F, Burnier M, Magnin JL, et al. Fractional excretion of trace lithium and uric acid in acute renal failure. J Am Soc Nephrol 1994;4:1429–37.

69. Kelton J, Kelley WN, Holmes EW. A rapid method for diagnosis of acute uric acid nephropathy. Arch Int Med 1978;138:612–15.

70. Tungsanga K, Boonwichit D, Lekhakula A, Sitprija V. Urine uric acid and urine creatinine ratio in acute renal failure. Arch Int Med 1984;144:934–7.

71. Gibey R, Dupond JL, Alber D, et al. Predictive value of urinary N-acetyl-beta-D-glucosaminidase (NAG), alanine–aminopeptidase (AAP) and beta-2–microglobulin (beta2M) in evaluating nephrotoxicity of gentamicin. Clin Chim Acta 1981;116:25–34.

72. Ichimura T, Bonventre JV, Bailly V, et al. Kidney injury molecule-1 (KIM-1), a putative epithelial cell adhesion molecule containing a novel immunoglobulin domain, is up-regulated in renal cells after injury. J Biol Chem 1998;273:4135–42.

73. Ichimura T, Hung CC, Yang SA, Stevens JL, Bonventre JV. Kidney injury molecule-1: a tissue and urinary biomarker for nephro-toxicant-induced renal injury. Am J Physiol 2004;286:F552–63.

74. Han WK, Bailly V, Abichandani R, Thadhani R, Bonventre JV. Kidney injury molecule-1 (KIM-1): a novel biomarker for human renal proximal tubule injury. Kidney Int 2002;62:237–44.

75. Zahedi K, Wang Z, Barone S, et al. Expression of SSAT, a novel biomarker of tubular cell damage, increases in kidney ischemia-reperfusion injury. Am J Physiol 2003;284:F1046–55.

76. Mishra J, Dent C, Tarabishi R, et al. Neutrophil gelatinase-associated lipocalin (NGAL) as a biomarker for acute renal injury after cardiac surgery. Lancet 2005;365:1231–8.

77. Amin RP, Vickers AE, Sistare F, et al. Identification of putative gene based markers of renal toxicity. Environ Health Perspect 2004;112:465–79.

78. O'Neill WC. Sonographic evaluation of renal failure. Am J Kidney Dis 2000;35(6):1021–38.

79. Mucelli RP, Bertolotto M. Imaging techniques in acute renal failure. Kidney Int 1998;53(suppl):S102–5.

80. Amis ES Jr, Cronan JJ, Pfister RC, Yoder IC. Ultrasonic inaccuracies in diagnosing renal obstruction. Urology 1982;19:101–5.

81. Webb JA. Ultrasonography in the diagnosis of renal obstruction. BMJ 1990;301:944–6.

82. Stevens S, Brown BD, McGahan JP. Nephrogenic diabetes insipidus: a cause of severe nonobstructive urinary tract dilation. J Ultrasound Med 1995;14:543–5.

83. Rascoff JH, Golden RA, Spinowitz BS, Charytan C. Nondilated obstructive nephropathy. Arch Int Med 1983;143:696–8.

84. Jeffrey RB, Federle MP. CT and ultrasonography of acute renal abnormalities. Radiol Clin North Am 1983;21:515–25.

85. Maillet PJ, Pelle-Francoz D, Laville M, Gay F, Pinet A. Nondilated obstructive acute renal failure: diagnostic procedures and therapeutic management. Radiology 1986;160:659–62.

86. Manley JA, O'Neill WC. Sonographic abnormalities in acute tubular necrosis and prerenal azotemia. J Am Soc Nephrol 2000;11:131A.

87. Hricak H, Cruz C, Romanski R, et al. Renal parenchymal disease: sonographic-histologic correlation. Radiology 1982;144:141–7.

88. Huntington DK, Hill SC, Hill MC. Sonographic manifestations of medical renal disease. Semin Ultrasound CT MR 1991;12:290–307.

89. Stevens PE. Doppler ultrasound in renal disease: not quite 'the answer to a maiden's prayer'. Ren Fail 1995;17:89–100.

90. Mason PD, Pusey CD. Glomerulonephritis: diagnosis and treatment. BMJ 1994;309:1557–63.
91. Vieweg J, Teh C, Freed K, et al. Unenhanced helical computerized tomography for the evaluation of patients with acute flank pain. J Urol 1998;160:679–84.
92. Conlon PJ, Kovalik E, Schwab SJ. Percutaneous renal biopsy of ventilated intensive care unit patients. Clin Nephrol 1995;43:309–11.
93. Wilson DM, Turner DR, Cameron JS, et al. Value of renal biopsy in acute intrinsic renal failure. BMJ 1976;2:459–61.
94. Mal F, Meyrier A, Callard P, et al. The diagnostic yield of transjugular renal biopsy. Experience with 200 cases. Kidney Int 1992;41:445–9.

7

Physiologic basis for pulmonary–renal syndromes

John Hotchkiss and Hamid Rabb

Kidney dysfunction is often accompanied by dysfunction of other organs in the critical care scenario. Lung dysfunction is particularly common, and astute clinicians have observed for some time that there seems to be a predisposition to combined lung and kidney dysfunction. Accordingly, an intimate knowledge of normal lung structure, as well as normal and pathologic lung function, aids in understanding the complex interactions between these organs. In this chapter, we cover those aspects of lung physiology most germane to the setting of renal compromise, and then turn to specific renal processes as archetypes for each potential pathway of adverse interaction. This 'physiology-based' approach will provide a broader context in which to view kidney–lung interactions.

Renal failure can induce or aggravate lung dysfunction; conversely, lung damage, particularly in the setting of mechanical ventilation, can worsen renal performance. The pathways of communication in these settings include 'pure' hemodynamic effects (decreased renal perfusion due to mechanical ventilation or pulmonary compromise due to elevated intravascular pressure). There may be communication via bloodborne mediators (including activated cells, bacteria/bacterial products, cytokines or hormones, and gas) that can operate in either direction. Finally, a given 'pulmonary renal syndrome' may represent simultaneous response to common antigens within both tissue beds (or erroneously targeted immunologic activity) arising from a specific underlying disease process, either autoimmune, infectious, or toxin-related (Table 7.1).

Table 7.1 Major nonmechanical processes associated with significant simultaneous pulmonary and renal compromise.

Rheumatologic	Infectious
Goodpasture's disease	Systemic inflammatory response to sepsis (SIRS)
ANCA-positive vasculitides:	Legionella
Wegener's granulomatosis	Bacterial endocarditis (especially right-sided)
Periarteritis nodosa	Cytomegalovirus
Churg–Strauss granulomatosis	Leptospirosis
Systemic lupus erythematosus	Human immunodeficiency virus
Scleroderma	Hantavirus
Rheumatoid arthritis	
Sjögren's syndrome	

LUNG PHYSIOLOGY AND PULMONARY INJURY

Normal lung structure and function

Airspaces

The lung's primary function is as an organ for the absorption of oxygen and elimination of CO_2, which mandates the presentation of a large airspace surface in intimate contact with an (equally large) vascular surface to afford maximally efficient diffusion. The arrangement of the airways and terminal airspaces as a repeatedly branching network with the predominance of exchange surfaces presented within the most distal generations is an extremely efficient mechanism for gas transport to a large contained surface area. The airways terminate in exchange surfaces within the alveoli and terminal alveolar ducts, which are lined with two cell populations responsible for much of the functional behavior of the lung. Alveolar type I cells, the predominant cell type by area, primarily serve a barrier function. Alveolar type II cells, a much smaller population, synthesize surfactant (vide infra), provide a precursor population for re-epithelialization of the alveolus, and serve transport functions. Resident macrophages within the alveoli serve important defensive functions and may promote inflammation or fibrosis in the setting of acute lung injury.

Pulmonary vasculature

Blood flows to the lungs across two distinct circulatory pathways: the pulmonary circulation and the bronchial circulation. The bronchial circulation arises from the systemic arterial blood supply, and constitutes a high-pressure nutrient circuit, particularly for the conducting airways. The bronchial circulation is a potential site of pulmonary hemorrhage (in the setting of mycobacterial disease, for instance), and an alternative source of blood flow in the setting of pulmonary circuit occlusion.

The pulmonary circulation, in contrast, is a low-pressure exchange circuit with a geometric arrangement suited to maximize contact surface area between the blood and air compartments.[1] Right ventricular output flows down a progressively branching vascular pathway and through an alveolar capillary network, which shares a common basement membrane with the alveolar epithelial cells and is in such close apposition to the pulmonary airspaces that it may properly be considered a capillary sheet. The capillary sheet then drains into the pulmonary venous circulation and left atrium. Smaller pulmonary arteries and veins pass through the pulmonary interstitial spaces, effectively 'between' the alveoli. The interstitial course of these smaller vessels has important implications for fluid balance, as will be discussed below.[2-6] The pulmonary vasculature is far from an inert conduit, however. Pulmonary vascular tone and metabolic activity are modulated by catecholamines, cytokines, arachidonic acid metabolites, nitric oxide, and acid–base status, among other factors.[7-10] Moreover, the large surface area of the endothelium presents a number of catalytic enzyme activities, the most familiar of which is the serine protease angiotensin-converting enzyme (ACE), which also plays an important role in kinin metabolism. Less familiar are steroid hormone activities for interconversion of androgens and environmental phytoestrogens, for example.[11]

As pulmonary fluid balance generally leads to ultrafiltration of plasma into the pulmonary interstitium, lymphatic drainage of the interstitium may assume considerable importance. Lymphatic flow can be substantially increased in the face of chronic 'ultrafiltration overload', a physiologic adaptation that may allow tolerance of vascular filtration pressures, which may threaten functional integrity if applied acutely.

Ventilation–perfusion matching

Efficient gas exchange by the lung is critically dependent on appropriate matching between the distribution of ventilation (V) and the distribution of perfusion (Q). In the absence of such matching, underventilated or unventilated lung regions that receive significant perfusion represent 'wasted' perfusion and compromise the efficiency of gas exchange.[12,13] In general, there is a reasonable matching between the regional levels of alveolar ventilation and perfusion. As 'V/Q mismatch' develops, underventilated regions of the lung receive more perfusion, while well-ventilated regions with more effective alveolar gas exchange receive less of the pulmonary blood flow. The overall effect is to decrease the effectiveness of the lung as an organ of gas exchange.[14-16] In the most extreme form, consolidated, atelectatic, or fluid-filled lung zones receive significant perfusion. Without exposure to 'fresh' gas, this blood effectively represents a direct right-to-left shunt ('venous admixture'); the sigmoidal shape of the oxyhemoglobin O_2 content curve precludes 'compensation' by well-ventilated but underperfused lung units, and the arterial oxygenation may deteriorate dramatically. The normal lung maintains proper V:Q matching at least in part through hypoxic vasoconstriction (pH also plays a role), processes which may be overcome by disease or drugs.

Resident nonpulmonary cells

An important consideration in pulmonary pathology is the sequestration within the lung of large numbers of defensive cells with immunologic or inflammatory potential. Although a high density of inflammatory/immune cells is teleologically reasonable in view of the lung's potential attack by inhaled pathogens, the presence of a large population of potentially pro-inflammatory cells also creates the potential for lung damage due to overexuberant induction of inflammatory responses. The clinical relevance of this concern is seen most clearly in the profound lung injury which may attend recovery from neutropenia in patients treated for malignancies.[17–19] Perhaps the most important populations are those sequestered within the pulmonary vasculature and alveolar macrophages. The pulmonary capillary 'sheet' is of a dimension and configuration such that leukocytes, particularly neutrophils, must 'deform' to pass through to the pulmonary venous circulation.[20–23] Activated neutrophils, by virtue of actin polymerization and cytoplasmic 'stiffening', are unable to deform adequately, and are trapped within the pulmonary circulation. Neutrophil–endothelial adhesion contributes further to such sequestration; approximately 50% of the 'circulation' leukocytes are sequestered within the pulmonary vasculature. Similarly, intra-alveolar macrophages, in addition to their role in pathogen clearance, may play a significant role in lung injury and/or maladaptive repair and fibrosis.

Pulmonary fluid handling: filtration

Perhaps the most important aspect of normal lung function from the standpoint of kidney–lung interaction revolves around the pulmonary handling of fluid. The massive surface area of the blood compartment – airspace interface – and its obligate anatomic 'thinness', place the interstitium and alveolar spaces at risk of flooding from fluid filtration. Many clinically relevant processes increase the hydrostatic pressure for ultrafiltration, increase barrier fluid permeability, or both. Ultrafiltration within the lung is governed by Starling's law; the relatively high permeability of the filtration barrier to albumin increases the influence of hydrostatic pressures, potentially obligating substantial lymphatic drainage. Pulmonary fluid filtration may

occur across alveolar capillaries, small, precapillary interstitial vessels, and postcapillary interstitial vessels. The latter pathways may assume relatively more importance in the setting of lung injury.[6] In general, the effective filtration pressure is taken as the pressure within the intermediate segment, a conceptual physiologic 'compartment' which includes the alveolar capillary bed. Intermediate segment filtration pressure, which drives fluid filtration, is most often estimated using the pulmonary double occlusion technique. The effective intravascular hydraulic filtration pressure is determined by left atrial pressure, pulmonary blood flow, and the relative resistances of the precapillary, capillary, and postcapillary segments.[24–26] Juxtavascular interstitial pressures may also contribute to fluid filtration dynamics, particularly under pathologic circumstances (vide infra).[2–6] Under normal circumstances, filtered fluid that is not actively reabsorbed generally passes predominantly into the interstitium, thence into lymphatics.

Pulmonary fluid handling: reabsorption

Given the propensity of the pulmonary vasculature to form ultrafiltrate, and the frequency of potentially deleterious increases in pulmonary microvascular pressures, pulmonary permeability, or both, the pathways for fluid reabsorption assume considerable importance. The initial 'line of defense' resides in the capacity for augmentation of lymphatic drainage, which is considerable. However, beyond a 'critical content' of lung water, interstitial overload and subsequent alveolar flooding occur; moreover, there may be activation of degradative enzymes, leading to directly weakened ground substance.[27] Alveolar fluid reabsorption is an energetically demanding process in which sodium enters alveolar epithelia via the amiloride-sensitive sodium channel, and is 'pumped' into the interstitium by the sodium–potassium ATPase. Water follows passively down an osmotic gradient.[28–30] Inhibition of the Na channel markedly increases effective pulmonary fluid permeability in the setting of ischemia–reperfusion lung injury.[31] As will be discussed below, 'flooding' has significant deleterious consequences beyond its direct effect to compromise pulmonary gas exchange.

Dynamics during lung inflation

Alveolar mechanics

With the exception of the heart, the lung is unique in the dynamic geometric changes it undergoes in the course of normal function. The lung's function as a gas exchange organ mandates a thin barrier between the alveolar airspaces and the blood compartment. The fluid phase covering the otherwise naked epithelial air side barrier creates an air–liquid interface, an entity introducing the effects of surface tension into the function of the lung.[32,33] If unimpeded, the effects of surface tension on pulmonary dynamics would promote airspace collapse at low lung volumes, and increase the pressure required to inflate the lung. Surfactant, synthesized by type II alveolar cells, substantially obviates these effects by reducing alveolar surface tension. The surfactant-induced reduction in surface tension has several salutary effects. It decreases the likelihood of airspace collapse at low lung volumes and decreases the pressure required to inflate the lung within the midrange of lung volumes. Moreover, the reduction in surface tension afforded by surfactant decreases negative interstitial and interfacial pressures across pulmonary vessels, lowering the transvascular gradient for fluid filtration.[33] Finally, under normal circumstances, a significant fraction of the energy expended in lung inflation is dissipated within the surfactant layer; surfactant and surface tension within the alveoli may actually act as a 'load-bearing' element within the lung. Often observed in the clinical setting, inactivation of surfactant can have significant consequences for lung mechanics, fluid dynamics, as well as alveolar and vascular stresses.

Vascular mechanics
Airspace inflation has profound effects on the pulmonary vasculature, effects which are significantly modulated by the presence and activity of surfactant.[32] Airspace inflation directly compresses the alveolar capillary compartment, with the exception of 'alveolar corner vessels', an effect which increases intermediate segment resistance.[24–26] Under certain circumstances, lengthening of pulmonary vessels may further elevate total pulmonary vascular resistance.[26] The effects of lung inflation on extra-alveolar/interstitial vessels differs markedly from the compressive effect observed in the capillary sheet. As the lung inflates, perivascular interstitial pressure declines, and may fall below pleural pressure.[2–5] This effectively negative perivascular pressure increases both vascular stress and the hydraulic gradient for fluid filtration by augmenting the transvascular pressure gradient. Decreased surfactant activity, common in the clinical setting, increases the trans-

mission of alveolar surface stress to the interstitial compartment, where it serves to drop interstitial pressure further below pleural pressure, thereby increasing transvascular stresses.[33] Paradoxically, then, airspace inflation may decrease the transvascular stress on the alveolar capillary membrane, but increase the stress and filtration pressure across extra-alveolar vessels.[34]

Many clinically relevant conditions directly affect pulmonary barrier function. These effects uniformly compromise pulmonary fluid handling, either by increasing pulmonary permeability, or through interference with salt and water reabsorption. A common clinical scenario is that of increased pulmonary fluid permeability that arises as a consequence of inflammation, either systemic (as in sepsis) or local (as with severe pneumonia or local inflammation).[35–37] Elevated intravascular pressures, attendant to markedly elevated cardiac output or left atrial pressures, have been shown to promote capillary rupture, epithelial cell delamination, and increases in erythrocyte, protein, and water permeability in animal models.[38–45] A possible human correlate of such hemodynamically induced structural damage is the observation of increased alveolar erythrocytes and protein in elite athletes undergoing maximal aerobic efforts.[46] Overt capillary rupture may also arise from elevated airspace pressures in the context of increased vascular pressure, as may occur in humans during mechanical ventilation.[47] Finally, compromised activity of alveolar fluid reabsorptive mechanisms may contribute to alveolar flooding; the ability to reabsorb alveolar fluid has been shown to correlate inversely with mortality in the clinical setting.[48] Whatever the underlying mechanism, the resulting accumulation of fluid and/or protein in alveolar spaces may inactivate surfactant, increase surface tension, promote inflammation, and accelerate further flooding, creating a vicious cycle of lung injury.[33,48–51] Moreover, the presence of alveolar 'rents' raises the possibility of direct transfer of bacteria, bacterial product, or even air into the systemic arterial circulation, with attendant deleterious consequences on remote organs.[52–54]

Abnormal mechanics
The injured lung displays a number of mechanical derangements which directly compromise pulmonary function and promote further lung injury. Acute lung injury and acute respiratory distress syndrome (ARDS) are surprisingly nonhomogeneous processes, with a predominance of consolidation and alveolar flooding observed in the

dependent lung zones.[55,56] These airless lung regions elevate the shunt fraction and compromise efficiency of oxygenation. In addition, much recent interest has focused on the phenomenon of pulmonary derecruitment/recruitment, in which alveolar airspaces collapse during expiration and are forcibly reopened during lung inflation.[57,58] Although not all authorities subscribe to the concept of derecruitment, its advocates have focused on the potential for repeated cycles of 'opening and collapse' to augment lung injury via increased mechanical stress loads and induction of inflammatory mediators; the latter may also compromise remote organs.[59–66] Even absent cyclic collapse and re-expansion of alveoli, the predominantly dependent consolidation or alveolar flooding (dorsal in the supine position) results in a 'baby lung' of decreased capacity to accept inflation volume; attempts to maintain normal blood gas tensions (especially CO_2) may expose the remaining normal lung to unacceptably high levels of mechanical stress and/or promote cytokine release.[64]

Pulmonary vascular compromise

In addition to derangements of barrier function and airspace mechanics, the injured or diseased lung may display functional abnormalities which arise primarily from interference with normal patterns of pulmonary perfusion. The most overt example of such a process is pulmonary thromboembolism. Here, both structural occlusion due to the thrombus and mediator release (such as serotonin) interfere with the normal pattern and regulation of pulmonary perfusion and ventilation–perfusion matching, producing V/Q mismatch and decreasing the efficiency of gas exchange.[67,68] Consolidative processes – pneumonia, hemorrhage, alveolar edema, or the dependent regions of ARDS-afflicted lungs – increase the shunt fraction, compromising oxygenation to a greater extent than CO_2 removal. Disordered regulation of vascular tone, with inappropriate perfusion of consolidated or underventilated lung regions may result from sepsis.[69–71] Deliberate manipulation of pulmonary vascular tone with inhaled nitric oxide or prostacyclin has been advocated as a technique to improve V:Q matching; conversely, administration of such pulmonary vasodilators from the blood side (as with intravenous nitrates or prostacyclin) can overcome hypoxic vasoconstriction and worsen V:Q matching.

Mechanisms of renal disease-associated lung dysfunction

Elevated vascular pressure

Of the multiple mechanisms by which renal disease may compromise lung integrity, the simplest relates to pulmonary vascular pressures. As noted above, marked elevations of pulmonary vascular pressures can directly damage the pulmonary filtration barrier. Severe left atrial/pulmonary venous hypertension may be observed with volume overload, diastolic dysfunction, or acute severe elevations in systemic vascular resistance. Even in the absence of pressure-induced vascular fracturing or delamination, increased vascular pressure and the attendant elevation in ultrafiltration may lead to alveolar flooding; if significant protein also enters the airspaces, surfactant may be inactivated with deleterious consequences on lung mechanics and fluid clearance.[49,50] The combination of surfactant inactivation, interstitial edema, and 'alveolar space filling' will diminish gas exchange efficiency, promoting dyspnea and hypoxia in the spontaneously breathing patient. In the mechanically ventilated patient, such effects may predispose to ventilator-induced lung injury.

Humoral/immunologic factors

Recent experimental evidence suggests a potential role for the uremic milieu in the development or excerbation of lung injury and dysfunction.[72,73] In animal models, acute renal failure increases pulmonary protein permeability and alveolar hemorrhage, an effect which may be partially blocked through macrophage pacification. Decreased activity of a number of important alveolar membrane channels – epithelial sodium channel (ENaC) aquaporin-1 and (AQ1) – is also seen in this setting; as noted above, decrements in ENaC increase susceptibility to ischemia–reperfusion injury.[31] Further, blockade of AQ activity increases susceptibility to ventilator-induced lung.[74] The elevated nitric oxide production attendant to severe renal failure may increase the potential for peroxynitrite-induced lung damage; increased bronchoalveolar lavage nitric oxide content appears to correlate with severity of lung injury in an animal model, although causality is uncertain.[75,76] Finally, the prooxidant environment prevalent in renal failure may predispose to lung injury from otherwise innocuous stimuli, and has the potential to interfere with surfactant activity, production, or both.

Immunologic and cellular processes affecting the kidney may also directly affect the lung. The large vascular surface areas common to both organs afford ample 'targets' for such overlap; moreover, the kidney and lung share important antigenic characteristics. This is most clear in the setting of Goodpasture's disease, in which immunologic attack on the NC-1 domain of type IV collagen (a shared kidney/lung antigen) leads to vascular damage in both organs. Similarly, antineutrophil cytoplasmic antibody (ANCA)-positive vasculitides, systemic lupus erythematosus (SLE), cryoglobulinemia, and antiphospholipid antibody syndrome may each injure vascular beds within both kidney and lung, although the mechanisms attendant to these processes are less clear than those in Goodpasture's disease. To the extent that acute or chronic renal failure increases leukocyte cytoplasmic 'stiffness', the uremic or azotemic patient may sequester relatively more leukocytes within the pulmonary vasculature and thus be predisposed to more dramatic inflammation-associated lung injury.[77]

Intradialytic changes

Critically ill patients with acute renal failure often require renal replacement therapy, either intermittent or continuous (CRRT). Such therapy can have significant detrimental effects on the lung. It has been known for many years that dialysis against complement inactivating, 'bioincompatible' membranes can promote pulmonary leukocyte sequestration and dysfunction. More recent evidence indicates that even biocompatible membranes, as used in CRRT, may activate platelets and macrophages.[78–83] Activated macrophages and/or platelets may subsequently contribute to injury of remote organs, including the lung. Because of its position within the circulation, the lung is the vascular bed most directly susceptible to cells activated within the venous circulation, small air emboli, or products derived from activation of the coagulation or kallikrein cascades.

SPECIFIC PULMONARY–RENAL SYNDROMES

Kidney–lung and ventilator–kidney interactions

The combination of acute renal failure and requirement for mechanical ventilation is known to be particularly lethal, with a mortality rate from 70 to 90%. As noted previously, acute renal failure itself may directly compromise pulmonary integrity. In addition, many of the same 'mechanisms' may increase the likelihood of structural damage arising from mechanical ventilation (ventilator-induced lung injury or VILI). Any of the factors increasing pulmonary vascular permeability or pulmonary vascular pressures, impairing clearance mechanisms, or affecting the inflammatory milieu of the lung will accentuate ventilator-induced mechanical damage. Moreover, patients with underlying metabolic acidosis may be exposed to excessive ventilatory pressures or frequencies in an attempt to normalize pH or pCO_2; such correction to 'normal' may also accentuate lung injury.[75,84]

Conversely, mechanical ventilation can significantly contribute to renal compromise. To the extent they are transmitted to the juxtacardiac region, elevated intrathoracic pressures due to positive airway pressure will compromise venous return, decreasing cardiac ouput and possibly arterial pressure, with deleterious effects on renal function.[85–89] Very high levels of airway pressure can also increase pulmonary vascular resistance, with similar effects on systemic hemodynamics. The elevation in juxtacardiac pressure also decreases left atrial transmural pressure and distension, lowering atrial natriuretic peptide (ANP) release and decreasing urinary flow.[90–93] As noted previously, the injured and mechanically ventilated lung may provide a portal of entry to the systemic circulation for bacteria, bacterial products, inflammatory mediators, or even air/gas embolism; such effects may further compromise renal function or exacerbate renal injury.[52–54]

Acute lung injury: physiology and consequences

Acute lung injury and its more severe manifestation, ARDS, are among the most common processes the nephrologist will encounter in the intensive care unit. The primary physiologic derangement underlying ARDS is increased pulmonary permeability to fluid and protein. Increased blood–air barrier permeability leads to alveolar flooding and surfactant inactivation; surfactant inactivation and flooding lead, in turn, to dependent consolidation, dramatically reduced pulmonary compliance, and shunt physiology. Mechanical stresses associated with ventilation and elevated pulmonary vascular pressure may further compromise barrier integrity.[94] Elevated intrathoracic pressures compromise renal hemo-dynamics and disorder the hormonal milieu. Finally, protracted periods of ventilatory support, with attendant risks of infection, nephrotoxic medications, and intercurrent hemodynamic com-promise, also increase the risk for development or exacerbation of renal injury.

Acute lung injury: treatment

The shunt physiology which underlies ARDS resists improvement with incremental FiO_2 (frac-tion of inspired oxygen), mandating the use of elevated airpace pressures to 'recruit,' or open, consolidated or collapsed lung regions and main-tain adequate oxygenation. However, current liter-ature strongly supports the use of a 'stretch limited ventilation strategy', often with quite small tidal volumes (about 6–7 ml/kg).[95,96] Unfortunately, without measures to maintain unstable but recruited alveolar units open, they may recollapse during expiration and reopen throughout inspira-tion, potentially augmenting structural lung injury.[55–63] Although the data supporting applica-tion of positive end-expiratory pressure (PEEP) adequate to avoid extensive end-expiratory collapse (high PEEP) are not as strong, or the mechanism(s) of action as clear, theoretical consid-erations, a wealth of animal data, and significant clinical data indicate that this is a reasonable strat-egy.[55,56,62,63,97] Similarly, there are preclinical data to suggest the utility of prone positioning (ventilation in the prone rather than supine position) in improving oxygenation and diminishing struc-tural lung injury.[98] Although the largest trial to date failed to demonstrate an overall benefit of prone positioning, even in that study there was improvement in the sickest patients, and the prone position was applied only for about 7 hours/day.[99] Numerous smaller studies have demonstrated sig-nificant oxygenation benefits.[100–105] The role and optimal implementation of 'recruitment maneu-vers' – generally a maneuver which transiently increases airway pressure exposure in an attempt to open collapsed lung units – is still under active investigation.[106–108]

High-pressure pulmonary edema syndromes

In their extreme manifestations, the high pul-monary vascular pressure injury syndromes con-stitute clinical counterparts to the alveolar epithelial delamination and fracturing seen in the laboratory setting. Less-severe elevations of pul-monary vascular pressure may induce edema for-mation with attendant lung dysfunction, and perhaps even injury from tidal excursions. In each case, a physiologic derangement leads to elevated left atrial pressure and concurrent elevation of pul-monary venous and pulmonary capillary pressure.

At present, many of the patients the nephrolo-gist sees in the intensive care unit have risk factors for coronary artery disease as well as renal disease; the potential contribution of intermittent myocar-dial ischemia in provoking respiratory failure mandates that these patients undergo evaluation for coronary artery disease prior to evaluation for other etiologies. Myocardial ischemia, which may be painless, is accompanied by an acute decline in left ventricular (LV) compliance; increased sympa-thetic tone due to pain or agitation from dyspnea may also elevate LV afterload. Both effects increase pulmonary venous and capillary pressures. Papil-lary muscle ischemia, if present, may also contribute to left atrial and pulmonary venous hypertension by inducing acute and often transient mitral regurgitation. In younger patients presenting with a suspicious history, sympath-omimetic abuse (such as cocaine) should be considered.

Renal artery stenosis can readily cause high-pressure pulmonary edema and lung dysfunction. Elevated afterload due to increased angiotensin II (AII) activity, and/or gross volume overload if the process is severe and bilateral, ultimately increase LV end-diastolic pressure. The subsequent eleva-tion of left atrial pressure increases pulmonary capillary pressure, promoting edema formation, suboptimal V:Q matching (and, in the extreme, shunt physiology), and decreased compliance. This entity should be strongly considered in patients presenting with repeated and paroxysmal episodes of pulmonary edema and hypertension who do not have demonstrable myocardial ischemia. Other diagnostic clues include abrupt decrements in renal function with AII axis block-ade, apparent 'extreme' volume sensitivity of renal function, and significant azotemia in the presence of a bland urinalysis with modest or no proteinuria (and no paraproteins). Of note, a significant percentage of patients with renal artery stenosis are normotensive; the absence of antecedent hypertension does not exclude the diagnosis.

Decreased LV compliance, often denoted 'LV diastolic dysfunction', may arise independent of active myocardial ischemia, and is commonly a consequence of long-standing hypertension and LV hypertrophy. The decrease in compliance renders LV pressure very sensitive to volume status; small changes in volume (due to dietary indiscretion or overexuberant fluid administration) may lead to marked increases in pulmonary vascular pressures, with concomitant edema formation and lung dysfunction.

Pulmonary thromboembolism

A pulmonary process commonly confronting the intensive care nephrologist is pulmonary thromboembolism (PTE). Parenthetically, PTE is a leading cause of 'undiagnosed' hospital deaths. PTE is characterized by marked derangement of V/Q matching, which elevates alveolar deadspace and decreases the efficiency of ventilation. Both mechanical occlusion of vascular channels and mediator release with deranged vascular tone contribute to the mismatch. Increased total minute ventilation, however, can often compensate for the increased alveolar deadspace – at least initially. For similar reasons, significant hypoxemia may not be observed in the absence of a massive pulmonary embolus. A major concern is that the initial, symptomatic, PTE episode will be followed by a lethal recurrent embolism; much of current therapy of non-massive PTE focuses on prevention of subsequent lethal embolism. Hemodynamic compromise from PTE can be severe – including pulseless electrical activity – and arises from acute pulmonary hypertension and right ventricular (RV) failure. The normal RV, when confronted with an acute resistive overload, dilates and becomes hypofunctional (at least in part due to acute RV strain and ischemia), lowering cardiac output and possibly arterial pressure. Additionally, the failing and dilating right ventricle, constrained within the fixed volume of the pericardium, can shift the interventricular septum further into the left ventricle. Such paradoxical septal shift can compromise LV end-diastolic 'stretch', further depressing cardiac output. Septal shift can be significantly exacerbated by overexuberant fluid administration in such patients, with dire consequences. Tachycardia is often an early and very worrisome sign in the context of PTE, and should prompt consideration of echocardiography. Hemodynamic support involves judicious fluid administration, and use of norepinephrine as a primary pressor (to preserve coronary perfusion in the face of compromised cardiac output). Aggressive thrombolytic, endovascular, or operative intervention may be warranted, and can be lifesaving.

Rapidly progressive glomerulonephritis (RPGN)

The rapidly progressive glomerulonephritides and related processes can present with life-threatening pulmonary injury. RPGN-associated pulmonary injury should be considered in the setting of pulmonary hemorrhage, with or without overt renal failure; a normal urinalysis does not 'rule out' an underlying systemic process in this setting. In these diseases, the pulmonary injury is primarily a hemorrhagic response to immune or vascular injury; the role of mechanical factors (such as vascular pressure or inflation stress) is much less clear. Multiple disease processes can present in this fashion, with the most common being Goodpasture's disease, Wegener's granulomatosis, SLE, cryoglobulinemia, and the antiphospholipid antibody syndrome. As noted above, the major issue in these processes is that they be considered; each of these diseases results in potentially irreversible end-organ damage due to vascular compromise, and prompt intervention is of paramount importance. Therapy often involves immunosuppression with accompanying plasmapheresis; acute initial suppression can often be obtained with 'pulse dose' steroids, which may be very useful while a definitive diagnosis is sought.

INITIAL CLINICAL APPROACH

When confronted with a patient suffering combined pulmonary and renal compromise, the initial approach should focus on elements of triage: Does the patient have life-threatening pulmonary compromise and/or are there electrolyte or volume abnormalities mandating emergent or invasive therapy, such as dialysis? Initial efforts should be focused on stabilization and assessing the severity of the problems.

Subsequently, evaluation of arterial blood gases will prove extremely useful. In addition to acid–base details, arterial blood gases usually allow differentiation of hypoxia due to hypoventilation from hypoxia attending V/Q mismatch and that arising from shunt physiology. Briefly, the alveolar arterial (Aa) gradient is defined by:

Aa gradient $\simeq$ FiO$_2$ * (PATM$-$PH$_2$O) * (PCO$_2$ arterial/respiratory quotient $-$ PO$_2$arterial)

In general, the respiratory quotient is approx. 0.8 and PH$_2$O at sea level is approx. 49 mmHg.

A normal Aa gradient suggests hypoventilation, whereas an elevated Aa gradient is consistent with either V/Q mismatch or shunt physiology. If the process is due to V/Q mismatch, application of a low level of supplemental oxygen can markedly improve blood gases, an outcome not observed if hypoxemia is due to shunt physiology. Moreover, on occasion, a blood gas may reveal unsuspected lung pathology. The most common examples of a blood gas uncovering unsuspected pathology are seen in chronic obstructive lung disease or COLD (CO$_2$ retention) or in a severely volume-depleted patient who may not have significant findings on examination or radiography until volume resuscitated (the Aa gradient is often elevated despite the paucity of other associated findings).

A chest radiograph may clarify the 'anatomic' basis for shunt physiology, if present, by revealing whether the underlying process is characterized by airspace filling. Following identification of an (air) space filling process, the clinician is obligated to determine if the fluid is due to hemorrhage (as in Goodpasture's disease or ANCA-positive vasculitides), composed of inflammatory cells (as in diffuse pneumonia), or is an ultrafiltrate of plasma (as in congestive heart failure). In this setting, associated clinical signs or symptoms, such as unexplained fever, rash, arthralgia, prior hemoptysis, or epistaxis, may be useful in assessing the potential presence of a rheumatologic process. Laboratory findings, such as hematuria, proteinuria, or evidence of additional multisystem involvement, suggest the need to consider a rheumatologic process which may require specific immunosuppressive therapy. Serologic studies which may be helpful include ANCA for ANCA-positive vasculitides (Wegener's granulomatosis, periarteritis nodosa (PAN), and Churg–Strauss granulomatosis); antiglomerular basement membrane (GBM) antibody titer (for anti-GBM disease); antinuclear antibodies (for SLE); cryoglobulins; and human immunodeficiency virus (HIV) titers. It is important to remember that a clinical presentation which includes both renal and respiratory compromise is by definition a multisystem disease, and substantially increases the probability that the patient has a disease process mandating specific immunosuppressive or antibiotic therapy. Early renal biopsy may be of great utility in this setting, providing diagnostic information in a more timely fashion than is common with serologic studies, and often being of higher yield than lung biopsy. In an acute and time-sensitive setting, a renal biopsy may provide crucial information required for initiation of therapy several days before serologic data are available.

Combined lung–kidney dysfunction is common and associated with a high mortality in the critically ill patient. Prior emphasis had been on classic immunologic associations occurring with autoimmune diseases. However, recent developments have vastly expanded our understanding of the multiple ways that lung and kidney dysfunction can entwine into a dangerous spiral. The physiologic framework presented here will hopefully allow the clinician and investigator to approach this problem in a rational fashion.

Interesting new data indicate that the renin-angiotensin system might play an important role in modulating pulmonary resistance to injury, insofar as angiotensin II (AII) increases susceptibility to acid aspiration and sepsis-induced lung injury. The modulation of lung injury by AII appears to be mediated by the AT1a receptor and is independent of its hemodynamic effects.[109]

REFERENCES

1. Hopkins SR, Powell FL. Ventilation-perfusion heterogeneity: insights from comparative physiology. In: Hlastala MP, Robertson HT, (eds). Complexity in structure and function of the lung. New York: Marcel Dekker; 1998:549–70.
2. Hida W, Hildebrandt J. Alveolar surface tension, lung inflation, and hydration affect interstitial pressure. J Appl Physiol: Respirat Exercise Physiol 1984;57(1):262–70.
3. Benjamin JJ, Murtagh PS, Proctor DF, Menkes HA, Permutt S. Pulmonary vascular interdependence in excised dog lobes. J Appl Physiol 1974;37(6):887–94.
4. Lai-Fook S. A continuum mechanics analysis of pulmonary vascular interdependence in isolated dog lobes. J Appl Physiol: Respirat Environ Exercise Physiol 1979;46(3):419–29.
5. Smith JC, Mitzner W. Analysis of pulmonary vascular interdependence in excised dog lobes. J Appl Physiol: Respirat Environ Exercise Physiol 1980;48(3):450–67.
6. Lamm WJE, Luchtel D, Albert RK. Sites of leakage in three models of acute lung injury. J Appl Physiol 1988;64(3):1079–83.
7. Schmeck J, Janzen R, Munter K, et al. Endothelin-1 and thromboxane A2 increase pulmonary vascular resistance in granulocyte-mediated lung injury. Crit Care Med 1998;26(11)1868–74.
8. Zamora CA, Baron DA, Heffner JE. Thromboxane contributes to pulmonary hypertension in ischemia reperfusion lung injury. J Appl Physiol 1993;74(1):224–9.
9. Puybasset L, Stewart T, Rouby JJ, et al. Inhaled nitric oxide reverses the increase in pulmonary vascular resistance induced by permissive hypercapnia in patients with acute respiratory distress syndrome. Anesthesiology 1994;80:1254–67.
10. Brimioulle S, Lejeune P, Vachiery JL, et al. Effects of acidosis and alkalosis on hypoxic pulmonary vasoconstriction in dogs. Am J Physiol 1990;258:H347–53.

11. Blomquist CH, Lima PH, Hotchkiss JR. Inhibition of 3α-hydroxysteroid dehydrogenase (3α-HSD) activity of human lung microsomes of genistein, daidzein, coumestrol and C18-, C19- and C21-hydroxysteroids and ketosteroids. Steroids 2005;70(8):507–14.

12. Hopkins SR, McKenzie DC, Schoene RB, Glenny RW, Robertson HT. Pulmonary gas exchange during exercise in athletes. I. Ventilation-perfusion mismatch and diffusion limitation. J Appl Physiol 1994;77(2):912–17.

13. Rice AJ, Thornton AT, Gore CJ, et al. Pulmonary gas exchange during exercise in highly trained cyclists with arterial hypoxemia. J Appl Physiol 1999;87(5):1802–12.

14. Lim LL. A statistical model of the VA/Q distribution. J Appl Physiol 1990;69(1):281–92.

15. Kapitan KS, Wagner PD. Linear programming analysis of VA/Q distributions: average distribution. J Appl Physiol 1987;62(4):1356–62.

16. Gale GE, Torre-Bueno JR, Moon RE, Saltzman HA, Wagner PD. Ventilation-perfusion inequality in normal humans during exercise at sea level and simulated altitude. J Appl Physiol 1985;58(3):978–88.

17. Rimensberger PC, Fedorko L, Cutz E, Bohn DJ. Attenuation of ventilator-induced acute lung injury in an animal model by inhibition of neutrophil adhesion by leumedins (NPC 15669). Crit Care Med 1998;26(3):548–55.

18. Imanaka H, Shimaoka M, Matsuura N, et al. Ventilator-induced lung injury is associated with neutrophil infiltration, macrophage activation, and TGF-beta 1 mRNA upregulation in rat lungs. Anesth Analg 2001;92(2):428–36.

19. Rinaldo JE, Henson JE, Dauber JH, Henson PM. Role of alveolar macrophages in endotoxin-induced neutrophilic alveolitis in rats. Tissue Cell 1985;17(4):461–72.

20. Doerschuk CM, Beyers N, Coxson HO, Wiggs B, Hogg JC. Comparison of neutrophil and capillary diameters and their relation to neutrophil sequestration in the lung. J Appl Physiol 1993;74(6):3040–5.

21. Wiggs BR, English D, Quinlan WM, et al. Contributions of capillary pathway size and neutrophil deformability to neutrophil transit through rabbit lungs. J Appl Physiol 1994;77(1):463–70.

22. Hogg JC, Coxson HO, Brumwell ML, et al. Erythrocyte and polymorphonuclear cell transit time and concentration in human pulmonary capillaries. J Appl Physiol 1994;77(4):1795–800.

23. Motosugi H, Graham L, Noblitt TW, et al. Changes in neutrophil actin and shape during sequestration induced by complement fragments in rabbits. Am J Pathol 1996;149(3):963–73.

24. De Bono EF, Caro CG. Effect of lung-inflating pressure on pulmonary blood pressure and flow. Am J Physiol 1963;205(6):1178–86.

25. Dawson CA, Grimm DJ, Linehan JH. Effects of lung inflation on longitudinal distribution of pulmonary vascular resistance. J Appl Physiol 1977;43(6):1089–92.

26. Hakim TS, Michel RP, Chang HK. Effect of lung inflation on pulmonary vascular resistance by arterial and venous occlusion. J Appl Physiol 1982;53;1110–15.

27. Miserocchi G, Negrini D, Passi A, De Luca G. Development of lung edema: interstitial fluid dynamics and molecular structure. News Physiol Sci 2001;16:66–71.

28. Dematte JE, Sznajder JJ. Mechanisms of pulmonary edema clearance: from basic research to clinical implication. Intensive Care Med 2000;26:477–80.

29. Mathay MA, Folkesson HG, Verkman AS. Salt and water transport across alveolar and distal airway epithelia in the adult lung. Am J Physiol 1996;270(Lung Cell Mol Physiol 14):L487–503.

30. Icard P, Saumon G. Alveolar sodium and liquid transport in mice. Am J Physiol 1999;277(Lung Cell Mol Physiol 21):L1232–8.

31. Khimenko PL, Barnard JW, Moore TM, et al. Vascular permeability and epithelial transport effects on lung edema formation in ischemia and reperfusion. J Appl Physiol 1994;77:1116–21.

32. Smith JC, Stamenovic D. Surface forces in lungs. I. Alveolar surface tension-lung volume relationships. J Appl Physiol 1986;60(4):1341–50.

33. Hida W, Hildebrandt J. Alveolar surface tension, lung inflation, and hydration affect interstitial pressure [Px(f)]. J Appl Physiol Respirat Exercise Physiol 1984;57(1):262–70.

34. Hotchkiss JR, Blanch L, Naviera A, et al. Relative roles of vascular and airspace pressures in ventilator induced lung injury. Crit Care Med 2001;29(8):1593–8.

35. Tassiopoulos AK, Carlin RE, Gao Y, et al. Role of nitric oxide and tumor necrosis factor on lung injury caused by ischemia/reperfusion of the lower extremities. J Vasc Surg 1997;26(4):647–5.

36. Vedder NB, Winn RK, Rice CL, et al. A monoclonal antibody to the adherence-promoting leukocyte glycoprotein, CD18, reduces organ injury and improves survival from hemorrhagic shock and resuscitation in rabbits. J Clin Invest 1988;81(3):939–44.

37. Sheridan BC, McIntyre RC Jr, Moore EE, et al. Neutrophils mediate pulmonary vasomotor dysfunction in endotoxin-induced acute lung injury. J Trauma 1997;42(3):391–6.

38. Costello ML, Mathieu-Costello O, West JB. Stress failure of alveolar epithelial cells studied by scanning electron microscopy. Am Rev Respir Dis 1992;145:1446–55.

39. Fu Z, Costello ML, Tsukimoto K, et al. High lung volume increases stress failure in pulmonary capillaries. J Appl Physiol 1992;73:123–33.

40. Tsukimoto K, Mathieu-Costello O, Prediletto R, Elliott AR, West JB. Ultrastructural appearances of pulmonary capillaries at high transmural pressures. J Appl Physiol 1991;71:573–82.

41. Bachofen H, Schurch S, Michel RP, Weibel ER. Experimental hydrostatic pulmonary edema in rabbit lungs. Morphology. Am Rev Respir Dis 1993;147:989–96.

42. Bachofen H, Schurch S, Weibel ER. Experimental hydrostatic pulmonary edema in rabbit lungs. Barrier lesions. Am Rev Respir Dis 1993;147:997–1004.

43. Broccard AF, Hotchkiss JR, Kuwayama N, et al. Consequences of vascular flow on lung injury induced by mechanical ventilation. Am J Respir Crit Care Med 1998;157:1935–42.

44. Hotchkiss JR Jr, Blanch L, Murias G, et al. Effects of decreased respiratory frequency on ventilator-induced lung injury. Am J Respir Crit Care Med 2000;161:463–8.

45. Guery BP, DeBoisblanc BP, Fialdes P, et al. Pulmonary stress injury within physiological ranges of airway and vascular pressures. J Crit Care 1998;13(2):58–66.

46. Hopkins SR, Schoene RB, Henderson WR, et al. Intense exercise impairs the integrity of the pulmonary blood-gas barrier in elite athletes. Am J Respir Crit Care Med 1997;155(3):1090–4.

47. Hotchkiss JR, Simonson D, Marek D, Marini JJ, Dries D. Pulmonary microvascular fracture in a patient with ARDS subjected to high-pressure mechanical ventilation. Crit Care Med 2002;30(10):2368–70.

48. Ware LB, Matthay MA. Alveolar fluid clearance is impaired in the majority of patients with acute lung injury and the acute respiratory distress syndrome. Am J Respir Crit Care Med 2001;163(6):1376–83.

49. Wang Z, Notter RH. Additivity of protein and nonprotein inhibitors of lung surfactant activity. Am J Respir Crit Care Med 1998;158(1):28–35.

50. Nitta K, Kobayashi T. Impairment of surfactant activity and ventilation by proteins in lung edema fluid. Respir Physiol 1994;95(1):43–51.

51. Humphrey H, Hall J, Sznajder I, Silverstein M, Wood L. Improved survival in ARDS patients associated with a reduction in pulmonary capillary wedge pressure. Chest 1990;97:1176–80.

52. Nahum A, Hoyt J, Schmitz L, et al. Effect of mechanical ventilation strategy on dissemination of intratracheally instilled *Escherichia coli* in dogs. Crit Care Med 1997;25(10):1733–43.

53. Murphy DB, Cregg N, Tremblay L, et al. Adverse ventilatory strategy causes pulmonary-to-systemic translocation of endotoxin. Am J Respir Crit Care Med 2000;162(1):27–33.

54. Marini JJ, Culver BH. Systemic gas embolism complicating mechanical ventilation in the adult respiratory distress syndrome. Ann Intern Med 1989;110(9):699–703.

55. Pelosi P, Goldner M, McKibben A, et al. Recruitment and derecruitment during acute respiratory failure: an experimental study. Am J Respir Crit Care Med 2001;164(1):122–30.

56. Crotti S, Mascheroni D, Caironi P, et al. Recruitment and derecruitment during acute respiratory failure: a clinical study. Am J Respir Crit Care Med 2001;164(1):131–40.

57. Hickling K. Recruitment greatly alters the pressure volume curve: a mathematical model of ARDS lungs. Am J Respir Crit Care Med 1998;158:194–202.

58. Hickling KG. Best compliance during a decremental, but not incremental, positive end-expiratory pressure trial is related to open-lung positive end-expiratory pressure: a mathematical model of acute respiratory distress syndrome lungs. Am J Respir Crit Care Med 2001;163(1):69–78.

59. Martynowicz MA, Walters BJ, Hubmayr RD. Mechanisms of recruitment in oleic acid-injured lungs. J Appl Physiol 2001;90(5):1744–53.

60. Matthay MA, Bhattacharya S, Gaver D, et al. Ventilator-induced lung injury: in vivo and in vitro mechanisms. Am J Physiol Lung Cell Mol Physiol 2002;283(4):L678–82.

61. Mead J, Takashima T, Leith D. Stress distribution in lungs: a model of pulmonary elasticity. J Appl Physiol 1970;28:596–608.

62. Muscedere JG, Mullen JB, Gan K, Slutsky AS. Tidal ventilation at low airway pressures can augment lung injury. Am J Respir Crit Care Med 1994;149:1327–34.

63. Tremblay L, Valenza F, Ribeiro SP, Li J, Slutsky AS. Injurious ventilatory strategies increase cytokines and c-fos m-RNA expression in an isolated rat lung model. J Clin Invest 1997;99:944–52.

64. Vlahakis NE, Schroeder MA, Limper AH, Hubmayr RD. Stretch induces cytokine release by alveolar epithelial cells in vitro. Am J Physiol 1999;277(1 Pt 1):L167–73.

65. Slutsky AS, Tremblay LN. Multiple system organ failure: is mechanical ventilation a contributing factor? Am J Respir Crit Care Med 1998;157:1721–5.

66. Ranieri VM, Suter PM, Tortorella C, et al. Effect of mechanical ventilation on inflammatory mediators in patients with acute respiratory distress syndrome: a randomized controlled trial. JAMA 1999;282(1):54–61.

67. Smulders YM. Pathophysiology and treatment of haemodynamic instability in acute pulmonary embolism: the pivotal role of pulmonary vasoconstriction. Cardiovasc Res 2000;48(1):23–33.

68. Huval WV, Mathieson MA, Stemp LI, et al. Therapeutic benefits of 5–hydroxytryptamine inhibition following pulmonary embolism. Ann Surg 1983;197(2):220–5.

69. Clavijo LC, Carter MB, Matheson PJ, et al. Platelet-activating factor and bacteremia-induced pulmonary hypertension. J Surg Res 2000;88(2):173–80.

70. Lambermont B, Kolh P, Detry O, et al. Analysis of endotoxin effects on the intact pulmonary circulation. Cardiovasc Res 1999;41(1):275–81.

71. Wang le F, Patel M, Razavi HM, et al. Role of inducible nitric oxide synthase in pulmonary microvascular protein leak in murine sepsis. Am J Respir Crit Care Med 2002;165(12):1634–9.

72. Rabb H, Wang Z, Nemoto T, Soleimani M. Downregulation of the water channel aquaporin 5 in the lung following renal ischemic reperfusion injury occurs independent of reperfusion products. J Am Soc Nephrol 1999;10:639A.

73. Rabb H, Wang Z, Nemoto T, et al. Acute renal failure leads to dysregulation of lung salt and water channels. Kidney Int 2003;63:600–6.

74. Hales CA, Du HK, Volokhov A, Mourfarrej R, Quinn DA. Aquaporin channels may modulate ventilator-induced lung injury. Respir Physiol 2001;124(2):159–66.

75. Broccard AF, Hotchkiss JR, Vannay C, et al. Protective effects of hypercapnic acidosis on ventilator-induced lung injury. Am J Respir Crit Care Med 2001;164(5):802–6.

76. Wang le F, Patel M, Razavi HM, et al. Role of inducible nitric oxide synthase in pulmonary microvascular protein leak in murine sepsis. Am J Respir Crit Care Med 2002;165(12):1634–9.

77. Skoutelis AT, Kaleridis VE, Goumenos DS, et al. Polymorphonuclear leukocyte rigidity is defective in patients with chronic renal failure. Nephrol Dial Transplant 2000;15(11):1788–93.

78. Kawabata K, Nakai S, Miwa M, et al. Platelet GPIIb/IIIa is activated and platelet-leukocyte coaggregates formed in vivo during hemodialysis. Nephron 2002;90(4):391–400.

79. Menegatti E, Rossi D, Chiara M, et al. Cytokine release pathway in mononuclear cells stimulated in vitro by dialysis membranes. Am J Nephrol 2002;22(5–6):509–14.

80. Kawabata K, Nakai S, Miwa M, et al. Changes in Mac-1 and CD14 expression on monocytes and serum soluble CD14 level during push/pull hemodiafiltration. Nephron 2002;90(3):273–81.

81. Cianciolo G, Stefoni S, Donati G, et al. Intra- and post-dialytic platelet activation and PDGF-AB release: cellulose diacetate vs polysulfone membranes. Nephrol Dial Transplant 2001;16(6):1222–9.

82. Pertosa G, Grandaliano G, Gesualdo L, Schena FP. Clinical relevance of cytokine production in hemodialysis. Kidney Int Suppl 2000;76:S104–11.

83. Pertosa G, Gesualdo L, Bottalico D, Schena FP. Endotoxins modulate chronically tumour necrosis factor alpha and interleukin 6 release by uraemic monocytes. Nephrol Dial Transplant 1995;10(3):328–33.

84. Shibata K, Cregg N, Engelberts D, et al. Hypercapnic acidosis may attenuate acute lung injury by inhibition of endogenous xanthine oxidase. Am J Respir Crit Care Med 1998;158(5 Pt 1):1578–84.

85. Fessler HE, Brower RG, Shapiro EP, Permutt S. Effects of positive end-expiratory pressure and body position on pressure in the thoracic great veins. Am Rev Respir Dis 1993;148:1657–64.

86. Schuster S, Erbel R, Weilemann LS, et al. Hemodynamics during PEEP ventilation in patients with severe left ventricular failure studied by transesophageal echocardiography. Chest 1990;97:1181–9.

87. Mitaka C, Nagura T, Sakanishi N, Tsunoda Y, Amaha K. Two-dimensional echocardiographic evaluation of inferior vena cava, right ventricle, and left ventricle during positive-pressure ventilation with varying levels of positive end-expiratory pressure. Crit Care Med 1989;17:205–10.

88. Shinozaki M, Muteki T, Kaku N, Tsuda H. Hemodynamic relationship between renal venous pressure and blood flow regulation during positive end-expiratory pressure. Crit Care Med 1988;16:144–7.

89. Culver BH, Marini JJ, Butler J. Lung volume and pleural pressure effects on ventricular function. J Appl Physiol 1981;50:630–5.

90. Ramamoorthy C, Rooney MW, Dries DJ, Mathru M. Aggressive hydration during continuous positive-pressure ventilation restores atrial transmural pressure, plasma atrial natriuretic peptide concentrations, and renal function. Crit Care Med 1992;20:1014–9.

91. Leithner C, Frass M, Pacher R, et al. Mechanical ventilation with positive end-expiratory pressure decreases release of alpha-atrial natriuretic peptide. Crit Care Med 1987;15:484–8.

92. Teba L, Dedhia HV, Schiebel FG, Blehschmidt NG, Lindner WJ. Positive-pressure ventilation with positive end-expiratory pressure and atrial natriuretic peptide release. Crit Care Med 1990;18:831–5.

93. Kharasch ED, Yeo KT, Kenny MA, Buffington CW. Atrial natriuretic factor may mediate the renal effects of PEEP ventilation. Anesthesiology 1988;69:862–9.

94. Dreyfuss D, Saumon G. Ventilator-induced lung injury. Lessons from experimental studies. Am J Respir Crit Care Med 1998;157:294–323.

95. Ney L, Kuebler WM. Ventilation with lower tidal volumes as compared with traditional tidal volumes for acute lung injury and the acute respiratory distress syndrome. The Acute Respiratory Distress Syndrome Network. N Engl J Med 2000;342(18):1301–8.

96. Amato MB, Barbas CS, Medeiros DM, et al. Effect of a protective-ventilation strategy on mortality in acute respiratory distress syndrome. N Engl J Med 1998;338:347–54.

97. Webb HH, Tierney DF. Experimental pulmonary edema due to intermittent positive pressure ventilation with high inflation pressures. Protection by positive end-expiratory pressure. Am Rev Respir Dis 1974;110(5):556–65.

98. Broccard A, Shapiro RS, Schmitz LL, et al. Prone positioning attenuates and redistributes ventilator-induced lung injury in dogs. Crit Care Med 2000;28(2):295–303.

99. Gattinoni L, Tognoni G, Pesenti A, et al. Prone-Supine Study Group. Effect of prone positioning on the survival of patients with acute respiratory failure. N Engl J Med 2001;345(8):568–73.

100. Michaels AJ, Wanek SM, Dreifuss BA, et al. A protocolized approach to pulmonary failure and the role of intermittent prone positioning. J Trauma 2002;52(6):1037–47.

101. Venet C, Guyomarc'h S, Migeot C, et al. The oxygenation variations related to prone positioning during mechanical ventilation: a clinical comparison between ARDS and non-ARDS hypoxemic patients. Intensive Care Med 2001;27(8):1352–9.

102. Voggenreiter G, Neudeck F, Aufmkolk M, et al. Intermittent prone positioning in the treatment of severe and moderate posttraumatic lung injury. Crit Care Med 1999;27(11):2375–82.

103. Curley MA, Thompson JE, Arnold JH. The effects of early and repeated prone positioning in pediatric patients with acute lung injury. Chest 2000;118(1):156–63.

104. Blanch L, Mancebo J, Perez M, et al. Short-term effects of prone position in critically ill patients with acute respiratory distress syndrome. Intensive Care Med 1997;23(10):1033–9.

105. Nakos G, Tsangaris I, Kostanti E, et al. Effect of the prone position on patients with hydrostatic pulmonary edema compared with patients with acute respiratory distress syndrome and pulmonary fibrosis. Am J Respir Crit Care Med 2000;161(2 Pt 1):360–8.

106. Cakar N, der Kloot TV, Youngblood M, Adams A, Nahum A. Oxygenation response to a recruitment maneuver during supine and prone positions in an oleic acid-induced lung injury model. Am J Respir Crit Care Med 2000;161(6):1949–56.

107. Villagra A, Ochagavia A, Vatua S, et al. Recruitment maneuvers during lung protective ventilation in acute respiratory distress syndrome. Am J Respir Crit Care Med 2002;165(2):165–70.

108. Richard JC, Maggiore SM, Jonson B, et al. Influence of tidal volume on alveolar recruitment. Respective role of PEEP and a recruitment maneuver. Am J Respir Crit Care Med 2001;163(7):1609–13.

109. Imai Y, et al. Angiotensin-converting enzyme 2 protects from severe acute lung failure. Nature 2005;436:112–116.

8

Acute renal failure – pharmacotherapies

Hugh R Brady and Niamh Kieran

OVERVIEW OF ETIOLOGY AND PATHOGENESIS OF ARF

Acute renal failure (ARF) is a common clinical syndrome defined as a rapid deterioration of renal function associated with accumulation of nitrogenous waste products and disturbances of extracellular volume, electrolyte, and acid–base homeostasis.[1-3] ARF complicates approximately 5% of hospital admissions and up to 30% of admissions to intensive care units (ICUs). ARF is usually asymptomatic and diagnosed when routine biochemical screening of hospitalized patients reveals a recent increase in the blood urea nitrogen (BUN) and serum creatinine levels. Critically ill patients with ARF are generally sicker, characterized by greater hemodynamic instability, longer length of ICU stay, and higher ICU and hospital mortality than patients without ARF. In a recent study, ICU and hospital mortality was almost fourfold higher in patients who developed ARF.[4] It is important to recognize that ARF can be prevented in many settings if predisposing conditions are recognized and promptly treated.

ARF may complicate a host of diseases that for purposes of diagnosis and management are conveniently divided into three categories:

1. prenal ARF (~55–60%), a physiologic response to renal hypoperfusion in which the integrity of renal parenchymal tissue is preserved
2. intrinsic renal ARF (~35–40%), in which ARF is caused by diseases of renal parenchyma
3. postrenal ARF (<5%) due to acute obstruction of the urinary tract (Table 8.1).

Most intrinsic renal ARF is caused by ischemia or nephrotoxins (often in combination) and is classically associated with acute tubular necrosis (ATN). Management is directed at prevention of ATN in high-risk individuals and control of uremic complications in patients with established ATN until spontaneous recovery of renal function.

Prerenal ARF

Prerenal ARF is the most common cause of ARF and is frequently diagnosed and treated by general physicians/internists without consultation of the nephrologist. It represents an appropriate physiologic response to renal hypoperfusion of sufficient magnitude to impair glomerular filtration and excretion of nitrogenous waste.[1] By definition, the integrity of renal parenchymal tissue is preserved and the reduction of glomerular filtration rate (GFR) associated with prerenal failure is rapidly and completely reversed when the underlying cause of glomerular hypoperfusion is corrected. Renal blood flow, though reduced in prerenal failure, is sufficient to provide adequate oxygen and metabolic substrates to sustain the viability of renal tubular cells. However, if prerenal failure is not appropriately treated, it can lead to ischemic injury to renal tubular cells and to the development of ATN. Thus, prerenal ARF and ischemic ATN are part of a spectrum of manifestations of renal hypoperfusion. Indeed, clinical and biochemical features of prerenal ARF and ischemic ATN may coexist in some patients in a condition known as 'the intermediate syndrome'. Definitive diagnosis of prerenal failure hinges on prompt recovery of GFR after restoration of renal perfusion.

Table 8.1 Classification and major disease categories causing acute renal failure (ARF).		
Disease category	**Disease/symptom**	**Percent of patients with ARF**
Prerenal ARF caused by acute renal hypoperfusion	Intravascular volume depletion	55–60
	Decreased cardiac output	
	Systemic vasodilatation	
	Renal vasoconstriction	
	Pharmacologic agents that acutely impair autoregulation and GFR in specific settings	
Intrinsic renal ARF caused by acute diseases of renal parenchyma		35–40
Diseases involving large renal vessels	Renal artery thrombosis	
	Atheroembolism	
	Renal vein thrombosis	
Diseases of small renal vessels and glomeruli	Glomerulonephritis or vasculitis	
	HUS or TTP	
	Malignant hypertension	
Acute injury to renal tubules mediated by ischemia or toxins*	Ischemia	
	Exogenous toxins	
	Endogenous toxins	
Acute diseases of the tubulointerstitium	Allergic interstitial nephritis	
	Acute bilateral pyelonephritis	
Postrenal ARF caused by acute obstruction of urinary collecting system		<5%

*Accounts for more than 90% of cases in the intrinsic renal ARF category in most series. GFR = glomular filtration rate; HUS = hemolytic uremic syndrome; TTP = thrombotic thrombocytopenic purpura.

Intrinsic renal ARF

From a clinicopathologic viewpoint, it is useful to categorize the causes of intrinsic renal ARF into:

1. diseases involving large renal vessels
2. diseases of the renal microvasculature and glomeruli
3. ischemic and nephrotoxic ATN
4. other acute processes involving the tubulo-interstitium.

Most intrinsic renal ARF is caused by ischemia or nephrotoxins (often in combination) and is classically associated with ATN. Thus, the terms ischemic and nephrotoxic ATN are commonly used to denote ischemic or nephrotoxic ARF in clinical practice. Ischemic ATN and toxic ATN account for about 90% of intrinsic renal ARF.

Ischemic ATN differs from prerenal ARF in that renal hypoperfusion has been severe enough to cause ischemic injury to renal parenchymal cells, particularly tubule epithelium, and ARF does not resolve spontaneously upon restoration of renal blood flow. The course of ATN can be divided into initiation, maintenance, and recovery phases, the pathogenesis of which is attributed to several interrelated pathologic processes that include enhanced vasomotor tone with reduction in renal blood flow, tubule epithelial cell injury often with necrosis and detachment from the tubule basement membrane, renal tubular obstruction by ATN casts composed of detached tubule epithelial cells and necrotic debris encased in Tamm–Horsfall protein produced by thick ascending limb cells, backleak of glomerular filtrate through an ischemic epithelium, and oxidant- and leukocyte-mediated injury on reperfusion.[1–3,5–7] Recent advances in cellular and molecular biology have identified a variety of molecules that underpin these key events. Many of these are potential targets for therapeutic intervention.[7]

Postrenal ARF

Urinary tract obstruction accounts for less than 5% of cases of ARF. Because one kidney has sufficient clearance capacity to excrete the nitrogenous waste products generated daily, ARF resulting from obstruction implies blockade of the urethra or bladder neck, bilateral ureteric obstruction, or unilateral ureteric obstruction in a patient with either one functioning kidney or pre-exisiting chronic renal insufficiency. It occurs in the absence of renal parenchymal disease and is potentially rapidly reversible when the cause of the urinary tract obstruction is treated. This syndrome is usually easily recognized by clinical assessment and ultrasonography of the urinary tract. If obstruction persists untreated, irreversible renal parenchymal injury and chronic renal failure can result.

PREVENTION OF ATN AND OTHER FORMS OF INTRINSIC RENAL ARF

Prevention of ischemic and nephrotoxic ATN

Identification of high-risk individuals
Hypovolemia is a major risk factor for ATN during major surgery, sepsis, or exposure to nephrotoxic drugs or radiocontrast, particularly in those individuals at increased risk of developing ATN. The risk associated with hypovolemia is accelerated in patients with pre-existing chronic renal insufficiency and in patients with pre-existing vascular disease such as patients with diabetes and atherosclerosis.[1] Specific algorithms have been designed and validated to identify patients at risk of developing renal failure after cardiac surgery.[8] Careful monitoring of intravascular volume and correction of hypovolemia can significantly reduce the incidence of ATN in this setting.

Optimization of intravascular volume
Optimization of intravascular volume and cardiovascular function is of pivotal importance in the prevention of prerenal ARF and ischemic ATN. This principle has been validated most convincingly in the context of contrast nephropathy where prophylactic infusion of half-normal saline (1 ml/kg for 12 hours pre- and post-procedure) dramatically reduces the risk of ARF by comparison with patients treated with mannitol and furosemide.[9,10]

Prompt correction of hypovolemia, using appropriate replacement fluids based on the source of fluid loss, is of key importance. Hypovolemia due to severe hemorrhage is best corrected with packed red blood cells if the patient is hemodynamically unstable or if the hematocrit is dangerously low. In the absence of hemodynamic instability or active bleeding, isotonic saline may be used. The choice of replacement for extrarenal, third space, or nonhemorrhagic renal losses is controversial. A review of randomized controlled trials comparing crystalloid with colloid replacement for the resuscitation of critically ill patients concluded that the routine use of colloids may be associated with an adverse outcome and is not justified.[11] Thus, isotonic saline is the replacement fluid of choice until systemic hemodynamics have stabilized. Serum potassium and acid–base status should be monitored in all subjects. Potassium supplementation of replacement fluids is rarely required unless sodium bicarbonate induces hypokalemia during treatment of metabolic acidosis. Cardiac failure may require aggressive management with positive inotropes, antiarrhythmic drugs, preload- and/or afterload-reducing agents, and mechanical aids such as an intra-aortic balloon pump or left ventricular assist devices. Invasive hemodynamic monitoring is useful for guiding therapy in complicated patients in whom clinical assessment of intravascular volume and cardiovascular function may be unreliable.

Cautious use of drugs that impair renal hemodynamic compensatory responses
Several classes of commonly prescribed drugs impair renal adaptive responses and can convert compensated renal hypoperfusion into overt prerenal ARF or indeed trigger progression of prerenal ARF to ischemic ATN. The most common offenders in this regard are nonsteroidal anti-inflammatory drugs (NSAIDs), angiotensin-converting enzyme (ACE) inhibitors, and angiotensin II receptor blockers (ARBs). NSAIDs inhibit renal prostaglandin biosynthesis; they do

not compromise GFR in normal individuals but may precipitate prerenal ARF in subjects with true hypovolemia or decreased effective arterial blood volume, or in patients with chronic renal insufficiency in whom GFR is being maintained in part by prostaglandin-dependent hyperfiltration through a few remaining nephrons. Similarly, ACE inhibitors and ARBs may trigger prerenal ARF in individuals in whom intraglomerular pressure and GFR are dependent on angiotensin II. This complication is classically seen in patients with bilateral renal artery stenosis or with unilateral stenosis in a solitary functioning kidney. Here, angiotensin II preserves glomerular filtration pressure distal to renal arterial stenosis by increasing systemic arterial pressure and by triggering selective constriction of efferent arterioles. ACE inhibitors or ARBs blunt these compensatory responses and lead to reversible ARF in approximately 30% of patients, particularly in patients also taking diuretics. ACE inhibitors or ARBs, like NSAIDs, may also precipitate prerenal ARF in patients with compensated renal hypoperfusion of other causes, thus requiring close monitoring of the serum creatinine level when these drugs are administered to high-risk individuals.

Monitoring doses of nephrotoxic antibiotics, chemotherapeutics, and other drugs

Careful monitoring of circulating drug levels appears to reduce the incidence of ARF associated with aminoglycoside antibiotics or calcineurin inhibitors (cyclosporine and tacrolimus), although as many as 33% of cases of aminoglycoside nephrotoxicity occur in patients with 'therapeutic' levels. The risk of aminoglycoside toxicity is lowered by limiting the cumulative dose and by maintaining serum levels within the therapeutic range. There is convincing evidence that once-daily dosing with these agents affords equal antimicrobial activity and less nephrotoxicity than conventional regimens.[12]

Lack of efficacy of low-dose dopamine, diuretics, and other targeted preventive strategies

In the past, there was a vogue for prophylactic use of mannitol and loop diuretics for prevention of nephrotoxic and ischemic ATN. It was proposed that loop diuretics would protect against ATN by increasing renal blood flow (through a weak vasodilatory action), by washing out intratubular casts, and reduce oxygen consumption in the tubular cells by blocking transcellular sodium trans-

port. Similarly, mannitol was postulated to prevent ATN by increasing renal blood flow, washing out intratubular casts, decreasing cell swelling, and scavenging free radicals. Unfortunately, these theoretic benefits were not borne out in subsequent controlled clinical trials, and there are insufficient data to support the use of these agents in humans, except to treat hypervolemia.[1,2]

'Renal-dose dopamine' (1–3 µg/kg/min) augments renal blood flow, sodium excretion and, to a lesser extent, GFR in healthy subjects and is widely used for the treatment of ATN. Despite the attractive theoretic rationale, low-dose dopamine has not been demonstrated to prevent or alter the course of ischemic or nephrotoxic ATN, in prospective controlled clinical trials. Indeed, the available evidence would suggest lack of efficacy.[13,14] Furthermore, dopamine, even at low doses, is potentially toxic in critically ill patients, can induce tachyarrhythmias, and myocardial and intestinal ischemia and may increase sudden cardiac death, among other side effects. The reasons for these adverse effects are multiple. The original dose–response curves that formed the rationale for using low-dose dopamine to achieve selective activation of dopamine receptors without activation of α- or β-adrenoceptors are derived from dopamine infusion into healthy subjects. In critically ill patients with pre-existing adrenergic activation and metabolic disturbances, low-dose dopamine is frequently associated with tachycardia and an increase in the cardiac index, suggesting further adrenoceptor activation. Furthermore, low-dose dopamine may suppress central respiratory drive and induce arteriovenous shunting in the pulmonary circulation, both of which may exacerbate hypoxemia and also transiently decrease T-cell function, impairing resistance to infection in compromised patients.[13,14] Thus, the routine administration of dopamine to patients with oliguric ARF is not justified and may be dangerous.

Prevention of other forms of ARF

Several other agents are used to prevent ARF in specific clinical settings. The prophylactic oral administration of the antioxidant acetylcysteine (600 mg twice daily, on the day before and on the day of administration of the contrast agent) has been shown to reduce the incidence of contrast-induced ARF in high-risk patients, with pre-existing chronic renal insufficiency (creatinine clearance <50 ml/min).[15] Acetylcysteine is also useful in limiting acetaminophen-induced renal injury if given within 24 hours of ingestion. Allopurinol limits uric acid generation and may reduce the incidence of ARF in patients receiving treatment for hematologic malignancy; however, occasional patients receiving allopurinol still develop ARF, probably through the toxic actions of hypoxanthine crystals on tubule function. Forced diuresis and alkalinization of urine may further attenuate renal injury caused by uric acid and may also reduce the incidence of ARF in patients receiving high-dose methotrexate or with severe rhabdomyolysis. Both ethanol and fomepizole (4-methylpyrazole) inhibit alcohol dehydrogenase, thus preventing ethylene glycol metabolism to the nephrotoxic metabolite glycolic acid, and fomepizole is an important adjunct to hemodialysis in the emergency management of this intoxication.[16]

PHARMACOTHERAPY TO ACCELERATE RECOVERY OF ESTABLISHED ATN

Several agents have been tested for their ability to attenuate injury or hasten recovery in ischemic and nephrotoxic ATN; however, none has consistently been shown to be of benefit. These include:

- vasodilators such as atrial natriuretic peptide (ANP), calcium channel blockers, and 'renal-dose' dopamine, which could potentially improve renal blood flow in ATN
- compounds such as mannitol and loop diuretics, which may theoretically relieve intratubular obstruction
- growth factors such as insulin-like growth factor-1 (IGF-1), administered in an attempt to accelerate regeneration and repair of tubule epithelium
- agents such as antibodies against intracellular adhesion molecule-1 (ICAM-1), given to target leukocyte-mediated renal injury during reperfusion (Table 8.2).

Unfortunately, none of these strategies has been proven to reduce the incidence of ATN or to reduce dialysis requirements or mortality in patients with established ATN when assessed in controlled clinical trials.[1-3,5-7,16] The management of ATN still hinges on measures to prevent and treat uremic complications until patients recover renal function spontaneously (Table 8.3). We shall address some of the more commonly employed or more promising strategies (Table 8.4).[6,7,17]

'Renal-dose dopamine' (1–3 µg/kg/min), as previously mentioned, augments renal blood flow, sodium excretion and, to a lesser extent, GFR in healthy subjects and is widely used for the treatment of ATN. Despite the attractive rationale, studies in humans do not support its use in the setting of established ATN, and suggest that low-dose dopamine may even increase sudden cardiac death in critically ill patients, among other side effects.[13,14]

Endothelin-1, the most potent vasoconstrictor peptide known in humans, appears to be a major contributor to the persistent intrarenal vasoconstriction that characterizes ATN. Endothelin-1 receptor antagonists improve renal function in many forms of experimental ATN. Unfortunately, initial human studies using a nonselective endothelin receptor antagonist for prevention of contrast nephropathy have been unsuccessful.[18]

ANP is a 28 amino acid polypeptide synthesized in cardiac atrial muscle. ANP augments GFR, renal blood flow, and sodium and water excretion, and confers protection in experimental models of ATN.[1-3] Unfortunately, a large multicenter trial in critically ill patients with ARF failed to show any clinically significant improvement in dialysis-free survival or overall mortality in ATN.[19]

Calcium channel antagonists, with attenuating effects on vascular smooth muscle tone, have been studied as renal vasodilators. In human renal transplantation, calcium antagonists afforded modest protection against ischemic ATN.[20] Calcium antagonists may reduce vasoconstriction associated with cyclosporine and radiocontrast media.[21,22] However, none of these agents has conferred benefit of sufficient magnitude to warrant their routine use.

The administration of high-dose intravenous loop blocker diuretics to individuals with oliguric ATN is commonly practiced, but should be done so cautiously in critically ill patients, solely for the treatment of hypervolemia. Although this strategy may reduce fluid overload, there is no evidence that it alters mortality or dialysis-free survival.[23] Indeed, a recent retrospective survey of critically ill patients with ARF demonstrated that diuretic use was associated with an increased risk of death and nonrecovery of renal function.[24] The adverse outcome in this study may reflect a 'masking' effect of diuretic use in delaying diagnosis and dialysis treatment for ARF or a direct toxic effect of diuretics.[24] On the balance of available evidence, high-dose loop diuretics should be used cautiously in patients with ARF and withdrawn promptly in patients who fail to respond to such treatment.

Table 8.2 Potential strategies to prevent or reverse acute tubular necrosis.	
Pathophysiologic event	**Therapeutic intervention**
Renal vasoconstriction	iNOS antisense oligonucleotides
	Endothelin receptor antagonists
	Atrial natriuretic peptide and related peptides
	Calcium channel blockers
	Leukotriene receptor antagonists
	PAF antagonists
Tubular obstruction	RGD peptides
Tubular regeneration	Epidermal growth factor
	Hepatocyte growth factor
	Insulin-like growth factor-1
Reperfusion injury	Anti-ICAM-1 mAb
	Anti-CD18 mAb
	Free radical scavengers
	Protease inhibitors
	α-MSH
	Lipoxin analogues
	Biocompatible membranes
	Adenosine (A_2) receptor agonists

iNOS = inducible nitric oxide synthase, PAF = platelet activating factor; RGD peptides = peptides bearing the arginine–glycine–aspartic acid motif; mAb = monoclonal antibodies; ICAM-1 = intercellular adhesion molecule-1; α-MSH = α-melanocyte-stimulating hormone.

Similarly, the available data do not support the routine administration of mannitol to oliguric patients.[6] Moreover, when administered to severely oliguric or anuric patients, mannitol may trigger expansion of intravascular volume and pulmonary edema, and severe hyponatremia due to osmotic shift of water from the intracellular to the extracellular and intravascular space.

In contrast to many organs where ischemia results in permanent cell loss, the kidney has a remarkable capacity to recover its structure and function. Several strategies have been employed in an effort to accelerate tubular repair and regeneration and to hasten recovery. Epidermal growth factor, hepatocyte growth factor, and IGF reduce the extent of renal dysfunction and accelerate renal recovery when administered to animals subjected to renal ischemia.[1–3] In human studies, IGF-1 administered postoperatively to patients who underwent renovascular surgery improved creatinine clearance but not overall mortality or dialysis-free survival.[25] Furthermore, there was no improvement in recovery of renal function in a randomized controlled trial of IGF-1 in patients with ATN in an ICU setting with higher comorbidities.[26]

Restoration of renal blood flow after ischemia is followed rapidly by infiltration of the kidney by monocytes and neutrophils, which in turn contribute to oxidant injury.[1] CD11/CD18 β2 integrins on neutrophils and ICAM-1 on renal endothelial cells appear to mediate neutrophil recruitment. Monoclonal antibodies against CD11/CD18 integrins and ICAM-1 protect in models of experimental ischemic ATN.[27] Mice deficient in ICAM-1 are protected against ARF.[27] Antibodies against ICAM-1 have been administered safely to humans in trials of renal allograft rejection and warrant further investigation in ischemic ATN.

Other experimental strategies for the treatment of established ATN include maneuvers to reverse intrarenal vasoconstriction (e.g. leukotriene and platelet activating factor (PAF) antagonists), prevent cast formation and relieve tubule obstruction (e.g. RGD peptides), replenish cell ATP

Table 8.3   Complications of acute renal failure.

Category	Condition
Metabolic	Metabolic acidosis
	Hypocalcemia
	Hypermagnesemia
	Hyponatremia
	Hyperphosphatemia
	Hyperuricemia
Cardiovascular	Pulmonary edema
	Pericarditis
	Hypertension
	Pulmonary embolism
	Arrhythmias
	Pericardial effusion
	Myocardial infarction
	Pneumonitis
Gastrointestinal	Nausea
	Malnutrition
	Gastrointestinal ulcers/bleeding
	Stomatitis or gingivitis
	Parotitis or pancreatitis
	Vomiting
	Gastritis
Neurologic	Neuromuscular irritability
	Mental status changes
	Somnolence
	Asterixis
	Seizures
	Coma
Hematologic	Anemia
	Bleeding
Other complications	Hiccups
	Decreased insulin catabolism
	Mild insulin resistance
	Elevated parathyroid hormone
	Reduced 1,25-dihydroxy- and 25-hydroxyvitamin D
	Low total triiodothyronine and thyroxine
	Normal free thyroxine

levels (e.g. MgATP), scavenge oxygen free radicals (e.g. superoxide dismutase, catalase), inhibit leukocyte–endothelial cell adhesion during reperfusion (e.g. anti-CD18, anti-P-selectin monoclonal antibodies and α-melanocyte stimulating hormone (α-MSH)), and stimulate cellular regeneration (e.g. amino acid infusions). Although many of these maneuvers afford some benefit in experimental

Table 8.4 Supportive management of intrinsic acute renal failure.

Complication	Treatment
Intravascular volume overload	Restrict salt (1–2 g/day) and water (usually <1 L/day)
	Diuretics (usually loop diuretics ± thiazides)
	Ultrafiltration or dialysis
Hyponatremia	Restrict free water intake (<1 L/day)
	Avoid hypotonic intravenous solutions (including dextrose solutions)
Hyperkalemia	Restrict dietary K^+ intake (usually <40 mmol/day)
	Eliminate K^+ supplements and K^+ sparing diuretics
	Potassium-binding ion exchange resins
	Glucose (50 ml of 50% dextrose) and insulin (10 units regular)
	Sodium bicarbonate (usually 50–100 mmol)
	β2 agonist inhaled
	Calcium gluconate (10 ml of 10% solution over 2–5 minutes)
	Dialysis (low K^+ dialysate)
Metabolic acidosis	Restrict dietary protein (usually 0.6 g/kg/day of high biologic value)
	Sodium bicarbonate (maintain serum bicarbonate >15 mmol/L and arterial pH >7.2)
	Dialysis
Hyperphosphatemia	Restrict dietary phosphate intake (usually < 800 mg/day)
	Phosphate-binding agents (calcium acetate, calcium carbonate, aluminum hydroxide and sevelamer)
Hypocalcemia	Calcium carbonate (if symptomatic or if sodium bicarbonate to be administered)
	Calcium gluconate (10–20 ml of 10% solution)
Hypermagnesemia	Discontinue Mg^{2+}-containing antacids
Hyperuricemia	Treatment usually not necessary (if urate <900 μmol/L)
Nutrition	Dietary protein (~0.8 g/kg/day) if not catabolic
	Carbohydrate (~100 g/day)
	Enteral or parenteral nutrition (if prolonged course or very catabolic)
Drug dosage	Adjust for GFR
	Avoid NSAIDs, ACE inhibitors, radiocontrast
Indications for dialysis	Uremia (signs and symptoms)
	Intractable volume overload
	Hyperkalemia or metabolic acidosis refractory to other measures

ACE = angiotensin-converting enzyme; GFR = glomerular filtration rate; NSAIDs = nonsteroidal anti-inflammatory drugs.

models of ischemic or nephrotoxic ARF (see Table 8.4), their efficacy has yet to be proven in clinical trials.[7,17]

Will monotherapy ever work?

It is noteworthy that so many agents have failed to prevent or accelerate recovery from ATN when used as monotherapies, despite attractive theoretical rationale and promising results in experimental animals. Given that ATN is a complex syndrome involving coexistent disturbances of renal blood flow, tubule integrity, and leukocyte trafficking, it seems logical that future studies should address the efficacy of combination regimens that simultaneously target two or more of the aforementioned steps in the pathophysiology of ATN. In this regard, a recent study demonstrated that an analogue of the lipoxygenase product lipoxinA$_4$ (LXA$_4$) is protective in experimental ischemic ARF.[28] LXA$_4$ has several potential beneficial actions in ARF, including intrarenal vasodilation, inhibition of neutrophil recruitment, stimulation of clearance of apoptotic neutrophils, and modulation of cytokine production.[29]

PHARMACOTHERAPY TO MAJOR COMPLICATIONS OF ATN

In health, the kidney regulates salt and water balance and intravascular volume, plays a key role in potassium, phosphate, and acid–base homeostasis, and is involved in drug excretion. The kidney is also an important source of erythropoietin and is the site for 1α-hydroxylation of vitamin D. As a result, ATN is frequently complicated by hypervolemia, hyperkalemia, hyperphosphatemia, metabolic acidosis, anemia, and hypocalcemia (see Table 8.3). The kidney also excretes nitrogenous waste generated from metabolism of dietary protein. Accumulation of nitrogenous waste during ATN may ultimately result in the life-threatening clinical uremic syndrome. The severity of these metabolic sequelae generally correlates with the degree of renal injury and the patient's catabolic state. For optimum management, these complications must be anticipated and preventive measures instituted from the time of diagnosis.

Diuretic regimens for management of hypervolemia

Expansion of the extracellular fluid volume is an almost inevitable consequence of oligoanuric ATN, and manifests clinically as elevation of the jugular venous pressure, third heart sound, basal lung crackles, pleural effusions or ascites, dependent edema, increased body weight, and pulmonary edema (see Table 8.3). If hypervolemia develops despite salt and water restriction, patients should initially receive a bolus injection of a loop diuretic such as furosemide or bumetanide (see Table 8.4). Although it is reasonable to begin with conventional doses, the dose should be increased rapidly in nonresponders (e.g. furosemide 200 mg, bumetanide 10 mg). Patients who fail to diurese with high-dose bolus injection of loop diuretics may respond if these agents are administered by continuous infusion (e.g. furosemide 10–40 mg/h), by intravenous bolus mixed in salt-poor albumin, or by intravenous bolus 30 minutes after a thiazide diuretic such as hydrochlorothiazide or metolazone orally or chlorothiazide intravenously. The latter approach is intended to block sodium reabsorption at multiple sites along the nephron (loop diuretic; loop of Henle; thiazide; distal cortical nephron). In practice, combination regimens rarely provide clinically significant augmentation in urine output by comparison with high-dose loop diuretic alone. Diuretic therapy should be stopped in resistant patients as prolonged administration may induce ototoxicity. Mannitol is still used in some centers to treat hypervolemia. However, its use is not without risk. Whereas mannitol is an effective osmotic diuretic, it may precipitate pulmonary edema in patients with established ATN if mannitol-induced expansion of intravascular volume is not associated with diuresis. Consequently, loop diuretics remain the diuretics of choice for most nephrologists. Where possible, loop diuretics should be avoided if aminoglycosides have been used within the last 48 hours as they appear to increase the risk of aminoglycoside-induced ATN and ototoxicity. Pulmonary edema is a life-threatening complication of hypervolemia. Whereas it may be possible to control pulmonary edema in ATN by fluid restriction and diuretics, many oliguric patients require fluid removal by ultrafiltration. The latter is usually performed as part of the dialysis procedure.

Treatment of hyperkalemia

Hyperkalemia is almost inevitable in patients with oliguric ATN. Serum potassium typically rises by 0.5 mmol/L/day in oligoanuric patients because of impaired excretion of potassium derived from diet, potassium-containing solutions, and potassium released from injured tubular epithelium or other cells (e.g. rhabdomyolysis, tumor lysis). Hyperkalemia may be compounded by metabolic acidosis, which triggers potassium efflux from cells. In the absence of clinical or electrocardiographic (ECG) evidence of hyperkalemia, mild hyperkalemia (5.0–6.0 mmol/L) can usually be controlled by restriction of dietary potassium or oral administration of potassium-binding ion-exchange resins such as sodium polystyrene sulfonate (15–30 g in 50–100 ml 20% sorbitol every 3–4 hours) or Calcium Resonium (15–30 g three or four times daily). Loop diuretics are used concomitantly to enhance potassium excretion in diuretic-responsive patients.

Hyperkalemia requires more aggressive treatment when its levels exceed 6.0 mmol/L. In the absence of ECG changes, dietary restriction, cation exchange resins and diuretics are supplemented by the administration of intravenous insulin (10 units soluble insulin) and glucose (50 ml 50% dextrose), which shifts potassium into cells within 30–60 minutes. The latter serves as a useful temporizing measure while total body potassium is reduced by loop diuretics. Sodium bicarbonate (~50 mmol over 5 minutes) also promotes rapid shift of potassium into cells (onset within 15 minutes, duration 1–2 hours) and is often administered with insulin-dextrose, particularly in acidotic patients. Frequent glucometer readings and monitoring of potassium levels are advisable. In patients with hyperkalemia of >7.0 mmol/L or with lesser degrees of hyperkalemia associated with ECG abnormalities or arrhythmias, calcium gluconate or calcium carbonate (10 ml of 10% solution over 5 minutes) should be given intravenously for cardioprotection. In reality, dialysis is initiated in most oliguric ATN patients once the serum potassium rises above 6.0 mmol/L, unless there is clear evidence of improving renal function and the measures described above serve to control the serum potassium until dialysis can be initiated.

Treatment of metabolic acidosis

The metabolism of dietary protein normally yields 50–100 mmol of fixed nonvolatile acids per day. These require renal excretion for preservation of acid–base homeostasis. Consequently metabolic acidosis with widening of the anion gap is a common complication in ATN. Metabolic acidosis does not usually require treatment unless the serum bicarbonate and pH fall below 15 mmol/L and 7.2, respectively. Acidosis is corrected by administration of sodium bicarbonate orally or intravenously (see Table 8.4). The initial rate of replacement should be based on the estimated bicarbonate deficit:

Bicarbonate deficit (mmol) = 0.4 × Lean body weight × (Desired serum bicarbonate − Measured serum bicarbonate)

and adjusted subsequently according to serum levels. In general, sodium bicarbonate is administered to maintain a serum bicarbonate concentration of 15–20 mmol/L. Patients should be monitored for complications of bicarbonate administration, as overzealous correction may result in overshoot metabolic alkalosis, hypocalcemia, hypokalemia, volume overload, and pulmonary edema. Other disturbances of acid–base homeostasis are less frequent in patients with ATN and may reflect comorbidities such as respiratory acidosis or alkalosis in patients requiring mechanical ventilation or metabolic alkalosis caused by loss of gastric acid through vomiting or nasogastric aspiration in patients with gastrointestinal dysfunction.

Treatment of hyperphosphatemia

Mild hyperphosphatemia is common in ATN and can usually be controlled by restriction of dietary phosphate and oral administration of dietary phosphate binders (e.g. calcium carbonate 500 mg three times/day, sevelamer hydrochloride 800–1600 mg three times/day), which inhibit absorption of phosphate from the gastrointestinal tract (see Table 8.4). Aluminum-containing phosphate binders should be avoided, except in cases of hypercalcemia, where calcium-containing phosphate binders are contraindicated. Metastatic deposition of calcium phosphate may develop as a consequence of severe hyperphosphatemia in highly catabolic patients, particularly when the product of serum calcium and serum phosphate levels (mg/dl) exceeds 70 (approximately 5.6 mmol/L). In this setting, dialysis is indicated if dietary intervention and phosphate binders cannot lower serum phosphate rapidly.

Nutritional management

Malnutrition is a frequent complication of ARF and contributes to high mortality seen in patients with ARF.[30] Many patients with ARF are catabolic, resulting in net protein breakdown and negative nitrogen balance. Malnutrition develops as a consequence of several factors, including:

- inability to eat or loss of appetite
- the catabolic nature of the underlying medical disorder (e.g. sepsis, rhabdomyolysis, trauma)
- nutrient losses in drainage fluids or dialysate
- increased protein breakdown due to insulin resistance that stimulates increased hepatic gluconeogenesis, using amino acids released from muscle as substrate
- reduced synthesis of amino acids in the kidney and muscle protein
- inadequate nutritional support, contributing to loss of lean body mass.[30]

Treatment requires a multidisciplinary approach that involves physicians, nurses, and dietitians (see Table 8.4). The objective of dietary modification during the maintenance phase of ARF is to provide sufficient calories to avoid protein catabolism and starvation ketoacidosis, while minimizing the generation of nitrogenous waste that may precipitate uremic syndrome. This is best achieved by providing a dietary protein intake of high biologic value (i.e. rich in essential amino acids) protein at approximately 0.8 g/kg/day and providing most calories in the form of carbohydrate (approximately 100 g/day). Higher protein intake is advisable in catabolic patients or those with a prolonged maintenance phase, even if it precipitates the need for dialysis. Enteral nutrition, the standard modality of nutritional support for critically ill patients, is available in specific formulas adapted to the metabolic alterations in uremia. Supplementation of water-soluble vitamins is advised, particularly in patients requiring dialysis.[30] Management of nutrition is easier in nonoliguric patients and after institution of dialysis.

Treatment of hematologic complications

Anemia, prolongation of bleeding time, and leukocytosis are common hematologic complications of ARF and are usually multifactorial in origin. Factors that contribute to anemia include hemodilution, inhibition of erythropoiesis, hemolysis, bleeding, reduced red cell survival time, and frequent phlebotomy. A bleeding diathesis usually reflects mild thrombocytopenia, platelet dysfunction, and/or clotting factor abnormalities. Anemia may require red cell transfusion in patients with symptoms or active bleeding. Erythropoietin is not useful in ARF, in contrast to chronic renal failure, because of its relatively delayed onset of action and bone marrow resistance in critically ill patients. The bleeding diathesis is typically mild and, if problematic, can be reversed temporarily by desmopressin, correction of anemia, or dialysis should hemorrhage develop or should patients require invasive procedures or surgery. Patients with ATN have an increased incidence of upper gastrointestinal hemorrhage caused by stress erosions and ulcers. This complication can be prevented by regular doses of antacids, histamine H_2 antagonists, and proton pump inhibitors. Gastric stress ulcer prophylaxis is not indicated unless the patient is intubated or has a concurrent coagulopathy. Neither magnesium- nor aluminum-based antacids should be used for extended periods in patients with ATN, as these cations may accumulate to toxic levels.

TREATMENT OF OTHER FORMS OF ARF

Treatment of other intrarenal causes of ARF must be tailored to the causative disease. Patients with glomerulonephritis or vasculitis may respond to corticosteroids, alkylating agents, and/or plasmapheresis, depending on the primary disease. Systemic anticoagulation should be considered in patients with ARF caused by renal artery or vein thrombosis or in those suffering thromboembolization to the kidney. Antiplatelet agents, plasma exchange, and plasma infusion are useful in treatment of hemolytic uremic syndrome (HUS) and thrombotic thrombocytopenic purpura (TTP). Allergic interstitial nephritis typically resolves spontaneously when the inciting drug is discontinued; however, corticosteroids appear to hasten recovery and may obviate the need for dialysis in some cases. Aggressive control of systemic arterial pressure is of paramount importance in limiting renal injury in malignant hypertensive nephrosclerosis, toxemia of pregnancy, and other vascular diseases. Hypertension and ARF associated with scleroderma may be exquisitely sensitive to treatment with ACE inhibitors. Prompt evaluation and diagnosis of renal transplant rejection with renal biopsy is indicated in renal transplant recipients with unexplained ARF.

SUMMARY

The management of ATN still hinges on measures to prevent and treat uremic complications until patients recover renal function spontaneously. It is of paramount importance to recognize those patients at risk and employ measures to prevent ATN and associated complications. Given the lack of effective therapy to prevent ATN or hasten renal recovery, there is an urgent need to develop new therapeutic strategies. It is likely that successful treatment of human ATN will require a multifaceted approach using combinations of agents that do not influence the course of human ATN when used alone.

REFERENCES

1. Brady HR, Brenner BM, Clarkson MR, Lieberthal W. Acute renal failure. In: Brenner BM, Rector FC, eds. The kidney, 6th edn. Philadelphia, PA: WB Saunders; 2000:1201–62.
2. Brady HR, Singer GG. Acute renal failure. Lancet 1995;346:1533–40.
3. Thadhani R, Pascual M, Bonventre JV. Acute renal failure. N Engl J Med 1996;334:1448–60.
4. Clermont G, Acker CG, Angus DC, et al. Renal failure in the ICU: comparison of the impact of acute renal failure and end-stage renal disease on ICU outcomes. Kidney Int 2002;62:986–96.
5. Fisch BJ, Linas SL. Prerenal acute renal failure. In: Brady HR, Wilcox CS, eds. Therapy in nephrology and hypertension. Philadelphia, PA: WB Saunders; 1998:17–20.
6. Goligorsky MS, Allgren RL, Hammerman MR. Medical management of ischemic acute tubular necrosis. In: Brady HR, Wilcox CS, eds. Therapy in nephrology and hypertension. Philadelphia, PA: WB Saunders; 1998:21–8.
7. Kieran NE, Brady HR. Treatment of acute renal failure: promising experimental strategies and new therapeutic challenges. Semin Dialysis 1999;12:275–7.
8. Fortescue EB, Bates DW, Chertow GM. Predicting acute renal failure after coronary bypass surgery: cross-validation of two risk-stratification algorithms. Kidney Int 2000;57:2594–602.
9. Barrett BJ, Parfrey PS. Contrast nephropathy. In: Brady HR, Wilcox CS, eds. Therapy in nephrology and hypertension. Philadelphia, PA: WB Saunders; 1998:41–4.
10. Solomon R, Werner C, Mann D, D'Elia J, Silva P. Effects of saline, mannitol, and furosemide to prevent acute decreases in renal function induced by radiocontrast agents. N Engl J Med 1994;331:1416–20.
11. Schierhout G, Roberts I. Fluid resuscitation with colloid or crystalloid solutions in critically ill patients: a systemic review of randomised trials. Br Med J 1998;316:961–4.
12. Prins JM, Buller HR, Kuijper EJ, Tange RA, Speelman P. Once versus thrice daily gentamicin in patients with serious infections. Lancet 1993;341:335–9.
13. Denton MD, Chertow G, Brady HR. 'Renal-dose' dopamine for the treatment of acute renal failure: scientific rationale, experimental studies and clinical trials. Kidney Int 1996;49:4–14.
14. ANZICS clinical trials group. Low dose dopamine in patients with early renal dysfunction: a placebo-controlled randomized trial. Lancet 2000;356:2139–43.
15. Tepel M, Van Der Giet M, Zidek W. Prevention of radiographic-contrast-agent-induced reductions in renal function by acetlycysteine. N Engl J Med 2000;343:180–4.
16. Brent J, McMartin K, Phillips S, et al. Fomepizole for the treatment of ethylene glycol poisoning. N Engl J Med 1999;340:832–38.
17. Rabb H, Bonventre J. Experimental strategies for acute renal failure – the future. In: Brady HR, Wilcox CS, eds. Therapy in nephrology and hypertension. Philadelphia, PA: WB Saunders; 1998:72–81.
18. Wang A, Holcslaw T, Bashore TM, et al. Exacerbation of radio-contrast nephrotoxicity by endothelin receptor antagonism. Kidney Int 2000;57:1675–80.
19. Allgren RL, Marbury TC, Rahman SN, et al. Anaritide in acute tubular necrosis. N Engl J Med 1997;336:828–34.
20. Neumayer HH, Kunzendorf U, Schreiber M. Protective effects of calcium antagonists in human renal transplantation. Kidney Int Suppl 1992;36:S87–93.
21. Ruggenenti P, Perico N, Mosconi L, et al. Calcium channel blockers protect transplant patients from cyclosporine-induced daily renal hypoperfusion. Kidney Int 1993;43:706–11.
22. Neumayer HH, Junge W, Kufner A, Wenning A. Prevention of radiocontrast-media-induced nephrotoxicity by the calcium channel blocker nitrendipine: a prospective randomized clinical trial. Nephrol Dial Transplant 1989;4:1030–6.
23. Brater DC. Diuretic therapy. N Engl J Med 1998;339:387–95.
24. Mehta RL, Pascual MT, Soroko S, Chertow G. Diuretics, mortality, and non recovery of renal function in acute renal failure. JAMA 2002;288:2547–53.
25. Franklin SC, Moulton M, Sicard GA, et al. Insulin-like growth factor 1 preserves renal function postoperatively. Am J Physiol 1997;272:F257.
26. Hirschberg R, Kopple J, Capra W, et al. Multicenter clinical trial of recombinant human insulin-like growth factor 1 in patients with acute renal failure. Kidney Int 1999;55(6):2423–32.
27. Rabb H, O'Meara YM, Maderna P, Coleman P, Brady HR. Leukocytes, cell adhesion molecules and ischemic acute renal failure. Kidney Int 1997;51:1463–8.
28. Kieran NE, Doran PP, Connolly SB, et al. Modification of the transcriptomic response to renal ischemia/reperfusion injury by lipoxin analog. Kidney Int 2003;64(2):480–92.
29. Kieran NE, Godson CG. Lipoxin bioactions. Kidney Int 2004;65:1145–54.
30. Druml W. Nutritional management of acute renal failure. Am J Kidney Dis 2001;37(S2):S89–94.

9

Indications for initiation, cessation, and withdrawal of renal replacement therapy

Shigehiko Uchino and Rinaldo Bellomo

INTRODUCTION

Acute renal failure (ARF) is a common complication in critical illness. The incidence of ARF in the intensive care unit (ICU) has been reported from 1.5% to 24%, depending on populations studied and criteria used.[1-5] Some of these patients do not have enough solute clearance and/or diuresis, accumulate uremic toxins and water, develop uremia and/or fluid overload, and require renal replacement therapy (RRT). One of the major problems related to RRT is that, although it supports kidneys like a mechanical ventilator does for the lungs, available randomized controlled evidence to guide clinical practice is limited. There is some consensus on how and when to initiate, cease, and withdraw mechanical ventilation.[6-9] On the other hand, because of limited evidence, there is little consensus on how and when to initiate, cease, and withdraw RRT. Thus, practice variation is significant.

In this chapter, we review the evidence and seek to make some suggestions concerning indications of initiation, cessation, and withdrawal of RRT that we feel are appropriate for critically ill patients.

INITIATION OF RRT IN ICU

Since intermittent hemodialysis (IHD) became available as a treatment for ARF, the timing of initiation of RRT has been controversial.[10-15] Initially, due to the technical inadequacies of IHD, it was not uncommon for RRT itself to contribute to morbidity and mortality by inducing bleeding, thrombosis, hypotension, arrhythmias, and infection. However, in 1960, Teschan et al reported good outcomes with 'prophylactic' hemodialysis in 15 patients with acute renal failure.[10] They used dialysis before clinical evidence of uremia developed or nonprotein nitrogen reached 200 mg/dl and maintained it below 150 mg/dl. These patients remained free from uremic symptoms or chemical imbalances, had no or liberalized restriction of fluid and nutrition, and 10 of these patients survived. In 1965, Kirkland et al argued against this approach, using 400 consecutive patient data sets.[12] These authors reserved hemodialysis and peritoneal dialysis until severe uremia developed despite conservative therapy and did not find significant difference in survival rate compared to previous results with 'prophylactic' hemodialysis. In 1972, Kleinknecht et al compared 221 patients treated with 'prophylactic' hemodialysis with 279 patients who were treated in a 'conservative way' before the introduction of the new more interventional approach.[13] Mortality was reduced from 42% to 29% after the institution of 'prophylactic' hemodialysis. Much controversy has continued to exist ever since on the timing of RRT and, 30 years later, such controversy still persists due to the lack of randomized controlled trials. Gettings et al, for example, analyzed 100 ARF patients admitted to their trauma center and treated with continuous RRT (CRRT).[14] Patients were characterized as 'early' or 'late' starters, based on whether blood urea nitrogen (BUN) was less than or greater than 60 mg/dl, prior to CRRT initiation. There was no difference between the two groups in terms of Injury Severity Score, admission Glasgow Coma Score, presence of shock at admission, age, gender, or trauma type. However, survival rate was significantly higher among 'early' starter (39% vs 20%, p = 0.041). Kresse et al compared ARF patients who were admitted to ICU between 1991 and 1993 (Group 1) and between 1994 and 1995 (Group 2).[15]

There was no difference in demographics or etiology of ARF between the two groups but RRT was started at an earlier stage of renal insufficiency (less elevated creatinine or reduced urine output) in Group 2. Compared to Group 1, mortality was improved from 78.9% to 59.6% in Group 2 (p <0.001).

Textbooks and the real world

Although these observational studies tend to suggest significant benefits for the 'early' initiation of RRT and no disadvantages, one of the most common textbooks of internal medicine,[16] even in the current edition, states that the indications of RRT for ARF are 'symptoms or signs of the uremic syndrome, management of refractory hypervolemia, hyperkalemia or acidosis' or a 'BUN level of greater than 100 mg/dl'.

Because of such long-standing confusion, lack of controlled randomized studies, unsupported dogma, local preferences, and the influence of traditional teaching, current practice for the initiation of RRT is, therefore, extremely varied. Figure 9.1A–C shows creatinine, urea, and urine output at the beginning of RRT in a recent but yet unpublished international epidemiologic study (the BEST kidney study).[17] Asian and South American study units seemed to initiate RRT later than the other regions (higher creatinine and/or urea and lower urine output). On the other hand, mean urine output was more than 1 L/day in Europe when RRT was started. The ranges of these values were wide: from 320 to 438 μmol/L in creatinine, from 23.2 to 31.1 mmol/L in urea, and from 609 to 1111 ml/day in urine output. Importantly, however, the upper limit for urea was 31.1 mmol/L, clearly below the 100 mg/dl described by textbooks. Put another way, essentially no one in this study of 52 units in 23 countries practices medicine as suggested in textbooks, which obviously appear outdated.

Why we should start early

The main reasons against early initiation of RRT are that bioincompatible dialysis membranes might induce increased inflammation and renal injury and that dialysis-associated hypotension can also further exacerbate renal injury and delay renal recovery.[18,19] However, such issues are not relevant to patients in modern ICUs. Biocompatible membranes are now widely available and have been shown to be less nephrotoxic.[18] CRRT is available, which is essentially free of treatment-induced hypotension. Thus, although studies which support early initiation are only epidemiologic, at the very least we are not aware of any evidence against the early initiation of modern forms of RRT.

We consider it important to take a more modern and physiology-based view of the timing of RRT in the ICU. Thus, we have published modern criteria for initiation of RRT (Box 9.1).[20,21] First, we think RRT should be started early to prevent rather than treat developing fluid overload. For critically ill patients, it is often difficult to restrict fluid intake because they require adequate nutrition and multiple drug administration. On top of such requirements, some patients have increased vascular permeability and tend to develop organ (especially lung) edema easily. For example, a patient with moderate left ventricular dysfunction and chronic renal impairment might have coronary bypass graft surgery, which is complicated by postoperative bleeding. He might require 'take-back' to the operating room and come back to ICU with a marked coagulopathy requiring the rapid transfusion of fresh frozen plasma, cryoprecipitate, and platelets. He might be hypotensive and oliguric. The central venous pressure might be 16 mmHg

---

Box 9.1 Criteria for initiation of continuous renal replacement therapy in the intensive care unit

1. Oliguria (urine output <200 ml/12 hours)
2. Anuria (urine output <50 ml/12 hours)
3. Severe acidemia (pH <7.1) due to metabolic acidosis
4. Azotemia ([urea] >30 mmol/L)
5. Hyperkalemia ([K^+] >6.5 mmol/L or rapidly rising [K^+])
6. Suspected uremic organ involvement (pericarditis/encephalopathy/neuropathy/myopathy)
7. Severe dysnatremia ([Na^+] >160 or <115 mmol/L)
8. Hyperthermia (core temperature >39.5°C)
9. Clinically significant organ edema (especially lung)
10. Drug overdose with dialyzable toxin
11. Coagulopathy requiring large amounts of blood products in patient at risk of pulmonary edema/ARDS

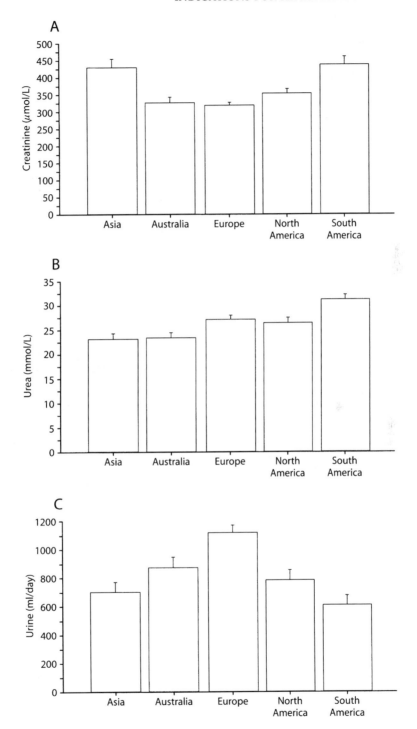

Figure 9.1 Creatinine output (A), urea output (B), and urine output (C) at the beginning of renal replacement therapy for the five regions.

and the pulmonary artery occlusive pressure (PAOP) 18 mmHg. Gas exchange might be significantly impaired and chest X-ray might already show upper lobe blood diversion. Such a patient would not be uremic, nor particularly fluid overloaded, nor hyperkalemic. Yet, in our opinion, it would be physiologically unsound and clinically dangerous to delay the initiation of RRT just because this patient doesn't fulfill 'conventional criteria' for such RRT. Preventing pulmonary edema/ARDS (acute respiratory distress syndrome) is physiologically 'safer' and can be easily achieved with CRRT by removing up to 1 L/h of fluid and without the need for anticoagulation. Such patient could then receive 2–4 L of clotting factors, blood, and platelets without developing fluid overload.

Secondly, RRT, in the form of CRRT, can be started to prevent or minimize significant biochemical abnormalities. It is not certain which level of azotemia can cause or contribute to complication (encephalopathy, coagulopathy, pericarditis, etc.) in ICU patients. It is also not certain how aggressively metabolic acidosis should be treated. However, it is known that toxins that accumulate during rising azotemia can induce immune dysfunction.[22] Severe acidemia may have negative inotropic and pulmonary vasoconstrictive effects.[23] Thus, considering the safety of recent technology (CRRT), it is at least physiologically reasonable to start RRT early to prevent such problems, rather than wait until they happen.

Nonrenal indications

Another 'current practice' issue that needs to be addressed in terms of initiation of RRT is that of so-called nonrenal indications for CRRT. Ronco et al conducted a questionnaire to 345 clinicians who attended one of two international meetings of critical care nephrology:[24] 52% of the respondents reported using CRRT for extended indications even in the absence of ARF and approximately 6% answered 'removal of septic mediators' as a reason for initiating CRRT in their ICU. In the BEST kidney database, 11.5% of patients had RRT for 'immunomodulation' as at least one of the reasons for initiating RRT. This practice is not in keeping with the available evidence. There have been many studies showing that CRRT can remove cytokines and other inflammatory factors from septic patients;[25–28] however, the molecular weights of such substances are too great for them to be

removed efficiently by currently available hemofilters. Cole et al conducted a randomized controlled trial to evaluate the ability of continuous venovenous hemofiltration (CVVH, 2 L/h exchange) to reduce plasma cytokine concentration in septic shock patients.[29] These investigators found that CVVH was not associated with an overall reduction in plasma cytokine concentrations. Although some new techniques (high-volume hemofiltration, large-pore-size filters, coupled plasma filtration with adsorption) seem promising,[30–32] CRRT used at current doses with commercially available filters cannot be recommended for patients with sepsis but no ARF.

In summary, the timing of initiation of RRT remains controversial and current practice varies widely. Although there is no high-quality evidence (i.e. multicenter randomized controlled trials), some epidemiologic studies and physiologic reasoning suggest that early initiation of RRT might achieve better outcomes for ARF patients and no evidence exists against such thinking. With current technology (biocompatible membranes and CRRT), early initiation is feasible and physiologically sound and we think it should be the approach of choice until one or more randomized controlled trials are conducted to provide clinicians with better-quality evidence to guide their practice.

CESSATION OF RRT IN ICU

Multiple published studies have looked at how and when to wean patients from mechanical ventilation.[33–36] However, although RRT is a way of supporting another crucial organ, there is no study that has specifically addressed how and when to cease RRT. This is partially because, with IHD, whether RRT should be performed or not is decided on a daily basis and a formal decision to stop is not always made. IHD is typically not given when a patient doesn't fulfill the criteria for the application of RRT, which, of course, are exactly same as those for the initiation of RRT. However, with CRRT, a physician needs to formally decide when to cease treatment. Appropriate cessation of CRRT is crucial for clinical and economic outcomes. Due to the lack of information, however, current practice in terms of cessation of CRRT is again extremely varied. Figure 9.2A–C shows creatinine, urea, and urine volume at the end of CRRT in the BEST kidney study. Study centers in South America (four in Brazil and one in Uruguay) seem

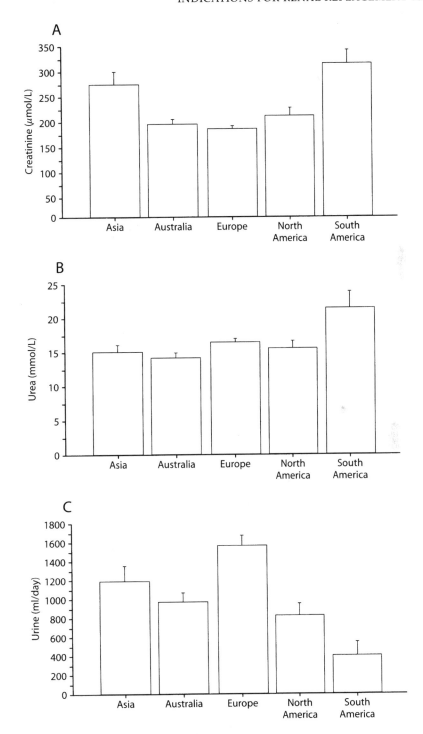

Figure 9.2 Creatinine output (A), urea output (B), and urine output (C) at the end of renal replacement therapy for the five regions.

to cease CRRT earlier than study centers in other regions.

We previously published criteria for weaning from CRRT (Box 9.2).[21] We believe that, on physiologic grounds, just as CRRT should be initiated early, it should be ceased late. When the criteria for cessation have been fulfilled, a trial of weaning from CRRT should be offered for 12–24 hours. If, during this period of time, the criteria for initiating CRRT become re-established, CRRT should be rapidly reinstituted for a period of at least 24 hours before the patient is reassessed once again. Once a patient has been stable to improving for 24 hours on a CRRT-free regimen, the double-lumen catheter can be removed.

Another issue concerning the cessation of CRRT is whether CRRT can be switched to IHD once a patient becomes hemodynamically stable. Again, due to the lack of information, current practice is variable. Figure 9.3 shows rates of switching from CRRT to IHD for five regions from the BEST (beginning and ending supportive therapy) kidney database. Approximately 40% of patients whose CRRT was ceased in Asia and North America were switched to IHD. On the other hand, more than 80% of patients in Australia continued CRRT until their renal function improved.

Mehta et al conducted a randomized controlled trial comparing CRRT and IHD[37] and showed that patients who received CRRT with no crossover to IHD had a 92.3% rate of renal recovery and that patients who crossed over from CRRT to IHD had a 44.7% rate of complete renal recovery. These two groups are not easily compared because such crossover was not conducted randomly and crossover groups might have had more severe renal injury and required longer duration of RRT.

Box 9.2   **Criteria for cessation of continuous renal replacement therapy (CRRT) in the intensive care unit**

1.   All criteria for initiating CRRT are absent
2.   Urine output averages 1 ml/kg/h over a 24-hour period
3.   Fluid balance can be kept approximately neutral with current urine output
4.   There is a complication related to CRRT

Nonetheless, IHD might cause intravascular fluid depletion and hypotension and delay renal recovery.[17] We believe that CRRT should be continued until a patient recovers dialysis-independent renal function.

In summary, the timing of cessation of CRRT varies among regions and clinicians. It is our view that CRRT should be continued as long as the criteria for initiation of CRRT are present. Once a patient fulfills all criteria for cessation of CRRT, the procedure can be ceased. However, clinicians should have a low threshold for recommencing CRRT to avoid the development of fluid overload or uremic complications. Switching from CRRT to IHD might cause delay of renal recovery and, in some patients, impede it altogether; in our view, it is not justifiable. A survey of physician and nurse opinion about current practice patterns, observational studies of the clinical decision-making process in relation to stopping or transition to a different modality, and observational studies of physiologic status at the time of cessation or transition are urgently needed.

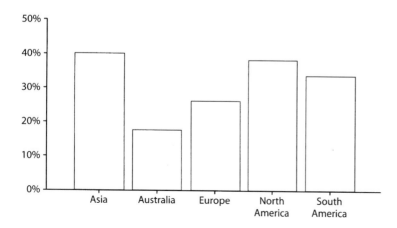

Figure 9.3 Rates of switching from continuous renal replacement therapy to intermittent hemodialysis for the five regions.

WITHDRAWAL OF RRT IN ICU

The mortality of ARF remains high, despite improved intensive care for critically ill patients.[1-5] For some patients, continuing RRT and other organ support might merely lead to an undignified delay in an inevitable death. Accordingly, there is a growing concern on issues surrounding the withholding or withdrawing of life-support treatments in such patients. Prendergast and Luce reported that recommendations to withhold or withdraw life support in their ICU preceded 179 of 200 deaths (90%) in 1992 and 1993, compared with 114 of 224 deaths (51%) in 1987 and 1988.[38] Woodrow and Turney analyzed the cause of death in 636 ARF patients during 1956 and 1989 and found that the rate of withdrawing treatment had increased from 5.7% in the 1950s to 15.4% in the 1980s.[39] According to the BEST kidney database, approximately 20% of all deaths in patients who had RRT were preceded by formal withdrawal of RRT. Patients' renal support treatment was withdrawn after a median of 4.1 (interquartile range (IQR), 1.4–10.4) days of RRT and patients typically died the next day (median, 1.0 day; IQR, 0.0–1.5).

The difference between withdrawing RRT and withdrawing other organ support technology (mechanical ventilation and vasopressors) is that patients usually don't die as rapidly when RRT alone is withdrawn. Zamperetti et al conducted a questionnaire of participants in the First International Course of Critical Care Nephrology.[40] Their aim was to examine the ethical approach of intensivists and nephrologists to the initiation or withdrawal of CRRT. Only 43% of responders thought that CRRT and other organ supports are equivalent and that every support should be withdrawn when futile. The responders were asked to give a score to determine the difficulty of terminating different vital supports. The highest score was for mechanical ventilation as the most difficult support to terminate. It was followed by CRRT, artificial feeding/hydration, vasoactive drugs, antibiotics, and blood transfusion.

Severity scores to guide decision-making

Both general and ARF-specific severity scoring systems have been applied for outcome prediction in ARF patients.[41-43] Parker et al calculated APACHE-II score[44] for patients with ARF at the time of initiation of dialysis and found that it was a statistically significant predictor of patient survival and recovery of renal function.[41] Fiaccadori et al[42] reported that predicted mortalities with APACHE-II and SAPS-II[45] were close to observed mortality (APACHE-II, 36.2%; SAPS-II, 39.3%; observed mortality, 39.1%). However, areas under the receiver operating characteristic (ROC) curve were 0.75 and 0.77, respectively, and they concluded that none of these scoring systems provided sufficient confidence for the prediction of outcome in individual patients. Douma et al examined the performance of seven general and four ARF-specific severity scoring systems.[43] With APACHE-III[46] and Liano's models,[47] although their ability to discriminate mortality from survival was poor (areas under the ROC curve were less than 0.78), the observed mortality in the highest quintiles of risk were 97% and 98%, respectively. These investigators concluded that the two models were able to identify a group of patients with a near 100% chance of mortality. As a whole, although severity scoring systems are more or less helpful to make the decision to withdraw RRT, they are far from ideal in guiding clinicians with individual decisions.

The current practice of withdrawing life support in ICU varies widely from clinician to clinician. Ethical, social, moral, and religious values of each clinician influence their medical decision-makings. Cook et al used a cross-sectional survey, submitting 12 hypothetical scenarios to ICU clinicians and nurses, in order to examine their attitudes regarding the management of life support.[48] They found that the same option was chosen by more than 50% of respondents in only 1 of 12 scenarios, and that opposite extremes of care were chosen by more than 10% of the respondents in 8 of 12 scenarios. The same patient may thus receive full aggressive intensive care treatment from one healthcare provider and only comfort measures from another. To reduce such confusion, appropriate guidelines or criteria for withdrawal of organ support are needed. Indeed, the questionnaire conducted by Zamperetti et al[40] showed that only 6% of responders thought that no such criteria were needed to guide them in withdrawing CRRT.

The Renal Physicians Association and the American Society of Nephrology formed a working group that completed the clinical practice guideline on shared decision-making in the appropriate initiation of and withdrawal from dialysis.[49] The guideline presents recommendations concerning withholding or withdrawing dialysis in adult patients with either ARF or end-stage renal failure (ESRF). They state that it is appropriate to withhold or withdraw dialysis for patients with ARF or ESRF for:

- patients with decision-making capacity who, being fully informed and making voluntary choices, refuse dialysis or request that dialysis be discontinued.
- patients who no longer possess decision-making capacity who have previously indicated refusal of dialysis in an oral or written advance directive.
- patients who no longer possess decision-making capacity and whose properly appointed legal agents refuse dialysis or request that it be discontinued.
- patients with irreversible, profound neurologic impairment such that they lack signs of thought, sensation, purposeful behavior, and awareness of self and environment.

Although the guideline is well written and clear-cut, it is most relevant to American clinicians and does not include consideration for religious and cultural differences. For example, the role of the family in end-of-life decision-making varies greatly among countries. In Mediterranean Europe, generally, the family plays a bigger role in decision-making than in the United States. In European countries, furthermore, physicians appear to also wield greater decisional power than in the USA.[50] Attitudes to 'patients with profound neurological impairment' are also varied. Asian countries tend to be conservative in this situation.[51]

In summary, death in ICU is often preceded by withdrawal of RRT and other organ support. Current practice on how and when to withdraw, however, is varied and the same patient might be treated in completely different ways in different units and in different countries. Current general and ARF-specific severity scoring models have limited clinical usefulness. Comprehensive evidence-based guidelines will be required to better inform current practice. Such guidelines will also need to be adjusted with cultural, religious, and legal difference among countries. A deeper understanding of the determinants of current behavior is needed to develop more sophisticated guidelines for ICU clinicians who must make crucial decisions for withdrawal of RRT and other forms of life support.

OVERALL SUMMARY AND CONCLUSION

In this chapter, we have presented the current evidence and practice for the initiation, cessation, and withdrawal of RRT. It is obvious from our analysis that lack of level I evidence is a fundamental problem and causes much uncertainty and confusion in daily practice. Both observational and randomized controlled studies with a sufficiently large sample size will be required. Nonetheless, the lack of level I data does not mean that all treatments are the same. Physicians must still carefully analyze what data are available and come to a judgment of what might be 'best practice' at this time. At present, we consider that such best practice is that RRT should be continuous[52] and should be started 'early' and stopped 'late'. We firmly believe that prevention of complications is better than treatment and that, with the availability of CRRT, artificial renal support can be offered with minimal morbidity to all patients. Finally, we believe that, as soon as it appears that the continuation of RRT might not be in the best interest of patients, sensitive, open, clear, and compassionate discussions should take place with patients or their legal representatives to ensure that the ethical principles of autonomy, nonmaleficence, and beneficence are respected at all times.

REFERENCES

1. Shaefer JH, Jochimsen F, Keller F, et al. Outcome prediction of acute renal failure in medical intensive care. Intensive Care Med 1991;17:19–24.
2. Brivet FG, Kleinknecht DJ, Philippe L, et al. Acute renal failure in intensive care units – causes, outcome, and prognostic factors of hospital mortality: a prospective, multicenter study. Crit Care Med 1996;24:192–8.
3. Paganini EP, Tapolyas M, Goormastic M, et al. Establishing a dialysis therapy/patient outcome link in intensive care unit acute dialysis for patients with acute renal failure. Am J Kidney Dis 1996;28:81–9.
4. Guerin C, Girard R, Selli JM, et al. Initial versus delayed acute renal failure in the intensive care unit. Am J Respir Crit Care Med 2000;161:872–9.
5. De Mendoca A, Vincent JL, Suter PM, Moreno R. Acute renal failure in the ICU: risk factors and outcome evaluated by the SOFA score. Intensive Care Med 2000;26:915–21.
6. Slutsky AS. Consensus conference on mechanical ventilation – January 28–30, 1993 at Northbrook, Illinois, USA. Part I. European Society of Intensive Care Medicine, the ACCP and the SCCM. Int Care Med 1994;20:64–79.
7. Slutsky AS. Consensus conference on mechanical ventilation – January 28–30, 1993 at Northbrook, Illinois, USA. Part 2. Int Care Med 1994;20:150–62.
8. Tobin MJ. Advances in mechanical ventilation. N Engl J Med 2001;344:1986–96.
9. Truog RD, Cist AF, Brackett SE, et al. Recommendations for end-of-life care in the intensive care unit: The Ethics Committee of the Society of Critical Care Medicine. Crit Care Med 2001;29:2332–48.
10. Teschan PE, Baxter CR, O'Brien CR, et al. Prophylactic hemodialysis in the treatment of acute renal failure. Ann Intern Med 1960;53:992–1016.

11. Whelton A, Danodio JV. Post-traumatic acute renal failure in Vietnam. A comparison with the Korean War experience. Johns Hopkins Med J 1969;124:95–105.
12. Kirkland K, Edwards KDG, Wyte HM. Oliguric renal failure: a report of 400 cases including classification, survival and response to dialysis. Austr Ann Med 1965;1:275–81.
13. Keinknecht D, Jungers P, Chanard J, et al. Uremic and non-uremic complications in acute renal failure: evaluation of early and frequent dialysis on prognosis. Kidney Int 1972;1:190–6.
14. Gettings LG, Reynolds HN, Scalea T. Outcome in post-traumatic acute renal failure when continuous renal replacement therapy is applied early vs. late. Intensive Care Med 1999;25:805–13.
15. Kresse S, Schlee H, Deuber HJ, et al. Influence of renal replacement therapy on outcome of patients with acute renal failure. Kidney Int 1999;56:S75–8.
16. Brady HR, Brenner BM. Acute renal failure. In: Fauci AS, Braunwald E, Isselbacher KJ, et al, eds. Harrison's principles of internal medicine, 14th edn. New York: McGraw-Hill;1998;1504–13.
17. Uchino S, Morimatsu H, Bellomo R, for the B.E.S.T. Kidney Investigators. A multinational, multicenter, prospective, epidemiological survey of acute renal failure in critical illness: the B.E.S.T (Beginning and Ending Supportive Therapy) Kidney Study. 27th Annual Scientific Meeting on Intensive Care, Perth, Australia, Oct. 2002 (abstract).
18. Hankim RM, Wingard RL, Parker RA. Effect of dialysis membrane in the treatment of patients with acute renal failure. N Engl J Med 1994;331:1338–42.
19. Conger JD, Schultz MF, Robinette JB. Responses to hemorrhagic arterial pressure reduction in different ischemic renal failure models. Kidney Int 1994;46:318–26.
20. Bellomo R, Ronco C. Indications and criteria for initiating renal replacement therapy in the intensive care unit. Kidney Int 1998;53(Suppl 66):S106–9.
21. Bellomo R, Ronco C. Continuous renal replacement therapy in the intensive care unit. Intensive Care Med 1999;25:781–9.
22. Haag-Weber M, Horl WH. The immune system in uremia and during its treatment. New Horizons 1995;3:669–79.
23. Marsh JD, Margolis TI, Kim D. Mechanism of diminished contractile response to catecholamines during acidosis. Am J Physiol 1988;254:H20–7.
24. Ronco C, Zanella M, Brendolan A, et al. Management of severe acute renal failure in critically ill patients: an international survey in 345 centers. Nephrol Dial Transplant 2001;16:230–7.
25. Sander A, Armbruster W, Sander B, et al. Hemofiltration increases IL-6 clearance in early systemic inflammatory response syndrome but does not alter IL-6 and TNFα plasma concentrations. Intensive Care Med 1997;23:878–84.
26. Kellum JA, Johnson JP, Kramer D, et al. Diffusive vs. convective therapy: effects on mediators of inflammation in patients with severe systemic inflammatory response syndrome. Crit Care Med 1998;26:1995–2000.
27. De Vriese AS, Colardyn FA, Philippe JJ, et al. Cytokine removal during continuous hemofiltration in septic patients. J Am Soc Nephrol 1999;10:846–53.
28. Van Bommel EFH, Hesse CJ, Jute NHPM, et al. Cytokine kinetics (TNFα, IL-1β, IL-6) during continuous hemofiltration: a laboratory and clinical study. Contrib Nephrol 1995;116:62–75.
29. Cole L, Bellomo R, Hart G, et al. A Phase II randomized controlled trial of continuous hemofiltration in sepsis. Crit Care Med 2002;30:100–6.
30. Uchino S, Bellomo R, Goldsmith D, et al. Super high flux hemofiltration: a new technique for cytokine removal. Intensive Care Med 2002;28:651–5.
31. Cole L, Bellomo R, Journois D, et al. High-volume haemofiltration in human septic shock. Intensive Care Med 2001;27:978–86.
32. Ronco C, Brendolan A, Lonnemann G, et al. A pilot study of coupled plasma filtration with adsorption in septic shock. Crit Care Med 2002;30:1250–5.
33. Brochard L, Rauss A, Benito S, et al. Comparison of three methods of gradual withdrawal from ventilatory support during weaning from mechanical ventilation. Am J Respir Crit Care Med 1994;150:896–903.
34. Esteban A, Frutos F, Tobin MJ, et al. A comparison of four methods of weaning patients from mechanical ventilation. N Engl J Med 1995;332:345–50.
35. Esteban A, Alia I, Tobin MJ, et al. Effect of spontaneous breathing trial duration on outcome of attempts to discontinue mechanical ventilation. Am J Respir Crit Care Med 1999;159:512–18.
36. Vitacca M, Vianello A, Colombo D, et al. Comparison of two methods for weaning patients with chronic obstructive pulmonary disease requiring mechanical ventilation for more than 15 days. Am J Respir Crit Care Med 2001;164:225–30.
37. Mehta RL, McDonald B, Gabbai FB, et al. A randomized clinical trial of continuous versus intermittent dialysis for acute renal failure. Kidney Int 2001;60:1154–63.
38. Prendergast TJ, Luce JM. Increasing incidence of withholding and withdrawal of life support from the critical ill. Am J Respir Crit Care Med 1997;155:15–20.
39. Woodrow G, Turney JH. Cause of death in acute renal failure. Nephrol Dial Transplant 1992;7:230–4.
40. Zamperetti N, Ronco C, Brendolan A, et al. Bioethical issues related to continuous renal replacement therapy in intensive care patients. Intensive Care Med 2000;26:407–15.
41. Parker RA, Himmelfarb J, Tolkoff-Rubin N, et al. Prognosis of patients with acute renal failure requiring dialysis: results of a multicenter study. Am J Kidney Dis 1998;32:432–43.
42. Fiaccadori E, Maggiore U, Lombardi M, et al. Predicting patient outcome from acute renal failure comparing three general severity of illness scoring systems. Kidney Int 2000;58:283–92.
43. Douma CE, Redekop WK, Van der Meulen JHP, et al. Predicting mortality in intensive care patients with acute renal failure treated with dialysis. J Am Soc Nephrol 1997;8:111–17.
44. Knaus WA, Draper EA, Wagner DP, Zimmerman JE. APACHE II: a severity of disease classification system. Crit Care Med 1985;13:818–29.
45. Le Gall J-R, Lemeshow S, Saulnier F. A new simplified acute physiology score (SAPS II) based on an European/North American multicentre study. JAMA 1993;270:2957–63.
46. Knaus WA, Wagner DP, Draper EA, et al. The APACHE III prognostic system. Risk prediction of hospital mortality for critically ill hospitalized adults. Chest 1991;100:1619–36.
47. Liano F, Gallego A, Pascual J, et al. Prognosis of acute tubular necrosis: an extended prospectively contrasted study. Nephron 1993;63:21–31.
48. Cook DJ, Guyatt GH, Jaeschke P, et al. Determinants in Canadian health care workers of the decision to withdraw life support from the critically ill. JAMA 1995;273:703–8.
49. Galla JH. Clinical practice guideline on shared decision-making in the appropriate initiation of and withdrawal from dialysis. J Am Soc Nephrol 2000;11:1340–2.
50. Vincent JL. Cultural differences in end-of-life care. Crit Care Med 2001;29:N52–5.
51. Asai A, Maekawa M, Akiguchi I, et al. Survey of Japanese physicians' attitudes towards the care of adult patients in persistent vegetative state. J Med Ethics 1999;25:302–8.
52. Phu NH, Hien TT, Mai NT, et al. Hemofiltration and peritoneal dialysis in infection-associated acute renal failure in Vietnam. N Engl J Med 2002;347:895–902.

10

Dose adequacy goals for acute renal replacement therapy

William R Clark and Michael A Kraus

INTRODUCTION

The primary aims of any dialysis therapy used in the acute renal failure (ARF) setting are minimizing patient intolerance and providing treatment adequacy. With respect to patient tolerance, hemodynamic stability[1] and a minimized inflammatory response due to interaction between the patient and the dialysis system[2] are the most important considerations. However, the factors influencing acute dialytic treatment adequacy are relatively poorly understood and, as opposed to chronic dialysis therapy,[3] the concept of treatment dose is not yet established firmly. Due to the complexity of the critically ill ARF patient, toxin removal, volume control, control of metabolic derangements, and nutritional provision may all influence treatment adequacy in acute dialysis.[4–8]

It is only recently that the nephrology community has begun to make a serious attempt to differentiate between the renal replacement needs of ARF patients and patients with end-stage renal disease (ESRD).[9] For example, the indications for initiation of acute dialysis therapy may differ significantly from those used in the ESRD setting.[10] In addition, that the management of the ARF patient with intermittent hemodialysis (IHD) cannot simply mimic the approach used for chronic HD patients is being acknowledged increasingly, along with the realization that dialytic requirements with respect to both solute and volume removal are significantly greater in the acute setting.[11] Indeed, for the typical scenario of ARF in the context of multi-organ failure, traditional therapies used in the ESRD setting such as HD (especially performed only thrice-weekly) and peritoneal dialysis may not be feasible or even contraindicated, based on physiologic and metabolic considerations.[12] Unlike the typical ESRD patient, patients with ARF are not at steady state and are unlikely to achieve acceptable azotemic control with a traditional thrice-weekly IHD schedule or peritoneal dialysis.[13]

FACTORS INFLUENCING TREATMENT DELIVERY IN ACUTE DIALYSIS THERAPIES

From the perspective of dialytic treatment adequacy for critically ill ARF patients, a number of general considerations are relevant. Similar to other therapeutic interventions, renal replacement therapy (RRT) should be implemented in such a manner as to minimize physiologic perturbations. Therefore, one aspect of adequate RRT is sufficiently early application that advanced hyperkalemia, azotemia, acidosis, and pulmonary edema are avoided. On the other hand, adequate therapy should not be so aggressive as to create derangements of its own. A second consideration in acute RRT adequacy is the degree to which a treatment mimics the flexibility, versatility, and efficacy of the native kidney. Finally, the renal substitutive therapy should not delay the recovery of kidney function and should have minimal or absent pro-inflammatory effects.

The importance of dialysis treatment-related parameters in determining outcome is gaining increasing recognition in the management of critically ill ARF patients. Specifically, recent studies suggest delivered dose, intensity, and timing of initiation influence the outcome of patients treated with both IHD and continuous renal replacement therapy (CRRT).[11,14–17] These outcome data have generated interest in developing techniques designed to quantify prescribed and delivered therapy in the acute setting.[4–6,12,13,18–26] As such, some of the same methodologies developed to quantify therapy in chronic dialysis have been adapted and extended for use in the ARF dialysis setting. The discussion below addresses the major factors determining therapy delivery in both intermittent and continuous therapies. Because IHD is largely diffusive in nature, the focus is on small solute removal for this therapy.

General factors influencing small solute removal and control in ARF

The primary patient-related factors influencing azotemia control in ARF are protein hypercatabolism, total body water, and body size. As opposed to most ESRD patients, critically ill patients with ARF are typically not in a steady state condition with respect to protein metabolism. In fact, urea generation rates and protein catabolic rates (PCRs) vary on a daily basis[18,19] and hypercatabolism is a very typical finding, with net normalized PCR (nPCR) values of 1.5 g/kg/day or greater and net nitrogen deficits of 6 g/day or greater routinely reported.[12,18,19,21,27,28] However, considerable interpatient variability has been reported and significant nPCR variations within individual patients may occur on a daily basis.

The ESRD literature is replete with studies demonstrating the importance of body size in dialysis dose determinations, and this is also an important consideration in the acute patient. Although not widely studied in ESRD patients, the potential effect of severe volume overload on solute distribution volumes is an additional consideration in ARF patients. For both nonuremics and patients with ESRD, numerous previous investigations have documented that total body water closely approximates urea distribution volume and that anthropometric formulae provide reasonable approximations of the latter parameter. However, Himmelfarb and colleagues have recently demonstrated that the relationship between V and lean body mass in ARF patients is not nearly as well defined.[6] Several factors in ARF make determination of this relationship quite difficult, including severe volume overload and ongoing catabolism of lean body mass. In a group of 11 critically ill ARF patients, Clark et al[29] reported a mean V of 65% of body weight, significantly greater than the 50–60% value typically reported for most patient populations. In concert with catabolism-induced loss of lean body mass, volume overload most likely

accounts for the markedly higher fractional urea distribution volumes in ARF.

As shown recently by Evanson et al,[22] failure to account for these volume disturbances may result in large discrepancies between prescribed and delivered dialysis doses. For a group of patients treated with IHD, these investigators used dialyzer KoA, prescribed blood flow rate and time, and a value of V equal to $0.60 \times$ pre-HD body weight to estimate prescribed Kt/V. Delivered Kt/V was estimated by an equation employing pre-HD and post-HD BUN values. A significant difference was observed between prescribed and delivered Kt/V per treatment (1.26 ± 0.45 vs 1.04 ± 0.49, respectively; mean $\pm$ SD). This difference appeared to be related primarily to the use of an estimated V, for prescription purposes, that was significantly less than the actual (kinetically derived) V. Our group has also highlighted the detrimental effect on expected small solute removal if volume overload is neglected.[30] In addition, the large discrepancy between prescribed and delivered ARF dialysis doses observed in the Evanson et al study has been corroborated by others.[14]

As is the case in chronic HD, vascular access function may also influence small solute clearance in acute dialysis, although the determinants of percutaneous access recirculation are not as well characterized in the latter setting. Percutaneous catheters designed for long-term use in chronic hemodialysis have been shown by Twardowski et al[31] to have very low (about 2%) degrees of recirculation, a finding corroborated by Kelber et al[32] in a study of ARF patients. However, these latter investigators reported a significantly higher degree of recirculation for femoral catheters, with mean values 10% and 18% for catheter lengths of 24 and 15 cm, respectively, at a blood flow rate of 250 ml/min. Consistent with data from Leblanc et al,[33] increasing blood flow rate resulted in a significant increase in recirculation.

Finally, dialyzer or filter function may also influence delivered dialysis dose in ARF patients. One of the major differences between stable ESRD and critically ill ARF patients is the severe bleeding diathesis frequently present in the latter population. Consequently, for many patients, dialysis either with no heparin or a markedly reduced heparin dose is prescribed. Sakiewicz et al[34] have recently assessed the effect of heparin-free dialysis on dialyzer function in ARF patients. In 29 ARF patients, some of whom received heparin-free dialysis, pre-treatment and post-treatment dialyzer fiber bundle volume (FBV) were measured using an ultrasound dilution technique. For the entire patient group, FBV decreased significantly despite no significant change in either arterial or pressure circuit pressure. However, subgroup analysis indicated that the FBV decrease was significant only in the patients treated with heparin-free dialysis. Although the extent of surface area loss did not influence measured dialysis dose in this particular study, these data still raise concerns about compromised dialyzer function during heparin-free dialysis.

Determinants of therapy delivery: IHD-specific

A treatment delivery factor specific to IHD is compartmentalization. During IHD, an inequality (dysequilibrium) in solute concentrations exists between various body compartments, with some solute being sequestered in certain relatively inaccessible compartments. This compartmentalization phenomenon has several clinical implications. First, it is responsible for the well-described rebound in plasma solute concentration that occurs postdialysis, during which time the solute dysequilibrium disappears.[35] Most importantly, compartmentalization reduces overall effective solute removal. For urea, many investigators have proposed that urea is distributed in the extracellular and intracellular spaces, with relative sequestration occurring in the latter during dialysis.[36] On the other hand, Daugirdas and Schneditz have proposed the regional blood flow model to account for intradialytic urea dysequilibrium.[37] In this model, urea dysequilibrium is related to the degree of mismatch between blood supply and urea content in different body compartments. Specifically, although skeletal muscle is a large reservoir for both water and urea, blood supply to this compartment, particularly during dialysis, is relatively low. This mismatch may be worsened in many critically ill ARF patients who have further impairment of skeletal muscle perfusion due to vasopressor dependence.

Determinants of therapy delivery: CRRT-specific

As opposed to IHD, the predominant mass transfer mechanism for different classes of solutes may differ significantly among the continuous therapies. Small solute removal can occur exclusively by con-

vection in continuous venovenous hemofiltration (CVVH),[38,39] predominantly by diffusion in continuous venovenous hemodialysis (CVVHD),[40,41] or by approximately equal contributions of both diffusion and convection in continuous venovenous hemodiafiltration (CVVHDF).[42] For a properly functioning filter, small solute sieving coefficients during CVVH are close to unity[43,44] such that clearances for these solutes are primarily determined by the ultrafiltration rate (UFR) and the mode of replacement fluid administration (predilution vs postdilution).[45] For the diffusion-based continuous therapies employing dialysate flow rates of approximately 3 L/h or less, urea and creatinine clearances approximate the effluent dialysate flow rate because of the existence of dialysis equilibrium.[24,40,41,46] For middle molecule removal, Jeffrey et al[47] have shown convection is more important than diffusion for a surrogate solute (vancomycin: molecular weight (MW), 1448) when the same ultrafiltration rate (CVVH) and effluent dialysate flow rate (CVVHD) of 25 ml/min (1.5 L/h) is used. As the relative importance of convection increases with solute MW, transmembrane removal of larger middle molecules (e.g. low-molecular weight proteins) occurs almost exclusively by this mechanism. However, adsorptive removal of inflammatory mediators in this class has also been demonstrated[48,49] and considerable controversy currently exists as to whether convection or adsorption should be employed preferentially to optimize mediator removal.

In light of recent survival data from Ronco et al,[15] there is increasing interest in the use of relatively high UFRs (>2 L/h) to achieve enhanced convective solute removal rates. One of the major determinants of convective solute removal, especially that pertaining to large molecules such as inflammatory mediators, is concentration polarization.[50] Concentration polarization specifically relates to an ultrafiltration-based process and applies to the kinetic behavior of an individual protein. Accumulation of a plasma protein that is predominantly or completely rejected by a membrane used for ultrafiltration of plasma occurs at the blood compartment membrane surface. This surface accumulation causes the protein concentration just adjacent to the membrane surface (i.e. the submembranous concentration) to be higher than the bulk (plasma) concentration. In this manner, a submembranous (high) to bulk (low) concentration gradient is established, resulting in 'back diffusion' from the membrane surface out into the plasma. At steady state, the rate of convective transport to the membrane surface is equal to the rate of back diffusion. The polarized layer of protein is the distance defined by the gradient between the submembranous and bulk concentrations. This distance (or thickness) of the polarized layer, which can be estimated by mass balance techniques, reflects the extent of the concentration polarization process.

Conditions which promote the process are high UFR (high rate of convective transport), low blood flow rate (low shear rate), and the use of postdilution (rather than predilution) replacement fluids (increased local protein concentrations).[51] The extent of the concentration polarization influences actual solute (protein) removal, but not in a predictable manner. In general, the degree to which the removal of a protein is influenced is directly related to that protein's extent of rejection by an individual membrane. In fact, concentration polarization actually enhances the removal of a molecular weight class of proteins (30–70 kDa) that otherwise would have minimal convective removal.[52,53] This is explained by the fact that the pertinent blood compartment concentration subjected to the ultrafiltrate flux is the high submembranous concentration primarily rather than the much lower bulk concentration. Therefore, the potentially desirable removal of certain proteins in this size range in ARF patients has to be weighed against concomitant albumin losses by the same mechanism.

On the other hand, the use of very high UFRs in conjunction with other conditions favorable to protein polarization may significantly impair overall membrane performance. The relationship between UFR and transmembrane pressure (TMP) is linear for relatively low UFRs and the positive slope of this line defines the ultrafiltration coefficient of the membrane. However, as UFR further increases, this curve eventually plateaus.[52] At this point, maintenance of a certain UFR is only maintained by a concomitant increase in TMP. At sufficiently high TMP, fouling of the membrane with denatured proteins may occur and an irreversible decline in solute and water permeability of the membrane ensues. Therefore, for optimal filter operation in the convective mode, the UFR (and associated TMP) need to fall on the initial (linear) portion of the UFR vs TMP relationship, with avoidance of the plateau region.

Convective solute removal can be quantified in the following manner:[54]

$$N = (1 - \sigma)J_v C_m$$

In this equation, N is the convective flux (mass removal rate per unit membrane area), J_v is the ultrafiltrate flux (ultrafiltration rate normalized to membrane area), C_m is the mean intramembrane solute concentration, and σ is the reflection coefficient, a measure of solute rejection. As Werynski and Waniewski have explained,[54] the parameter $(1-\sigma)$ can be viewed as the membrane resistance to convective solute flow. If σ equals 1, no convective transport occurs, whereas a value of 0 implies no resistance to convective flow. Of note, the appropriate blood compartment concentration used to determine C_m is the submembranous concentration rather than the bulk phase concentration. Therefore, this parameter is significantly influenced by the effects of concentration polarization.

It is useful to assess individually the parameters on the right-hand side of the above equation and the manner in which changes in these parameters may affect the rate of convective solute transport. During an RRT, changes in the permeability properties of the hemofilter membrane or in the operating conditions may alter these parameters. However, a complex interplay exists between these parameters and the net effect of changes in hemofilter membrane permeability or RRT operating conditions may be difficult to predict. To illustrate this point, the effect of a progressive decrease in membrane permeability as a membrane becomes fouled with proteins can be assessed. As a membrane becomes fouled with plasma proteins, the resistance to convective solute flow (σ) increases such that the parameter $(1-\sigma)$ decreases. In addition, fouling may result in a decrease in ultrafiltrate flux (J_v) despite attempted increases in TMP. This phenomenon is most relevant for CRRT systems operated without a blood pump, such as continuous arteriovenous hemofiltration (CAVH) and continuous arteriovenous hemodialysis (CAVHD). However, when the membranes become irreversibly fouled (i.e. gel formation occurs), even a hemofilter used in a venovenous system loses ultrafiltration capabilities. Finally, polarization of solute at the membrane surface due to the fouling causes an increase in the submembranous blood compartment concentration but a decrease in the filtrate concentration. The net effect on C_m, which essentially is a mean of the submembranous and filtrate concentrations, is difficult to predict and depends on the specific solute–membrane combination in question. In general, however, except for relatively large proteins capable of only minimal convective transport (e.g.

albumin), fouling results in a decrease in C_m because the decrease in filtrate concentration is predicted to be greater than the increase in the submembranous concentration.

UREA-BASED APPROACHES TO GUIDE PRESCRIPTION AND DELIVERY OF ACUTE DIALYSIS

In ESRD patients, several investigations have indicated survival varies directly with delivered HD dose,[55,56] although the point at which further increases in dose result in no additional survival benefit continues to be debated.[57] A number of urea-based quantification methods that differ greatly in complexity and usefulness are used in this setting[3] and some of these methodologies are now being applied to acute dialysis therapies.

Clark et al have recently developed a urea-based computer model designed to permit individualized RRT prescription for ARF patients.[13] The critical input parameter is the desired level of metabolic control, which is the time-averaged blood urea nitrogen (BUN_a) or steady-state BUN (BUN_s) for IHD or CRRT, respectively. For nPCR values over a range of approximately 1.5–2 g/kg/day, the model produced BUN vs time curves by the direct quantification method for simulated patients of varying dry weights (50–100 kg) who received variable CRRT clearances (500–2000 ml/h). Steady-state BUN vs time profiles for the same simulated patient population treated with IHD regimens (K = 180 ml/min, t = 4 hours per treatment) of variable frequency were generated by use of the variable-volume single-pool kinetic model. From these profiles, regression lines of required IHD frequency (per week) vs patient weight for desired BUN_a values of 60, 80, and 100 mg/dl were obtained. Regression lines of required CRRT urea clearance (ml/h) vs patient weight for desired BUN_s values of 60, 80, and 100 mg/dl were also generated. The required amounts of IHD (treatment frequency) and CRRT (urea clearance) at these three levels of azotemic control were compared.

For the attainment of intensive metabolic control (BUN_a = 60 mg/dl) at steady state, a required treatment frequency of 4.4 dialyses per week is predicted for a 50 kg patient. However, the model predicts that the same degree of metabolic control cannot be achieved even with daily IHD therapy in hypercatabolic ARF patients weighing more than 90 kg. Conversely, for the attainment of intensive

CRRT metabolic control (BUN_s = 60 mg/dl), required urea clearances of approximately 900 and 1900 ml/h are predicted for 50 kg and 100 kg patients, respectively. Therefore, this model suggests that, for many patients, rigorous azotemia control equivalent to that readily attainable with most CRRTs can only be achieved with intensive IHD regimens. Therefore, these modeled data suggest that the complication of inadequate azotemic control is less likely to occur in hypercatabolic ARF patients if a CRRT is used. Recent data from Schiffl et al[11] have corroborated the predictive validity of the IHD modeling. It is expected that the recent clinical dose–outcome data (vide infra) will generate further interest in therapy quantification in this setting.

Use of urea kinetic methods to guide delivery of acute dialysis

A number of recent investigations have extended urea kinetic methodologies, initially used in the ESRD population, to acute dialysis patients. In 28 ARF patients receiving 46 intermittent HD treatments, Evanson and colleagues[23] used cross-dialyzer clearance determinations to make several urea kinetic estimates of delivered therapy. The mean treatment parameters were dialysis duration of 223 minutes, blood flow rate of 260 ml/min, and dialysate flow rate of 533 ml/min. Applying immediate and 30-minute post-HD BUN values to the Daugirdas II formula,[58] these investigators determined estimates of delivered single-pool and double-pool urea Kt/V, respectively, while the Daugirdas rate equation was employed to estimate equilibrated Kt/V. These estimates of dose delivery were compared to prescribed Kt/V, estimated from anthropometric values of urea volume and manufacturer-derived in-vitro clearances. Mean (±SD) values for prescribed, single-pool, double-pool, and equilibrated Kt/V were 1.11 ± 0.32, 0.96 ± 0.33, 0.84 ± 0.28, and 0.84 ± 0.30, respectively. These data indicate a significant difference between prescribed and delivered dialysis dose and corroborate prior results[14,22] from the acute dialysis population. In addition, these results confirm findings from the chronic hemodialysis population that a significant difference exists between delivered single-pool and double-pool or equilibrated urea Kt/V.

In a more recent study, Schiffl and colleagues assessed the effect of thrice-weekly vs daily HD on urea kinetic parameters in 160 ARF patients.[11]

Single-pool Kt/V, derived from the Daugirdas II equation,[58] was used to estimate delivered HD dose. The treatment characteristics of the two patient groups are shown in Table 10.1. The cumulative (weekly) Kt/V delivered to the daily group was nearly twice that of the alternate-day group, on a mean basis. As there are kinetic benefits related solely to increased frequency, use of a more rigorous 'continuous-equivalent' kinetic approach, such as the equivalent renal clearance (EKR)[36,59] or the standard urea clearance,[60] would actually have increased the difference in delivered dose between the two groups.

Finally, in a very rigorous kinetic analysis, Marshall et al[26] recently employed urea-based kinetic techniques to quantify therapy delivery to ARF patients treated with sustained low-efficiency dialysis (SLED).[61,62] These investigators employed a direct dialysate quantification (DDQ) approach to estimate several patient-related and treatment-related urea kinetic parameters. The following were measured: dialyzer clearance (K), distribution volume (V), generation rate (G), protein catabolic rate (PCR), Kt/V solute removal index (SRI), and EKR (Table 10.2). In addition, urea rebound, based on a BUN sample obtained 60 min post-SLED, was estimated to have a mean value of only 4.1%. This finding, considerably lower than values reported for IHD, suggests the extracorporeal urea clearance provided by the chosen operating parameters (blood flow rate, 200 ml/min; dialysate flow rate, 100 ml/min) results in minimal dysequilibrium. In addition, based on the dialyzer urea clearance determined in the kinetic analyses and the above dialysate flow rate, the dialysis equilibrium characteristic of CVVHD at conventional dialysate flow rates (2 L/h or less) is not achieved in SLED.

THERAPY DOSE AND INTENSITY EFFECTS ON PATIENT OUTCOME IN ACUTE DIALYSIS

Intermittent hemodialysis

Based on presently available data, precise targets for optimal metabolic control are not able to be provided for ARF patients treated with either IHD or CRRT. However, at least for IHD, rough guidelines exist. Kjellstrand has suggested that IHD should be initiated before the BUN reaches 100 mg/dl and that therapy should be delivered at a level to maintain the predialysis BUN below 100 mg/dl.[63] Support for these recommendations is found in early comparative studies in which groups of patients received substantially different levels of IHD therapy.[64-66] In these investigations, survival was directly correlated with IHD intensity as measured by predialysis BUN, which ranged from approximately 90–150 mg/dl.

In a more contemporary study, Gillum et al[67] reported results from a multicenter, prospective study in which the effect of dialysis intensity on survival in patients with ARF was investigated. In this trial, a total of 34 patients with diverse ARF etiologies received either 'intensive' or 'non-intensive' dialysis. Daily dialysis for 5–6 hours per treatment was generally prescribed in the intensive group, whereas the regimen in the nonintensive group consisted of 5-hour treatments administered daily to every third day. Mean predialysis

---

Table 10.1 Treatment parameters in IHD dose study.

Characteristic	Alternate-day hemodialysis	Daily hemodialysis
Duration of session (hours)	3.4 ± 0.5	3.3 ± 0.4
Blood flow rate (ml/min)	243 ± 25	248 ± 45
Dose (Kt/V):		
Prescribed	1.21 ± 0.09	1.19 ± 0.11
Delivered	0.94 ± 0.11	0.92 ± 0.16
Weekly delivered	3.0 ± 0.6	5.8 ± 0.4
Time-averaged BUN (mg/dl)	104 ± 18	60 ± 20*
Ultrafiltrate volume (L/session)	3.5 ± 0.3	1.2 ± 0.5*

* $p < 0.001$ vs alternate-day group.

Source: adapted from Schiffl et al.[11] For further explanation of symbols used, please see text.

Table 10.1 Treatment parameters in IHD dose study.

Characteristic	Alternate-day hemodialysis	Daily hemodialysis
Duration of session (hours)	3.4 ± 0.5	3.3 ± 0.4
Blood flow rate (ml/min)	243 ± 25	248 ± 45
Dose (Kt/V):		
Prescribed	1.21 ± 0.09	1.19 ± 0.11
Delivered	0.94 ± 0.11	0.92 ± 0.16
Weekly delivered	3.0 ± 0.6	5.8 ± 0.4
Time-averaged BUN (mg/dl)	104 ± 18	60 ± 20*
Ultrafiltrate volume (L/session)	3.5 ± 0.3	1.2 ± 0.5*

[a] Hemodialyzer plasma water urea clearance.

[b] Volume of distribution of urea.

[c] Urea nitrogen generation rate.

[d] Protein catabolic rate normalized to body size.

Source: adapted from Marshall et al.[26] For further explanation of symbols used, please see text.

azotemia control achieved in the two groups was very close to the target BUN and serum creatinine values of 60 and 5 mg/dl, respectively (intensive group), and 100 and 9 mg/dl, respectively (nonintensive group). However, prescribed blood and dialysate flow rates were not provided. In addition, data permitting an estimation of the rate of interdialytic urea generation were not reported. Therefore, neither dialysis dose nor PCR could be estimated. Nevertheless, survival in the intensively treated group (41%) did not differ significantly from that in the nonintensive group (52%).

An even more recent investigation assessed outcome in 842 intensive care unit (ICU) ARF patients who received RRT between 1988 and 1994.[14] The Cleveland Clinic Foundation (CCF) ARF scoring system[68] was employed to estimate illness severity. In this system, 23 different demographic, clinical, and laboratory parameters are used to produce a score ranging from 0 (low mortality) to 20 (high mortality). Eight factors were found to be associated strongly with poor patient outcome, including need for mechanical ventilation, leukopenia, thrombocytopenia, number of nonrenal organ system failures, and a low rate of increase in the serum creatinine level. When patient outcome was adjusted for the CCF outcome score, survival was correlated with delivered IHD (Kt/V >1.0 per treatment).

The primary focus of the Schiffl et al study[11] was not kinetic determinations but rather the effect of

different IHD frequencies on patient survival. With respect to this, it should be noted that patients who had severe hemodynamic instability were considered to be candidates only for CRRT and were not eligible for the study. In addition, the mean time-averaged BUN was 60 mg/dl in the daily HD group, whereas the same parameter in the alternate-day group was 104 mg/dl. Although insufficient information was provided to determine precisely the mean predialysis BUN in the alternate-day group, it was very likely in the 140–145 mg/dl range. Consequently, although rigorous guidelines regarding azotemia control do not exist currently, it is clear that the control group received marginally adequate treatment at best.

With respect to outcome, the overall mortality was 37%, with the alternate-day HD group having a significantly ($p = 0.01$) higher mortality (46%) than the daily HD group (28%). Recovery of renal function and frequency of intradialytic hypotension were also favorably impacted by daily HD. The increased frequency (and total weekly duration) of treatment in the daily HD group resulted in significantly lower ultrafiltration requirements per treatment, the most likely explanation for the decreased frequency of hypotension. The authors also reported significantly lower development of oliguria, sepsis, respiratory failure, and gastrointestinal bleeding in the daily HD group. Finally, in the logistic regression analysis, alternate-day HD (vs daily HD) was one of four clinical factors that were predictive of increased mortality. The other factors were increasing APACHE III score, oliguria, and sepsis.

Multiple benefits of increased therapy frequency have been proposed. From a kinetic perspective, increasing frequency results in more efficient utilization of small solute depuration curves because long treatment periods in which solute concentrations are relatively low are avoided. In addition to the benefits specifically pertaining to the kinetics of solute removal, increased IHD frequency may result in decreased ultrafiltration requirements per treatment. The avoidance of hypotensive episodes related to rapid UFRs may also indirectly improve solute removal by decreasing the risk of therapy interruptions.

Both of the above studies have employed a single-pool quantification technique developed specifically for the ESRD population. The equation used in these studies contains constants accounting for the effects of intradialytic urea generation and ultrafiltration on delivered dose. However, these constants were generated from ESRD patients. Therefore, extrapolation of this or any other equation developed specifically for ESRD patients to ARF patients may be problematic.

Continuous therapies

Recent studies also suggest that the intensity or dose of CRRT influences outcome. Data from Storck et al[69] suggest that greater intensity of CRRT is associated with better patient outcome. In this study, patients were treated with either CAVH or CVVH such that a wide range of ultrafiltration rates was obtained. Survival was found to be significantly higher in the CVVH group than in the CAVH group, in which the mean ultrafiltration rates were 15.5 and 7.5 L/day, respectively. Whether the superior survival in the patients treated with CVVH rather than CAVH was related to the former's greater convective removal of small solutes or larger substances could not be determined from the data provided.

In a study performed by Ronco and colleagues,[15] the effect of dose on outcome was assessed in 425 patients treated with CVVH. Patients were randomized to one of three groups based on dose, for which the surrogate was UFR normalized to body weight. The prescribed doses were 25, 35, and 45 ml/h/kg, whereas mean delivered ultrafiltrate volumes were 31, 56, and 68 L/day. CVVH was performed in the postdilution mode with lactate-based substitution fluids. Survival was found to be significantly improved in the two higher-dose groups, relative to that in the lowest-dose group, whereas no survival difference between the two higher-dose groups was reported (Fig. 10.1). Although not prospectively defined as an outcome determinant, this same dose parameter appeared to influence outcome in a similar manner in a study published by Honore et al.[17]

An additional finding of the Ronco et al study related to the effect of the timing of dialysis initiation on outcome. For all three dose groups, the mean BUN at the time of CVVH initiation was significantly lower among survivors vs nonsurvivors. This latter finding has been corroborated by a retrospective study performed by Gettings et al.[16] These investigators found that patients whose BUN was less than 60 mg/dl at the time of CRRT initiation had a significantly higher survival than those patients whose BUN was greater than 60 mg/dl. Finally, suggestive evidence for a beneficial effect of relatively early initation of RRT was reported in a study recently published by Mehta et al.[70]

SUMMARY AND CONCLUSIONS

This chapter has addressed the issue of treatment dose in acute dialytic therapies. Dose determinants for intermittent, semicontinuous, and continuous therapies have been reviewed. In addition, recently proposed urea kinetic-based approaches to guide both therapy prescription and delivery have been discussed. Finally, the available clinical

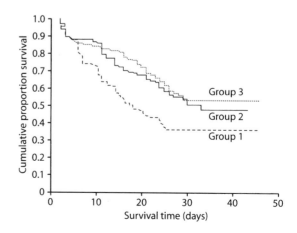

Figure 10.1 Effect of CVVH dose on survival. (Reprinted with permission from Ronco et al.[15])

data correlating dialytic treatment dose or intensity with outcome have been presented. It is expected that this latter issue will be assessed rigorously in the next few years.

REFERENCES

1. Manns M, Sigler MH, Teehan BP. Intradialytic renal hemodynamics: potential consequences for the management of the patient with acute renal failure. Nephrol Dial Transplant 1997;12:870–2.
2. Clark WR, Hamburger RJ, Lysaght MJ. Effect of membrane composition and structure on solute removal and biocompatibility in hemodialysis. Kidney Int 1999;56:2005–15.
3. Clark WR, Rocco MV, Collins AJ. Quantification of hemodialysis: analysis of methods and relevance to clinical outcome. Blood Purif 1997;15:92–111.
4. Clark WR, Mueller BA, Kraus MA, Macias WL. Solute control in acute renal failure: prescription and delivery of adequate extracorporeal therapy. Semin Dial 1996;9:133–9.
5. Clark WR, Mueller BA, Kraus MA, Macias WL. Dialysis prescription and kinetics in acute renal failure. Adv Ren Replace Ther 1997;4:64–71.
6. Himmelfarb J, Evanson J, Hakim RM, et al. Urea volume of distribution exceeds total body water in patients with acute renal failure. Kidney Int 2002;61:317–23.
7. Macias WL. Choice of replacement fluid/dialysate anion in continuous renal replacement therapy. Am J Kidney Dis 1996;28 (Suppl 3):S15–20.
8. Macias WL, Murphy MH, Alaka KJ, et al. Impact of the nutritional regimen on protein catabolism and nitrogen balance in patients with acute renal failure. J Parenter Enteral Nutr 1996;20:56–62.
9. Kanagasundaram NS, Paganini EP. Critical care dialysis – a Gordian knot. Nephrol Dial Transplant 1999;14:2590–4.
10. Bellomo R, Ronco C. Indications and criteria for initiating renal replacement therapy in the intensive care unit. Kidney Int 1998;53 (Suppl 66):S106–9.
11. Schiffl H, Lang SM, Fischer R. Daily hemodialysis and the outcome of acute renal failure. N Engl J Med 2002;346:305–10.
12. Clark WR, Mueller BA, Alaka KJ, Macias WL. A comparison of metabolic control by continuous and intermittent therapies in acute renal failure. J Am Soc Nephrol 1994;4:1413–20.
13. Clark WR, Mueller BA, Kraus MA, Macias WL. Extracorporeal therapy requirements for patients with acute renal failure. J Am Soc Nephrol 1997;8:804–12.
14. Paganini EP, Tapolyai M, Goormastic M, et al. Establishing a dialysis therapy/patient outcome link in intensive care unit acute dialysis for patients with acute renal failure. Am J Kidney Dis 1996;28(Suppl 3):S81–9.
15. Ronco C, Bellomo R, Homel P, et al. Effects of different doses in continuous veno-venous haemofiltration on outcomes of acute renal failure: a prospective randomised trial. Lancet 2000;356:26–30.
16. Gettings LG, Reynolds HN, Scalea T. Outcome in post-traumatic acute renal failure when continuous renal replacement therapy is applied early vs. late. Intensive Care Med 1999;25:805–13.
17. Honore PM, Jamez J, Wauthier M, et al. Prospective evaluation of short-term, high-volume isovolemic hemofiltration on the hemodynamic course and outcome in patients with intractable circulatory failure resulting from septic shock. Crit Care Med 2000;28:3581–7.
18. Clark WR, Murphy MH, Alaka KJ, et al. Urea kinetics in continuous hemofiltration. ASAIO J 1992;38:664–7.
19. Chima CS, Meyer L, Hummell AC, et al. Protein catabolic rate in patients with acute renal failure on continuous arteriovenous hemofiltration and total parenteral nutrition. J Am Soc Nephrol 1993;3:1516–21.
20. Canaud B, Bosc JY, Leblanc M, et al. On-line dialysis quantification in acutely ill patients: preliminary clinical experience with a multi-purpose urea sensor monitoring device. ASAIO J 1998;44:184–90.
21. Leblanc M, Garred LJ, Cardinal J, et al. Catabolism in critical illness: estimation from urea nitrogen appearance and creatinine production during continuous renal replacement therapy. Am J Kidney Dis 1998;32:444–53.
22. Evanson JA, Himmelfarb J, Wingard R, et al. Prescribed versus delivered dialysis in acute renal failure patients. Am J Kidney Dis 1998;32:731–8.
23. Evanson JA, Ikizler TA, Wingard R, et al. Measurement of the delivery of dialysis in acute renal failure. Kidney Int 1999;55:1501–8.
24. Brunet S, Leblanc M, Geadah D, et al. Diffusive and convective solute clearances during continuous renal replacement therapy at various dialysate and ultrafiltration flow rates. Am J Kidney Dis 1999;34:486–92.
25. Kanagasundaram NS, Larive AB, Paganini EP. A fractional dialysate collection method to estimate solute removal in continuous venovenous hemodialysis. Kidney Int 2000;58:2579–84.
26. Marshall MR, Golper TA, Shaver MJ, Alam MG, Chatoth DK. Urea kinetics during sustained low-efficiency dialysis in critically ill patients requiring renal replacement therapy. Am J Kidney Dis 2002;39:556–70.
27. Feinstein EI, Blumenkrantz MJ, Healy M, et al. Clinical and metabolic responses to parenteral nutrition in acute renal failure. Medicine 1981;60:124–37.
28. Feinstein EI, Kopple JD, Silberman H, Massry SG. Total parenteral nutrition with high or low nitrogen intakes in patients with acute renal failure. Kidney Int 1883;26:S319–23.
29. Clark WR, Alaka KJ, Mueller BA, Macias WL. Comparison of metabolic control by intermittent vs continuous renal replacement therapy in patients with acute renal failure [abstract]. Trans Am Soc Artif Intern Organs 1993;39:95.
30. Clark WR, Mueller BA, Kraus MA, Macias WL. Solute control by extracorporeal therapies in acute renal failure. Am J Kidney Dis 1996;28 (Suppl 3):S21–7.
31. Twardowski Z, Van Stone J, Jones M, Klusmeyer M, Haynie J. Blood recirculation in intravenous catheters for hemodialysis. J Am Soc Nephrol 1993;3:1978–81.
32. Kelber J, Delmez J, Windus D. Factors affecting delivery of high-efficiency dialysis using temporary vascular access. Am J Kidney Dis 1993;22:24–9.
33. Leblanc M, Fedak S, Mokris G, Paganini E. Blood recirculation in central temporary catheters for acute hemodialysis. Clin Nephrol 1996;45:315–19.
34. Sakiewicz PG, Kanangasundaram NS, Shore S, et al. On-line measurement of hemodialyzer volume in intermittent hemodialysis for acute renal failure [abstract]. J Am Soc Nephrol 1999;10:196A.
35. Pedrini L, Zereik S, Rasmy S. Causes, kinetics, and clinical implications of post-hemodialysis urea rebound. Kidney Int 1988;34:817–24.
36. Clark W, Leypoldt JK, Henderson L, et al. Quantifying the effect of changes in the hemodialysis prescription on effective solute removal with a mathematical model. J Am Soc Nephrol 1999;10:601–10.
37. Daugirdas JT, Schneditz D. Overestimation of hemodialysis dose depends on dialysis efficiency by regional blood flow but not by conventional two pool urea kinetic analysis. ASAIO J 1995;41:M719–24.

38. Macias WL, Mueller BA, Scarim SK, Robinson M, Rudy D. Continuous venovenous hemofiltration: an alternative to continuous arteriovenous hemofiltration and hemodiafiltration in acute renal failure. Am J Kidney Dis 1991;18:451–8.

39. Canaud B, Garred L, Christol J, et al. Pump-assisted continuous venovenous hemofiltration for treating acute uremia. Kidney Int 1988;33:S154–6.

40. Relton S, Greenberg A, Palevsky P. Dialysate and blood flow dependence of diffusive solute clearance during CVVHD. ASAIO J 1992;38:691–6.

41. Ifedoria O, Teehan B, Sigler M. Solute clearance in continuous venovenous hemodialysis. ASAIO J 1992;38:697–701.

42. Mehta RL. Therapeutic alternatives to renal replacement for critically ill patients in acute renal failure. Semin Nephrol 1994;14:64–82.

43. Golper T, Erbeck K, Roberts P, Price J. Small solute sieving coefficients using hemodialyzers as filters in continuous venovenous hemofiltration [abstract]. J Am Soc Nephrol 1992;3:367.

44. Schaeffer J, Olbricht CJ, Koch KM. Long-term performance of hemofilters in continuous hemofiltration. Nephron 1996;72:155–8.

45. Ofsthun NJ, Colton CK, Lysaght MJ. Determinants of fluid and solute removal rates during hemofiltration. In: Henderson L, Quellhorst E, Baldamus C, Lysaght M, eds. Hemofiltration. Berlin: Springer-Verlag; 1986:17–39.

46. Sigler MH, Teehan BP. Solute transport in continous hemodialysis: a new treatment for acute renal failure. Kidney Int 1987;32:562–71.

47. Jeffrey RF, Khan AA, Prabhu P, et al. A comparison of molecular clearance rates during continuous hemofiltration and hemodialysis with a novel volumetric continuous renal replacement system. Artif Organs 1994;18:425–8.

48. De Vriese A, Colardyn F, Philippe J, et al. Cytokine removal during continuous hemofiltration in septic patients. J Am Soc Nephrol 1999;10:846–53.

49. Gasche Y, Pascual M, Suter P, et al. Complement depletion during haemofiltration with polyacrylonitrile membranes. Nephrol Dial Transplant 1996;11:117–19.

50. Henderson LW. Biophysics of ultrafiltration and hemofiltration. In: Jacobs C, ed. Replacement of renal function by dialysis, 4th edn. Dortdrecht: Kluwer Academic Publishers; 1995:114–18.

51. Henderson LW. Pre vs post dilution hemofiltration. Clin Nephrol 1979;11:120–4.

52. Kim ST. Characteristics of protein removal in hemodiafiltration. Contrib Nephrol 1994;108:23–37.

53. Ono M, Taoka M, Takagi T, Ogawa H, Saito A. Comparison of types of on-line hemodiafiltration from the standpoint of low-molecular weight protein removal. Contrib Nephrol 1994;108:38–45.

54. Werynski A, Waniewski J. Theoretical description of mass transport in medical membrane devices. Artif Organs 1995;19:420–7.

55. NKF-DOQI Hemodialysis Work Group. NKF-DOQI clinical practice guidelines for hemodialysis adequacy. Am J Kidney Dis 1997;30(Suppl 2):S12–64.

56. Szczech LA, Lowrie EG, Li Z, et al. Changing hemodialysis thresholds for optimal survival. Kidney Int 2001;59:738–45.

57. Eknoyan G, Beck GJ, Cheung AK, et al. Effect of dialysis dose and membrane flux in maintenance hemodialysis. N Engl J Med 2002;347:2010–19.

58. Daugirdas JT. Second generation logarithmic estimates of single-pool variable volume Kt/V: an analysis of error. J Am Soc Nephrol 1993;4:1205–13.

59. Casino FG, Lopez T. The equivalent renal urea clearance: a new parameter to assess dialysis dose. Nephrol Dial Transplant 1996;11:1574–91.

60. Gotch FA. The current place of urea kinetic modeling with respect to different dialysis modalities. Nephrol Dial Transplant 1998;13(Suppl 6):10–14.

61. Marshall MR, Golper TA, Shaver MJ, Alam MG, Chatoth DK. Sustained low-efficiency dialysis for critically ill patients requiring renal replacement therapy: clinical experience. Kidney Int 2001;60:777–85.

62. Kumar V, Craig M, Depner TA, Yeun J. Extended daily dialysis: a new approach to renal replacement therapy for acute renal failure in the intensive care unit. Am J Kidney Dis 2000;36:294–300.

63. Kjellstrand C, Jacobson S, Lins L. Acute renal failure. In: Maher J, ed. Replacement of renal function by dialysis, 3rd edn. Dordrecht: Kluwer Academic Publishers; 1989:616–49.

64. Gornick C, Kjellstrand C. Acute renal failure complicating aortic aneurysm surgery. Nephron 1983;35:145–57.

65. Matas M, Payne W, Simmons R, Buselmeier T, Kjellstrand C. Acute renal failure following blunt civilian trauma. Ann Surg 1977;185:301–6.

66. Kleinknecht D, Jungers P, Chanard J, Barbanel C, Ganeval D. Uremic and non-uremic complications in acute renal failure: evaluation of early and frequent dialysis on prognosis. Kidney Int 1972;1:190–6.

67. Gillum DM, Dixon BS, Yanover MJ, et al. The role of intensive dialysis in acute renal failure. Clin Nephrol 1986;25:249–55.

68. Paganini EP, Halstenberg WK, Goormastic M. Risk modeling in acute renal failure requiring dialysis. Clin Nephrol 1996;46:206–11.

69. Storck M, Hartl W, Zimmerer E, Inthorn D. Comparison of pump-driven and spontaneous hemofiltration in postoperative acute renal failure. Lancet 1991;337:452–5.

70. Mehta RL, Pascual MT, Soroko S, Chertow GM. Diuretics, mortality, and nonrecovery of renal function in acute renal failure. JAMA 2002;288:2547–53.

11

Vascular access for renal replacement therapy

Jack Work

The choice of hemodialysis vascular access for renal replacement therapy in the intensive care unit (ICU) setting is determined by a number of factors, including patient acuity, which determines the need for immediate vascular access, dialysis modality, and anticipated duration of hemodialysis support. For the patient requiring immediate dialysis, a temporary noncuffed catheter may be placed at the bedside; on the other hand, if it were anticipated that the patient requires long-term dialysis support, placement of a cuffed tunneled catheter would be more appropriate. The hemodialysis catheter is a unique venous access device. Unlike other central venous catheters, the hemodialysis catheter supports both blood infusion and withdrawal at relatively high flow rates. Continuous renal replacement therapies require blood flow rates on the order of 50–150 ml/min, whereas intermittent hemodialysis therapies generally necessitate blood flow rates in the 300–500 ml/min ranges.

Most hemodialysis catheters are made of either silicone or polyurethane. Silicone is a soft and flexible material. Because of these properties, silicone catheters require a thicker wall to minimize lumen collapse and avoid kinking. Silicone has been used primarily for cuffed tunneled catheters; however, several temporary silicone catheters are available that require a stiffening inner stylet during insertion. Silicon is compatible with most ointments, but is degraded by iodine and is slightly degraded by povidone-iodine solutions.[1] Polyurethane is more rigid than silicone, allowing thinner catheter walls. Most central venous catheters are made of polurethane. The primary drawback to polyurethane catheters is that alcohol or ointments containing polyethylene glycol such as Betadine (povidone-iodine) ointment or mupirocin weaken the catheter wall, over time, leading to blistering and breakdown of the catheter. Newer composites such as polyurethane/polycarbonate copolymers have the same physical properties as polyurethane and are resistant to iodine and alcohol.[1] Unfortunately, it is frequently difficult to identify the particular catheter material in order to avoid using an incompatible agent.

Hemodialysis central venous catheters generally have two lumens. Hemodialysis catheters are available with a third lumen specifically designed for fluid or medication administration or blood sampling without compromising the dialysis lumens. Blood flow is directly proportional to the fourth power of the luminal diameter; thus, flow is doubled when the diameter is increased by only 19%. The catheter diameter and number of lumens selected should be based on the hemodialysis modality blood flow requirements and the need for a third lumen.

Acute or temporary catheters are noncuffed and nontunneled dual- or triple-lumen catheters. Most temporary catheters are usually composed of polyurethane, which owing to the relative strength of the material, permits a larger internal lumen for a given outer diameter. The catheter tip inserted in the neck or groin should be located in the superior vena cava or inferior vena cava, respectively. The relatively rigid temporary catheter tip should not be placed in the right atrium in order to minimize the possibility of catheter erosion through the cardiac wall. Temporary catheters' outer diameter ranges between 11 and 14 French (3F = 1 mm). The choice of catheter length is site-dependent. Common catheter lengths, by site of location, are listed in Table 11.1.

The tunneled cuffed catheter, frequently referred to as the PermCath, may be used as a temporary vascular access for patients with acute renal failure,

Table 11.1   Temporary catheter length by location of insertion.

Site of insertion	Length (cm)
Right internal jugular vein	12–15
Left internal jugular vein	15–20
Femoral vein	19–24

a backup vascular access, and a bridge access to allow time for maturation of a permanent access such as an autogenous fistula or graft. The cuffed tunneled catheter is a better first choice for vascular access in the patient who is likely to require more than 1–3 weeks of dialysis support because of the significantly lower infection rate compared to the temporary catheter (Table 11.2). Although the cuffed tunneled catheter can be placed successfully without fluoroscopic guidance,[2] fluoroscopic imaging increases safety, accuracy, and successful placement of central venous hemodialysis catheters. The difference in placing a cuffed tunneled catheter compared with the temporary catheter is the creation of the subcutaneous tunnel and catheter tip position. The cuffed tunneled catheter tip should be positioned in the right atrium for optimal flow.[3] The cuffed tunneled catheter may be used immediately after placement. Unfortunately, the cuffed tunneled catheter also has several disadvantages, albeit less frequent than the noncuffed temporary catheter, including high frequency of both infection and thrombosis (see Table 11.2).

SITE SELECTION FOR CATHETER INSERTION

The choice of access location influences the function of the catheter, the long-term complications associated with the catheter, and future sites for permanent access surgery in those patients who will require long-term dialysis support. The right internal jugular is generally accepted as the preferable site for upper body placement for both the temporary and the cuffed tunneled catheter because the rate of complications encountered during and after placement is lower than other upper body locations.[4,5] The right internal jugular location is important in lessening the development of central venous stenosis, which occurs more frequently with placement in the subclavian vein.[6,7]

Several studies have examined the incidence of central vein stenosis associated with either the subclavian or internal jugular venous access site. With temporary catheter placement, a 50% incidence of stenosis associated with the subclavian insertion site was reported compared to no stenosis with the internal jugular insertion site.[6] Another study reported a 42% incidence of stenosis with subclavian insertion sites and 10% with internal jugular insertion sites.[7] A retrospective study, comparing the incidence of symptomatic venous thrombosis by site of insertion in 774 catheter placements, found a 13% incidence of venous thrombosis with the subclavian catheters vs 3% with the internal jugular catheters.[8] The true incidence of venous stenosis secondary to central venous hemodialysis catheters is probably underestimated. Two studies have found that asymptomatic thrombosis occurs in approximately 65% of subclavian central venous catheters.[9,10]

The second choice for catheter insertion is not as clearly established, and site selection is dependent upon the patient's individual circumstances. This is particularly important in the patient who will require long-term dialysis support. The left or right subclavian vein appears to have less flow-related problems and less thrombosis compared to the left internal jugular vein or left external jugular vein.[8]

Table 11.2   Infection from temporary hemodialysis catheters compared to cuffed tunneled hemodialysis catheters.

Type of infection	Temporary catheter (No. per 1000 catheter days)	Cuffed tunneled catheter (No. per 1000 catheter days)
Bacteremia	6.2	1.8
Exit site infection	3.6	1.4
Tunnel infection	Not applicable	0.02
Distant infection	1.1	0.4

Source: modified from Oliver,[5] with permission.

For example, if a patient has exhausted the left upper extremity in terms of future vascular access sites, then the left subclavian vein would be the preferred insertion site when the right internal or external jugular vein are occluded. On the other hand, if the left upper extremity has a potential vascular access site, then the right subclavian vein would be the site of choice.

For conventional intermittent hemodialysis, a catheter should be able to deliver over 300 ml/min blood flow to provide adequate dialysis. To consistently obtain a blood flow greater than 300 ml/min, the cuffed tunneled catheter tip should be placed in the mid-right atrium. Catheter tip position was the only factor predictive of malfunction.[3] Adequate blood flow was more frequently found in a prospective study of 25 dialysis patients with central venous catheters with the catheter tip in the right atrium.[11] Because the cuffed tunneled catheter is placed with the patient in the supine position and is secured to the subcutaneous tissue by the cuff, when the patient is sitting up for treatment, the tip of the catheter may retract up by as much as 1–4 cm, depending upon the patient's body build.[12,13]

IMAGING TECHNIQUES FOR CATHETER INSERTION

Ultrasound guidance to assist cannulation of the internal jugular vein was first reported in a series of studies in the mid 1980s.[14] Indeed, unsuccessful insertion of central venous catheters may occur in 20% of cases.[15–17] The 1997 Dialysis Outcomes Quality Initiatives recommended 'real-time ultrasound guided insertion to reduce insertion related complications' based on both evidence and opinion.[4] Subsequently, several studies have further documented the importance of using ultrasound guidance for internal jugular vein cannulation. A prospective study evaluated an ultrasound-guided method for internal jugular vein cannulation in 302 patients compared to an external landmark technique in the same number of patients.[18] Successful cannulation was achieved in 100% of the ultrasound-guided group and in 88.1% of the landmark technique group. Importantly, the vein was punctured on the first attempt in 78% of the ultrasound-guided group but in only 38% of the landmark-guided group. Complications were significantly less in the ultrasound-guided group, with carotid artery puncture occurring in 1.7%, brachial plexus irritation in 0.4%, and hematoma in

0.2%, compared with the landmark-guided group, with carotid artery puncture occurring in 8.3%, brachial plexus irritation in 1.7%, and hematoma in 3.3%. Finally, the average time taken to access the vein was less in the ultrasound-guided group.[18] These observations have recently been confirmed in another prospective study of 100 patients undergoing routine internal jugular vein cannulation. Access time, failure rates, and complications were significantly fewer with the ultrasound-guided technique compared with the anatomic landmark group.[19] A number of other studies have examined the ultrasound-guided approach compared with the landmark-guided approach and established the ultrasound-guided method as the standard of care for insertion of cuffed tunneled catheters.[20]

The higher failure rate in the landmark-guided group may be explained by the anatomic variations of the internal jugular vein location. Several studies have documented the degree of anatomic variation in the location of the internal jugular vein.[20] As illustrated in Figure 11.1, anatomic variation occurs frequently. Ultrasound examination prior to placement of catheters is particularly important in patients with a previous history of central vein catheters. In 100 consecutive hemodialysis catheter placements in 79 patients who had been on dialysis for a mean of 19.6 months, a significant ultrasound finding of altered access approach was noted in 35% of the patients. These findings included total occlusion, nonocclusive thrombus, stenosis, and anatomic variation.[21] Ultrasound-guided cannulation of the femoral vein has also been shown to be effective. In approximately one-fourth of individuals, the femoral vein at the groin is directly posterior to the artery. Cannulation of the femoral vein was successful in 100% of patients using the ultrasound-guided technique compared with 89.5% of patients

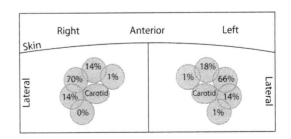

Figure 11.1 Anatomic variability of the internal jugular vein with respect to the carotid artery. (Reproduced from Caridi JG, venousaccess.com, with permission.)

using the landmark-guided technique. Using ultrasound, femoral artery puncture occurred in 7.1% and hematoma in 0% of patients compared with 15.8% femoral artery puncture and 2.6% hematoma in the external landmark group of patients.[22]

The DOQI guidelines state: 'fluoroscopy is mandatory for insertion of all cuffed dialysis catheters'.[4] Although there is little published evidence to support this recommendation, the use of fluoroscopy during catheter insertion does allow for placement of the guide wire into the inferior vena cava, decreasing the possibility for arrhythmias and ensuring proper catheter tip placement. In a study of 188 cuffed tunneled catheter placements, the use of fluoroscopy was compared to an external landmark technique, using the right fourth intercostal space as the landmark. All catheter insertions used ultrasound guidance. There were no differences in procedure success, complications, or catheter function with or without the use of fluoroscopy. Comparing postprocedure upright chest X-rays for tip position, 97% of the fluoroscopy group achieved a right atrial position compared with 92% in the landmark group.[2] Fluoroscopy may not be necessary for cuffed tunneled catheter insertion in selected patients without a history of prior catheters or venous abnormalities.

A postprocedure chest X-ray should be obtained if fluoroscopy is not used. Indeed, the necessity of the postprocedure chest X-ray has been questioned when the cuffed tunneled catheter is placed using fluoroscopy. Only seven procedural complications were identified in 937 consecutive central venous access procedures, of which 670 were cuffed tunneled catheters. All of the complications were noted with fluoroscopy. Postprocedure radiography failed to reveal any unknown complications, but did detect one malpositioned catheter.[23] This suggests that postprocedure radiography is of minimal benefit if fluoroscopy is used during cuffed tunneled catheter insertion. If fluoroscopy is used during central vein catheter insertion, obtaining a routine chest X-ray postprocedure should be an individual or institutional decision.

COMPLICATIONS OF CENTRAL VENOUS DIALYSIS CATHETER INSERTION

Significant immediate complications with central venous dialysis catheter insertion are almost entirely associated with the use of the anatomic landmark technique. The success of landmark-guided catheter placement depends on the target vein being in its expected position, being patent, and being of normal caliber. Frequently, the target vein fails to meet these requirements in a significant number of patients. The most common complications for either temporary or chronic dialysis catheters include inadvertent puncture of the carotid artery, air embolism, hemothorax, and pneumothorax.[24] Other significant complications include hemopericardium,[25] phrenic nerve palsy,[26] thyrocervical trunk pseudoaneurysm,[27] right atrial endocarditis,[28] and pulmonary abscess.[29]

Catheter insertion

Central venous dialysis catheters should be placed in a maximum barrier protection environment. Prior to surgical scrub, it is helpful to examine the selected site using an ultrasound to ensure that the patient has a suitable vein in the selected location. The insertion site and surrounding areas should be cleansed with surgical scrub and draped appropriately (include shoulder and chest wall if a cuffed tunneled catheter is to be inserted). The ultrasound probe should be covered with a sterile sheath, and the insertion site should be insonated to identify the vein. The ultrasound probe may be placed parallel to the long axis of the vessel and the cannulation needle inserted adjacent to the end or short axis of the probe. Alternatively, the probe may be placed perpendicular to the long axis of the vessel. This approach gives the vein the more typical appearance of a circle but limits the visualization of the needle. The vein typically collapses with gentle pressure of the probe, whereas the artery does not. A Valsalva or sniffing maneuver by the patient will enlarge or decrease, respectively, the size of the vein, further enabling one to distinguish the vein from the artery.[30] Occasionally, it is necessary to start high in the neck and follow down to the clavicular groove to optimally identify the vein. Using the right internal jugular vein cannulation as an example, the ultrasound probe is placed parallel and superior to the clavicle, over the groove between the sternal and clavicular heads of the sternocleidomastoid muscle. It is important to avoid inserting the catheter through the muscle, as this is uncomfortable for the patient on a chronic basis.

The site for insertion is infiltrated with local anesthesia. Using real-time ultrasound guidance, a 21-gauge micropuncture needle with an attached syringe is inserted into the vein (Fig. 11.2).

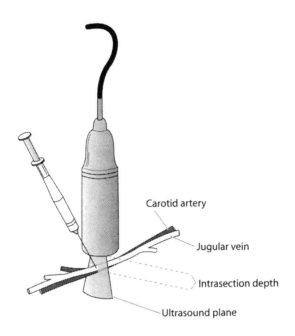

Figure 11.2 Ultrasound probe with needle guide used to localize central vein for cannulation.

Available from several commercial sources, the typical micropuncture kit consists of a 21-gauge needle, an 0.018-inch guide wire, and a 4F or 5F coaxial dilator, as illustrated in Fig. 11.3. The small needle limits potential complications if the carotid

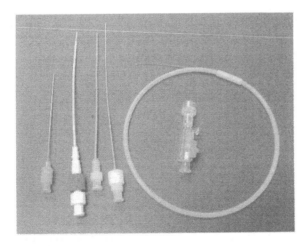

Figure 11.3 Micropuncture set with 21-gauge needle, coaxial 5F dilator with inner 3F dilator assembled, coaxial 5F dilator for 0.035-inch guide wire, 3F for 0.018-inch guide wire, 0.018-inch guide wire, flowswitch with Leur lock connections, and pinch valve for 0.035-inch guide wire.

artery is inadvertently punctured compared to a larger 18-gauge needle, which is included in commercially available dialysis catheter trays. In addition, using the smaller-gauge needle makes it more likely that only the anterior wall of the vein is punctured.[31] Under direct visualization, the vein will be seen to gently push in before penetrating the anterior vein wall. If the needle guide is being used, the ultrasound probe is peeled away, carefully maintaining the needle position. The syringe is removed, and an 0.018-inch guide wire is inserted through the needle. The guide wire is advanced. Using fluoroscopy, the position of the guide wire is confirmed. The needle is then removed and, if necessary, a small stab wound is made at the insertion site where the guide wire enters the skin. The coaxial 5F dilator is then advanced over the guide wire. The guide wire and 3F inner translational dilator are removed, leaving the 5F outer dilator in place. In order to prevent the possibility of an air embolism, a flow switch or stopcock is attached to the dilator.

In the critically ill ICU patient, a noncuffed temporary or cuffed tunneled catheter may be inserted under local anesthesia with minimal patient discomfort. If a peripheral intravenous (IV) access is available and conscious sedation is going to be given, it is advantageous to administer agents such as midazolam and fentanyl, which in combination provide adequate amnesic and analgesic, prior to cannulation of the vein. If a peripheral IV access is not available, one can administer conscious sedation through the dilator. When conscious sedation is used, the patient should be monitored according to institutional policy.

The next step depends on whether one is placing a noncuffed temporary or cuffed tunneled catheter. For temporary catheter placement, a standard 0.035-inch guide wire is advanced into the vein and then a 5F dilator is removed, leaving the guide wire. In stepwise fashion, dilators of increasing size are passed over the guide wire in order to progressively dilate the soft tissue and venous tract; the dilator should move freely on the guide wire. The dilator should not be forcefully advanced, as it is possible for the dilator to get off axis and impinge on the guide wire and perforate the vein and/or the mediastinum. If there is any doubt as to location of the dilator or if there is hesitancy or difficulty in dilating the tract, imaging techniques should be used to assist in placement. The last dilator is then exchanged for the temporary catheter, which is advanced over the guide wire into position. After securing the catheter in place, a chest X-ray should be obtained for confirmation of correct positioning and to check for any complications, if a fluoroscope was not available during insertion. If the patient requires long-term dialysis support, the temporary noncuffed catheter, when located in the internal jugular vein, may be safely converted to a cuffed tunneled catheter if there is no evidence of an exit-site infection.

For cuffed tunneled catheter insertion, one can either proceed to place a guide wire and then create the tunnel or create the tunnel first. The latter course of action minimizes the amount of time that a guide wire is in the circulation and permits immediate access to the central circulation during the procedure. A 1 cm skin incision is made from the dilator, extending laterally. The subcutaneous tissue is then exposed with blunt dissection, creating a subcutaneous pocket so that the catheter bend will be kink-free. Further dissection is made to ensure that the soft tissue around the 5F dilator is free. The catheter exit site is then identified by using landmark technique[2] or by laying the catheter on the patient's chest to approximate the final position in the right atrium. The catheter length may be selected based on patient's body build and type of catheter that will be used. The desired length of the subcutaneous tunnel may be determined more precisely by using a guide wire to measure the distance from the insertion site to the mid right atrium. Using this measurement as a guide, the length of tunnel may then be determined, so that the cuff is within the tunnel approximately 1–2 cm from the exit site.

Once the exit site for the catheter is identified, the area is infiltrated with local anesthesia; a puncture is made through the skin using a knife blade. A No. 11 knife blade inserted parallel to the skin and to the widest point of the blade accommodates most dual-lumen catheters. A long needle such as the micropuncture needle is used to infiltrate the tunnel tract, extending from the exit site to the venotomy insertion site. The catheter is mounted on the end of the tunneling device and the tunneling device is pulled from the exit site subcutaneously to the insertion site. Alternatively, an appropriately sized dilator with sheath can be used to create the subcutaneous tunnel and the catheter passed through the sheath.[32] The cuff of the catheter is pulled into the tunnel and the tunneling device is then carefully removed from the catheter.

A guide wire such as a Benson is now passed through the dilator into the inferior vena cava. Placement of the guide wire into the inferior vena cava decreases the likelihood of cardiac arrhythmias. The guide wire provided with most catheter trays may also be used. These guide wires typically are inexpensive J wires. ICU patients who have pacemaker wires or inferior vena cava filters should have their catheters placed under fluoroscopic guidance in order to avoid entanglement of the guide wire.[33] The 5F dilator is then removed and, in stepwise fashion, dilators of increasing size are passed over the guide wire in order to progressively dilate the soft tissue and venous tract. The dilator should move freely on the guide wire. It is possible for the dilator to get off axis and impinge on the guide wire and perforate the vein and/or the mediastinum. If there is any doubt as to location of the dilator or if there is hesitancy or difficulty in dilating the tract, the fluoroscope should be used to verify proper positioning.

After the final dilation, insert the dilator with Peel-Away sheath. As one inserts the sheath, a resistance is felt as the sheath goes through the soft tissue and then a final resistance as it enters the vein. The Peel-Away sheath is then advanced slightly. For the right internal jugular vein, which permits direct placement of the catheter into the right atrium, the dilator and guide wire may be removed together. The guide wire should be left in place to ensure access is available if there are any difficulties. It is always safest to leave the guide wire in place. For catheter placement on the left side or other alternative sites, the guide wire is left in place so that the catheter may be inserted over the guide wire and thereby tracts directly into the right atrial position. The sheath should be grasped between the finger and thumb of one's hand in order to occlude the sheath. This prevents bleeding and/or aspiration of air while leaving enough length of the sheath to insert the catheter. Alternatively, the catheter may be threaded over the guide wire without using a sheath and advanced through the venous tract into final position. One may need to slightly torque the catheter in order to advance it through the tract. This maneuver decreases the possibility of air embolism and may result in a smaller venotomy and therefore may result in less postprocedure bleeding.

Once the dilator and guide wire have been removed, the catheter tip is inserted into the opening of the sheath in such a way as to avoid twisting the catheter. The catheter is fed through the sheath. The catheter is pushed further into the sheath and the sheath is peeled downward toward the skin. As soon as the catheter is advanced maximally, the sheath is pulled out and then pealed down outside of the venotomy. This avoids the sheath creating a larger venous tract. Once the sheath has been completely removed, the catheter is pulled back into the tunnel so that the cuff is now approximately 1–2 cm from the exit site. The catheter is now checked to ensure that it is functioning properly. A 10 ml syringe should be rapidly pulled back without any shuttering to ensure blood flow greater than 300 ml/min.

The venotomy insertion site is closed using appropriate suture after confirmation of adequate flow. The exit site is closed using a purse-string suture wrapped around the catheter to provide a harness for the catheter at the skin surface. Additional suture is used to hold the catheter at the hub. Using 'air knots' to secure the catheter hub increases patient comfort and decreases the likelihood of skin necrosis. Topical antibiotic ointment may be applied to the incisions and needle puncture sites, and a gauze dressing is applied. Alternatively, a transparent semipermeable (nonocclusive) adhesive dressing may be used to secure the catheter. However, several studies have demonstrated higher bacterial colonization rates at the exit site when transparent dressings are used instead of gauze.[34] Routine dressing changes should be performed as per institutional policy, usually every 2 days or sooner if the dressing is moist or soiled. The need for prophylactic antibiotics for this procedure has never been established. The catheter lumen are filled or 'locked' with the appropriate designated amounts of heparin for each catheter lumen using 1000 units/ml concentration. Using positive intermittent flushing while filling the lumen with heparin and removing the needle while under positive pressure will reduce backflow of blood into the distal portion of the catheter. Use appropriate sterile technique, including wearing a mask, when connecting and disconnecting lines to the dialysis catheter.

Catheter removal

Catheter removal should be done with the patient in a supine position to minimize the possibility of air embolization. Various maneuvers have been recommended that increase intrathoracic pressure such as breath-hold, humming, or Valsalva during catheter placement or removal that have the potential for preventing air embolism. The potential usefulness of these physiologic maneuvers has recently been evaluated. The Valsalva maneuver

had the higher average positive central venous pressure and therefore would be more likely to prevent air embolism.[35] However, it may be difficult to get a patient to perform the maneuver at the correct time. If the cuffed tunneled catheter has been in place for more then 10 days, the fibrin growth around the Dacron cuff must be removed in order to remove the catheter. After sterile prep of the external part of the catheter and the chest wall, local anesthesia is administered at the exit site and blunt dissection is used to free the cuff. The tenacious fibrin sheath that is adherent to the cuff should be removed carefully using a hemostat. The catheter is removed and pressure is applied to the venotomy site. One may use an ointment with gauze dressing to occlude the exit site.

REFERENCES

1. Ash SR. The evolution and function of central venous catheters for dialysis. Semin Dial 2001;14:416–24.
2. Saad T. Tunneled-cuffed venous hemodialysis catheter insertion with or without use of fluoroscopy. J Am Soc Nephrol 2000;11:196 [abstract].
3. Petersen J, Delaney JH, Brakstad MT, et al. Silicone venous access devices positioned with their tips high in the superior vena cava are more likely to malfunction. Am J Surg 1999;178:38–41.
4. Schwab S, Besarab A, Beathard G, et al. NKF-DOQI clinical practice guidelines for vascular access. Am J Kidney Dis 1997;30: S150–90.
5. Oliver MJ. Acute dialysis catheters. Semin dialysis 2001;14:432–5.
6. Cimochowski GE, Worley E, Rutherford WE, et al. Superiority of the internal jugular over the subclavian access for temporary dialysis. Nephron 1990;54:154–61.
7. Schillinger F, Schillinger D, Montagnac R, et al. Post catheterization vein stenosis in haemodialysis: comparative angiographic study of 50 subclavian and 50 internal jugular accesses. Nephrol Dial Transplant 1991;6:722–4.
8. Trerotola SO, Kuhn-Fulton J, Johnson MS, et al. Tunneled infusion catheters: increased incidence of symptomatic venous thrombosis after subclavian versus internal jugular venous access. Radiology 2000;217(1):89–93.
9. Haire WD, Liegerman RP, Lund GB, et al. Thrombotic complications of silicone rubber catheters during autologous marrow and peripheral stem cell transplantation: prospective comparison of Hickman and Groshong catheters. Bone Marrow Transplant 1991;7:57–9.
10. DeCicco M, Matovic M, Balestreri, et al. Central venous thrombosis: an early and frequent complication in cancer patients bearing long-term silastic catheter – a prospective study. Thromb Res 1997;86:101–13.
11. Jean G, Chazot C, Vanel T, et al. Central venous catheters for haemodialysis: looking for optimal blood flow. Nephrol Dial Transplant 1997;12:1689–91.
12. Nazarian GK, Bjarnason H, Dietz CA, et al. Changes in tunneled catheter tip position when a patient is upright. J Vasc Interv Radiol 1997;8:437–41.
13. Kowalski CM, Kaufman JA, Rivita SM, et al. Migration of central venous catheters: implications for initial catheter tip positioning. J Vasc Interv Radiol 1997;8:443–7.

14. Denys BG, Uretsky BF. Anatomical variations of internal jugular vein location: impact on central venous access. Crit Care Med 1991;19:1516–19.

15. Mansfield PF, Hohn DC, Fornage BD, et al. Complications and failures of subclavian-vein catheterization. N Engl J Med 1994;331:1735–8.

16. Sznajder JI, Zveibil FR, Bitterman H, et al. Central vein catheterization. Failure and complication rates by three percutaneous approaches. Arch Intern Med 1986;146:259–61.

17. Bernard RW, Stahl WM. Subclavian vein catheterization: a prospective study. I. Non-infectious complications. Ann Surg 1971;173:184–90.

18. Denys BG, Uretsky BF, Reddy PS. Ultrasound-assisted cannulation of the internal jugular vein. Circulation 1993;87:1557–62.

19. Teichgraber UKM, Benter T, Gebel M, et al. A sonographically guided technique for central venous access. AJR Am J Roentgenol 1997;169:731–3.

20. Caridi JG, Hawkins IF, Weichmann BN, et al. Sonographic guidance when using the right internal jugular vein for central vein access. AJR Am J Roentgenol 1998;171:1259–63.

21. Forauer AR, Glockner JF. Importance of US findings in access planning during jugular vein hemodialysis catheter placements. J Vasc Interv Radiol 2000;11:233–8.

22. Kwon TH, Kim YL, Cho DK. Ultrasound-guided cannulation of the femoral vein for acute haemodialysis access. Nephrol Dial Transplant 1997;12:1009–12.

23. Caridi JG, West JH, Stavropoulos SW, et al. Internal jugular and upper extremity central venous access in interventional radiology: is a postprocedure chest radiography necessary? AJR Am J Roentgenol 2000;174:363–6.

24. Skolnick ML. The role of sonography in the placement and management of jugular an subclavian central venous catheters. AJR Am J Roentgenol 1994;163:291–5.

25. Jean G. Haemopericardium associated with disruption of a clot using a flexible J-guide-wire in a haemodialysis catheter. Nephrol Dial Transplant 1998;13:1898.

26. Islek G, Akpolat T, Danaci M. Phrenic nerve palsy caused by subclavian vein catheterization. Nephrol Dial Transplant 1998; 13:1023–5.

27. Peces R, Navascues RA, Baltar J, et al. Pseudoaneurysm of the thyrocervical trunk complicating percutaneous internal jugular-vein catheterization for haemodialysis. Nephrol Dial Transplant 1998;13:1009–11.

28. Tarng D, Huang T. Internal jugular vein haemodialysis catheter-induced right atrium endocarditis – case report and review of the literature. Scand J Urol Nephrol 1998;32:411–14.

29. Dittmer I, Tomson C. Pulmonary abscess complicating central venous hemodialysis catheter infection. Clin Nephrol 1998;49:66.

30. Longley DG, Finlay DE, Letourneau JG. Sonography of the upper extremity and jugular veins. AJR Am J Roentgenol 1993;160: 957–62.

31. Hull JE, Hunter CS, Luiken GA. The Groshong catheter: initial experience and early results of imaging-guided placement. Radiology 1992;185:803–7.

32. Caridi JG, Grundy LS, Ross EA, et al. Interventional radiology placement of twin Tesio catheters for dialysis access: review of 75 patients. J Vasc Interv Radiol 1999;10:78–83.

33. Loehr SP, Hamilton C, Dyer R. Retrieval of entrapped guide wire in an IVC filter facilitated with use of a myocardial biopsy forceps and snare device. J Vasc Interv Radiol 2001;12:116–19.

34. Conly JM, Grieves K, Pteres B. A prospective, randomized study comparing transparent and dry gauze dressings for central venous catheters. J Infect Dis 1989;159:310–19.

35. Wysoki MG, Covey A, Pollak J, et al. Evaluation of various maneuvers for prevention of air embolism during central venous catheter placement. J Vasc Interv Radiol 2001;12:764–6.

12

Extracorporeal anticoagulation for intermittent and continuous forms of renal replacement therapy in the intensive care unit

Andrew Davenport

INTRODUCTION

Traditionally, the coagulation pathways are divided into the intrinsic or contact pathway and the extrinsic pathway (Fig. 12.1). Activation of these serine protease cascades results in the creation of the tenase and prothrombinase complexes, which form on platelet surface membranes, and the subsequent generation of thrombin (Fig. 12.2), and platelet thrombi (Fig. 12.3). To control these procoagulant cascades, there are a series of natural anticoagulants, including antithrombin, heparin cofactor II, proteins S and C, and tissue factor pathway inhibitor (TFPI). Antithrombin, a serine pro-

tease inhibitor, formerly termed antithrombin III, is the major natural anticoagulant that not only inhibits thrombin but also factors Xa, IXa, XIa, XIIa, and kallikrein. Heparin cofactor II also inhibits thrombin. Protein C inactivates factors Va and VIIIa in reactions catalyzed by protein S. Similarly, there is a natural inhibitor for the extrinsic system, tissue factor pathway inhibitor (TFPI), which is mainly produced by the endothelium, and its release is stimulated by heparin.[1]

Studies in intensive care unit (ICU) patients have shown that the majority have evidence of both intrinsic and extrinsic coagulation cascade activation, as shown by reduced plasma levels of

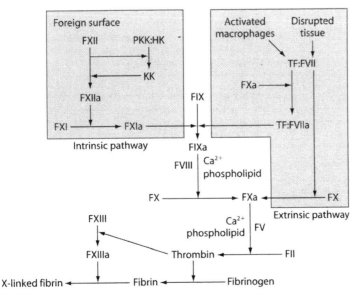

Figure 12.1 The intrinsic coagulation pathway starts with the activation of factor XII, which is accelerated by the conversion of prekallikrein (PK) and high molecular weight kallikrein (HK) to kallikrein (KK), leading to increased XIIa generation. By contrast, the extrinsic pathway starts with the release of tissue factor (TF) from disrupted endothelium and activated mononuclear phagocytes.

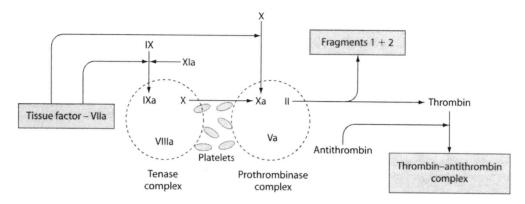

Figure 12.2 Intravascular coagulation can be assessed by measuring thrombin–antithrombin complexes and prothrombin fragments 1+2, as indirect markers of thrombin generation. Activation of the contact (extrinsic) coagulation cascade results in generation of factor XI, whereas activation of the intrinsic system leads to tissue factor release and cleavage of factor VII.

prekallikrein, factors XII, VII, and II, and increased XIIa, TF, and thrombin–antithrombin (TAT) complexes.[2] In keeping with coagulation cascade activity, the majority of ICU patients also have reduced levels of the natural anticoagulants antithrombin, heparin cofactor II, and proteins S and C. Similarly, the majority of ICU patients with multiple organ failure have reduced peripheral platelet counts. In

![Figure 12.3](platelet activation schematic)

Resting platelet

Inactive αIIbβ3
GP IIb/IIIa
receptor

GPIb/IX
receptor

Agonist,
e.g. thrombin

Vascular access
Dialyzer membrane
Blood lines

Platelet activation

Soluble
fibrinogen

Platelet aggregation

Figure 12.3 Schematic representation of platelet activation, which can occur not only by thrombin generation but also by contact activation during passage through the extracorporeal circuit.

addition to the changes in the coagulation cascade and platelet activity, ICU patients are often prescribed human albumin and other colloid expanders such as dextrans, gelatins, and high molecular weight starches. Repeated administration of these solutions, especially the higher molecular weight species which are slowly metabolized, can potentially increase the risk of bleeding, not only by diluting the plasma concentrations of clotting factors and platelets but also by reducing vonWillebrand factor and platelet adhesiveness.[3]

WHY DO EXTRACORPOREAL CIRCUITS CLOT?

The hemodialysis circuit represents a large extracorporeal surface area, and the simple passage of blood through the circuit could potentially lead to the deposition and activation of plasma coagulation proteins, and as the greatest surface area in the circuit is the dialyzer membrane, most studies have reported that this is the most important site for clotting.[4] In pediatric practice, the relative surface area of the extracorporeal circuit is increased, due to the use of smaller lumen diameter lines, leading to greater surface contact.

However, when investigators have attempted to study activation of the contact coagulation pathway during intermittent or continuous modes of dialysis (continuous renal replacement therapy or CRRT), they have failed to demonstrate any significant activation.[5] One ex-vivo hemodialysis study has shown that TAT complexes formed equally when factor XII-deficient plasma was used, so preventing activation of the extrinsic or contact coagulation cascade.[6] However, one study reported an increased incidence of very premature circuit clotting in those patients with low antithrombin levels.[7] Although, the release of TFPI does increase during hemodialysis, this appears to be a direct effect of the glycosaminoglycan heparin on endothelial release of TFPI, as it is not found with other anticoagulants.[8] This would suggest that activation of the clotting cascades, and in particular the contact pathway, is not the major determinant of thrombosis in the extracorporeal circuit.

For many years it has been well recognized that passage of blood through the extracorporeal circuit, and in particular across the dialyzer membrane, results in activation of leukocytes, macrophages, lymphocytes, complement proteins, and platelets.[9] However, it has only recently been recognized that monocyte activation can result in the surface expression and local release of tissue factor (see Fig. 12.1).[10] This process is accelerated by the presence of activated platelets, and thus generates thrombin and promotes local thrombosis in the extracorporeal circuit.

CIRCUIT DESIGN

The key with any extracorporeal circuit design is to minimize the risk of thrombus formation. The greatest pressure drop in the CRRT circuit occurs across the access catheter. Therefore, the choice of vascular access is important, not only in terms of insertion site but also of catheter design, composition, and coating.[11] When anticoagulant free or regional anticoagulants are used for CRRT, clotting of the vascular access catheter becomes a more common cause of circuit clotting.[12] In pediatric practice, vascular access is even more critical, especially in very small infants when special catheters, with internal lumens of 1.6–2.6 mm are used. The pressure required to generate flow through these catheters will be proportionately greater than that for comparable flows through larger-diameter catheters, as the resistance to flow depends upon Poiseuille's law. This is more likely to produce turbulent flow, and so activate leukocytes, monocytes, and platelets within the access catheter, and so increase subsequent dialyzer membrane interaction and predispose to clotting. Heparin-coated venous access catheters have been reported to cause less circuit clotting than conventional uncoated catheters.[13]

In any extracorporeal hemodialysis circuit, the dialyzer membrane represents the largest surface area. Clotting starts in the outer fibers. This is due to the blood flow velocity profile through the membrane, such that the blood flow is slower in the outer fibers than the central core. Thus, thought should be given to membrane design, composition, surface, and geometry to try and ensure an equal flow through the dialyzer and minimize dialyzer bioincompatability.[14] Similarly, a dialyzer with a large surface area will be more likely to result in thrombus deposition than a more efficient or porous membrane of smaller surface area. In addition, there is an effect due to membrane composition. Thus, cuprophane-based membranes generate more prothrombin fragments (PF) 1+2, and TATs than polycarbonate–polyether membranes,[14] but coating cellulosic dialyzers with vitamin E has been reported to reduce thrombin formation.[15] Other studies have shown greater thrombin generation with polyacrylonitrile membranes than either cuprophane or polysulfone, and this may relate to the negatively charged surface,[6] with increased factor XII adsorption and bradykinin formation.[9] Other clinicians have reported successfully running CRRT intraoperatively without anticoagulation when ethylene vinyl alcohol (EVAL) dialyzers were utilized.[16]

In a pure hemofiltration circuit, the convective movement of plasma water out through the hemofilter leads to hemoconcentration. If ultrafiltration rates are high, this may additionally result in increased protein deposition or fouling of the hemofilter membrane and the combination with hemoconcentration increases the risk of filter clotting. Thus, administration of the hemofiltration substitution fluid prefilter minimizes hemoconcentration within the fiber bundles and reduces membrane clotting.[11]

Most current dialysis machines use a roller pump as the blood pump. Even with a dual-lumen access catheter, blood flow is not constant, and there can be wide pressure swings, both positive and negative, which increase with faster blood pump speeds.[4] These pressures are not recorded by the machine, which simply displays a time-averaged pressure rather than a dynamic pressure profile.[17] These pressure swings can cause mechanical trauma to red blood cells and also result in leukocyte, macrophage, and platelet activation. Some machine manufacturers have developed a different pump technology, using a bellows-type action such as the Fresenius Accumen (Fresenius, Walnut Creek, CA), and this may help to reduce the propensity for extracorporeal thrombus formation.[11]

As with all extracorporeal circuits, dialysis lines need to be of a minimum length to prevent dependent loops and minimize cooling of blood in the circuit. The lines need to be inspected at regular intervals to make sure that there are no mechanical kinks following turning the patient.

ANTICOAGULANT-FREE DIALYSIS/HEMOFILTRATION

Interestingly, some studies have shown no difference in peripheral platelet counts, fibrinogen, or fibrinogen turnover when anticoagulant-free intermittent hemodialysis was compared to standard heparin treatments.[18] Anticoagulant-free dialysis is much more difficult in pediatric practice than in the adult, due to technical problems with access and the relatively disproportionate larger surface area of the extracorporeal circuit. Typically, in adult practice, the key to success is careful priming of the circuit, with special emphasis on removing all air from the dialyzer and lines, and ensuring tight connections to prevent air entry. A blood–air interface leads to premature clotting and, in anticoagulant-free circuits, the venous bubble trap is often the cause of circuit clotting.[19] Newer designs for CRRT have replaced the traditional venous air detector chamber with an air-porous device (Fresenius Accumen, Fresenius, Walnut Creek, CA), and this may allow more successful anticoagulant-free therapies. Most centers utilizing anticoagulant-free CRRT or intermittent dialysis prime the circuit with heparinized saline, and then flush the circuit with normal saline prior to connecting the patient. The dose of heparin in the priming fluid varies from center to center, from 1000 to 5000 IU/L with a priming volume of 1.0–2.0 L.[20] Other priming techniques for anticoagulant-free CRRT circuits have employed human albumin solutions that have been shown to reduce platelet adhesion to negatively charged polyacrylonitrile membranes. In clinical practice the results of albumin priming have been variable, with some centers reporting improved circuit survival and others no benefit.[20]

In adult practice, successful anticoagulant-free intermittent hemodialysis is associated with higher blood pump speeds,[19] and regular predilutional saline boluses. Similarly, for CRRT, many centers have not shown a major difference in circuit half-life when anticoagulant-free circuits have been compared with those using systemic heparinization, especially when fluid replacement has been predilutional.[11] In pediatric practice, blood pump speeds may be limited by the size of the patient, and predilutional volumes by the relative size of the extracorporeal circuit.

UNFRACTIONATED HEPARIN

Unfractionated heparin remains the standard extracorporeal anticoagulant throughout the world, and studies have shown that heparin reduces PF 1+2 production during dialysis.[21] Unfractionated heparin is a series of glycosaminoglycans (MW range 5–100 kDa), which predominately interact with antithrombin. After its reaction with heparin, antithrombin undergoes conformational change that increases its ability to inactivate the serine proteases thrombin, factor Xa, and factor IXa. Thrombin is most sensitive to this interaction, with heparin binding to both thrombin and antithrombin. Heparin cofactor II is also catalyzed by heparin, but the anticoagulant effect is only achieved at high levels of heparin, and is specific for thrombin. Although heparin can reduce coagulation cascade activation and thrombin generation, it can also directly activate platelets, and result in the formation of circulating platelet aggregates, or microthrombi, which deposit on the dialyzer.[22]

Heparin is a systemic anticoagulant, with an action time of 3–5 minutes. It is not removed by dialysis or hemofiltration but is eliminated in a dose-dependent manner, mainly by hepatic heparinase activity. The half-life is increased in renal failure to 40–120 minutes, as normally some 35% is renally excreted.

Heparin is a highly negatively charged molecule, that can be adsorbed on plastic. Thus, when using heparin it is important to use a diluted solution to minimize any adsorption during infusion through the narrow-lumen anticoagulant tubing, and then also to maximize thorough mixing with the passing blood.

Provided there is no risk of bleeding, for intermittent hemodialysis a loading dose of 10–20 IU/kg can be administered,[20] followed by a maintenance dose of 10–20 IU/kg, and then the infusion terminated 30 minutes prior to the end of dialysis. The dosage schedule for CRRT is similar, with a loading dose of heparin (10–20 IU/kg) at the start of CRRT, followed by a maintenance infusion of 3–20 IU/kg/h.[23]

It is important that the effect of heparin is monitored, as individual patients differ in their response, due to differences in baseline antithrombin levels, other natural anticoagulants (such as proteins S and C), and even the dialyzer used will affect heparin requirements. Not all the heparin molecules in unfractionated heparin contain the pentasaccharides unit which binds to antithrombin; thus, the anticoagulant potency may vary from batch to batch. The whole blood clotting time (WBCT) and the activated coagulation time (ACT) are the most common bedside tests of heparin anticoagulation. Fresh unanticoagulated whole blood samples should be rapidly delivered into a glass tube at 37°C. The ACT is similar, but contains an activator of the intrinsic coagulation system. Both are prone to error, due to sampling errors, volumes tested, and test tube sizes, and require regular quality control. In addition, the results are dependent upon the level of coagulation factors, platelets, and hematocrit. Thus, the results of WBCT and ACT taken from the same patient will differ, during hemofiltration with postdilutional fluid replacement, if taken prior to and postfilter, simply due to ultrafiltration increasing hematocrit and platelet concentration, causing shorter times postfilter. The activated partial thromboplastin time (APTT) is a laboratory test on plasma separated from citrated blood, and should be measured in conjunction with a prothrombin time, which although little affected by heparin, provides valuable information about the levels of coagulation factors. Centers differ not only in which monitoring tests are performed and their frequency but also in the site at which samples are taken.[24,25] Sampling immediately prior to the arterial port of the hemofilter/hemodialyzer targets whole blood ACT of around 140–180 seconds or a laboratory APPT of 100–140 seconds.

Filter patency has not been proven to be determined either by the total heparin dose or by APPT or other clotting studies.[20] Very few studies have reported that either increased heparin administration resulted in increased filter patency or that increased APTT was associated with prolonged circuit life. Although van der Wetering and colleagues reported a reduced filter patency rate with systemic APTT times less than 35 seconds,[26] they also reported that with a systemic APTT of 15–35 seconds the incidence of de-novo patient hemorrhage was 2.9 per 1000 hours CRRT, which increased to 7.4 at an APTT of 45–55 seconds.[26]

In patients at risk of hemorrhage, the dose of heparin for intermittent hemodialysis can be reduced to provide minimal heparinization. Most centers give a single loading dose, and then, if thrombus forms in the dialyzer or venous air detector, give a second small bolus of about 50% original load, aiming for a prefilter/dialyzer whole blood ACT of 120 seconds and APPT of 80 seconds, although other clinicians have omitted the bolus dose but given an infusion of 15 IU/kg/h without provoking hemorrhage.[27] Even using low-dose heparin (500 IU/h) for CRRT in patients at risk of hemorrhage has not been proven to reduce the risk of bleeding complications.[28]

The main complication of heparin is hemorrhage. Fortunately, the half-life is relatively short, and heparin activity can be quickly reversed with protamine, 1 mg given for every 1000 IU heparin. Rarely, heparin administration can result in an acute allergic reaction, usually due to pork sensitivity. Occasionally, patients can develop heparin-induced thrombocytopenia (HIT; Table 12.1). The more severe antibody-mediated syndrome usually develops following cardiac or vascular surgery, when the patient has been exposed to large doses of heparin. The standard laboratory method for detecting heparin-dependent antibodies uses a platelet aggregation assay, utilizing platelets from normal healthy donors, the patient's plasma, and the same heparin preparation, as administered to the patient. This screening test may be negative in up to 50% of cases, and if HIT type II is clinically suspected, then a more sensitive ELISA test using PF4 complexed with heparin should be performed.

REGIONAL HEPARINIZATION

Regional heparinization was developed to achieve maximum anticoagulation during passage

Table 12.1 Heparin-induced thrombocytopenia (HIT).

Characteristic	HIT type I	HIT type II
Frequency	10–20%	2–3%
Timing	1–4 days	5–10 days
Platelet count	100×10^{12}/L	$30–50 \times 10^{12}$/L
Antibody	No	Yes
Thrombosis	No	Yes
Skin necrosis	No	Yes
Repeated circuit clotting	No	Yes
Access thrombosis	No	Yes
Management	Observe	Withdraw heparin

through the hemofilter/dialyzer but with minimum systemic effects, thereby reducing the risk of patient hemorrhage yet achieving prolonged membrane patency and extracorporeal life. Protamine is a small basic protein which binds to the anionic heparin, and the complex is then taken up by the reticuloendothelial system, broken down, and the protamine released. This results in an increase in protamine half-life with dose and duration of therapy.

As regional heparinization is designed for patients at risk of hemorrhage, start with a loading dose of heparin (5–10 IU/kg) at the beginning of CRRT, followed by a maintenance dose of 3–12 IU/kg/h.[29] Protamine infusion postfilter starts at a rate calculated on the basis of 1 mg of protamine neutralizes 100 IU of standard heparin. Monitoring is more complex, as the APTT must be measured both before and after the heparin infusion and then after protamine. Then, based on these times, the dose of heparin or protamine and/or both must be adjusted:[30] too little protamine and the patient is at risk of hemorrhage and, conversely, too much protamine and the CRRT circuit may clot or the patient adversely react to protamine.

Comparison of regional heparinization, during spontaneous CRRT, and standard low-dose heparin (500 IU/h), was reported to result in a mean 33% increase in filter life and 29% for a pumped CRRT circuit.[28] These data would favor the use of regional heparinization in increasing circuit patency.

Unfortunately, in clinical practice the half-life of heparin is dose-dependent and increases with prolonged administration. The heparin–protamine complex is taken up by the reticuloendothelial system and broken down, with the release of heparin back into the circulation.[29] Thus, the protamine infusion has to be adjusted to the needs of the individual patient. In clinical practice, the variability in the amount of protamine required to neutralize 100 IU heparin varies by more than threefold, making it difficult to successfully establish regional heparinization with simple standardized protocols.[30]

Protamine has a number of potentially adverse clinical effects, including hypotension due to the combination of reduced cardiac output and decreased systemic vascular resistance, increased pulmonary vascular resistance, bronchospasm, and decreased platelet function.[30] When given in large boluses to reverse heparin-associated hemorrhage, protamine can also cause severe anaphylactic reactions, but these are unlikely when infused during CRRT at the low doses used in clinical practice (0.6–2 mg/100 IU heparin).[28]

Regional heparinization cannot be used with heparin-coated hemofilters/dialyzers, as the protamine binds to the heparin coating, so neutralizing its effect. Protamine has less effect on neutralizing low molecular weight heparins (LMWHs) than standard heparin, due to the smaller size of the molecule and reduced charge. In view of the increased half-life of the LMWHs, regional heparinization with protamine is not recommended.

As patients are given standard heparin, they can still develop the side effects of heparin (see above). Indeed, in some series there has been no proven reduction in the incidence of hemorrhagic events during regional heparinization compared with standard heparin anticoagulation during CRRT.[28]

RECOMBINANT ANTITHROMBIN AND HEPARIN

Heparin is an ineffective anticoagulant in patients with congenital antithrombin deficiency, and very premature clotting of the extracorporeal circuit has been reported in critically ill patients with low levels of antithrombin.[7] Now that recombinant antithrombin is available, several studies have looked at the effect of administering both antithrombin and unfractionated heparin.

For intermittent dialysis, a loading dose of 3000 IU provides normal antithrombin levels for at least 4 hours.[31] In CRRT, a lower loading dose of 1000 IU, with a continuous infusion of 250–500 IU/h, has been suggested. Standard unfractionated heparin is then given as a loading dose (5–10 IU/kg) at the start of CRRT, followed by a reduced maintenance dose of 3–5 IU/kg/h, and adjusted to WBCT or ACTT.[20]

Most studies have failed to show that a bolus of antithrombin failed to reduce PF 1+2 or TAT production during dialysis,[31] although it may prolong CRRT circuit life in the ICU patient with low antithrombin levels.[32] Most studies have failed to show any significant duration of extracorporeal circuit life, and/or small molecular weight solute clearance, suggesting no improvement in membrane patency.[20] Thus, recombinant antithrombin provides increased complexity and greatly increased cost for no major clinical advantage.

LOW MOLECULAR WEIGHT HEPARINS

LMWHs are glycosaminoglycans with a molecular weight of around 5 kDa. As LMWHs comprise fewer than 18 saccharides, they cannot bind to both antithrombin and thrombin simultaneously, thus losing antithrombin activity compared to standard heparin. As inactivation of factor Xa does not require direct heparin binding, by activating antithrombin, LMWH retains anti-Xa activity.

The currently available LMWHs – dalteparin, enoxaparin, nadroparin, reviparin, and tinzaparin – differ in size, half-life, and biologic activity. The terminal half-life is much greater for the LMWHs than unfractionated heparin, with enoxaparin having the longest half-life at 27.7 hours.[33] Compared with standard heparin, LMWHs have been reported to be more effective in reducing fibrin deposition on dialyzer membranes, and extracorporeal clotting,[34] but also with less hemorrhagic complications.[35] This appears to be due to both a quicker onset of action than standard heparin, and also less leukocyte and platelet activation.[36]

For intermittent dialysis, most adult and pediatric centers use a single loading dose, as this lasts for up to 4 hours, or even longer.[37,38] Similarly, the doses of LMWHs used in clinical practice are reducing – e.g. the recommended loading dose for enoxaparin is 1 mg/kg – but many centers use an average dose of 0.7 mg/kg, or 40 mg,[39] and in our own clinical practice some patients use as little as 20 mg. LMWHs have been successfully used for intermittent dialysis in patients at risk of hemorrhage using a loading dose of 0.5 mg/kg, after first priming the circuit with 3500 IU anti-Xa LMWH in 2.0 L saline, and then continuing an infusion of 100–400 anti-Xa U/h.[35]

When LMWHs were first used in CRRT, most centers either used a loading dose followed by a continuous infusion, or gave further bolus doses 6 hourly.[40,41] Although LMWHs are relatively small molecules, they are not significantly cleared during CRRT.[7] More recently, LMWHs have been shown to be effective when started as a continuous infusion without a loading dose (e.g. dalteparin 600 IU/h, tinzaparin 400–800 IU/h), achieving a mean anti-Xa activity of 0.49 IU/ml (therapeutic range for systemic anticoagulation 0.3–0.8 IU/ml) within 1 hour of starting CRRT.[28,42] However, most studies have shown that when low doses of LMWH are used for CRRT, although the risk of hemorrhage has been reduced, filter life and/or patency has similarly been reduced,[40] whereas if higher doses are used the risk of hemorrhage is increased.[43] Thus, LMWH when used either as a fixed or variable dose regimen for CRRT does not offer any benefit over standard unfractionated heparin.[43]

As stated earlier, by activating antithrombin, LMWH retains anti-Xa activity. Thus, when monitoring the effect of anticoagulation with LMWH, there is only a modest effect on the APTT, and special assays are required to determine the inhibition of factor Xa. Some commercial kits for testing factor Xa activity include purified antithrombin. Thus, although they are an assay of heparin, or LMWHs, these kits are a poor indicator of heparin anticoagulation. Hence, it is most important that when LMWHs are used, an assay which omits exogenous antithrombin is sought, so that the LMWH dose can be titrated against anticoagulant activity, otherwise anti-Xa activity and the effect of LMWH on anticoagulation may not correlate. The recommended anti-Xa activity range for standard intermittent hemodialysis is 0.2–0.4 IU/ml, and this has been reported to allow successful treatment of patients at risk of hemorrhage[44,45] (Table 12.2).

Table 12.2 Dosing schedule for intermittent pediatric hemodialysis using LMWH dalteparin.

Condition	Dose
Dalteparin bolus dose	
Weight <15 kg	1500 anti-Xa units
Weight 15–30 kg	2500 anti-Xa units
Weight 30–50 kg	5000 anti-Xa units
Monitor postdialysis anti-Xa activity:	
<0.2 IU/ml	↑ bolus dose by 500 anti-Xa units
0.3–0.5 IU/ml	↓ bolus dose by 500 anti-Xa units
>0.5 IU/ml	↓ bolus dose by 1000 anti-Xa units

If bleeding does occur, then this may be more severe than standard heparin, due to the prolonged half-life. Protamine may only have a moderate effect; this will depend upon the individual LMWH used, and in severe cases fresh frozen plasma may be required. HIT type II may rarely develop with LMWHs,[44] but if it does LMWHs must be discontinued.

HEPARIN-COATED EXTRACORPOREAL CIRCUITS

Heparin bonding of cardiopulmonary and extracorporeal oxygenation circuits has been shown to result in a reduction in heparin requirement and risk of hemorrhage. Currently, there are heparin-coated venous access catheters and heparin-bonded dialyzer membranes (Duraflo, Baxter, Deerborne, IL), but no completely heparin-coated extracorporeal circuit for intermittent hemodialysis and/or CRRT.

Heparin binds to extracorporeal lines and/or dialyzer, and is designed to reduce extracorporeal platelet, leukocyte activation, and thrombogenesis.[46] The amount of heparin released from the membrane is very small (<1%), and we and others have not noted any change in APTT during treatment. In our experience, anticoagulant-free circuits utilizing heparin-bonded dialyzers can operate in excess of 48 hours. Other groups using heparin-coated CRRT circuits in patients with liver disease have also reported circuit lives in excess of 40 hours.[47] Initial results in ICU patients again suggest less platelet activation and both prolonged filter patency and circuit life.[48] Most centers have used low-dose heparin, as the circuit half-life was not different from anticoagulant-free circuits due to problems with access clotting.

DERMATAN SULFATE AND HEPARINOIDS

Dermatan sulfate is a proteoglycan that acts as a direct thrombin inhibitor by binding to heparin cofactor II. Trials using either a single bolus dose of 6 mg/kg, or smaller bolus of 4 mg/kg coupled with a continuous infusion of 0.65 mg/kg/h, reported that dermatan sulfate was an effective anticoagulant for intermittent hemodialysis, although when polyacrylonitrile membranes were used, greater doses were required compared to cuprophane.[49]

Subsequently, dermatan sulfate has been superseded by danaparoid, which is a mixture of glycosaminoglycans (84% heparan sulfate, 12% dermatan sulfate and 4% chondroitin sulfate) and is derived from porcine intestinal mucosa. Danaparoid exerts its anticoagulant effect predominantly by activating antithrombin, primarily against factor Xa but also against thrombin. As danaparoid has a minimal effect on platelets, it has been successfully used in the management of patients with heparin-induced thrombocytopenia, although there is a potential cross reactivity of <5%.[50] Prior to starting danaparoid in cases of HIT type II, laboratory testing should be undertaken to exclude cross reactivity. The main disadvantage of danaparoid is the prolonged half-life of around 30 hours in renal failure; thus monitoring and adjusting of the loading dose is often based not on the anti-Xa activity at the end of the dialysis session but on the anti-Xa activity prior to the start of the subsequent dialysis session. In adult practice, an initial loading dose of 3750 IU is recommended (reduced to 2500 IU in patients <55 kg), providing there is no additional hemorrhagic risk, and then 2500 IU prior to the subsequent dialysis (2000 IU if <55 kg), or alternatively start at 35 IU/kg. Thereafter, the dose is adjusted on the basis of the predialysis anti-Xa activity and/or the presence of fibrin threads in the dialysis chamber, aiming for intradialytic anti-Xa activity of 0.5–0.8 IU/ml.[51] In pediatric practice, it has been suggested that a loading dose of 1000 IU + 30 IU/kg is used for children under 10 years old, and 1500 IU + 30 IU/kg for older children. The loading dose is then titrated against the subsequent predialysis anti-Xa activity (<0.3, same bolus; 0.3–0.4, reduce bolus by 2500 IU, and if >0.4, omit bolus dose).[51] If the same loading dose is continuously used, then the predialysis anti-Xa activity will increase over time due to the prolonged half-life.

For CRRT, an initial bolus dose is required, and if there is no hemorrhagic risk then administer 2500 IU (35 IU/kg) of danaparoid followed by an initial infusion of 400 IU/h, then adjusted (usually between 200 and 400 IU/h) to the desired anti-Xa activity (0.4–0.6).[7,20] The major problem with danaparoid is the prolonged half-life. If bleeding occurs, there is no simple antidote, and patients may require activated factor VII concentrate or fresh frozen plasma.

Fondaparinux is a newer heparinoid, a synthetic pentasaccharide which selectively inhibits activated factor X, so can be used for anticoagulating patients with HIT type II. As with danaparoid, the half life is increased in renal failure, but as the molecular weight is only 1.7 kDa, there is some removal by hgh flux membranes. the dose should be titrated to achieve a therapeutic anti-factor Xa time of between 70 and 110 s. There is very limited data for CRRT, but for hemodialysis a dose of 2.5 mg prior to treatment, for alternate day treatment has been suggested

PROSTACYCLIN

Prostacyclin (PGI$_2$) is a natural anticoagulant produced by endothelial cells, by the breakdown of arachidonic acid. PGI$_2$, and its analogue epoprostenol, are potent antiplatelet agents blocking cAMP, and have been shown to reduce platelet microthrombi during hemodialysis and CRRT compared with standard heparin and LMWH.[52] Although both agents are potent arterial vasodilators, most patients do not develop symptomatic hypotension at the doses used (PGI$_2$, 5 ng/kg/min; range, 2.5–10 ng/kg/min), as some 40% of the dose is lost during passage through the dialyzer.[23] Hypotension can be avoided by ensuring that patients are not hypovolemic, and by infusing PGI$_2$, starting at 0.5 ng/kg/min prior to dialysis, and increasing the dose over a few minutes. Fortunately, as the half-life is in minutes, any hypotensive episode can readily be reversed by stopping the infusion. As platelet microthrombi are reduced, membrane fouling is less, and dialyzer efficiency increased.[53]

Other prostanoids, such as PGE$_1$ (alprostadil), PGE$_2$, and PGD also have antiplatelet effects and can be used as extracorporeal anticoagulants. As PGE$_1$ is metabolized in the lung, it has less systemic vasodilatory properties compared to prostacyclin, and does not cause hypotension.[1] These prostanoids are not as potent as PGI$_2$, and thus the dose of alprostadil required is 5–20 ng/kg/min.

PGI$_2$ does not have any direct effect on the plasma coagulation pathways, so its anticoagulant activity cannot be readily assessed, even by thromboelastography.[54] Thrombin generation does occur during dialysis with PGI$_2$, and some authors have advocated a combination of reduced doses of both heparin and PGI$_2$.[55] Some groups have found PGI$_2$ and prostanoids to be equally effective as heparin in maintaining CRRT circuit life, with better filter patency.[52,56,57]

When used as the sole extracorporeal anticoagulant, PGI$_2$ has been shown to significantly reduce the incidence of hemorrhage in patients at risk of bleeding.[57,58] PGI$_2$ and its analogues are essentially regional rather than systemic anticoagulants.

Although PGI$_2$ has been used in cases of heparin-associated thrombocytopenia, it does not prevent thrombosis and should not be used in cases which require systemic anticoagulation.[50]

COMBINATION OF HEPARIN AND PROSTACYCLIN

Some groups have added PGI$_2$ to patients anticoagulated with standard heparin who had repeated clotting of the CRRT circuit, to good effect.[7,59] Using a combination of anticoagulants, some centers have reduced both the absolute dose of both prostacyclin (2–6.5 ng/kg/min) and/or alprostadil (2.5–10 ng/kg/min) with standard heparin (200–500 IU/h).[5,53,59,60]

The combination of heparin and PGI$_2$ has been reported to achieve CRRT circuit lives >48 hours.[59] Other studies observed that the combination increased hemofilter/dialyzer patency when compared to heparin and PGI$_2$ alone, with filter patency maintained for up to 80 hours.[24]

Apart from the additional cost and complexity of the circuit, careful comparison of the combination of heparin and PGI$_2$ showed either no increase in the overall incidence of hemorrhage,[52] or less than that for heparin alone.[24]

DIRECT THROMBIN INHIBITORS: HIRUDIN AND ARGATROBAN

The direct thrombin inhibitors are now the agents of choice in managing patients with HIT. Hirudin, originally obtained from leeches, is an irreversible thrombin inhibitor, and is now available in recombinant form, lepirudin (6.9 kDa). As hirudin is renally excreted, the biological half-life is increased to more than 35 hours in renal failure. After diluting the lepirudin solution to a concentration of 2 mg/ml, the loading doses used in clinical practice for intermittent hemodialysis have varied from 0.02 to 0.15 mg/kg.[61] The dose of hirudin in the dialysis patient depends upon several factors. First, hirudin can pass through plasma filters and also high-flux and high-efficiency dialyzers, and therefore in these cases a higher loading dose is required to compensate for dialyzer losses.[61] Whereas cellulosic and polysulfone low-flux dialyzers are relatively impermeable, low-flux hemophan is partially permeable, and cellulose acetate almost completely permeable.[62] On the other hand, approximately one-third of patients regularly treated with hirudin develop so-called hirudin antibodies; these reduce hirudin clearance, so potentiating the effect of hirudin, and thus the loading dose needs to be reduced.[63]

The dosing for CRRT is more problematical, as hirudin will be cleared during hemofiltration and/or dialysis, and patients are more likely to develop hirudin antibodies. Both continuous infusions (6–25 µg/kg/h), and repetitive boluses (5–40 µg/kg) have been used.[64]

Most centers monitor hirudin by using the APTT, aiming for a ratio of 1.5–2.5 × normal. When hirudin was first used, with a target APTT of 1.5–2.5, several cases of bleeding were reported.[65] The relationship between plasma hirudin concentration and the APTT is not linear, and what may appear to be small increases in the APTT can correspond to much larger increases in the hirudin concentration, and so increase the risk of hemorrhage.[7] The manufacturer of lepirudin has advocated the use of a direct test of thrombin activation – the ecarin clotting time – to monitor the anticoagulant effect of hirudin. Ecarin activation of prothrombin is independent of cofactors, does not require phospholipid, calcium, or factor Va, and can be performed at the bedside. Other clinicians measure the plasma hirudin, aiming for a concentration between 500 and 1200 µgL. Bivalirudin, which has only recently been released, is a new reversible direct thrombin inhibitor, and as yet there are no data for intermittent dialysis and/or CRRT.

As hirudin is an irreversible thrombin inhibitor, overdosage and consequent hemorrhage are serious risks, especially when most centers rely on the APTT to adjust dosages. Not surprisingly major bleeding has been reported in patients anticoagulated for CRRT with hirudin infusions of 5–10 µg/kg/h.[7,64]

Argatroban is a synthetic reversible thrombin inhibitor, derived from L-arginine. Unlike hirudin, argatroban is hepatically metabolized, and the recommended starting dose is 2 µg/kg/min, reduced to 0.5 µg/kg/min in patients with liver disease, aiming for a target APTT of 1.5–2.0 × normal.[66] Argatroban is not significantly removed by high-flux dialyzers and/or hemofilters. In preliminary studies for intermittent hemodialysis, the average starting dose was 0.9 µg/kg/min, reducing to a maintenance dose of 0.7 µg/kg/min.[67] More recently, one study investigated three dosing regimens in patients with normal liver function: (1) a 250 µg/kg bolus, with a second additional 250 µg/kg bolus allowed; (2) compared with a 250 µg/kg bolus, followed by 2 µg/kg/min infusion; and (3) a steady-state, 2 µg/kg/min infusion initiated 4 hours predialysis.[68] The results from this study suggest that the preferable argatroban treatment regimen for hemodialysis was the 250 µg/kg bolus, followed by a 2 µg/kg/min infusion. However, if patients were already on an argatroban infusion for treatment of venous thrombosis, then continuing at 2 µg/kg/min was satisfactory. If postdialysis systemic anticoagulation is not required, the infusion could be stopped up to 1 hour in advance of the anticipated completion of the hemodialysis session. In patients with liver disease then, these doses would need to be reduced, and more careful monitoring of APTT required.

In critically ill patients with liver dysfunction and acute renal failure requiring CRRT, the steady-state argatroban dose associated with APTTs of 1.5–2.5 × baseline was approximately 0.5 µg/kg/min.[67]

NAFAMOSTAT MESILATE AND APROTININ

Nafamostat and aprotinin are serine protease inhibitors, which, although they potentially inhibit broad enzymatic systems (including coagulation cascades, platelet and complement activation, and kinin and fibrinolysis cascades), essentially act as regional anticoagulants.

Gabexate mesilate is a short-acting (half-life 80 seconds) serine protease inhibitor that acts at the same sites as antithrombin, but is not dependent on it for effect.[1] Gabexate has now been superseded by nafamostat mesilate, which again has a short half-life of 5–8 minutes, and some 40% is cleared during passage through the dialyzer.[69] By inhibiting thrombin, factor Xa, and XIIa, nafamostat prolongs the WBCT, ACT, and APTT, thus allowing bedside monitoring. Most experience comes from Japan, where the circuit is primed with 20 mg of nafamostat in 1.0 L normal saline, and the nafamatostat initially infused at 40 mg/h during intermittent hemodialysis, to maintain a target APPT ratio of 2.0 × normal.[70] Nafamostat contains a cationic portion which binds to negatively charged polyacrylonitrile (PAN) membranes, and also to some extent to polymethylmethacrylate membranes; if these membranes are used, the nafamostat dose has to be increased, and may not be as effective with PAN 69 dialyzers.[69]

As nafamostat is a regional anticoagulant, it has been successfully used to dialyze patients at risk of bleeding.[70,71] In these cases, the circuit was either primed with 40 mg nafamostat, followed by an infusion of 20–40 mg/h, or primed with 20 mg of nafamostat, and then an infusion of 40 mg/h.[70,71] Similar doses of nafamostat are used for CRRT.

The reported complications of nafamostat include myalgia, arthralgia, eosinophilia, and, rarely, anaphylactoid reactions and agranulocytosis.[20]

Aprotinin is obtained from bovine lung, and is a nonspecific serine protease inhibitor, with an elimination half-life of around 2 hours. The effects of aprotinin on the coagulation cascade depend upon the circulating plasma concentrations, as the affinity of aprotinin is far greater for plasmin than kallikrein. At a plasma level of 125 kIU/ml (kallikrein inactivation units), aprotinin inhibits fibrinolysis and complement activation.[72] At higher levels, 250–500 kIU/ml, plasma kallikrein will be inhibited, so reducing blood coagulation mediated via contact with anionic surfaces.[73] More importantly, aprotinin can prevent platelet activation by reducing polymorphonuclear leukocyte degranulation and release of myeloperoxidase. In addition, aprotinin may be viewed as an antithrombin substitute for generalized antiprotease activity in conditions of systemic inflammation. Reduced kinin activation will also improve circulatory stability.

Cardiopulmonary bypass circuits and extracorporeal oxgenators use an initial loading dose of 2×10^6 kIU of aprotinin, followed by a maintenance infusion of 500 000 kIU/h. Aprotinin, at doses of 800 000 kIU, has been used for hemodialysis and, as with nafamostat, binds to PAN membranes.[73] For CRRT, lower doses have been used, 50 000 kIU/h, as the anticoagulant effect is primarily due to prevention of complement, platelet, and polymorphonuclear leukocyte activation rather than kallikrein inhibition.

CITRATE

Although regional citrate anticoagulation has been used for more than 20 years, only a few centers regularly use citrate for intermittent hemodialysis.[74] Anticoagulation with citrate induces a degree of complexity, and if trisodium citrate is used, then a specialized calcium-free, low or zero magnesium and reduced or bicarbonate-free dialysate is required. Calcium then has to be infused centrally to restore the plasma ionized calcium concentration.[34] By complexing calcium and reducing calcium concentration, citrate not only prevents activation of the coagulation cascades but also platelets, during passage through the dialyzer,

but not complement or leukocyte activation.[75] Thus, membrane fouling and deposition of fibrin and platelets are much reduced when citrate is used compared with LMWH and standard heparin.[34] The half-life of citrate complex is minutes, and thus citrate is a regional anticoagulant, allowing the successful dialysis of patients at risk of bleeding.[74,76]

Citrate has been used as the anticoagulant for CRRT since the late 1980s, initially for continuous dialysis/hemodiafiltration,[77] and more recently for venovenous hemofiltration.[78] As initially there were no commercially available calcium-free fluids for dialyzate or replacement solutions, a variety of protocols have been developed by different institutions (Table 12.3).[77–80] In essence, all protocols titrate the citrate infusion against the blood flow, using a calcium-free dialyzate and/or replacement solutions, and then reinfusion of calcium at a central site (Fig. 12.4). More recently, several investigators have reported that it is possible to use commercial calcium-containing solutions when performing continuous hemodiafiltration (see Table 12.3).[81–83] Citrate has been shown to be a highly effective regional anticoagulant for CRRT that also reduces the risk of potential hemorrhage.[76–80] Indeed, as citrate is a regional anticoagulant, access problems are a more common cause of circuit clotting, especially if the calcium infusion is returned into the venous dialysis line. Thus, some centers have now altered the extracorporeal circuit to infuse citrate as close to the venous catheter arterial port as possible.

Bedside monitoring is possible by using whole blood ACT (200–250 seconds); however, most centers adjust the citrate infusion according the postdialyzer calcium concentration (target 0.25–0.35 mmol/L).[80] The rate of the citrate infusion is dependent upon the blood flow. Thus, during hemodialysis and/or hemodiafiltration with blood flows of 300 ml/min or greater a citrate infusion of 50–60 mmol/h would be appropriate,[84] whereas during CRRT, with lower blood flow rates, citrate infusion is correspondingly lower (see Table 12.3). Thereafter, the rate of citrate infusion is adjusted according to the calcium concentration, being reduced if the calcium is less than 0.25 mmol/L, and correspondingly increased when greater than 0.36 mmol/L.[80]

Citrate dialysis has been reported to result in citrate intoxication, either when citrate is not metabolized rapidly, if there is hepatic failure, or muscle hypoperfusion, or during isolated ultrafiltration, when citrate is not being dialyzed out. Failure to

Table 12.3   CRRT citrate anticoagulation protocols.

Reference (main author)	Modality	Blood flow rate (ml/min)	Citrate infusion (mmol/h)	Dialysate composition (mmol/L)	Substitution fluid mmol/L
Mehta[77]	CAVHD	52–125	23.8	Na^+ 117 Cl^- 122.5 Mg^{++} 0.75 Dextrose 2.5%	Na^+ 145 Cl^- 145 Na^+ 145
Tolwani[79]	CVVHD	125–150	17.5	Na^+ 145 Cl^- 145 Mg^{++} 1.0	None
Bunchman[81]	CVVHD	100	17	Na^+ 140 Cl^- 105 Mg^{++} 0.75 $NaHCO_3^-$ 35	None
Kutsogiannis[80]	CVVHDF	125	25	Na^+ 110 Cl^- 110 Mg^{++} 0.75	Na^+ 110 Cl^- 110 Mg^{++} 0.75 Vary $NaHCO_3^-$
Gupta[82]	CVVHDF	150	16.9	Na^+ 132 Mg^{++} 0.75 Lactate 40	Na^+ 154
Cointault[83]	CVVHDF	125	28.3	Na^+ 140 Cl^- 109.5 Ca^{++} 1.75 Mg^{++} 0.50 $NaHCO_3^-$ 32 Lactate 3.0	Na^+ 140 Cl^- 109.5 Ca^{++} 1.75 Mg^{++} 0.50 $NaHCO_3^-$ 32 Lactate 3.0
Palsson[78]	CVVH	180	18.6	None	Na^+ 140 Cl^- 101.5 Mg^{++} 0.75 Citrate 13.3 Dextrose 0.2%

CAVHD = continuous arteriovenous hemodialysis; CVVHD = continuous venovenous hemodialysis; CVVHDF = continuous venovenous hemodiafiltration; CVVH = continuous venovenous hemofiltration.

adequately metabolize citrate results in an increased total calcium to ionized calcium ratio (>2.5), due to the accumulation of the calcium citrate complex. Not surprisingly, this has been most commonly reported in patients with liver failure,[85] and should be managed by decreasing the citrate infusion.[80] In addition, citrate has been reported to cause hyperalbuminemia, hyperammonemia, and hyper-natremia during sorbent-based dialysis. During CRRT, hypernatremia can occur due to the sodium load if trisodium citrate is used, and thus many centers have developed specialized hyponatremic dialysates.[77] Similarly, as each citrate molecule is metabolized through to three bicarbonates, patients are at risk of developing a metabolic alkalosis.[86] To reduce this complication, many centers use special-

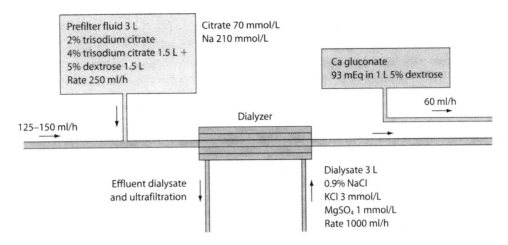

Figure 12.4 Schematic representation of a CRRT circuit for hemodiafiltration using citrate anticoagulation based on Palsson and Niles.[78]

ized dialysates and/or replacement solutions with a high chloride load.[77] If bicarbonate dialysate has been used, then, during intermittent hemodialysis, patients can potentially develop profound alkalosis, with parethesiae, arrhythmia, and even cardiac arrest. Now that there is a commercially available zero calcium bicarbonate-based dialysate, all patients treated by CRRT in one study developed metabolic alkalosis after 7 days.[81] To overcome some of these problems, some centers have used citrate dextrose-A rather than 4% trisodium citrate, or reduced the citrate concentration, in combination with a reduced bicarbonate dialysate concentration, to 25 mmol/L.[81,86] Other centers have reported that when citrate is used for high-flux dialysis, additional calcium supplementation is required compared to standard intermittent dialysis.[87] Hypomagnesemia has also been observed in children treated by CRRT using citrate anticoagulation.[81]

Despite the apparent complexity of using citrate, and the potential array of metabolic disturbances, citrate use is growing in popularity for CRRT, as it is a very effective regional anticoagulant, especially in patients at risk of hemorrhage. More recently special citrate based replacement solutions/dialysates have been commercially developed, and are currently undergoing clinical trials, and will soon be available for general use.

DEFIBROTIDE

Defibrotide is a naturally occurring polydesoxyribonucleotide that has both antithrombotic and profibrinolytic properties. More recently, it has been used to treat thrombotic microangiopathy following bone marrow transplantation. Although there are no reports of its use in CRRT, defibrotide has been successfully used for intermittent hemodialysis in patients at risk of hemorrhage. Patients were given a loading dose of 400 mg at the start of dialysis, and then a further bolus of 400 mg after 2 hours of dialysis.[88]

SUMMARY

Anticoagulation for the patient with acute renal failure in the ICU is more problematic than that for the patient with chronic renal failure attending for routine hemodialysis. As part of the generalized inflammatory process, coagulation cascades, platelets, complement, and mononuclear leukocytes are all activated and will promote thrombus formation in the extracorporeal circuit. Thus, more careful thought is required in designing the extracorporeal circuit, particularly for CRRT. In addition, the pediatric patient poses greater problems than the adult, due to the relative increase in the extracorporeal surface area, coupled with smaller vascular access devices and lower blood pump speeds. A dialyzer/hemofilter should be chosen to minimize bioincompatibility, maximize laminar blood flow, and minimize surface area available for contact activation. Similar thought is required for the site and choice of vascular access, and the circuit design for hemofiltration in terms of site of fluid replacement and filtration fraction.

Although standard unfractionated heparin remains the most commonly used anticoagulant, for both acute intermittent hemodialysis and CRRT, it does not prevent platelet microthrombi formation, and still carries a significant risk of bleeding. LMWHs have an earlier onset of action, reduce membrane fibrin and platelet deposition compared to standard heparin during intermittent hemodialysis, but have increased half-lives and require specialist monitoring, and as a consequence do not have any clinical advantage over standard unfractionated heparin for CRRT. Regional anticoagulants have the advantage of reducing the risk of bleeding, but also tend to reduce membrane fouling. Most of these drugs – prostacyclin and other prostanoids, nafamostat, and aprotinin – are very expensive and are not for everyday practice. Citrate, although more expensive than heparin, is an effective alternative. Anticoagulation with citrate does requires a degree of complexity, with a specialized dialysate, and monitoring to regulate both the rate of citrate and calcium infusions.

In cases of heparin-induced thrombocytopenia type II that require systemic anticoagulation, the choice lies between danaparoid and the direct thrombin inhibitors hirudin and argatroban. There is a small risk of cross-reactivity with danaparoid, but the main drawback of danaparoid is the prolonged half-life in renal failure, which can make dosing problematic for CRRT. Hirudin is an irreversible thrombin antagonist, which also has a prolonged half-life. Monitoring can be difficult, as there is no linear relationship between plasma concentration and APTT, and hemorrhage is a potential and serious problem. Despite the introduction of hirudin analogues, which are reversible thrombin antagonists, argatroban will probably supersede hirudin for dialysis patients, as it is a reversible thrombin antagonist, and is not affected by renal failure.

REFERENCES

1. Webb AR, Mythen MG, Jacobson D, Mackie IJ. Maintaining blood flow in the extracorporeal circuit: hemostasis and anticoagulation. Intensive Care Med 1995;21:84–93.
2. Davenport A. The coagulation system in the critically ill patient with acute renal failure and the effect of an extracorporeal circuit. Am J Kidney Dis 1997;30:(Suppl 4):S20–7.
3. de Jonge E, Levi M. Effects of different plasma substitutes on blood coagulation. Crit Care Med 2001;29:1261–7.
4. Holt AW, Bierer P, Berstein AD, Bury LJ, Vedig AE. Continuous renal replacement therapy in critically ill patients: monitoring circuit function. Anaesth Intensive Care 1996;24:423–4.
5. Salmon J, Cardigan R, Mackie I, et al. Continuous venovenous hemofiltration using polyacrylonitrile filters does not activate contact system and intrinsic system coagulation pathways. Intensive Care Med 1997;23:38–43.
6. Frank RD, Weber J, Dresbach H, et al. Role of contact system activation in hemodialyzer-induced thrombogenicity. Kidney Int 2001;60:1972–81.
7. Shulman RI, Singer M, Rock J. Keeping the circuit open: lessons from the lab. Blood Purif 2002;20:275–81.
8. Kario K, Matsuo T, Yamada T, Matsuo M. Increased tissue factor pathway inhibitor levels in uremic patients on regular hemodialysis. Thromb Haemostat 1994;71:275–9.
9. Olbricht C, Lonnemann G, Frei U, Koch KM. Hemodialysis, hemofiltration, and complications of technique. In: Davison AM, Cameron JS, Grunfeld JP, et al, eds. Oxford textbook of clinical nephrology, 2nd edn. Oxford: Oxford University Press; 1997: 2023–47.
10. Gorbet MB, Sefton MV. Leukocyte activation and leukocyte procoagulant activities after blood contact with polystyrene and polyethyleneglycol immobilized polystyrene beads. J Lab Clin Med 2001;137:345–55.
11. Davenport A. Anticoagulation in patients with acute renal failure treated with continuous renal replacement therapies. Home Hemodial Int 1998;2:41–60.
12. Laliberte-Murphy K, Palsson R, Williams WW, Tolkoff-Rubin N, Niles JL. Continuous venovenous hemofiltration as a bridge to liver transplantation. Blood Purif 2002;20:318–19.
13. Davenport A. Central venous catheters for hemodialysis: how to overcome the problems. Home Hemodial Int 2000;2:43–5.
14. Sperschneider H, Deppisch R, Beck W, Wolf H, Stein G. Impact of membrane choice and blood flow pattern on coagulation and heparin requirement – potential consequences on lipid concentrations. Nephrol Dial Transplant 1997;12:2638–46.
15. Huraib S, Tanimu D, Shaheen F, et al. Effect of vitamin E modified dialysers on dialyser clotting, erythropoietin and heparin dosage: a comparative crossover study. Am J Nephrol 2000;20:364–8.
16. Wake M, Sanagawa Y, Tanaka Y. [Management of intraoperative anticoagulantless CHD with EVAL-dialyzer in four patients on maintenance dialysis]. Masui 2002;51:250–4 [in Japanese].
17. Davenport A, Will EJ, Davison AM. The effect of the direction of dialysate flow on the efficiency of continuous arteriovenous hemodialysis. Blood Purif 1990;8:329–36.
18. Romao JE Jr, Fadil MA, Sabbaga E, Marcondes M. Hemodialysis without anticoagulant: hemostasis parameters, fibrinogen kinetic, and dialysis efficiency. Nephrol Dial Transplant 1997; 12:106–10.
19. Keller F, Seeman J, Preuschof L, Offermann G. Risk factors of system clotting in heparin free hemodialysis. Nephrol Dial Transplant 1990;5:802–7.
20. Davenport A. Problems with anticoagulation. In: Lameire N, Mehta R, eds. Complications of dialysis: recognition and management. Boston: Marcel Dekker; 1999:215–40.
21. Ambuhl PM, Wuthrich RP, Korte W, Schmid L, Krapf R. Plasma hypercoagulability in hemodialysis patients: impact of dialysis and anticoagulation. Nephrol Dial Transplant 1997;12:2355–64.
22. Matsuo T, Matsuo M, Kario K, Suzuki S. Characteristics of heparin-induced platelet aggregates in chronic hemodialysis with long-term heparin use. Haemostasis 2000;30:249–57.
23. Zobel G, Ring E, Kuttnig M, Grubbauer HM. Continuous arteriovenous hemofiltration versus continuous venovenous hemofiltration in critically ill pediatric patients. Contrib Nephrol 1991; 93:257–60.
24. Favre H, Martin Y, Stoermann C. Anticoagulation in continuous extracorporeal renal replacement therapy. Semin Dial 1996;9: 112–18.

25. Ward DM. The approach to anticoagulation in patients treated with extracorporeal therapy in the intensive care unit. Crit Care Nephrol 1997;4:160–73.
26. van der Wetering J, Westendorp RGJ, van der Hoeven JG, et al. Heparin use in continuous renal replacement therapies: the struggle between filter coagulation and patient hemorrhage. J Am Soc Nephrol 1996;7:145–50.
27. Ozen S, Saatci U, Bakkaloglu A, Uyumaz H, Kavukcu S. Tight heparin regimen for hemodiaysis in children. Int Urol Nephrol 1993;25:499–501.
28. Bellomo R, Teede H, Boyce N. Anticoagulant regimens in acute continuous hemodiafiltration: a comparative study. Intensive Care Med 1993;19:329–32.
29. Mehta RL. Anticoagulation strategies for continuous renal replacement therapies: what works? Am J Kidney Dis 1996:28: (Suppl 3):S8–14.
30. Kaplan AA. Continuous arteriovenous hemofiltration- and related therapies. In Jacobs C, Kjellstrand KE, Koch KM, Winchester JF, eds. Replacement of renal function by dialysis, 4th edn. Kluwer; Dordrecht: 1996:390–417.
31. Langley PG, Keays R, Hughes RD, et al. Antithrombin III supplementation reduces heparin requirement and platelet loss during hemodialysis of patients with fulminant hepatic failure. Hepatology 1991;14:251–6.
32. Schrader J, Kostering H, Kramer P, Scheler F. Antithrombin III substitution in dialysis dependent renal insufficiency. Dtsch Med Wochenschr 1982;107:1847–50.
33. Stiekema JC, Van Griensen JM, Van Dinther TG, Cohen AF. A cross over comparison of the anti-clotting effects of three low molecular weight heparins and glycosaminoglycuron. B J Clin Pharmacol 1993;36:51–6.
34. Hofbauer R, Moser D, Frass M, et al. Effect of anticoagulation on blood membrane interactions during hemodialysis. Kidney Int 1999;56:1578–83.
35. Hafner G, Klingel R, Wandel E, et al. Laboratory control of minimal heparinization during hemodialysis in patients with a risk of hemorrhage. Blood Coagul Fibrinolysis 1994;5:221–6.
36. Leitienne P, Fouque D, Rigal D, et al. Heparins and blood polymorphonuclear stimulation in hemodialysis: an expansion of the biocompatibility concept. Nephrol Dial Transplant 2000;15: 1631–7.
37. Bianchetti MG, Speck S, Muller R, Oetliker OH. [Simple coagulation prophylaxis using low molecular heparin enoxaparin in pediatric hemodialysis.] Schweiz Rundsch Med Prax 1990;79: 730–1 [in German].
38. Van Biljon I, van Damme-Lombaerts R, Demol A, et al. Low molecular weight heparin for anticoagulation during hemodialysis in children – a preliminary study. Eur J Pediatr 1996;155:70.
39. Saltissi D, Morgan C, Westhuyzen J, Healy H. Comparison of low molecular weight heparin (enoxaparin sodium) and standard fractionated heparin for hemodialysis. Nephrol Dial Transplant 1999;14:2698–703.
40. Jeffrey RF, Khan AA, Douglas JT, Will EJ, Davison AM. Anticoagulation with low molecular weight heparin (fragmin) during continuous hemodialysis in the intensive care unit. Artif Organs 1993;17:717–20.
41. Wynckel A, Bernieh B, Toupance O, et al. Guidelines to the use of enoxaparin in slow continuous dialysis. Contrib Nephrol 1991; 93:221–4.
42. Voiculescu M, Ismail G, Ionescu C, Micu D, Szigeti A. Anticoagulation efficacy and safety with a low molecular weight heparin – tinzaparin in continuous real replacement therapies. Blood Purif 2002;20:313.
43. Schepens D, De Keulenaer B. Efficacy and safety of nadropine as anticoagulant therapy in continuous venovenous hemofiltration. Blood Purif 2002;20:314.
44. Reeves JH, Cumming AR, Gallagher L, O'Brien JL, Santamaria JD. A controlled trial of low molecular weight heparin (dalteparin) versus unfractionated heparin as anticoagulant during continuous venovenous hemodialysis with filtration. Crit Care Med 1999;27:2224–8.
45. Leu JG, Chiang SS, Lin SM, Pai JK, Jiang WW. Low molecular weight heparin in hemodialysis patients with a bleeding tendency. Nephron 2000;86:499–501.
46. Bannan S, Danby A, Cowan D, Ashraf S, Martin PG. Low heparinization with heparin-bonded bypass circuits: is it a safe strategy? Ann Thorac Surg 1997;63:663–8.
47. Ellis A, Wendon JA, Williams R. Effect of albumin priming on hemofiltration circuits. 13th European Crit Care Meeting, Athens, 1996:362.
48. Sieffert E, Matéo J, Deligeon N, Payen D. Continuous venovenous hemofiltration using heparin coated or non heparin coated membranes in critically ill patients. Proc Continuous Hemofiltration Therapies, Paris, 1996:14–15.
49. Ryan KE, Lane DA, Flynn A, et al. Antithrombotic properties of dermatan sulphate (MF 701) in hemodialysis for chronic renal failure. Thromb Haemostat 1992;10:563–9.
50. Davenport A. Management of heparin-induced thrombocytopenia during continuous renal replacement therapy. Am J Kidney Dis 1998;32:E3.
51. Neuhaus TJ, Goetschel P, Schmugge M, Leumann E. Heparin induced thrombocytopenia type II on hemodialysis: switch to danaparoid. Pediatr Nephrol 2000;14:713–6.
52. Journois D, Safran D, Castelain MH, et al. [Comparison of the antithrombotic effects of heparin, enoxaparin and prostacycline in continuous hemofiltration.] Ann Fr Anesth Reanim 1990;9: 331–7 [in French].
53. Langenecker SA, Felfernig M, Werba A, et al. Anticoagulation with prostacyclin and heparin during continuous venovenous hemofiltration. Crit Care Med 1994;22:1774–81.
54. Davenport A, Will EJ, Davison AM. The effect of prostacyclin on intracranial pressure in patients with acute hepatic and renal failure. Clin Nephrol 1991;25:151–7.
55. Turney JH, Fewell MR, Williams LC, Parsons V, Weston MJ. Platelet protection and heparin sparing with prostacyclin during regular dialysis therapy. Lancet 1980;ii:219–22.
56. Rylance PB, Gordge MP, Ireland H, Lane DA, Weston MJ. Hemodialysis with prostacyclin (epoprostenol) alone. Proc EDTA-ERA 1984;21:281–6.
57. Davenport A, Will EJ, Davison AM. Comparison of the use of standard heparin and prostacyclin anticoagulation in spontaneous and pump driven extracorporeal circuits in patients with combined acute renal and hepatic failure. Nephron 1994;66:431–7.
58. Swartz RD, Flamenbaum W, Dubrow A, et al. Epoprostenol (PGI$_2$, prostacyclin) during high-risk hemodialysis: preventing further bleeding complications. J Clin Pharmacol 1988;28:818–25.
59. Stevens PE, Davies SP, Brown EA, et al. Continuous arteriovenous hemodialysis in critically ill patients. Lancet 1988;ii:150–2.
60. Zobel G, Ring E, Rödel S. Prognosis in pediatric patients with multiple organ system failure and continuous extracorporeal renal support. Contrib Nephrol 1995;116:163–8.
61. Davenport A. Anticoagulation in patients with acute renal failure treated with continuous renal replacement therapies. Home Hemodial Int 1998;2:41–60.
62. Willey ML, de Denus S, Spinler SA. Removal of lepirudin, a recombinant hirudin, by hemodialysis, hemofiltration, or plasmapheresis. Pharmacotherapy 2002;2:492–9.
63. Eichler P, Friesen HJ, Lubenow N, Jaeger B, Greinacher A. Antihirudin antibodies in patients with heparin induced thrombocytopenia treated with lepirudin: incidence, effects on aPTT, and clinical relevance. Blood 2000;96:2373–8.

64. Fischer KG, Loo van de A, Bohler J. Recombinant hirudin (lepirudin) as anticoagulant in intensive care patients treated with continuous hemodialysis. Kidney Int 1999;72(Suppl S):46–50.

65. Kern H, Ziemer S, Kox WJ. Bleeding after intermittent or continuous r-hirudin during CVVH. Intensive Care Med 1999;11: 1311–14.

66. Davenport A. The management of heparin induced thrombocytopenia during renal replacement therapy. Hemodial Int 2001; 3:81–5.

67. Reddy BV, Nahlik L, Trevino S, Murray PT. Argatroban anticoagulation during renal replacement therapy. Blood Purif 2002;20: 313–14.

68. Murray PT, Reddy BV, Grossman EJ, et al. A prospective comparison of three argatroban treatment regimens during hemodialysis in end-stage renal disease. Kidney Int 2004;66:2446–53.

69. Akizawa T. Beneficial characteristics of protease inhibitor as an anticoagulant for extracorporeal circulation. Rinsho Ketsueki 1990;31:782–6.

70. Matsuo T, Kario K, Nakao K, Yamada T, Matsuo M. Anticoagulation with nafamostat mesilate, a synthetic protease inhibitor, in hemodialysis patients with a bleeding risk. Haemostasis 1993;23: 135–41.

71. Akizawa T, Koshikawa S, Ota K, et al. Nafamostat mesilate: a regional anticoagulant for hemodialysis in patients at high risk for bleeding. Nephron 1993;64:376–81.

72. Himmelfarb J, Holbrook D, McMonagle E. Effects of aprotinin on complement and granulocyte activation during ex-vivo hemodialysis. Am J Kidney Dis 1994;24:901–6.

73. Matata BM, Wark S, Sudaram S, et al. In vitro contact phase activation with hemodialysis membranes: role of pharmaceutical agents. Biomaterials 1995;16:1305–12.

74. Pinnick RV, Wiegmann TB, Diederich DA. Regional citrate anticoagulation for hemodialysis in the patient at high risk for bleeding. N Engl J Med 1983;3:258–61.

75. Dhondt A, Vanholder R, Tielmans C, et al. Effect of regional citrate anticoagulation on leukopenia, complement activation, and expression of leukocyte surface molecules during hemodialysis with unmodified cellulose membranes. Nephron 2000;85:334–42.

76. Flanigan MJ, Vo Brecht J, Freeman RM, Lim VS. Reducing the hemorrhagic complications of hemodialysis: a controlled trial of low dose heparin and citrate antcoagulation. Am J Kidney Dis 1987;9:147–53.

77. Mehta RL, McDonald BR, Aguilar MM, Ward DM. Regional citrate anticoagulation for continuous arterio-venous hemodialysis in critically ill patients. Kidney Int 1990;38:976–81.

78. Palsson R, Niles JR. Regional citrate anticoagulation in continuous venovenous hemofiltration in critically ill patients with a high risk of bleeding. Kidney Int 1999;55:1991–7.

79. Tolwani AJ, Campbell RC, Schenk MB, Allon M, Warnock DG. Simplified citrate anticoagulation for continuous renal replacement therapy. Kidney Int 2001;60:370–4.

80. Kutsogiannis DJ, Mayers I, Chi WD, Gibney RT. Regional citrate anticoagulation in continuous venovenous hemodiafiltration. Am J Kidney Dis 2000;35:802–11.

81. Bunchman T, Maxvold NJ, Barnett J, Hutchings A, Benfield MR. Pediatric hemofiltration: normocarb dialysate solution with citrate anticoagulation. Pediatr Nephrol 2002;17:150–4.

82. Gupta M, Wadhwa NK, Bukovsky R. Regional citrate anticoagulation for continuous venovenous hemodiafiltration using calcium-containing dialysate. Am J Kidney Dis 2004;43:67–73.

83. Cointault O, Kamar N, Bories P, et al. Regional citrate anticoagulation in continuous venovenous haemodiafiltration using commercial solutions. Nephrol Dial Transplant 2004;19:171–8.

84. Apsner R, Buchmayer H, Lang T, et al. Simplified citrate anticoagulation for high flux hemodialysis. Am J Kidney Dis 2001;38: 979–87.

85. Meier-Kriesche H-U, Gitomer J, Finkel K, DuBose T. Increased total to ionized calcium ratio during continuous venovenous hemodialysis with regional citrate anticoagulation. Crit Care Med 2001;29:748–52.

86. Davenport A. CRRT in the management of patients with liver disease. Semin Dial 1996;9:78–84.

87. Flanigan MJ, Pillsbury L, Sadewasser G, Lim VS. Regional hemodialysis anticoagulation: hypertonic trisodium citrate or anticoagulation citrate dextrose-A. Am J Kidney Dis 1996;27: 519–24.

88. Filimberti E, Cinotti S, Salvadori M, et al. Hemodialysis with defibrotide: effects on coagulation parameters. Int J Artif Organs 1992;15:590–4.

13

Intermittent hemodialysis

Mark R Marshall and Tom Golper

Intermittent hemodialysis (IHD) has been a clinical reality for critically ill acute renal failure (ARF) patients for half a century. The fundamental therapeutic objectives underlying these early efforts continue to form the basis for modern practice.[1] Over this period, there have been refinements in the technology of vascular access, hemodialyzers, and supporting machinery as well as a clearer understanding of patient response to IHD. As a result, the application of IHD treatments has become safer and easier. Although the mortality of critically ill ARF patients remains high, there is evidence that outcomes are gradually improving despite a higher degree of prevalent illness severity.[2,3]

IHD is overall the most common renal replacement therapy for critically ill ARF patients.[4] Practice patterns are determined mostly by logistic concerns such as cost and access to technology, and follow predictable geographic patterns that can be in most part related to reimbursement patterns and clinical responsibility for the respective modalities. In the United States, IHD is far more commonly utilized than continuous renal replacement therapy (CRRT), and managed by nephrologists.[5] In Australia, the converse is true.[6] European practice patterns vary by region, and both CRRT and IHD on balance appear equally common, with responsibility for therapy equally split between intensivists and nephrologists.[7]

This chapter has the following aims: (1) to provide a description and assessment of practical aspects of IHD for critically ill ARF patients and (2) to provide strategies for the avoidance of common complications.

THERAPEUTIC OBJECTIVES FOR IHD

There is uncertainty as to optimal physiologic targets in critically ill ARF patients. Studies to resolve key issues have often been hampered by difficulties in study design and execution, or poor standardization of definitions.[8] Consequently, clinicians often rely on default reasoning extrapolated from the end-stage renal disease (ESRD) setting. The usual minimum recommendation is that renal replacement therapy be used to treat the occurrence of threatening acidosis or hyperkalemia, refractory hypervolemia, and features of the uremic syndrome such as pericarditis or coma. These criteria, however, do not constitute therapeutic objectives that will optimize patient outcomes in this setting.

Critically ill ARF patients in the modern era generally die from their original disease or pre-existing conditions. The concept of *corrected* mortality was originally developed by Kennedy et al,[9] and can be defined as the mortality attributable to ARF itself. While corrected mortality is low in noncritically ill ARF patients, it rises sharply with illness severity and may exceed 50% for those at the severe end of the spectrum. The main contributors to corrected mortality in these studies are infection, nonresolving shock, and hemorrhage.[10] These conditions therefore can be considered to define the endpoints of uremic toxicity as mediated by retained substances in ARF: i.e. a uremic syndrome for the critically ill as opposed to the typical description for the ESRD setting.[11]

The object of renal replacement therapy in this setting therefore goes beyond optimization of fluid status and correction of the usual biochemical abnormalities, and should be broadened to address the specific requirements of critically ill ARF patients. First, the process of maintaining fluid and solute control should not compromise other aspects of the clinical condition by exacerbating hemodynamic instability, increasing end-organ damage, or delaying renal recovery.

Secondly, blood purification in this setting can be applied to mediators of damage that are either absent or not given emphasis within the traditional list of potential uremic toxins described in the ESRD literature. In critically ill ARF patients, there is activation of humoral pro-inflammatory cytokine systems, characterized by a variety of medium (300 Da to 12 kDa) and large (>12 kDa) molecules (shown in Table 13.1[12–14]). These are essential for the local host response to a microbiological challenge. However, their uncontrolled production and systemic release may lead to indiscriminate tissue damage and the exacerbation of multiple organ failure due to their cardiodepressant, vasodilatory, and immunomodulatory properties.[15] Several studies have found correlations between circulating levels of pro-inflammatory cytokines and outcomes of patients with sepsis, which has in turn led to increasing experimentation to determine whether facilitated clearance of these inflammatory mediators results in improved patient outcomes.[13] These mediators can therefore be considered as potential uremic toxins in this population, and the impact of IHD upon their clearance is included in subsequent discussions.

Therapeutic objectives and therapy prescription for IHD should be individualized according to the requirements of the clinical situation. Dehydration may be required for patients with threatening pulmonary edema, whereas fluid loading may be desirable for the aggressive optimization of oxygen delivery during septic shock. Serum

Table 13.1   Properties of selected putative mediators of tissue injury and physiologic antagonists.[12–14]

Mediators	Approx molecular weight (Da)	Sieving coefficient	Effect
Pro-inflammatory			
Amino acid metabolites	600	0.5–0.91	Neurotoxicity, hypocoagulability
Bradykinin	1,100		Vasodilatation and increased vascular permeability
Endothelin	2,500	0.19	End-organ ischemia
C3a/C5a	11,000	0.11–0.77	Pro-inflammatory cytokines synthesis, neutrophil activation, vasodilatation, increased vascular permeability
Factor D	24,000		Complement activation
LPS	67,000		Pro-inflammatory cytokines synthesis
LPS fragments	<1000–20,000		
TNF-alpha	17,000 (54,000)	0–0.2	Fever, hypercoagulability, neutrophil activation, suppression of bone marrow stem cell maturation, hypotension from vasodilatation and myocardial depression, wasting and negative nitrogen balance, B-cell growth factor
IL-1	17,500	0.07–0.42	
IL-6	22,000	0.01–0.32	
IL-8	8,000	0–0.48	
Anti-inflammatory			
sTNFr	30,000–50,000	<0.1	Reduces ability of TNF-α to activate cells
IL-1ra	24,000	0.28–0.45	Reduces ability of IL-1 to activate cells
IL-10	18,000	0	Inhibits pro-inflammatory cytokine synthesis

LPS, lipopolysaccharide; IL, interleukin; TNF, tumor necrosis factor; sTNFr, soluble TNF receptor.

electrolyte and bicarbonate concentrations should be maintained in the normal range. Targets for uremic solute control are discussed later in the chapter.

EQUIPMENT

Vascular access

Angioaccess for IHD is usually via single- or double-lumen polyurethane or silicone temporary catheters in the internal jugular (IJ), subclavian (SC), or femoral (FE) veins. Tunneled cuffed catheters used in the ESRD setting may also be used, and probably perform better than temporary catheters.[16] They are, however, more difficult to insert and exchange, and discussion here will be limited to the more commonly used temporary catheter. SC catheters are associated with a higher incidence of procedural complications, as well as stenosis and thrombosis in the vein.[17] This vascular damage is of less importance to critically ill ARF patients than to ESRD patients, since a minority of the former group survive without recovery of renal function to require maintenance IHD.

Catheter performance is more important for IHD than for CRRT. Higher blood flows are necessary during IHD to provide sufficient overall solute clearance, whereas lower blood flows are sufficient to achieve adequate clearance by CRRT due to its continuous nature. In general, blood flow rate can be safely increased during IHD until the venous and arterial pressures are plus and minus 350 mmHg, respectively, after which hemolysis can occur.[18] Left-sided IJ and SC catheters tend to provide unreliable blood flow, at a rate that is typically up to 100 ml/min lower than elsewhere because their tips abut the walls of either the superior vena cava

or innominate vein. FE and right-sided IJ or SC catheters provide the best blood flow.[19] There are significant differences between blood flows achieved with different catheter brands, and larger-bore lines are preferred.[17]

Access recirculation (AR) has not been as well defined for temporary as for tunneled cuffed catheters. Using ultrasound dilution, AR for all sites is approximately 10% at blood flow rate (QB) 250–350 ml/min, and may rise to as much as 35% at QB greater than 500 ml/min.[19,20] AR depends on the design and site of the catheter. For instance, AR has been shown to be negligible in IJ catheters. AR is higher in FE catheters as opposed to elsewhere, especially if the catheter is shorter than 20 cm.[19,20] Up to half of treatments will require catheters to be utilized with inflow and outflow lines in reversed configuration, such that the original 'venous' line is used as for blood inflow (relative to dialyzer), and the original 'arterial' line for outflow. AR in this situation is approximately doubled therefore, in the order of 20% at 250–350 ml/min.[17] Figure 13.1 models the impact of AR on urea clearance as a function of catheter location. The impact of AR on dialysis dose is illustrated by the study of Leblanc and colleagues, in which the urea reduction ratio was significantly higher with SC (62.5%) vs FE (54.5%) catheters despite identical IHD operating parameters.[21]

Infection of temporary catheters is common, with rates several times that of tunneled cuffed catheters. Bacteremia, exit-site infection, and distant infection in one series occurred at 6.2, 3.6, and 1.1 episodes per 1000 catheter days, respectively.[17] In one study, the risk of bacteremia was increased after 1 and 3 weeks at the FE and IJ sites, respectively, and increased threefold by the use of the FE vs IJ site.[22] In another study, this risk was increased

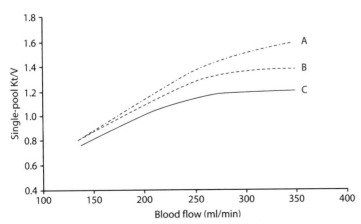

Figure 13.1 The relationship between delivered dialysis dose (expressed as single-pool Kt/V) and blood flow as a function of temporary catheter performance with respect to access recirculation (AR). Intermittent hemodialysis treatments are modeled under the following conditions: duration = 240 min, dialysate flow = 500 ml/min, hemodialyzer mass transfer coefficient = 911 ml/min, V = 40 L, nPCR = 0.8 g/kg/day. (A) Internal jugular catheter with no recirculation; (B) 20 cm femoral catheter assumed to have AR of 0% at 150 ml/min, 8.5% at 250 ml/min, and 17% at 350 ml/min; (C) 15 cm femoral catheter assumed to have AR of 5% at 150 ml/min, 20% at 250 ml/min and 30% at 350 ml/min.

sixfold by the use of the IJ vs SC site (no FE catheters used in this study).[23] Both polysporin and mupirocin ointments have been shown in randomized controlled trials to significantly reduce the risk of bacteremia from tunneled cuffed catheters.[24,25] There are generally less data for temporary catheters, although both povidone and mupirocin ointments with dry gauze exit-site dressings are reported to be similarly useful.[26,27] There is also increasing interest in the use of antimicrobial solutions to lock catheters between treatments, but this technique is yet to be studied for temporary catheters. In general, the study of such antimicrobial strategies has been sketchy in ARF as opposed to ESRD settings, and their benefit is therefore uncertain for critically ill patients.

Machines

IHD in the intensive care unit (ICU) is usually performed using machines transported from maintenance dialysis facilities. As such, machines need to be robust and mobile. Commercial IHD machines vary a great deal in technical complexity. Increasing sophistication usually reflects greater accuracy of treatment monitoring, a broader range of operating functions, and a larger degree of procedural automation. It should be recognized, however, that experienced operators can undoubtedly perform very safe and efficacious IHD treatments with relatively basic equipment.

In general, the technical attributes of IHD machines depend on the requirements of the clinical situation. The hemodynamic stability of critically ill patients during IHD is facilitated by precise and predictable fluid removal. This is especially relevant for procedures where the ultrafiltration rate is greater than that required for the restoration of euvolemia, such as for plasma exchange and hemodiafiltration. Machines with computerized flow or volumetric ultrafiltration control are therefore preferred for the ICU.

The capability for sodium profiling, ultrafiltration profiling, and blood temperature monitoring may be desirable (see below), and should be considered by clinicians establishing IHD programs in the ICU. Some manufacturers are providing IHD machines with integrated functions for sustained low-efficiency dialysis (SLED) that can be selected from start-up without any manual adjustments, and this flexibility will be desirable.

Most IHD machines reconstitute dialysate from electrolyte concentrate and purified water in a single-pass arrangement. Alternatively, machines can utilize a batch delivery system where the dialysate is already reconstituted.[28] The Genius machine (Fresenius AG, Hamburg, Germany) is the most popular system, and over 2000 treatments are reported in the literature. The technical elements of the machine and reported patient outcomes appear to be satisfactory.[29] A disadvantage to this machine may be the fixed volume of dialysate and hence limited clearance. Furthermore, batch dialysate increases its weight: single-pass machines weigh 70–90 kg, whereas the Genius weighs 160 kg, 75 kg of which is dialysate.

Hemodiafiltration (HDF) is usually performed for critically ill ARF patients as CRRT, with substitution fluid and dialysate in commercially prepared bags. However, intermittent treatments have been performed in this setting with standard IHD machinery, using sterile substitution fluid generated online from ultrapure dialysate, which is then diverted by a separate pump to be infused directly into the extracorporeal blood circuit either in predilution or postdilution mode.[30] Ultrapurification is by a series of ultrafilters placed strategically along the dialysate pathway, and studies have consistently shown that endotoxin levels, sterility, and chemical composition are indistinguishable from the commercial fluid preparations.[31]

Dialysate composition

The IHD prescription should specify the composition of reconstituted dialysate. Dialysate [K+] and (ionized) [Ca^{2+}] range from 0 up to 4 and 1.75 mmol/L, respectively. These concentrations can only be changed by physically exchanging the canister of concentrate. In general, a dialysate [K+] concentration of 3 or 4 mmol/L is required for potassium homeostasis in this setting, unless intake or efflux from the intracellular pool is substantial and uncontrollable. If lower dialysate [K+] is used, it is often prudent to recheck serum [K+] either during or immediately post-IHD to ensure that hypokalemia has not occurred. A dialysate [Ca^{2+}] of around 1.25 mmol/L is usually adequate for most patients, although dialysis against a low or [Ca^{2+}]-free dialysate is an invaluable tool for the treatment of threatening hypercalcemia in the ARF patient.[32] Postdialysis serum [Ca^{2+}] should be monitored for hypocalcemia if reduced [Ca^{2+}] dialysate is being used.

Acetate is more stable than bicarbonate in solution, and was previously preferred as buffer in commercial dialysate concentrates. However, hyperacetatemia may supervene if the rate of acetate uptake from dialysate is greater than its metabolic conversion to bicarbonate (see Bicarbonate-buffered dialysate section). Most contemporary IHD machines use bicarbonate as buffer in the dialysate, and this should be standard for critically ill ARF patients. Dialysate generally needs to be alkalotic to maintain normal acid–base status in the patient. Bicarbonate concentration can be varied according to need by the proportioning system of the IHD machine, from approximately 24 up to 40 mmol/L (default ~35 mmol/L). A similar situation exists with sodium, with concentrations possible between approximately 130 and 150 mmol/L and the default being around 140 mmol/L. Once again, this can be titrated to the clinical situation, with the caution that changes in patient sodium mass balance can lead to water shifts with quite marked changes in extracellular fluid volume and therefore hemodynamic stability (see Sodium and ultrafiltrate profiling section).

Water treatment

Water can be delivered either by a central purification plant, a portable purification system incorporated into the dialysis machine, or by a batch system. Water purification itself is achieved by reverse osmosis (RO). If water is soft (<0.1 dH, 1.8 ppm $CaCO_3$) then only a particle filter and charcoal cartridge are needed with the RO treatment to purify water, whereas a water softener is needed to pretreat harder water to protect the RO membranes.[33] Most ICUs do not have a central water purification plant, although this is an increasing practice amongst units who perform online HDF for either conventional or sustained low-efficiency treatments. The ICU may be able to share a water loop from a maintenance dialysis facility, although an auxiliary pump is often needed if the loop is extended more than 100 meters from the plant.

Hemodialyzer membranes

During hemodialysis, complement is activated by contact between blood and components of the extracorporeal blood circuit. The degree of this activation is largely determined by hemodialyzer membrane composition. Membranes made of unsubstituted cellulose (e.g. cuprophane, CU) have exposed hydroxyl groups that activate complement efficiently via the alternative pathway. These hydroxyl groups can be substituted with tertiary amino groups (hemophan) or acetate (cellulose acetate, CA; cellulose diacetate, CDA; cellulose triacetate, CTA). Alternatively, hemodialyzers can be made entirely from synthetic plastics such as polysulfone (PS), polyamide (PA), polyacrylonitrile (PAN), polymethylmethacrylate (PMMA), and acrylonitrile 69 (AN69). In general, hemodialyzers other than those made of unsubstituted cellulose activate less complement, although there is a wide degree of overlap in that some synthetic membranes such as PMMA still have a substantial capacity to activate complement.[33]

Following complement activation, there is an increased expression of leukocyte adhesion molecules, which leads to retention of leukocytes in lungs, renal parenchyma, and other organs. Subsequently, products of leukocyte activation are released (e.g. reactive oxygen species, proteases, leukotrienes, and pro-inflammatory cytokines).[34] Activation of a variety of other cellular pathways has also been documented. These immune mechanisms have been most clearly defined in ESRD, although there are some data in the critically ill ARF population.[35,36]

Biocompatibility is a membrane attribute that includes amongst other things the activating capacity of the membrane on complement and leukocytes: a membrane with a high activating capacity is regarded as *bioincompatible*, a low capacity *biocompatible*. This property is usually attributed by consensus of opinion leaders, due to the lack of formal criteria to constitute a definition.

These immune processes are known to accelerate the decline in residual renal function in ESRD patients, and are postulated to be determinants of mortality and recovery of renal function in critically ill ARF patients. Table 13.2 summarizes the results of appropriate clinical studies,[36-44] while excluding frequently quoted series that were not specifically designed to evaluate the role of membrane design in outcomes.[45-48] The divergent results require explanation. It is clear that investigators are not consistent in their selection of hemodialyzers for each of the two arms. Studies demonstrating outcome differences mostly used unsubstituted cellulose as the bioincompatible hemodialyzer. Those demonstrating no difference mostly used substituted cellulose as the bioincompatible hemodialyzer, or PMMA as the biocompatible hemodialyzer. As mentioned above, modification of cellulose will improve biocompatibility, whereas

Table 13.2 Pivotal studies evaluating the role of membrane design on overall mortality and renal recovery in critically ill ARF patients.

Reference No.	Design (N)	BCM hemodialyzers				BICM hemodialyzers				p	ARF recovery
		Material	Flux	Size (m²)	Survival (%)	Material	Flux	Size (m²)	Survival (%)		
36	RCT (52)	AN69	High	1.0	62	CU	Low	1.0	35	0.052	BCM>BICM
37	RCT (51)	PMMA	N/A	N/A	58	CA	Low	1.1	64	NS	ND
38	RCT (160)	PMMA	Low	1.2	60	CU	Low	1.2	58	NS	ND
39	CT (66)	PS	High	1.2	73	CA	Low	1.1	76	NS	ND
40*	CT (153)	PMMA/PS	Low	1.5/1.2	57	CU	Low	1.2	46	0.03	BCM>BICM
41	RCT (124)	PS	High	1.3	43	CDA	Low	1.4	45	NS	ND
		PS	Low	1.3	36	CDA	Low	1.4	45	NS	ND
42	CT (57)	PA	High	1.3	64	CU	Low	1.3	72	NS	ND
43	RCT (76)	AN69/PAN	High	1.0	63	CU	Low	1.0	34	0.01	BCM>BICM
44	CT (72)	PMMA	Low	1.5	57	CU	Low	1.2	37	NS	BCM>BICM

AN69, acrylonitrile and sodium methallyl sulfonate copolymer; ARF, acute renal failure; BICM, bioincompatible membrane; BCM, biocompatible membrane; CA, cellulose acetate; CDA, cellulose diacetate; CT, controlled trial; CU, cuprophane; PA, polyamide; PAN, polyacrylonitrile; PMMA, polymethylmethacrylate; PS, polysulfone; RCT, randomized controlled trial.

* Includes patients from Reference 44.

PMMA is not as biocompatible as other synthetic membranes.

Statistical criticisms have also been made in a number of these studies in relation to insufficient power, imbalance in the randomization process, and lack of intention to treat analysis.[49–51] Results may also be confounded by performance characteristics of the hemodialyzers independent of biocompatibility. As can be seen in Table 13.2, the hemodialyzers chosen for the biocompatible arm frequently had high flux characteristics and a larger surface area than the corresponding hemodialyzers chosen for comparison. Several meta-analyses have recently been undertaken to empower statistical analyses, all with results as divergent as the original studies, since the criteria for study inclusion in these analyses do not eliminate the confounding factors mentioned above. For instance, one report on 722 patients determined the relative survival advantage for those treated with a biocompatible hemodialyzer to be 1.09 (95% CI 0.88–1.32),[52] whereas another study on 649 patients determined it to be 1.37 (95% CI 1.02–1.83).[53]

Although more studies are needed to fully resolve the issue of biocompatibility, a general recommendation can be made against the use of unsubstituted cuprophane in view of reasonable doubt regarding a deleterious effect. This maneuver adds little to the total cost of care for any individual critically ill patient, but may of course amount to a substantial cumulative cost given many patients over time.[54]

HDF and high-flux IHD

Uremic solute removal can occur by two separate processes. Solutes can be dragged with plasma water across the membrane during ultrafiltration (convection). Blood purification is subsequently achieved by the infusion of crystalloid substitution fluid that dilutes solutes remaining in the body. Solutes can also be removed during dialysis, with blood purification by movement of the solute through the membrane down its concentration gradient (diffusion).

In the literature pertaining to ESRD patients, there is still debate as to whether convective clearance as provided by HDF or high-flux IHD confers additional clinical benefit over conventional IHD. This debate extends to critically ill ARF patients, where interest in HDF and high-flux IHD stems from the potential for therapeutic removal of cytokines such as those in Table 13.1. Although many of these mediators are water soluble, their

molecular weight precludes mass transfer during low-flux IHD. The diameter of pores in the skin (as opposed to support) layer of low-flux membranes is about 1.0–2.0 nm, and in high-flux membranes about 3.0–5.0 nm. The relationship between membrane pore size and molecular weight cut-off (MWCO, the minimum molecular weight at which rejection of solutes is 90%) varies according to conditions other than pore size alone, although these pore sizes generally equate to MWCO of approximately 10 kDa and 50 kDa, respectively. Diffusion through these pores is the main mechanism for mass transfer of small solutes, whereas convection is more important for middle-sized and larger solutes.[55] This paradigm has been the rationale for experimental therapeutic strategies such as 'super high flux'[56,57] (membranes with MWCO of 100–150 kDa) and high-volume[58,59] (convective fluid clearance of 100 ml/kg/h or greater) hemofiltration.

However, it is also increasingly apparent that mass transfer across the membrane may play a relatively minor role in the removal of these mediators. Their sieving coefficient (proportionality constant between the rate of solute movement and fluid movement across the membrane) is frequently well below 1, and removal by convection therefore trivial in comparison to their endogenous clearance.[12,14] Studies have nevertheless confirmed extracorporeal removal of a range of cytokines with a significant fall in their circulating levels, and this has been due to an adsorptive mechanism resulting in up to a tenfold higher removal of such mediators in comparison to convective removal alone.[60] Accordingly, negligible amounts of cytokines are observed in filtrate and dialysate, until such time as the membrane becomes saturated.[61] Adsorption is critically dependent on membrane composition and structure; an open pore structure and hydrophobic (e.g. synthetic) membrane is necessary for binding to the hydrophobic amino acids in the polypeptide structure of cytokines.[62]

There is therefore potential for therapy to remove such mediators using high-flux membranes or HDF with high ultrafiltration rates, although it is likely that removal will be as much by adsorption as by convection. These considerations are theoretical at present, and a review of the literature examining the effects of renal replacement therapy on the mediators of septic shock found that benefits remain unclear.[63] In humans, the only studies conclusively showing benefit were uncontrolled, whereas controlled reports failed to reveal consistent improvement. Furthermore, it has been shown that such therapies are unselective in the removal of pro- vs anti-inflammatory cytokines, raising the potential for exacerbation of the patient inflammatory milieu. The limited clinical data concerning intermittent HDF for critically ill ARF patients have demonstrated no clinical or laboratory advantage over conventional IHD.[30] Similarly, what data there are suggest that high-flux dialysis in this setting does not influence outcomes.[41,64] At the present time, more studies are needed before a recommendation can be made with regard to HDF and high-flux IHD.

STRATEGIES FOR THE AVOIDANCE OF COMMON COMPLICATIONS

Extracorporeal blood circuit clotting

Anticoagulation is required for IHD, and this topic is covered in Chapter 12.

Intradialytic hypotension

Hypotension is detrimental for end-organ function and recovery in critically ill patients. Renal vascular reactivity is abnormal in postischemic ARF and, consequently, there is reduced autoregulation and paradoxical vasoconstriction in response to reduced renal perfusion pressure during hypotension.[65] Recurrent renal injury has been demonstrated to prolong the course of ARF in animal models, whereas morphologic studies in humans have shown fresh ischemic lesions in kidney biopsy specimens from patients with ARF of over 3 weeks' duration.[66] This has specific relevance to renal replacement therapy, and hypotension associated with IHD has been shown to reduce residual native renal function as measured by creatinine clearance.[67,68]

A frequent schedule of IHD and substantial treatment times will minimize ultrafiltration goals and rates, and are the most effective measures to minimize hypotension. The following specific technical strategies can also be applied.

Bicarbonate-buffered dialysate
Hyperacetatemia has a peripheral vasodilating effect,[69] a myocardial depressant effect,[70] and is able to increase oxygen consumption as a result of acetate metabolism.[71] Consequently, acetate-buffered dialysate is associated with an increased frequency of hypotension relative to bicarbonate-buffered dialysate.[72] Bicarbonate-buffered dialysate should be routinely used in critically ill ARF patients.

Sodium and ultrafiltration profiling
Solute removal during IHD leads to a rapid reduction in serum osmolarity. The intercompartmental transfer of these solutes is not instantaneous, and osmotic forces therefore promote water movement into cells, leading to a reduction in extracellular volume and effective circulating volume. Sodium profiling ameliorates hemodynamic instability from this process during maintenance IHD in the ESRD setting. This intervention involves higher dialysate sodium concentration at the start of dialysis, with decrements thereafter in a stepped, exponential or linear manner until the base concentration is achieved at the end of the treatment. The increased serum osmolarity facilitates fluid transfer from the interstitial to vascular compartment, thereby maintaining effective circulating volume during ultrafiltration.[73] Another widespread practice with much anecdotal support amongst technical and nursing staff directly performing treatments is ultrafiltration profiling, which involves variation in ultrafiltration rates during the treatment. The commonest practice uses a higher rate at the start of the treatment when serum osmolarity is greatest, with a lower rate later in the treatment. This technique has not been shown to have a clinical benefit when used in isolation, although it may be useful when combined with sodium profiling.[74] A large number of protocols have been empirically developed to be available as a standard function on most commercial dialysis machinery.

There are sparse data on the subject of either technique in the critically ill. Paganini and colleagues randomized patients to conventional IHD or an intervention comprising sodium profiling (160 mmol/L at the start of treatment, 140 mmol/L base concentration) combined with ultrafiltration profiling (50% of ultrafiltration volume removed in the first one-third of the treatment, the rest removed over the remainder). Delivered dialysis dose was equal between the groups, although hemodynamic stability was better in the interventional group despite a larger ultrafiltration volume.[75] This approach seems to be safe and effective, although further study is needed to determine the exact value of the individual interventions, and the value of simpler approaches such as the use of high sodium dialysate without profiling.

Blood volume monitoring

Blood volume monitoring involves a biofeedback system that automatically adjusts ultrafiltration rate and dialysate sodium content in response to a fall in circulating blood volume. Blood volume is determined using principles of mass conservation from real-time hematocrit (or plasma protein) monitoring by a device placed on the extracorporeal blood circuit. A number of automated systems are now available as standard features in hemodialysis machinery. Systems such as these have now been convincingly shown to reduce the occurrence of intradialytic hypotension in ESRD patients on maintenance hemodialysis who are prone to this complication.[76] However, in a prospective observational study of 20 critically ill ARF patients, it has been shown that hypotension still occurred in up to 30% of treatments, suggesting no benefit with this technique.[77] The probable reason for this discrepancy is the different relationship between blood volume and hypotension in two settings. Autonomic function and circulating humoral agents all mediate and mitigate this relationship, and these factors are not comparable between ESRD and critically ill ARF patients.

Dialysate calcium

There are encouraging data that high dialysate calcium (1.75 mmol/L) preserves left ventricular function in patients with cardiomyopathy during IHD, and improved blood pressure in patients prone to severe intradialytic hypotension.[78] This technique is limited by the development of hypercalcemia, however, and has not been studied in the critically ill ARF patient cohort.

Blood temperature monitoring

Vasoconstriction due to lower body temperatures has been used to increase vascular resistance and improve hemodynamic stability during IHD. Ample data have demonstrated a clinically useful effect during maintenance IHD in the ESRD setting.[79] There are some data that strongly suggest that thermal energy transfer is the main reason for the superior hemodynamic tolerability of isolated ultrafiltration and HDF.[80,81] Hypothermia, however, is often undesirable in critically ill patients due to the adverse effect on myocardial function, end-organ perfusion, blood clotting, and probably renal recovery.[82] Blood temperature monitoring is a technique whereby the patient's blood temperature is maintained precisely at the target value by a series of feedback loops controlling thermal transfer to and from the dialysate.[83] This function is available as an integrated module in commercially available IHD machines and is effective in ameliorating hemodynamic instability for susceptible ESRD patients.[84] Blood temperature monitoring might conceivably allow for controlled cooling in critically ill ARF patients without the risk of hypothermic damage. However, to our knowledge, this hypothesis remains untested.

Modality

A number of studies in the late 1970s and early 1980s demonstrated superior cardiovascular stability during HDF for maintenance treatments in ESRD patients, although these earlier studies involved comparisons with those receiving acetate-buffered IHD. However, observational reports suggest an advantage also in comparison to historical controls treated with bicarbonate-buffered IHD.[85]

In comparison to bicarbonate-buffered IHD, HDF has other attributes that theoretically enhance cardiovascular stability. The infusion of substitution fluid has a cooling effect due to heat loss in the circuit.[81] In addition, sodium removal may be lower relative to IHD when the sodium concentration in the substitution fluid or bicarbonate solution is equal to that in the dialysate.[86] Expansion of the vascular volume may therefore develop over the course of treatment. It has also been suggested that convection during these treatments may remove antihypertensive agents or endogenous vasoactive substances more efficiently from the circulation, leading to increased peripheral vasoconstriction.[87] Finally, high fluxes of calcium during HDF may contribute to increased cardiac output and peripheral vascular resistance.[88]

Two prospective controlled trials involving ESRD patients have arrived at diametrically opposed conclusions regarding the superior hemodynamic stability of HDF,[89,90] and both have been criticized for methodologic inadequacy.[91] Appropriately designed and powered studies are required to resolve these uncertainties.

IHD DOSE

Dialysis prescription has traditionally been reactive to the patient's clinical or biochemical state. As such, dialysis treatments have usually been scheduled according to pragmatic assessments of the patient's progress and logistic considerations such as staff and machinery availability. More recently, data have been reported that provide a basis for rational prescription using a urea-based approach, which will narrow the focus of the remainder of this section. A more expansive discussion of issues pertaining to dose adequacy is provided in Chapter 10.

The concept of clearance is fundamental to the understanding of dialysis dose, and relates solute removal during renal replacement therapy to blood purification in the patient. Targets for optimal IHD dose have usually been developed as clearance-based expressions using urea kinetic modeling (UKM) techniques developed in stable ESRD populations.

As a consequence, Kt/V is consequently also the most popular expression for dialysis dose in the critically ill ARF population.[92,93] However, the calculation of this expression by popular simplified formulae (e.g. method of Daugirdas,[94] etc.) may be inappropriate due to empirical rather than determined values for urea nitrogen generation rate and distribution volume within the formulae that may limit accuracy in critically ill ARF patients.[95] While impractical, formal iterative multicompartment UKM undoubtedly provide more accurate values.[96] A promising alternative is online dialysis quantification using urea and conductivity sensors.[97,98]

Most importantly, however, Kt/V realistically reflects only the effect of a single IHD treatment upon solute control. Cumulative Kt/V does not change proportionally to cumulative solute removal when IHD schedules are altered by changes to treatment frequency rather than to individual treatment operating parameters.[99] For instance, Figure 13.2 illustrates the increased removal of urea by a schedule that delivers a given cumulative weekly Kt/V through a greater number of treatments.

There are several competing UKM methods for quantifying different renal replacement therapies in a manner that accounts for schedule. Gotch recently derived an expression termed 'standard Kt/V' (stdKt/V),[100] while Keshaviah and Star derived the 'solute removal index' (SRI) about a decade ago.[101] Both expressions are similar from a UKM perspective, and each has been argued to provide a superior definition of treatment equivalency in the ESRD setting by being numerically equal for clinically equivalent regimens of IHD and continuous ambulatory peritoneal dialysis (CAPD). For example, if one considers expert consensus about minimum standards for delivered Kt/V for each therapy,[102,103] IHD delivering an equilibrated Kt/V of 1.05 three times a week and CAPD delivering a weekly Kt/V of 2.0 will both

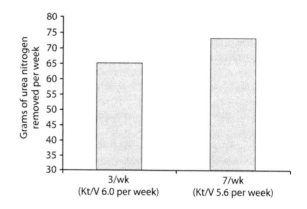

Figure 13.2 A comparison of urea nitrogen removed per week during two dialysis regimens where residual renal function is absent, net protein catabolic rate (nPCR) is 0.8 g/kg/day, and the starting blood urea nitrogen (BUN) for the week is 93 mg/dl. Regimen A: 3 treatments per week, duration of treatment 240 minutes, V = 40 L, and Kd = 333 ml/min. Regimen B: 7 treatments per week, duration 120 minutes, V = 40 L, and Kd = 267 ml/min.

correspond to a stdKt/V of 2.0.[104] A similar situation exists for SRI, where IHD delivering an equilibrated Kt/V of 0.97 three times a week and CAPD delivering a weekly Kt/V of 1.75 will both correspond to a SRI of 1.75.[105]

Both methods are problematic in the critically ill ARF population. As originally described, stdKt/V is calculated using urea mass removal rate extrapolated from G, which requires the patient to be in urea steady state. In contrast, SRI as originally described is calculated using urea mass removal rate from direct dialysate quantification, which remains valid during urea nonsteady state and irregular dialysis schedules so long as measurements are undertaken for every treatment. This cumbersome requirement can be avoided by the calculation of SRI from blood-sided measurements using a number of formulae, although these variably do not account for urea generation and/or ultrafiltration during dialysis, or multicompartment effects.[101,106]

An additional problem lies with the reliance of stdKt/V and SRI on peak urea concentrations. Kinetically equivalent therapy prescriptions will be those that produce the same urea mass removal rate at the same predialysis BUN. The peak concentration hypothesis defines the peak predialysis BUN for use in calculations as the maximum after the longest interdialytic break,[107] although for stdKt/V this peak has been redefined as the average of all predialysis BUN in the week.[104] Urea concentrations may be very asymmetrical and variable in the critically ill ARF population, and these arbitrary definitions may have accordingly less significance. The arguments supporting the peak concentration hypothesis in the ESRD setting cannot be extrapolated to the critically ill ARF population, where the rudimentary nature of dose–outcome relationships precludes validation of any one hypothesis over its competitors.

We believe the most appropriate UKM expression for this purpose is the equivalent renal urea clearance (EKR).[108] EKR expresses the dose of any renal replacement therapy as the continuous urea clearance that will result in the same steady-state time-averaged urea concentration for a given amount of urea removal. EKR is modeled using time-averaged as opposed to peak urea concentration, which has more validity and is easier to define for patients in urea nonsteady state or with irregular IHD schedules. EKR is usually corrected to a V of 40 L to account for different body sizes (cEKR). It is to be emphasized that cEKR is not simply time-averaged hemodialyzer urea clearance. By way of an example, cEKR would not triple if hemodialyzer clearance were to be tripled for a given IHD regimen. cEKR is a mass balance parameter that accounts for inefficiency of intermittent therapies.

Caution must be exercised when calculating cEKR for the patient who is in urea nonsteady state. Even for a regular schedule of identical IHD treatments, the traditional formula for cEKR will provide falsely low values if calculations are made when the time-averaged BUN is falling, and falsely high values when it is rising. For instance, a study of nine patients on a consistent prescription of SLED documented cEKR to be 34% lower when treatment was initiated, compared with when the BUN had fallen to a steady state level.[109] A recent study of acute dialysis therapies based on simulations documented cEKR to progressively rise by 35% after the initiation of CRRT and the subsequent fall in BUN from 150 mg/dL to a steady state level of 50 mg/dL.[110] In both of these examples, cEKR values were unrealistically variable when clearly there had been no change in treatment operating parameters and in particular treatment clearance. A number of alternative UKM formulae have been developed to calculate cEKR avoiding such inaccuracy in the setting of urea nonsteady state, and any one of them can be used depending on the degree of precision required and the data available.[109,111,112] However, in busy clinical settings a previously published nomogram is convenient, although it loses accuracy with variation of dialysis prescription and/or delivery within the weekly interval (Fig. 13.2).[108,113]

The importance of defining valid UKM methods for dose measurement has increased due to studies that have shown delivered IHD dose to be low compared to targets established for ESRD, and substantially lower than that prescribed.[114] Three recent reports have supported a relationship between IHD dose and mortality. The first study to demonstrate the influence of dialysis dose upon outcomes was a retrospective observational report from the Cleveland Clinic Foundation. A higher dose of IHD per treatment was associated with significantly improved outcome in patients with intermediate illness severity (see Fig. 13.3).[92] This study did not attempt to relate outcomes to the frequency of IHD or total dose. The second study was a prospective controlled study, and demonstrated

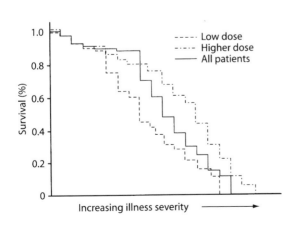

Figure 13.3 Dose–outcome relationship (mortality versus illness severity stratified by dialysis dose treatment) for 842 critically ill ARF patients from the Cleveland Clinic Foundation requiring either IHD or CRRT. IHD patients are shown. Those with intermediate illness severity were most affected by IHD dose, with higher dose (single-pool Kt/V >1.0, urea reduction ratio >58%) being associated with a significantly lower mortality.[92]

that a cumulative single pool Kt/V of 6.0 per week (by simple addition) was associated with improved outcomes relative to 3.0 per week, and that daily treatments were associated with better outcomes than alternate-day treatments.[93] This study did not attempt to define the optimal dialysis dose beyond which no further benefit was accrued, and was not able to separate the effect of IHD treatment frequency from that of dose. The third study was a prospective randomized controlled study examining dose–outcome relationships in CRRT, and demonstrated that a clearance of 35 ml/kg/h was necessary to optimize patient outcomes.[115]

Figure 13.4 can be used to compare these IHD and CRRT regimens. It can be seen that daily dialysis achieving a single pool Kt/V of 1.5 would be necessary to achieve the small solute clearance that was defined as optimal in the CRRT study. Although no study has assessed IHD dose separately from IHD treatment frequency, it is hard to conceive of a practical situation where this dose of dialysis could be delivered on a schedule other than daily.

At the present time, IHD should deliver a cEKR of at least 23 ml/min. It is possible and indeed likely there would be additional clinical benefit in achieving higher clearances such as that defined as optimal in the CRRT study. It is not appropriate,

however, to make this recommendation without having replicated the results of that study with IHD. The proposed cEKR target of 23 ml/min corresponds well to those of other investigators. For instance, daily IHD delivering a Kt/V of 0.9–1.0 per treatment has been proposed as adequate by one opinion leader[116] (cEKR ~ 25 ml/min), and a steady-state time-averaged blood urea nitrogen (BUN) concentration of 60 mg/dl by another[117] (cEKR ~ 25 ml/min assuming G between 10 and 20 mg/min, which is usual in this setting).

A separate feature of solute control is time-averaged deviation in concentration. Figure 13.5 illustrates this principle, with BUN time–concentration profiles for two IHD regimens delivering the same small solute removal (as determined by cEKR), but using a different number of treatments. The large unphysiologic swings in solute concentrations during the three times a week regimen may be detrimental, as might be excessive peak concentrations of uremic solutes. The clinical impact of this time-averaged deviation in solute concentrations remains unknown. The stability of solute control remains an often-quoted advantage to CRRT, and also IHD regimens using frequent treatments.

The conclusions from all UKM data must be approached in a circumspect manner. Uncertainty arises from the lack of a robust marker of uremic

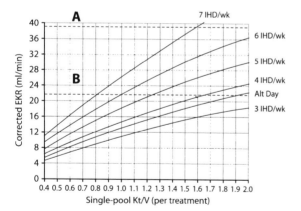

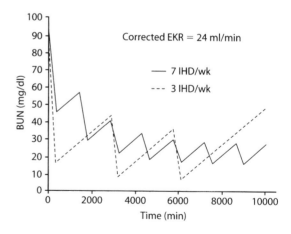

Figure 13.4 The relationship between continuous urea clearance corrected to a V of 40 L (cEKR) and variable volume single-pool Kt/V. The solid lines relate cEKR to single-pool Kt/V for a given intermittent hemodialysis schedule. The dotted lines indicate cEKR associated with superior outcomes in two recent studies. (A) Continuous renal replacement therapy (CRRT) delivering a clearance of 35 ml/kg/h corrected to a V of 40 L (assumed to equal a weight of 66 kg).[103] (B) Intermittent hemodialysis (IHD) delivering a single-pool Kt/V of 0.92 per treatment at a frequency of 6.2 per week.[91]

Figure 13.5 A comparison of blood urea nitrogen (BUN) time–concentration profiles between two intermittent hemodialysis (IHD) regimens delivering a corrected equivalent renal clearance (cEKR) of 24 ml/min. The solid line reflects solute removal over 3 treatments per week, the dotted solute removal over 7 treatments per week.

solute burden or clinical toxicity. Although serum urea and UKM are the usual tools for this purpose in the ESRD setting, it is important to remain open to their possible imprecision, especially in the critically ill ARF patient where the inverse correlation between urea removal and uremic toxicity is still emerging. Better markers of uremic toxicity are needed. For instance, a recent study demonstrated better outcomes with CRRT vs CAPD in critically ill ARF patients.[118] These outcomes did not correlate with urea clearance (CRRT ~ CAPD), but instead correlated with creatinine clearance (CRRT >CAPD), suggesting in this study the latter may be a better uremic marker.[119] Finally, it seems that high IHD dose principally benefits patients with illnesses of intermediate severity. Patient outcomes at either extremes of illness are much less influenced: patients who are mildly ill tend to survive whereas those who are severely ill tend to die, irrespective of IHD dose.[92]

THE PRACTICE OF IHD IN THE ICU

Currently there are no unequivocal data that demonstrate the superiority of any one renal replacement therapy for critically ill ARF patients. It has been claimed that CRRT provides better hemodynamic stability and improved mortality relative to IHD, but this has not been corroborated by randomized controlled prospective studies.[120] Most published experience is largely redundant: no studies have compared regimens that reflect optimal modern practice (i.e. IHD providing adequate dose using biocompatible membranes and bicarbonate dialysate vs CRRT with a filtration rate of 35 ml/kg/h).

Undoubtedly, CRRT offers specific advantages over IHD under some circumstances. On the basis of current evidence, it is likely that CRRT will not translate to overall clinical benefit if applied indiscriminately to all patients. Therapy choice depends on the patient's condition and the clinical objectives of the prescribing clinician. IHD can provide safe and efficacious renal replacement therapy in most cases, with recourse to other therapies as the individual situation dictates. For example, CRRT will be more appropriate for a patient unable to achieve ultrafiltration goals using IHD because of hemodynamic instability, and intermittent high-efficiency postdilution HDF may be more appropriate than IHD for a highly catabolic patient.

The sentiments recently expressed by Lameire and colleagues highlight an important counterpart to these technical aspects: the skill and experience of staff providing any renal replacement therapy probably influence patient outcomes as much as the type of therapy per se.[121]

The majority of data relating the outcomes of critically ill ARF patients to IHD practice patterns are inconclusive. A pragmatic and individualized approach is therefore warranted. In certain areas, however, there are enough published data to allow the following recommendations:

- IHD angioaccess via the right IJ is preferable, with recourse to the left side and femorals as needed. Suitable catheter lengths should be chosen to allow the catheter tip to reach the lower superior vena cava (SVC) for IJ and SC catheters (~15 cm on the right, 20 cm on the left), and the inferior vena cava (IVC) for FE catheters (>20 cm). Catheters may be dressed with polysporin, povidone, or mupirocin ointment and dry gauze to minimize infection.
- IHD machinery should be equipped with computerized flow or volumetric ultrafiltration control. The option for sodium/ultrafiltration profiling and SLED is preferable.
- Dialysate should be buffered with bicarbonate rather than acetate.
- Hemodialyzer membranes composed of substituted cellulose or synthetic plastics are preferable to those composed of unsubstituted cellulose. There are not enough data to make recommendations with regard to membrane flux and adsorption characteristics.
- Hypotension should be avoided, and hemodynamic stability can be improved by any of the measures shown in Box 13.1.

Box 13.1 Measures to improve hemodynamic stability during treatments

---

Minimize ultrafiltration rate requirements by:
- Increased frequency of treatments (up to daily)
- Increased duration of treatments (up to 6–8 hours, then consider SLED or CRRT)

Bicarbonate-buffered dialysate

Sodium/ultrafiltration profiling

? HDF

? Blood temperature monitoring

? Increase dialysate [Ca^{2+}]

For abbreviations, see text.

- IHD dose should be monitored to ensure prescribed dialysis is delivered, and cEKR is the preferred expression of dialysis dose. We propose the cEKR–spKt/V nomogram as a useful prescriptive tool. A cEKR >23 ml/min should be achieved by any given combination of spKt/V and frequency. Small solute removal per treatment can be increased by any of the measures shown in Box 13.2.
- There are not enough data to make recommendations with regard to the optimal frequency of IHD treatments independent of dose. However, it is likely that a minimum of alternate day and, more likely, daily treatments will be necessary to achieve adequate dialysis dose.

Box 13.2   Measures to increase dialysis dose

Maximize hemodialyzer surface area (up to 2.0–2.2 m^2)

Maximize hemodialyzer porosity (high-flux)

Maximize blood flow rate by:

- Maximization of internal lumen diameter of catheter (up to 2.0–2.2 mm)
- Titration of blood flow to maximum arterial and venous pressures (up to minus and plus 300–350 mmHg, respectively)
- Correct positioning of catheter tip in SVC and IVC as appropriate
- Right-sided IJ and SC >left-sided IJ and SC

Minimize access recirculation by:

- Correct positioning of catheter tip in SVC and IVC as appropriate
- IJ and SC >FE catheters

Maximize dialysate flow (up to 800–1000 ml/min)

Postdilution HDF

Optimize anticoagulation to reduce hemodialyzer fiber bundle clotting

Optimize circulation to reduce compartmental urea sequestration

Increased treatment frequency (up to daily)

Increased treatment duration (up to 6–8 hours, then consider SLED or CRRT)

For abbreviations, see text.

REFERENCES

1. Teschan PE, Baxter CR, O'Brien TF, Freyhof JN, Hall WH. Prophylactic hemodialysis in the treatment of acute renal failure. Ann Int Med 1960;53:992–1016.

2. McCarthy J. Prognosis of patients with acute renal failure in the intensive care unit: A tale of two eras. Mayo Clin Proc 1996;71:117–26.

3. Druml W. Prognosis of acute renal failure. Nephron 1996;73:8–15.

4. Ronco C, Zanella M, Brendolan A, et al. Management of severe acute renal failure in critically ill patients: an international survey in 345 centres. Nephrol Dial Transplant 2001;16:230–7.

5. Mehta R. Continuous renal replacement therapies in the acute renal failure setting: current concepts. Adv Ren Replace Ther 1997;4:81–92.

6. Silvester W. Prospective survey of renal replacement therapy for acute renal failure in 21 hospitals in state of Victoria, Australia. Blood Purif 1997;15:147 [Abstract].

7. Lameire N, Van Biesen W, Vanholder R, Colardijn F. The place of intermittent hemodialysis in the treatment of acute renal failure in the ICU patient. Kidney Int 1998;66(Suppl):S110–19.

8. Silvester W. Outcome studies of continuous renal replacement therapy in the intensive care unit. Kidney Int 1998;53(Suppl): S138–41.

9. Kennedy A, Burton J, Luke R, et al. Factors affecting the prognosis in acute renal failure. A survey of 251 cases. Q J Med 1973;42:73–86.

10. Liano F, Junco E, Pascual J, Madero R, Verde E, and the Madrid Acute Renal Failure Study Group. The spectrum of acute renal failure in the intensive care unit compared with other settings. Kidney Int 1998;53(Suppl):S16–24.

11. Levy EM, Viscoli CM, Horwitz RI. The effect of acute renal failure on mortality. A cohort analysis. JAMA 1996;275:1489–94.

12. Sieberth HG, Kierdorf HP. Is cytokine removal by continuous hemofiltration feasible? Kidney Int 1999;72(Suppl):S79–83.

13. Schetz M. Non-renal indications for continuous renal replacement therapy. Kidney Int 1999;72(Suppl):S88–94.

14. Lonnemann G, Linnenweber S, Burg M, Koch KM. Transfer of endogenous pyrogens across artificial membranes? Kidney Int 1998;66(Suppl):S43–6.

15. Hack CE, Aarden LA, Thijs LG. Role of cytokines in sepsis. Adv Immunol 1997;66:101–95.

16. Canaud B, Leray-Moragues H, Leblanc M, et al. Temporary vascular access for extracorporeal renal replacement therapies in acute renal failure patients. Kidney Int 1998;66(Suppl):S142–50.

17. Oliver M. Acute dialysis catheters. Semin Dial 2001;14:432–5.

18. Twardowski Z, Haynie J, Moore H. Blood flow, negative pressure, and hemolysis during hemodialysis. Home Hemodialysis International 1999;3:45–50.

19. Little M, Conlon P, Walshe J. Access recirculation in temporary hemodialysis catheters as measured by saline dilution technique. Am J Kidney Dis 2000;36:1135–9.

20. Kanagasundaram N, Larive B, Garcia M, Depner T, Daugirdas J. Intermittent hemodialysis in ICU acute renal failure—access recirculation in temporary veno-venous catheters. J Am Soc Nephrol 2001;12:451 [Abstract].

21. Leblanc M, Fedak S, Mokris G, Paganini EP. Blood recirculation in temporary central catheters for acute hemodialysis. Clin Nephrol 1996;45:315–9.

22. Oliver MJ, Callery SM, Thorpe KE, Schwab SJ, Churchill DN. Risk of bacteremia from temporary hemodialysis catheters by site of insertion and duration of use: a prospective study. Kidney Int 2000;58:2543–5.

23. Kairaitis LK, Gottlieb T. Outcome and complications of temporary haemodialysis catheters. Nephrol Dial Transplant 1999;14:1710–4.

24. Johnson D, MacGinley R, Kay T, et al. A randomised controlled trial of topical exit site mupirocin application in patients with tunnelled, cuffed haemodialysis catheters. Nephrol Dial Transplant 2002;17:1802–7.

25. Lok C, Stanley K, Hux J, et al. Hemodialysis infection prevention with polysporin ointment. J Am Soc Nephrol 2003;13:169–79.

26. Levin A, Mason AJ, Jindal KK, Fong IW, Goldstein MB. Prevention of hemodialysis subclavian vein catheter infections by topical povidone-iodine. Kidney Int 1991;40:934–8.

27. Sesso R, Barbosa D, Leme IL, et al. Staphylococcus aureus prophylaxis in hemodialysis patients using central venous catheter: effect of mupirocin ointment. J Am Soc Nephrol 1998;9:1085–92.

28. Fassbinder W. Renaissance of the batch method? Nephrol Dial Transplant 1998;13:3010.

29. Lonnemann G, Floege J, Kliem V, Brunkhorst R, Koch K. Extended daily veno-venous high flux haemodialysis in patients with acute renal failure and multiple organ dysfunction syndrome using a single path batch dialysis system. Nephrol Dial Transplant 2000;15:1189–93.

30. Pettila V, Tiula E. Intermittent hemodiafiltration in acute renal failure in critically ill patients. Clin Nephrol 2001;56:324–31.

31. Vaslaki L, Karatson A, Voros P, et al. Can sterile and pyrogen-free on-line substitution fluid be routinely delivered? A multicentric study on the microbiological safety of on-line haemodiafiltration. Nephrol Dial Transplant 2000;15(Suppl):74–8.

32. Kaye M. Dialysate calcium loss using a calcium free dialysate. Int J Artif Organs 1994;17:365–72.

33. Dhondt A, Van Biesen W, Vanholder R, Lameire N. Selected practical aspects of intermittent hemodialysis in acute renal failure patients. Contrib Neph 2001;132:222–35.

34. Modi G, Pereira B, Jaber B. Hemodialysis in acute renal failure: Does the membrane matter? Semin Dial 2001;14:318–21.

35. Jaber BL, Cendoroglo M, Balakrishnan VS, et al. Impact of dialyzer membrane selection on cellular responses in acute renal failure: a crossover study. Kidney Int 2000;57:2107–16.

36. Schiffl H, Lang SM, Konig A, et al. Biocompatible membranes in acute renal failure: prospective case-controlled study. Lancet 1994;344:570–2.

37. Assouad M, Tseng S, Dunn K, et al. Biocompatibility of dialyzer membranes is important in the outcomes of acute renal failure. J Am Soc Nephrol 1996;7:1437 [Abstract].

38. Jorres A, Gahl GM, Dobis C, et al. Haemodialysis-membrane biocompatibility and mortality of patients with dialysis-dependent acute renal failure: a prospective randomised multicentre trial. Lancet 1999;354:1337–41.

39. Albright RC, Jr., Smelser JM, McCarthy JT, et al. Patient survival and renal recovery in acute renal failure: randomized comparison of cellulose acetate and polysulfone membrane dialyzers. Mayo Clinic Proc 2000;75:1141–7.

40. Himmelfarb J, Tolkoff Rubin N, Chandran P, et al. A multicenter comparison of dialysis membranes in the treatment of acute renal failure requiring dialysis. J Am Soc Nephrol 1998;9:257–66.

41. Gastaldello K, Melot C, Kahn R-J, et al. Comparison of cellulose diacetate and polysulfone membranes in the outcome of acute renal failure: A prospective randomized study. Nephrol Dial Transplant 2000;15:224–30.

42. Kurtal H, von Herrath D, Schaefer K. Is the choice of membrane important for patients with acute renal failure requiring hemodialysis? Artif Organs 1995;19:391–4.

43. Schiffl H, Sitter T, Lang S, et al. Bioincompatible membranes place patients with acute renal failure at increased risk of infection. ASAIO J 1995;41:M709–12.

44. Hakim RM, Wingard RL, Parker RA. Effect of the dialysis membrane in the treatment of patients with acute renal failure. N Engl J Med 1994;331:1338–42.

45. Cosentino F, Chaff C, Piedmonte M. Risk factors influencing survival in ICU acute renal failure. Nephrol Dial Transplant 1994;9:179–82.

46. Liano F, Pascual J, Group at MARFS. Epidemiology of acute renal failure: a prospective, multicenter, community-based study. Kidney Int 1996;50:811–18.

47. Neveu H, Kleinknecht D, Brivet F, Loirat P, Landais P, and the French Study Group on Acute Renal Failure. Prognostic factors in acute renal failure due to sepsis. Results of a prospective multicenter study. Nephrol Dial Transplant 1996;11:293–9.

48. Schiffl H, Lang SM, Haider M. Bioincompatibility of dialyzer membranes may have a negative impact on outcome of acute renal failure, independent of the dose of dialysis delivered: a retrospective multicenter analysis. ASAIO J 1998;44:M418–22.

49. Vanholder R, De Vriese A, Lameire N. The role of dialyzer biocompatibility in acute renal failure. Blood Purif 2000;18:1–12.

50. Karsou S, Jaber B, Pereira B. Impact of intermittent hemodialysis variables on clinical outcomes in acute renal failure. Am J Kidney Dis 2000;35:980–91.

51. Shaldon S. Biocompatible membranes in acute renal failure: Prospective case-controlled study. Nephrol Dial Transplant 1997;12:235–6.

52. Jaber B, Lau J, Schmid C, et al. Effect of biocompatibility of hemodialysis membranes on mortality in acute renal failure: a meta-analysis. Clin Nephrol 2002;57:274–82.

53. Subramanian S, Venkataraman R, Kellum JA. Influence of dialysis membranes on outcomes in acute renal failure: a meta-analysis. Kidney Int 2002;62:1819–23.

54. Jacobs C. Membrane biocompatibility in the treatment of acute renal failure: what is the evidence in 1996? Nephrol Dial Transplant 1997;12:38–42.

55. Leypoldt JK. Solute fluxes in different treatment modalities. Nephrol Dial Transplant 2000;15(Suppl):3–9.

56. Lee PA, Weger GW, Pryor RW, Matson JR. Effects of filter pore size on efficacy of continuous arteriovenous hemofiltration therapy for Staphylococcus aureus-induced septicemia in immature swine. Crit Care Med 1998;26:730–7.

57. Uchino S, Bellomo R, Goldsmith D, et al. Super high flux hemofiltration: a new technique for cytokine removal. Intensive Care Med 2002;28:651–5.

58. Honore PM, Jamez J, Wauthier M, et al. Prospective evaluation of short-term, high-volume isovolemic hemofiltration on the hemodynamic course and outcome in patients with intractable circulatory failure resulting from septic shock. Crit Care Med 2000;28:3581–7.

59. Cole L, Bellomo R, Journois D, et al. High-volume haemofiltration in human septic shock. Intensive Care Med 2001;27:978–86.

60. De Vriese AS, Colardyn FA, Philippe JJ, et al. Cytokine removal during continuous hemofiltration in septic patients. J Am Soc Nephrol 1999;10:846–53.

61. Schetz M. Removal of cytokines in septic patients using continuous veno-venous hemodiafiltration. Crit Care Med 1994;22:715–6.

62. Goldfarb S, Golper TA. Proinflammatory cytokines and hemofiltration membranes. J Am Soc Nephrol 1994;5:228–32.

63. De Vriese AS, Vanholder RC, De Sutter JH, Colardyn FA, Lameire NH. Continuous renal replacement therapies in sepsis: where are the data? Nephrol Dial Transplant 1998;13:1362–4.

64. Ponikvar J, Russ R, Kenda R, Bren A, Ponikvar R. Low-flux versus high-flux synthetic dialysis membranes in acute renal failure: prospective randomized study. Artif Organs 2001;25:946–50.

65. Conger J, Robinette J, Hammond W. Difference in vascular reactivity in models of ischemic acute renal failure. Kidney Int 1991;39:1087–95.

66. Solez L, Morel-Maronger L, Sraer J. The morphology of acute tubular necrosis in man: analysis of 57 renal biopsies and comparison with the glycerol model. Medicine 1979;58:362–7.

67. Manns M, Sigler M, Teehan B. Renal function changes during intermittent hemodialysis (IHD) vs continuous hemodialysis (CVVHD) in acute renal failure (ARF). ASAIO J 1996;42:78 [Abstract].

68. Sigler M, Manns M, Teehan B. Effects of intermittent hemodialysis on residual renal function in critically ill patients with acute renal failure. J Am Soc Nephrol 1994;5:477 [Abstract].

69. Herrero JA, Trobo JI, Torrente J, et al. Hemodialysis with acetate, DL-lactate and bicarbonate: a hemodynamic and gasometric study. Kidney Int 1994;46:1167–77.

70. Wizemann V, Soetanto R, Thormann J, Lubbecke F, Kramer W. Effects of acetate on left ventricular function in hemodialysis patients. Nephron 1993;64:101–5.

71. Kishimoto T, Tanaka H, Maekawa M, et al. Dialysis-induced hypoxaemia. Nephrol Dial Transplant 1993;8(Suppl):25–9.

72. Man N, Fournier G, Thireau P, Gaillard J, Funck-Brentano J. Effect of bicarbonate-containing dialysate on chronic hemodialysis patients: a comparative study. Artif Organs 1982;6:421–8.

73. Stiller S, Bonnie-Schorn E, Grassmann A, Uhlenbusch-Korwer I, Mann H. A critical review of sodium profiling for hemodialysis. Semin Dial 2001;14:337–47.

74. Oliver MJ, Edwards LJ, Churchill DN. Impact of sodium and ultrafiltration profiling on hemodialysis-related symptoms. J Am Soc Nephrol 2001;12:151–6.

75. Paganini E, Sandy D, Moreno L, Kozlowski L, Sakai K. The effect of sodium and ultrafiltration modeling on plasma volume and haemodynamic stability in intensive care patients receiving haemodialysis for acute renal failure: a prospective, stratified, randomized, cross-over study. Nephrol Dial Transplant 1996;11(Suppl):32–7.

76. Santoro A, Mancini E, Basile C, et al. Blood volume controlled hemodialysis in hypotension-prone patients: a randomized, multicenter controlled trial. Kidney Int 2002;62:1034–45.

77. Tonelli M, Astephen P, Andreou P, et al. Blood volume monitoring in intermittent hemodialysis for acute renal failure. Kidney Int 2002;62:1075–80.

78. Alappan R, Cruz D, Abu-Alfa A, Mahnensmith R, Pezarella M. Treatment of severe intradialytic hypotension with the addition of high dialysate calcium concentration to midodrine and/or cool dialysate. Am J Kidney Dis 2001;37:294–9.

79. Dheenan S, Henrich W. Preventing dialysis hypotension: A comparison of usual protective maneuvers. Kidney Int 2001;59:1175–81.

80. van der Sande FM, Gladziwa U, Kooman JP, Bocker G, Leunissen KM. Energy transfer is the single most important factor for the difference in vascular response between isolated ultrafiltration and hemodialysis. J Am Soc Nephrol 2000;11:1512–17.

81. van der Sande FM, Kooman JP, Konings CJ, Leunissen KM. Thermal effects and blood pressure response during postdilution hemodiafiltration and hemodialysis: the effect of amount of replacement fluid and dialysate temperature. J Am Soc Nephrol 2001;12:1916–20.

82. Zager RA, Gmur DJ, Bredl CR, Eng MJ. Temperature effects on ischemic and hypoxic renal proximal tubular injury. Lab Invest 1991;64:766–76.

83. Schneditz D. Temperature and thermal balance in hemodialysis. Semin Dial 2001;14:357–64.

84. Maggiore Q, Pizzarelli F, Santoro A, et al and The Study Group of Thermal Balance and Vascular Stability. The effects of control of thermal balance on vascular stability in hemodialysis patients: results of the European randomized clinical trial. Am J Kidney Dis 2002;40:280–90.

85. Pizarelli F, Cerrai T, Dattalo P, Tetta C, Maggiore Q. Convective treatments with on-line production of replacement fluid: a clinical experience lasting 6 years. Nephrol Dial Transplant 1998;13:363–9.

86. Pedrini LA, Ponti R, Faranna P, Cozzi G, Locatelli F. Sodium modeling in haemodiafiltration. Kidney Int 1991;40:525–32.

87. Arese M, Cristol JP, Bosc JY, et al. Removal of constitutive and inducible nitric oxide synthase-active compounds in a modified hemodiafiltration with on-line production of substitution fluid: the contribution of convection and diffusion. Int J Artif Organs 1996;19:704–11.

88. Canaud B, Bosc JY, Leray H, et al. On-line haemodiafiltration: State of the art. Nephrol Dial Transplant 1998;13(Suppl):3–11.

89. Movilli E, Camerini C, Zein H, et al. A prospective comparison of bicarbonate dialysis, hemodiafiltration, and acetate-free biofiltration in the elderly. Am J Kidney Dis 1996;27:541–7.

90. Locatelli F, Mastrangelo F, Redaelli B, et al. Effects of different membranes and dialysis technologies on patient treatment tolerance and nutritional parameters. Kidney Int 1996;50:1293–1302.

91. Maggiore Q, Pizzarelli F, Dattolo P, Maggiore U, Cerrai T. Cardiovascular stability during haemodialysis, haemofiltration and haemodiafiltration. Nephrol Dial Transplant 2000;15(Suppl):68–73.

92. Paganini EP, Tapolyai M, Goormastic M, et al. Establishing a dialysis therapy/patient outcome link in intensive care unit acute dialysis for patients with acute renal failure. Am J Kidney Dis 1996;28(Suppl):S81–9.

93. Schiffl H, Lang S, Fischer R. Daily hemodialysis and the outcomes of acute renal failure. N Engl J Med 2002;346:305–10.

94. Daugirdas JT. Second generation logarithmic estimates of single-pool variable volume Kt/V: an analysis of error. J Am Soc Nephrol 1993;4:1205–13.

95. Clark WR, Mueller BA, Kraus MA, Macias WL. Dialysis prescription and kinetics in acute renal failure. Adv Ren Replace Ther 1997;4(Suppl):64–71.

96. Leblanc M, Tapolyai M, Paganini EP. What dialysis dose should be provided in acute renal failure? A review. Adv Ren Replace Ther 1995;2:255–64.

97. Canaud B, Bosc J, Leblanc M, et al. On-line dialysis quantification in acutely ill patients. Preliminary clinical experience with a multipurpose urea sensor monitoring device. ASAIO J 1998;44:185–90.

98. Ronco C, Brendolan A, Bellomo R. Online monitoring in continuous renal replacement therapies. 1999;72(Suppl):S8–14.

99. Clark W, Leypoldt L, Henderson L, et al. Quantifying the effect of changes in the hemodialysis prescription on effective solute removal with a mathematical model. J Am Soc Nephrol 1999;10:601–9.

100. Gotch F. The current place of urea kinetic modelling with respect to different dialysis modalities. Nephrol Dial Transplant 1998;13(Suppl):10–4.

101. Keshaviah P, Star R. A new approach to dialysis quantification: an adequacy index based on solute removal. Semin Dial 1994;7:85–90.

102. II. NKF-K/DOQI clinical practice guidelines for peritoneal dialysis adequacy: update 2000. Am J Kidney Dis 2001;37(Suppl 1):S65–136.

103. I. NKF-K/DOQI clinical practice guidelines for hemodialysis adequacy: update 2000. Am J Kidney Dis 2001;37(Suppl 1):S7–64.

104. Gotch F. Is Kt/V urea a satisfactory measure for dosing the newer dialysis regimens? Semin Dial 2001;14:15–17.

105. Keshaviah P. The solute removal index—A unified basis for comparing disparate therapies. Perit Dial Int 1995;15:101–4.

106. Bankhead M, Toto R, Star R. Accuracy of urea removal estimated by kinetic models. Kidney Int 1995;48:785–93.

107. Keshaviah PR, Nolph KD, Van Stone JC. The peak concentration hypothesis: a urea kinetic approach to comparing the adequacy of continuous ambulatory peritoneal dialysis (CAPD) and hemodialysis. Peritoneal Dialysis International 1989;9:257–60.

108. Casino F, Lopez T. The equivalent renal urea clearance: a new parameter to assess dialysis. Nephrol Dial Transplant 1996;11:1574–81.
109. Marshall MR, Golper TA, Shaver MJ, Alam MG, Chatoth DK. Urea kinetics during sustained low-efficiency dialysis in critically ill patients requiring renal replacement therapy. Am J Kidney Dis 2002;39:556–70.
110. Liao Z, Zhang W, Hardy P, et al. Kinetic comparison of different acute dialysis therapies. Artif Organs 2003;27:802–7.
111. Casino F, Marshall M. EKRmb—Simple and accurate quantification intermittent hemodialysis (IHD) dose in acute renal failure (ARF) patients by a mass balance method. J Am Soc Nephrol 2002;13:249A [Abstract] .
112. Casino F, Marshall M. Simple and accurate quantification of dialysis in acute renal failure patients during either the urea non-steady state or treatment with irregular or continuous schedules. Nephrol Dial Transplant 2004;19:1454–66.
113. Casino F. The EKRc graph: A simple method to estimate the time averaged urea clearance. Semin Dial 1999;12:11–14.
114. Evanson JA, Himmelfarb J, Wingard R, et al. Prescribed versus delivered dialysis in acute renal failure patients. Am J Kidney Dis 1998;32:731–8.
115. Ronco C, Bellomo R, Homel P, et al. Effects of different doses in continuous veno-venous haemofiltration on outcomes of acute renal failure: a prospective randomised trial. Lancet 2000;356:26–30.
116. Sigler M. Critical care nephrology: transport characteristics of the slow therapies: implications for achieving adequacy of dialysis in acute renal failure. Adv Renal Replace Ther 1997;4:68–80.
117. Clark WR, Mueller BA, Kraus MA, Macias WL. Extracorporeal therapy requirements for patients with acute renal failure. J Am Soc Nephrol 1997;8:804–12.
118. Phu NH, Hien TT, Mai NT, et al. Hemofiltration and peritoneal dialysis in infection-associated acute renal failure in Vietnam. N Engl J Med 2002;347:895–902.
119. Daugirdas J. Peritoneal dialysis in acute renal failure—why the bad outcome? N Engl J Med 2002;347:933–5.
120. Vanholder R, Van Biesen W, Lameire N. What is the renal replacement method of first choice for intensive care patients? J Am Soc Nephrol 2001;12(Suppl):S40–3.
121. Lameire N, Van Beisen W, Vanholder R. Dialysing the patient with acute renal failure in the ICU: The emperor's clothes? Nephrol Dial Transplant 1999;14:2570–3.

14

Continuous renal replacement therapies

Neesh I Pannu and Ravindra L Mehta

INTRODUCTION

Acute renal failure (ARF) is a common problem in the intensive care unit (ICU) and, despite significant improvements in the care of critically ill patients, the mortality from this complication remains over 50%. Over the last two decades there has been an evolution in the field of hemodialysis and, consequently, our approach to the treatment of ARF. The use of new devices and techniques has allowed us to achieve better-tolerated and more efficient renal replacement therapy (RRT).

Over 20 years ago continuous arteriovenous hemofiltration was reported as a treatment for ARF in critically ill patients.[1] This technique, which used mean arterial pressure to drive blood flow through an extracorporeal circuit and required both arterial and venous cannulation, had obvious advantages over intermittent renal replacement therapies, but had a limited capacity for solute clearance. The addition of a blood pump, ultrafiltration control and countercurrent dialysate have made modern continuous renal replacement therapy (CRRT) techniques both safer and easier to use. In this chapter, we will review the current literature about CRRTs and how they may be used in the ICU.

WHAT IS CONTINUOUS RENAL REPLACEMENT THERAPY?

CRRT is any extracorporeal blood purification therapy that is intended to substitute for impaired renal function; it is applied for 24 hours per day in an ICU. The term CRRT describes a variety of blood purification techniques, which may differ significantly according to the mechanism of solute transport, the type of membrane, the presence or absence of dialysate solution and the type of vascular access (Fig. 14.1). Recognizing the diversity of CRRT techniques, an international group of experts (the Acute Dialysis Quality Initiative) have proposed standardized terms for these therapies,[2] which are outlined in Table 14.1.

The basic premise in the development of these terms is to link the nomenclature to the operational characteristics of the different techniques. The letter C in all the terms describes the continuous nature of the methods, the next two letters (AV or VV) describe the driving forces through the circuit, and the remaining letters (UF, H, HD, HDF) represent the operational characteristics. The only exception to this is the acronym SCUF (slow continuous ultrafiltration), which remains as a reminder of the initiation of these therapies as simple techniques harnessing the power of AV circuits.[1]

Access

Arteriovenous (AV) refers to the use of an arterial catheter that allows blood flow into the extracorporeal circuit by virtue of the systemic blood pressure. The blood is returned via a central venous catheter. This technique of CRRT has fallen out of favor in recent years because of a high morbidity related to the placement and maintenance of large-bore arterial lines. Venovenous (VV) modalities use a single dual-lumen central venous catheter to access blood supply for the extracorporeal circuit as well as blood return. An extracorporeal blood pump is required to move blood through the circuit.

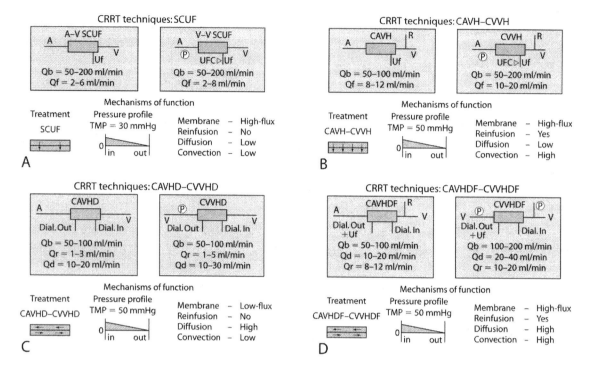

Figure 14.1 Schematics of different CRRT techniques. (A) Schematic representation of SCUF therapy. (B) Schematic representation of continuous arteriovenous or venovenous hemofiltration (CAVH–CVVH) therapy. (C) Schematic representation of continuous arteriovenous/venovenous hemodialysis (CAVHD–CVVHD) therapy. (D) Schematic representation of continuous arteriovenous/venovenous hemodiafiltration (CAVHDF–CVVHDF) therapy. A = artery; V = vein; Uf = ultrafiltrate; R = replacement fluid; P = peristaltic pump; Qb = blood flow; Qf = ultrafiltration rate; TMP = transmembrane pressure; in = dialyzer inlet; out = dialyzer outlet; UFC = ultrafiltration control system; Dial = dialysate; Qd = dialysate flow rate. Reproduced with permission from Bellomo R, Ronco C, Mehta RL. Nomenclature for continuous renal replacement therapies. Am J Kidney Dis 1996;28(5):S3:2–7.

Solute clearance

Solute removal in CRRT techniques is achieved either by convection, diffusion or a combination of both these methods (Fig. 14.2).

Hemodialysis (HD) is an extracorporeal therapy that achieves solute clearance primarily through diffusion. Solute moves down its concentration gradient across a semipermeable membrane from one fluid compartment to another. During this process, low molecular weight (MW) substances such as urea, creatinine, and potassium move from the blood compartment to the dialysate, whereas other solutes such as calcium and bicarbonate move in the opposite direction. The concentration differences between the two solutions are maximized with the use of countercurrent flow.

Hemofiltration (HF) is a process that achieves solute clearance primarily through convection, with the use of hydrostatic pressure to induce the filtration of plasma across a hemofilter membrane. Solutes are dragged across the membrane along with the plasma, resulting in convective transport of small and middle MW solutes in the same direction as water. Middle and larger MW substances are more efficiently removed using this technique than with dialysis. This process requires the use of replacement fluid to prevent iatrogenic acidosis and electrolyte depletion as well as excessive fluid removal. The solutes in the filtrate are in the same concentrations as those in the plasma, and solute removal is achieved by diluting the remaining plasma with substitution fluid. Plasma dilution can occur prefilter or postfilter. Solute clearance is entirely determined by ultrafiltration rate with hemofiltration techniques. If no replacement fluid is used and hydrostatic pressure is used for plasma water removal, the process is called ultrafiltration (UF).

Abbreviation	Definition	Description
Table 14.1	**Continuous renal replacement therapy nomenclature.**	
CAVH	Continuous arteriovenous hemofiltration	Driving force is patient's blood pressure Circuit is arteriovenous Ultrafiltrate produced is replaced with a replacement solution Ultrafiltration in excess of replacement results in patient volume loss Solute removal is through convection
CVVH	Continuous venovenous hemofiltration	Driving force is external pump Circuit is venovenous Other features similar to CAVH
SCUF	Slow continuous ultrafiltration	Form of CAVH or CVVH not associated with fluid replacement Primary aim is to achieve fluid removal in fluid overloaded states
CAVHD	Continuous arteriovenous hemodialysis	Driving force is patient's blood pressure Circuit is arteriovenous Dialysate solution is delivered across membrane countercurrent to blood flow at a rate substantially slower than blood flow rate. Typical dialysate flow rates are 1–2 L/h Fluid replacement is not routinely administered Solute removal is by diffusion
CVVHD	Continuous venovenous hemodialysis	Driving force is external pump Circuit is venovenous Other features similar to CAVHD
CAVHDF	Continuous arteriovenous hemodiafiltration	Driving force is patient's blood pressure Circuit is arteriovenous Dialysate solution is delivered across membrane countercurrent to blood flow at a rate substantially slower than blood flow rate. Typical dialysate flow rates are 1–2 L/h Ultrafiltration volumes are optimized to exceed desired weight loss and enhance solute clearance from convection Fluid losses are replaced in part or completely with replacement solution Solute removal is both diffusive and convective
CVVHDF	Continuous venovenous hemodiafiltration	Driving force is external pump Circuit is venovenous Other features similar to CAVHDF

Source: from Kellum et al.[10]

Hemodiafiltration (HDF), a modality that simultaneously incorporates both diffusion and convection techniques, markedly improves clearances and retains the simplicity of the procedure. Combining convection and diffusion allows flexibility in enhancing clearances by increasing the volume of ultrafiltrate or the dialysate flow rates. Using these methods, blood urea nitrogen (BUN) clearances in the range of 23–30 ml/min can be achieved, even in hypotensive patients.[3]

The choice of modality is dependent on several factors, including availability, physician expertise, hemodynamic stability, and the primary purpose of the procedure (fluid removal vs solute clearance).

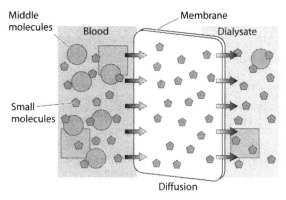

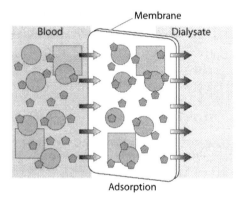

A Concentration gradient based transfer
Small molecular weight substances (<500 Da)
are transferred more rapidly

B Movement of water across the membrane
carries soultion across the membrane
Middle molecules are removed more efficiently

C Several solutes are removed from circulation by
adsorption to the membrane. This process is
influenced by the membrane structure and charge

Figure 14.2 Mechanisms of solute removal in dialysis. The success of any dialysis procedure depends on an understanding of the operational characteristics that are unique to these techniques and on appropriate use of specific components to deliver the therapy. Solute removal is achieved by (A) diffusion (hemodialysis), (B) convection (hemofiltration), or (C) combination of diffusion and convection (hemodiafiltration).

There is currently only limited information comparing diffusive vs convective blood purification techniques; results with CRRT techniques should be compared with those obtainable with intermittent hemodialysis (IHD), which remains the gold standard therapy.

WHAT ARE THE INDICATIONS FOR RENAL REPLACEMENT THERAPY IN PATIENTS WITH ACUTE RENAL FAILURE?

Patients with ARF require RRT when they have an acute fall in glomerular filtration rate and have developed, or are at risk of, clinically significant solute imbalance/toxicity or volume overload. The precise timing of RRT initiation is usually a matter of clinical judgment. The classic indications for dialysis include diuretic-resistant pulmonary edema, hyperkalemia, metabolic acidosis, uremic complications (pericarditis, encephalopathy, and bleeding), and certain dialyzable intoxications (e.g. lithium, toxic alcohols, salicylates). Although many of these indications are typically used in the setting of chronic renal failure, the consequences of these complications are likely to be more severe in critically ill patients; therefore, there has been a growing trend to start dialysis prior to the development of these indications. Delays in the initiation of treatment have often been based on a concern that dialysis itself may delay recovery of renal function. These fears have been largely dispelled by a recent study by Schiffl et al, which compared outcomes in patients with ARF treated with daily vs alternate-day dialysis for patients with acute renal failure.[4] Daily dialysis was not associated with a delay in renal recovery or an adverse effect on patient outcome.

WHEN SHOULD RENAL REPLACEMENT THERAPIES BE STARTED?

There is no commonly accepted definition for the timing of initiation of RRT in the setting of ARF. It has been suggested that patient outcome can be improved by early or more intensive dialysis to keep the BUN under 80–100 mg/dl (29–36 mmol/L). Recent nonrandomized studies have not been able to document significant benefit of prophylactic dialysis.[5,6] It is interesting to note that the average urea concentration at initiation of CRRT in a recent study of dialysis dosage was 17 mmol/L;[7] however, there is considerable variation in practice. A recent American survey of ICU dialysis practices found that the mean BUN and creatinine values at the initiation of dialysis were 98 mg/dl and 4.5 mg/dl, respectively.[8] However, because the BUN may reflect many factors other than the timing of initiation, no absolute value for BUN or creatinine should be used to determine when to initiate dialysis.

Only one randomized controlled trial has looked at the effect of timing of initiation of RRT on outcome. Bouman et al randomized 106 critically ill patients with ARF to early vs late initiation of dialysis. Early initiation was started within 12 hours of patients meeting the following criteria: low urine output (<30 ml/h) × 6 hours refractory to optimization of hemodynamics and diuretics, and creatinine clearance of <20 ml/min.[9] The late initiation group was started on dialysis when the classic indications for dialysis were met (volume overload, hyperkalemia, urea greater than 40 mmol/L). There was no significant difference between the groups in terms of ICU or hospital mortality, and no difference with respect to recovery of renal function. The results of this study must be interpreted with some caution, however: the study was underpowered to detect a clinically significant difference and the mortality rate in all treatment groups was very low.

The Acute Dialysis Quality Initiative (ADQI) consensus statement on dialysis treatment[10] makes no recommendations on the timing of initiation of RRT beyond those defined by the conventional criteria that apply to chronic renal failure.

ARE THERE NONRENAL INDICATIONS FOR CONTINUOUS RENAL REPLACEMENT THERAPY?

Although the use of CRRT in critically ill patients with ARF is widely accepted, CRRT has also been used for some nonrenal indications – most notably for the treatment of septic shock. Studies of high-volume hemofiltration (HVHF) in canine[11] and porcine models[12] of sepsis showed significant improvement in cardiac output (CO), mean arterial pressure (MAP), stroke volume (SV), and hepatic arterial flow; however these findings have not been replicated in human studies.

There are case reports and case series of CRRT use in a variety of conditions, including intoxication, cardiac failure, acute respiratory distress syndrome (ARDS), rhabdomyolysis, tumor lysis syndrome, and postcardiac surgery, but few if any prospective studies for many of these conditions.[13] At present, there are no established nonrenal indications for CRRT.

STARTING CONTINUOUS RENAL REPLACEMENT THERAPY: OPERATIONAL CHARACTERISTICS

It is important to recognize that although they utilize the same forces for solute and fluid removal, CRRT techniques are operationally different from intermittent forms of renal replacement therapy. The blood flow rate (100–200 ml/min) and dialysate flow rate (1–2 L/h) are usually lower, resulting in complete saturation of the dialysate, which becomes a limiting factor in diffusive clearance capacity. Continuous ultrafiltration results in the loss of significant amounts of plasma water, and requires the administration of replacement fluids. One of the unique features of CRRT techniques is the separation of solute removal from fluid removal. Variations in the composition of the dialysate and the dialysate flow rate can be used to control solute balance; water balance is achieved by varying the rate of replacement fluid. Time is not a limiting factor for fluid or solute removal with CRRT techniques. Several other key differences include vascular access, anticoagulation, and the composition of dialysate and replacement fluids. The operational characteristics of the most commonly used CRRT techniques are summarized in Table 14.2.

Access

Access to blood supply for the extracorporeal circuit varies with CRRT techniques. Arteriovenous techniques, which have largely fallen out of favor, have variable blood flow rates and lead to a higher

Table 14.2 Comparison of continuous renal replacement therapy modalities.

	SCUF	CAVH	CVVH	CAVHD	CAVHDF	CVVHD	CVVHDF	PD
Access	AV	AV	VV	AV	AV	VV	VV	Peritoneal catheter
Pump	No	No	Yes	No	No	Yes	Yes	No[b]
Filtrate (ml/h)	100	600	1000	300	600	300	800	500
Dialysate flow (L/h)	0	0	0	1	1	1	1	2.0[c]
Replacement fluid (L/day)	0	12	21.6	4.8	12	4.8	16.8	0
Urea clearance (ml/min)	1.7	10	16.7	21.7	26.7	21.7	30	8.5
Simplicity[a]	1	2	3	2	2	3	3	2
Cost[a]	1	2	4	3	3	4	4	3

For definitions of acronyms, see Table 14.1 and the text.

[a]l = most simple and least expensive; 4 = most difficult and most expensive.

[b]Cycler can be used to automate exchanges; however, it adds to the cost and complexity.

[c]2.0 L exchanges.

Source: reprinted with permission from Abdeen O, Mehta RL. Dialysis modalities in the intensive care unit. Crit Care Clin 2002;18(2):223–47.

risk of thrombosis. In general, large-bore, small-length catheters are preferable for AV procedures (CAVH, CAVHD, CAVHDF: see Table 14.1 for definitions) to permit a high blood flow rate. In pumped systems (CVVH, CVVHD, CVVHDF; see Table 14.1 for definitions), double-lumen venous catheters are commonly used; the size should be selected based on the site of insertion to optimize flow. A reduction in delivered blood flow will influence overall clearance and also promote clotting of the circuit.

Membranes

Membrane characteristics that should be considered when selecting membranes for CRRT techniques include small, middle, and large MW solute removal, water permeability and biocompatibility. Generally speaking, the efficiency of small solute clearance is largely determined by dialysate/ultrafiltration flow rate; therefore, filter surface area is not an important factor in choosing a dialysis membrane. High-flux membranes, which are designed to provide high water permeability, are generally recommended for hemofiltration procedures. Finally, although there is no conclusive evidence that membrane biocompatibility affects patient outcome, there is general consensus[10] that the use of synthetic membranes is preferable over cellulose-based membranes.

Pumps

CRRT circuits require the use of pumps to regulate flow of replacement fluid, dialysate, and anticoagulant, and in pumped CRRT, to regulate blood flow (Fig. 14.3). Until recently, most CRRT systems utilized standard intravenous pumps to deliver replacement fluid, dialysate, anticoagulant and control ultrafiltration.[14] Newer systems have been developed specifically for CRRT, which have integrated pumps to control blood flow, infusion of replacement fluid, dialysate and ultrafiltrate. As the pumps are linked, an alarm condition in one of the pumps results in all the pumps stopping simultaneously thereby reducing the potential for circuit problems. Although the newer CRRT systems resemble existing dialysis machines, the regulation of blood and dialysate flow are significantly different, making it difficult to adapt a dialysis machine for CRRT. However, many centers have adapted the REDY (REcirculating DialYsis sorbent system and the blood pump modules of existing dialysis machines to deliver CVVH because of the prohibitive cost of new technologies.

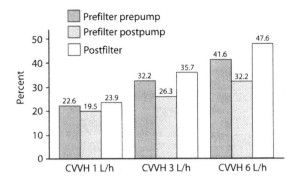

Figure 14.3 Pre- versus postfilter replacement fluid: effect on filtration fraction. Prefilter replacement tends to dilute the blood entering the circuit and enhances filter longevity by reducing the filtration fraction; however, in continuous venovenous hemofiltration (CVVH) circuits the overall clearance may be reduced as the amount of solute delivered to the filter is reduced.

Replacement/dialysate solutions

All CRRT techniques, other than slow continuous ultrafiltration (SCUF), require the use of sterile replacement fluids to compensate for the ultrafiltrate removed. Hemodialysis and hemodiafiltration techniques also require the used of a sterile dialysate. The optimal replacement solution approximates normal plasma water composition, replacing electrolytes and minerals in physiologic concentrations without replacing the metabolic solutes that accumulate in renal failure. The composition of these solutions can be varied extensively to achieve specific metabolic goals (e.g. bicarbonate-based solutions can be used to correct acidemia and the electrolyte content can be altered to correct electrolyte imbalance).[15,16] Table 14.3A and B shows the composition of the most commonly used solutions for replacement and dialysate. Most centers have used standard peritoneal dialysis (PD) solutions as dialysate; although commercial hemofiltration solutions are now available in Europe, only Baxter hemofiltration solution is available in the USA. A limitation of all these solutions is that they are acetate- or lactate-based, and the capacity to convert these buffers to bicarbonate may be limited in multiple organ failure.[17] More recently, bicarbonate-based solutions have become commercially available (Normocarb), which may be better tolerated than lactate- or acetate-based solutions.[18]

When citrate anticoagulation is used, modifications are necessary in both the replacement fluid and dialysis solution. Trisodium citrate is metabolized to bicarbonate by the liver; therefore, buffer is not generally required in the dialysate or the replacement fluid. Similarly, replacement solutions and dialysate are generally hyponatremic and calcium-free in order to prevent hypernatremia and filter clotting.

The volume of replacement solutions used largely depends upon the goals for fluid management and can be tailored for each individual patient, as described in fluid management below. In general, hemodialysis techniques (CAVHD/CVVHD) have no need for replacement solutions, whereas hemofiltration techniques (CAVH/CVVH) and hemodiafiltration methods (CAVHDF/CVVHDF) utilize moderate to large amounts of replacement fluid. Dialysate fluids in CRRT have a similar composition to replacement fluids and should generally approximate the desired plasma water composition.

Anticoagulation

Anticoagulation is an essential component of all extracorporeal therapies, including CRRT. The passage of blood through an extracorporeal circuit causes platelet activation and induces a variety of inflammatory and prothrombotic mediators, resulting in fibrin deposition on filter membranes. This not only affects filter longevity but also may decrease dialyzer efficacy in terms of water and solute removal. If anticoagulation is insufficient, filtration performance deteriorates and the filter may clot, contributing to blood loss. Excessive anticoagulation may result in bleeding complications, reported to occur in 5–26% of treatments.[19] Several methods of anticoagulation are now available and the key features of the most common methods are summarized in Table 14.4.

Standard unfractionated heparin is still the most common form of anticoagulation used with CRRT techniques. Heparin is generally administered as a bolus, followed by a continuous infusion into the arterial limb of the dialysis circuit, to maintain a partial thromboplastin time (PTT) of 1.5 to 2× normal. Systemic anticoagulation is relatively contraindicated in patients at high risk of bleeding, although the heparin dose can be modified in these circumstances; however, its use is associated with a high incidence of bleeding and in some instances heparin-induced thrombocytopenia.[20]

Table 14.3A Composition of replacement fluids for continuous renal replacement therapy.					
Replacement fluid	Golper	Kierdorf	Lauer-Paganini	Mehta (heparin)	Mehta (citrate)
Na (mEq/L)	147	140	140	140.5	154
K (mEq/L)	0	0	2	0	
Cl (mEq/L)	115	110	0	115.5	154
HCO_3 (mEq/L)	36	34	0	25	
Ca (mEq/L)	1.2	1.75	3.5	4	
Mg (mEq/L)	0.7	0.5	1.5	0	
Glucose (g/dl)	6.7	5.6	0	0	
Acetate (mEq/L)	0	41	40	0	

Source: modified with permission from Mehta RL. Supportive therapies: intermittent hemodialysis, continuous renal replacement therapies, and peritoneal dialysis. In: Berl T, Bonventre JV, eds. Atlas of diseases of the kidney. Philadelphia, Current Medicine. 1999.

Table 14.3B Composition of dialysate for continuous renal replacement therapy.								
Dialysate	1.5% Dianeal	Hemosol AG 4D	Hemosol LG 4D	Baxter	UCSD citrate	Prismasate BKO/3.5	Plasmalyte A	Normocarb
Na (mEq/L)	132	140	140	140	117	140	140	140
K (mEq/L)	0	4	4	2	4	0	5	0
Cl (mEq/L)	96	119	109.5	117	121	109.5	98	106.5
Lactate (mEq/L)	35	0	40	30	0	3	0	0
Acetate (mEq/L)	0	30	0	0	0	0	27	0
HCO_3 (mEq/L)	0	0	0	0	Variable	32	0	35
Ca (mEq/L)	3.5	3.5	4	3.5	0	3.5	0	0
Mg (mEq/L)	1.5	1.5	1.5	1.5	1.5	1	1.5	0
Dextrose (g/dl)	1.5	0.8	0.11	0.1	0.1–2.5	0.1–0.5	0	

Source: modified with permission from Mehta RL. Supportive therapies: intermittent hemodialysis, continuous renal replacement therapies, and peritoneal dialysis. In: Berl, T, Bonventre JV, eds. Atlas of diseases of the kidney. Philadelphia, Current Medicine. 1999.

In newly postoperative patients and others with a contraindication to systemic anticoagulation, regional anticoagulation of the circuit is preferred. Regional heparinization, with prefilter administration of heparin, and a postfilter protamine infusion has been used,[21] but regional citrate anticoagulation has become increasingly popular. Regional citrate anticoagulation is achieved using a continuous citrate infusion through the arterial limb of the CRRT circuit, which chelates free calcium and inhibits the coagulation cascade. The citrate–calcium complex is removed by a combination of dialysis clearance against calcium-free dialysate and endogenous processes. In patients with normal liver function, levels of citrate and ionized cal-

cium return to normal values within 30 minutes of discontinuing a citrate infusion.[22] Plasma calcium levels are restored with the use of a continuous calcium infusion at the site of blood return to the patient. The infusion rate of citrate is adjusted to keep the activated clotting time (ACT) above 160 seconds. Regional citrate anticoagulation requires the use of a specialized dialysis solution and frequent monitoring of ionized calcium.[23] Potential complications arising from this technique include metabolic alkalosis, hyponatremia, hypocalcemia, and citrate toxicity in patients with liver dysfunction. If properly monitored, the complication rate associated with this technique is quite low.[24] Filter longevity in excess of 96 hours is fairly common

Table 14.4   Anticoagulation modalities for continuous renal replacement.

Method	Filter prime	Initial dose	Maintenance dose	Monitoring	Advantages	Disadvantages
Saline solution	2 L saline	150–250 ml prefilter	100–250 ml/h prefilter	Visual check	No anticoagulant	Poor filter patency
Heparin	2 L saline 2500–10 000 U	5–10 U/kg	3–12/kg/h	ACT 200–250; PTT 1.5–2.0 × normal	Standard method; easy to use; inexpensive	Bleeding risk; thrombocytopenia
LMW heparin	2 L saline	40 mg	10–40 mg/6 h	Factor Xa levels; maintained between 0.1 and 0.41 U/ml	Decreased risk of bleeding	Special monitoring; not available everywhere; expensive
Regional heparin	2500 U/2 L saline	5–10 U/kg	3–12 U/kg/h; + protamine postfilter	PTT: postfilter ACT 200–250	Reduced bleeding risk	Complex; risk of thrombocytopenia; protamine effects; hypotension
Regional citrate	2 L saline	4% trisodium citrate 150–180 ml/h	100–180 ml/h 3–7% of BFR, Ca replaced by central line	ACT: 200–250 maintain ionized calcium 0.96–1.2 mmol/L	No bleeding; no thrombocytopenia; improved filter efficacy, longevity	Complex; needs Ca monitoring; alkalosis
Prostacyclin	2 L saline + heparin	Heparin 2–4 U/kg 4–8 ng/kg/min	4–8 ng/kg/min	ACT, PTT, platelet aggregation	Reduced heparinization	Needs heparin addition; hypotension
Hirudin	2 L saline	625 µg/kg/h	6–25 µg/kg/h	PTT	Alternative to heparin	Bleeding risk no reversal agent
Danaparoid	2 L saline	2500 IU bolus	400 IU/h	PTT Antifactor Xa	Alternative to heparin	Bleeding
Nafamostat mesylate	2 L saline	–	0.1 mg/kg/h	ACT	Alternative to heparin	Bleeding

ACT, activated clotting time; BFR, blot flow rate; PTT, partial thromboplastin time.

Source: modified with permission from Mehta RL. New developments in continuous arterio-venous hemofiltration/dialysis. In: Andreucci VE, Fine LG, eds. International yearbook of nephrology, New York, Springer: 1992.

with citrate anticoagulation, whereas 36–48 hours patency is usually the norm with heparin.[25]

Low MW heparin,[26,27] prostacyclin analogues[28] and other anticoagulants such as Orgaran (dana-paroid)[29] and high MW dextrans[30] have had limited experience.

At the current time, none of these methods is ideal, and selection is usually influenced by patient factors. Technical factors and experience with anticoagulants are important determinants of the success of any anticoagulant regimen.

HOW IS DOSE MEASURED WITH CONTINUOUS RENAL REPLACEMENT THERAPY?

The notion of dialysis dose quantification in ARF has been controversial, due in part to the lack of convincing evidence that azotemia control affects outcome in patients with ARF. In the end-stage renal failure population, where delivered dialysis dose positively correlates with outcome, dialysis dose has been quantified using a technique called urea kinetic modeling (UKM). Absolute concentrations of urea and creatinine are difficult to interpret; however, clearance of these marker substances appears to be the best measurement of therapy dose as it considers generation rates as well as plasma clearance. Whereas quantification of dialysis dose using UKM is intuitive with intermittent therapies, methods for measuring clearance in CRRT are variable, hampered in part by a lack of understanding of what parameters should be used to compute dialysis dosage.

Generally speaking, the total solute clearance in CRRT techniques is the sum of the convective and diffusive clearances.[31] Since the MW cut off for the membranes is >20 000 Da, most low and middle MW substances have sieving coefficients (SCs) of 1. Convective clearance is therefore directly proportional to the amount of filtrate produced. Small molecules are less dependent on convective clearance and are more effectively transferred by diffusion. Slow dialysate flow rates (1–2 L/h) allow for complete saturation of the dialysate fluid with solutes. Thus, the limiting factor for diffusive clearance is the dialysate flow rate, not the blood flow rate as it is with conventional hemodialysis.

At the present time, a UKM-based calculation of plasma solute clearance is the most common method of measuring dialysis dosage with both intermittent and continuous forms of dialysis, although it is not entirely clear that the calculated clearance values can be directly compared.[10] This calculation is called Kt/V, where K is clearance, t is duration of dialysis, and V is the volume of distribution of urea. The limitation of this method rests in the observation that critically ill patients with ARF are frequently catabolic and have highly variable fluid volumes; both conditions violate several of the assumptions implicit in UKM. Quantification of solute clearance using dialysate concentrations of clearance markers (calculation of a solute removal index, SRI) avoids some of the limitations of blood-based clearance calculations. There is no consensus as to which method should be used in all clinical situations.

At the present time, there is no consensus as to what the minimal dialysis dose should be in patients with acute renal failure. Extrapolating data from the end-stage renal disease (ESRD) population,[32] it seems reasonable to suggest a minimum Kt/V of 1.2 should be delivered at least three times a week in patients with ARF. However, several recent studies support the belief that more intensive dialysis may be beneficial in this patient group. A dose intensity study of CVVH in 425 critically ill patients demonstrated a significant decrease in patient mortality when ultrafiltration rates of 35 ml/kg/h (approx 3 L/h in a 70 kg male) were used as compared to 20 ml/kg/h.[33] A randomized trial of intermittent hemodialysis comparing daily vs alternate-day dialysis showed a reduction in mortality from 46% to 28% ($p < 0.05$).[4] Unfortunately, the delivered dialysis dose in the alternate-day group as measured by weekly Kt/V was less than 3.6; thus, the issue of minimal adequate dose remains unresolved.

DOES CONTINUOUS RENAL REPLACEMENT THERAPY CONFER AN ADVANTAGE OVER INTERMITTENT HEMODIALYSIS IN THE MANAGEMENT OF ACUTE RENAL FAILURE?

CRRT has several theoretical advantages over intermittent blood purification techniques, including better hemodynamic tolerability, more efficient solute clearance, better control of intravascular volume, and better clearance of middle and large MW substances.

Hypotension is one of the most common complications associated with IHD, occurring in approximately 20–30% of all treatments. Some of the causes are dialysis-specific, such as excessive or rapid volume removal, changes in plasma osmolality, and autonomic dysfunction. In critically ill patients who may be hemodynamically unstable, it would be desirable to minimize this complication, as it may lead to further organ ischemia and injury. Several prospective and retrospective studies have demonstrated better hemodynamic stability associated with CRRT;[34,35] however, this observation has not been validated in a randomized controlled trial.

Another advantage of CRRT is the improved efficiency of solute removal. Although the clearance rate of small solutes is slower per unit time with CRRT (17 ml/min vs more than 160 ml/min with conventional hemodialysis), CRRT is continuously administered; therefore, urea clearance is more efficient after 48 hours than with alternate-day IHD. Clark et al developed a computer model based on 20 critically ill patients to compare solute clearance in intermittent and continuous renal replacement therapies, and found that for a 50 kg male, an average of 4.4 dialysis sessions/week would be required to achieve equivalent uremic control. In patients with a weight >90 kg, equivalent uremic control could not be achieved with intermittent therapies even if daily dialysis was prescribed.[36]

Fluid management is often a difficult issue in the ICU, where nutritional requirements (total parenteral nutrition or TPN) and the use of intravenous medications necessitate the administration of large amounts of fluid to critically ill patients. The inability to severely restrict fluid intake in ICU patients results in excessive volume overload, which may compromise tissue perfusion and has been associated with adverse outcomes.[37] Attempts to restrict fluid in this setting may additionally compromise adequate nutrition.[38] The capacity to adjust fluid balance on an hourly basis, even in hemodynamically unstable patients, is in large part responsible for the growing popularity of CRRT amongst intensivists.

CRRT may also have an immunomodulatory effect. The rationale for the use of CRRT for the treatment of sepsis arises from the observed association between sepsis severity, mortality rate and serum concentrations of various cytokines, including tumor necrosis factor (TNF), and the interleukins IL-1, IL-6, and IL-8. Most of these middle MW molecules are water-soluble and are theoretically removable by plasma water purification. At the present time, the immunomodulatory effects of CRRT remain theoretical, and have not been shown to affect outcome in human studies.[39,40]

Despite its apparent advantages over intermittent therapies, superiority of CRRT with respect to mortality or recovery of renal function has not been demonstrated. In the largest randomized controlled trial to date (n = 166), IHD was associated with significantly lower inhospital (48% vs 65%) and ICU mortality (42% vs 60%). However, patients with hypotension were excluded from participating in the study, and there was a significant difference in severity scores between the treatment arms despite randomization.[41] A recently published meta-analysis comparing intermittent vs continuous renal replacement therapies concluded that CRRT did not improve survival or renal recovery in unselected critically ill patients. Moreover, the sample size required to show a 20% mortality difference between IHD and CRRT would be in excess of 1200 patients.[42] Further studies are needed to define the subset of patients with ARF who benefit from this therapy.

WHAT ARE THE DISADVANTAGES OF USING CONTINUOUS RENAL REPLACEMENT THERAPY?

There are a number of potential disadvantages associated with the use of CRRT. One-to-one nursing is generally required with patients on CRRT in order to manage fluid balance and monitor metabolic parameters, often resulting in increased nursing costs. Independent of nursing cost considerations, CRRT is roughly twice as expensive as alternate-day IHD.[43] CRRT requires some form of continuous anticoagulation. Regional anticoagulation circumvents the risk of prolonged systemic anticoagulation; however, it is labor-intensive and requires additional monitoring. Finally, because CRRT is administered continuously, patient mobility is restricted. In cases where a patient needs to be moved from the bedside, it may be difficult to perform CRRT. Disconnecting patients from CRRT deprives them of dialysis and ultrafiltration time, which decreases treatment efficacy.

WHAT PATIENTS SHOULD RECEIVE CONTINUOUS RENAL REPLACEMENT THERAPY?

Apart from the patients who are hemodynamically intolerant of IHD, the decision to use CRRT in critically ill patients with ARF is based on physician preference. There are large variations in physician practice both regionally and internationally. A recent survey of 2000 nephrologists across the United States by Mehta et al found that less than 25% of patients with ARF are treated with CRRT.[44] Continuous therapies are commonly used in Europe and particularly Australia, where more than 90% of critically ill patients with dialysis-dependent renal failure are treated with CRRT.[45] Patient characteristics such as age, comorbidity, hemodynamic stability, indications for dialysis, and the presence of other organ failures may be factors, as well as the type of physician, familiarity with and availability of this technique, and the cost of therapy.

LOOKING TO THE FUTURE

As experience with these techniques grows, innovations in technology will probably keep pace. Over the last 3 years, most of the major manufacturers of dialysis equipment have developed new pumps dedicated for the use of these therapies. Most of these devices (Hospal/Cobe PRISMA, Fresenius Acumen, Baxter BM14) offer automated fluid balancing and sophisticated controls that are similar to those in regular dialysis machines. Membrane technology is also evolving and antithrombogenic membranes are on the horizon.[46] Finally, the application of these therapies is likely to expand to other arenas, including the treatment of sepsis, congestive heart failure, multiorgan failure, as a form of liver support, and in cardiopulmonary bypass for cytokine manipulation. It remains to be seen how these therapies will change our current management of these patient groups.

REFERENCES

1. Kramer P, Wigger W, Rieger J, et al. Arteriovenous hemofiltration: a new and simple method for treatment of over-hydrated patients resistant to diuretics. Klin Wochenschr 1997;55:1121–2.
2. Palevsky PM, Bunchman T, Tetta C. The acute dialysis quality initiative – Part V: operational characteristics of CRRT. Adv Ren Replace Ther 2002;9(4):268–72.
3. McDonald BR, Mehta RL. Transmembrane flux of IL-1B and TNF in patients undergoing continuous arteriovenous hemodialysis (CAVHD). J Am Soc Nephrol 1990;1:368.
4. Schiffl H, Lang SM, Fischer R. Daily hemodialysis and the outcome of acute renal failure. N Engl J Med 2002;346(5)305–10.
5. Gillum DM, Kelleher SP, Dillingham MA, et al. The role of intensive dialysis in acute renal failure. Clin Nephrol 1986;25:249.
6. Conger JD. Interventions in clinical acute renal failure: What are the data? Am J Kidney Dis 1995;26:565.
7. Ronco C, Bellomo R, Homel P, et al. Effects of different doses in continuous veno-venous hemodialysis on outcomes of acute renal failure: a prospective randomized trial. Lancet 2000; 355:26–30.
8. Lewis J, Chertow GM, Paginini E, et al. A multi-center survey of patient characteristics, practice patterns, and outcomes in critically ill patients with ARF. J Am Soc Nephrol 1997;8:A0673.
9. Bouman C, Oudemans-van Straaten HM, Tijssen J, et al. Effects of early high-volume continuous venovenous hemofiltration on survival and recovery of renal function in intensive care patients with acute renal failure: a prospective , randomized trial. Crit Care Med 2002;30(10):2205–11.
10. Kellum JA, Mehta RL, Angus DC, Palevsky P, Ronco C. The first international consensus conference on continuous renal replacement therapy. Kidney Int 2002;62:1855–63.
11. Silvester W. Mediator removal with CRRT: complement and cytokines. Am J Kidney Dis 1997;30(5 Suppl 4):S38–43.
12. Grootendorst AF, van Bommel EF, van der Hoven B, van leengoed LA, van Osta AL. High-volume hemofiltration improves hemodynamics of endotoxin-induced shock in the pig. Intensive Care Med 1992;18:235–40.
13. Schetz M. Non-renal indications for continuous renal replacement therapy. Kidney Int suppl 1999;5(S72):S88–94.
14. Golper TA , Jacobs AA. Pumps utilized during continuous renal replacement therapy. Semin Dial 1996;9:119–24.
15. Palevsky PM. Continuous renal replacement therapy component selection: replacement fluid and dialysate. Semin Dial 1996; 9:107–11.
16. Macias WA, Clark WR. Acid base balance in continuous renal replacement therapy. Semin Dial 1996;9:145–51.
17. Levraut J, Ciebiera JP, Jambou P, et al. Effect of continuous venovenous hemofiltration with dialysis on lactate clearance in critically ill patients. Crit Care Med 1997;25:58–62.
18. Zimmerman D, Cotman P, Ting R, Karanicolas S, Tobe S. Continuous veno-venous hemodialysis with a novel bicarbonate dialysis solution: prospective cross-over comparison with a lactate buffered solution. Nephrol Dial Transplant 1999;14:2387–91.
19. Webb AR, Mythen MG, Jacobson D, Mackie IJ. Maintaining blood flow in the extracorporeal circuit. Intensive Care Med 1995; 21:84–93.
20. Mehta RL, Dobos GJ, Ward DM. Anticoagulation in continuous renal replacement procedures. Semin Dial 1992;5:61–8.
21. Abramson S, Niles JL. Anticoagulation in continuous renal replacement therapy. Curr Opin Nephrol Hypertens 1999;8(6): 701–7.
22. Mehta RL, McDonald BR, Aguilar MM. Regional citrate anticoagulation for continuous arteriovenous hemodialysis in critically ill patients. Kidney Int 1990;38:976–81.
23. Mehta RL, McDonald BR, Aguilar MM. Regional citrate anticoagulation for continuous arteriovenous hemodialysis in critically ill patients. Kidney Int 1990;38:976–81.
24. Flanigan MJ, Von Brecht JH, Freeman RM, et al. Reducing the hemorrhagic complications of dialysis: a controlled comparison of low dose heparin and citrate anticoagulation. Am J Kidney Dis 1987;9:147–51.
25. Bellomo R, Teede H, Boyce N. Anticoagulant regimens in acute continuous hemofiltration: a comparative study. Intensive Care Med 1993;19:329–32.
26. Hory B, Cachoux A, Toulemonde F. Continuous arteriovenous hemofiltration with low-molecular-weight heparin. Nephron 1985;42:125.
27. Wynckel A, Bernieh B, Toupance O, et al. Guidelines in using enoxaparin in slow continuous hemodialysis. In: Sieberth HG, Mann H, Stummvoll HK, eds. Continuous hemofiltration. Contrib Nephrol Basel: Karger; 1991;93:221–4.
28. Davenport A, Will EJ, Davison AM. Comparison of the use of standard heparin and prostacyclin anticoagulation in spontaneous and pump driven extracorporeal circuits in patient with combined acute renal and hepatic failure. Nephron 1994;66:431–7.
29. Chong BH, Magnani HN. Organan in heparin-induced thrombocytopenia. Haemostasis 1992;22:85–91.
30. Palevsky PM, Burr R, Moreland L, Tokiwa Y, Greenberg A. Failure of low molecular weight dextran to prevent clotting during continuous renal replacement therapy. ASAIO J 1995;24:847–9.
31. Siegler MH, Teehan BP. Solute transport in continuous hemodialysis: a new treatment for acute renal failure. Kidney Int 1987;32:562–71.

32. Gotch FA, Sargent JA. A mechanistic analysis of the National Cooperative Dialyis Study (NCDS). Kidney Int 1985;28(3)526–34.

33. Ronco C, Bellomo R, Homel P, et al. Effects of different doses in continuous veno-venous hemodialysis on outcomes of acute renal failure: a prospective randomized trial. Lancet 2000;355: 26–30.

34. Paganini E, O'Hara P, Nakamoto S. Slow continuous ultrafiltration in hemodialysis resistant oliguric renal failure. Trans Am Soc Artif Intern Organs 1984;30:173–8.

35. Davenport A, Will E, Davidson A. Improved cardiovascular stability during continuous modes of renal replacement therapy in critically ill patients with acute hepatic and renal failure. Crit Care Med 1993;21:328–38.

36. Clark WR, Mueller B, Kraus A, Macias WL. Extracorporeal therapy requirements for patients with acute renal failure. J Am Soc Nephrol 1997;8:804–12.

37. Mehta RL, Clark WC, Schetz M. Techniques for assessing and achieving fluid balance in acute renal failure. Curr Opin Crit Care 2002;8(6):535–43.

38. Campbell IT. Limitations of nutrient intake. The effect of stressors: trauma, sepsis and multiple organ failure. Eur J Clin Nutr 1999;53(Suppl 1):S143–7.

39. Honore PM, Jamez J, Wauthier M, et al. Prospective evaluation of short-term, high-volume isovolumic hemofiltration on the hemodynamic course and outcome in patients with intractable circulatory failure resulting from septic shock. Crit Care Med 2000;28(11):3581–7.

40. Cole L, Bellomo R, Hart G, et al. A phase II randomized, controlled trial of continuous hemofiltration in sepsis. Crit Care Med 2002;30(1):100–6.

41. Mehta RL, McDonald B, Gabbai F, and the Acute Renal Failure Collaborative Study Group. Continuous vs. intermittent hemodialysis for acute renal failure in the ICU: results from a randomized multicenter trial. JASN 1996;5:1457.

42. Tonelli M, Manns B, Feller-Kopman D. Acute renal failure in the intensive care unit: a systematic review of the impact of dialytic modality or mortality and renal recovery. Am J Kidney Dis 2002; 40(5):875–85.

43. Manns B, Doig CJ, Lee H, et al. Cost of acute renal failure requiring dialysis in the intensive care unit: clinical and resource implications of renal recovery. Crit Care Med 2003;31(1):449–55.

44. Mehta RL, Letteri JM. Current status of renal replacement therapy for acute renal failure. Am J Nephrol 1999;19:377–82.

45. Cole L, Bellomo R, Silvester W, Reeves JH. A prospective, multicenter study of the epidemiology, management, and outcome of severe acute renal failure in a "closed" ICU system. Am J Respir Crit Care Med 2000;162:191–6.

46. Yang VC, Fu Y, Kim JS. A potential thrombogenic hemodialysis membranes with impaired blood compatibility. ASAIO Trans 1991;37:M229–32.

15

Slow low-efficiency daily dialysis and hybrid renal replacement therapies for acute renal failure in the intensive care unit

Wim Van Biesen and Norbert Lameire

TERMINOLOGY AND DEFINITIONS OF HYBRID THERAPIES

Acute renal failure (ARF) with need for renal replacement (RRT) in the intensive care unit (ICU) is a complex and devastating condition, with a reported mortality rate as high as 50–80%.[1,2] Although gross mortality rates have only declined slightly over the past decades, it is accepted that survival is increased by improvement in overall care, since the comorbidity of patients and the severity of the underlying diseases treated have also dramatically increased.[3,4] Although ARF by itself contributes to the overall mortality of critically ill patients, ARF mostly develops as a consequence of other underlying diseases, and patients often do not die of ARF but from these underlying conditions. Thus, the idea that by inventing 'the perfect RRT machine', no more patients with ICU-related ARF will die, will of course remain an illusion. Because renal function mostly recovers if the ARF patient survives, RRT in ARF should thus be seen as a bridging therapy that allows the patient to survive while the native kidneys recover. The main objective of RRT is to avoid additional harm to the patient as much as possible during the spontaneous recovery of renal function.

Despite much debate, some very important and relevant questions regarding the treatment of ARF remain unanswered. This is mainly because it is hard, if not impossible, to conduct prospective randomized studies with a fair and equal distribution of all risk factors in different treatment arms because of the rather high mortality, and the wide scatter in underlying comorbidities. The contro-versy between continuous renal replacement therapy (CRRT) and intermittent hemodialysis (IHD) is an excellent example where the situation is still further complicated by the lack of clear definitions of the treatments used and the polarization and conflicts of interest between intensivists and nephrologists.[5,6] This has led to the situation that in countries such as Australia, where intensivists are in charge of the treatment of ICU-related ARF, 100% of RRT is performed as CRRT, whereas in other countries such as the United States or France, where the nephrologist is most often in charge, the majority of these patients are treated with IHD. Only a limited number of centers have a docu-mented balanced distribution of treatment modal-ities[2,5,7] (Fig. 15.1). A recent survey showed that resource availability, convenience, and practical limitations are more decisive in the choice of a given RRT modality than the conviction that one therapy is superior to another.[6] An RRT modality for ICU-related ARF should be easy to use and convenient, but nevertheless be able to deliver a broad range of different therapy modalities while trying as much as possible to reduce the workload to the end user (the ICU nurse). Both IHD and CRRT have their own limitations, and by trying to improve both techniques, it is apparent that both become more and more similar (Fig. 15.2). This has resulted in the development of 'hybrid techniques' such as SLEDD (slow low-efficiency daily dialysis or slow extended daily dailysis). Although the dose of dialysis for an ARF patient in the ICU is still not definitely established, it is quite accepted that for most ARF patients at the ICU, three times a week IHD is not a suitable blood purification

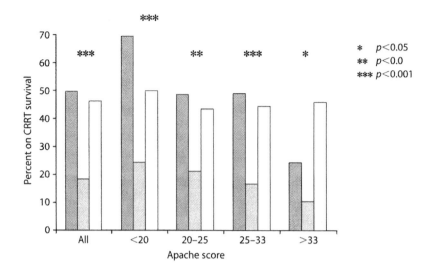

Figure 15.1 Distribution of continuous renal replacement therapy (CRRT) and intermittent hemodialysis/slow low-efficiency daily dialysis (IHD/SLEDD) in the intensive care unit (ICU) of the University Hospital Ghent. The percentage of ICU-related ARF patients on CRRT (gray box) is stratified per category of Apache score. The dark boxes indicate survival in the IHD/SLEDD group and the white boxes in the CRRT group. It appears that in all categories of severity of disease, as assessed by the Apache score, mortality is higher in the CRRT group.

technique, and that daily treatment is usually needed in critically ill patients.[8–10] Nephrologists with ICU experience also realized that some potential modifications of the IHD technique, such as hemodiafiltration (HDF), have been underused in the ICU. On the other hand, CRRT has become progressively complex, and the original concept of an

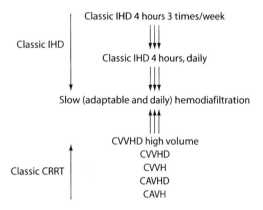

Figure 15.2 Evolution of intermittent hemodialysis (IHD) and continuous renal replacement therapy (CRRT) to a hybrid regimen. CAVH, continuous arteriovenous hemofiltration; CAVHD, continuous arteriovenous hemodialysis; CVVH, continuous venovenous hemofiltration; CVVHD, continuous venovenous hemodialysis.

'easy-going technique' without need for high-tech equipment has long since been replaced by high-volume, double-pump CRRT machines. Despite much effort, no study has ever been able to prove that one modality is superior over the other.[11,12]

Although the difference in treatment duration, being so-called continuous for CRRT and intermittent for IHD, is the most obvious difference between the two modalities, other additional differences might be more important to distinguish both modalities. From a physiological point of view, the major difference is that intermittent therapies rely mostly on diffusion, whereas the continuous techniques rely mostly on convection (Fig. 15.3). From a practical point of view, IHD is almost always performed with a 'dialysis machine' with need for a water treatment system that delivers online, high-quality dialysate fluid.[13] This system allows high dialysate flows and efficient removal of small solutes. In contrast, CRRT is mostly performed with a special device, without a separate water treatment system, and the substitution and dialysate fluids are delivered in industrially prepared, sterile bags. Today, bicarbonate-buffered substitution fluid is recommended, which has to be mixed from a two-compartment bag just before use.[14] These fluids are expensive, and their handling and storage is cumbersome. In addition, bags have to be replaced every 2 hours, which can

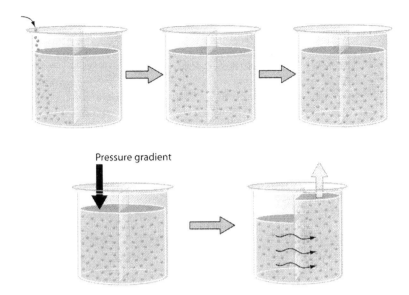

Pressure gradient

Figure 15.3 Schematic representation of diffusive (upper panel) and convective (lower panel) transport over a semipermeable membrane. The molecules move at random in the solvent, and the probability that they will hit and pass a pore is linearly related to their concentration. Therefore, more molecules will be transported from compartment A (with the higher concentration) to compartment B than vice versa. The net result is called 'diffusive transport'. This diffusive transport is thus driven by a concentration gradient. In addition, the amount of solute transfer is also dependent on the geometric size of the molecule, as the probability that a molecule hitting the membrane can actually pass through the pore decreases with the size of the molecule. In dialysis, a high concentration gradient between the blood and the dialysate compartment is maintained by increasing the dialysate flow: in this way, the concentrations of the different solutes in the dialysate at the level of the membrane are kept low, and the concentration difference high. If there is also water flux over the membrane, this water flux will drag other molecules with it through the pores. This solute drag is called 'convective transport'. This convective transport depends on the water flux over the membrane, and thus on the porosity of the membrane for water. The actual driving force is a pressure gradient over the membrane that forces the water over the membrane. This pressure gradient can be hydrostatic or osmotic. In contrast with diffusive transport, the amount of solute transported is independent on the size of the solute, as long as the smallest diameter of the molecule is lower than the pore size (the so-called cut-off level of the membrane). For convective treatments, the membrane must have a high hydraulic conductivity, to allow large water fluxes over the membrane.

potentially lead to touch contamination and increases the work load of the ICU nurse. Therefore, the flow rates of blood and of dialysate and/or substitution fluid are mostly limited in CRRT, necessitating the continuity of the treatment to obtain adequate efficiency.[15]

In this chapter, we will consider all those techniques that have no separate water treatment system as 'CRRT', whereas all techniques that have some form of local water treatment will be considered as 'IHD', independent of the treatment duration. Note that this definition does not specify whether the solute removal is convective or diffusive, although CRRT techniques, in general, will have a major component of (convective) hemofiltration. 'Hybrid therapies' such as SLEDD are those techniques where a conventional dialysis monitor with online fluid preparation is used for treatments that extend the usual duration of a 'conventional intermittent dialysis' session of 3–4 hours/treatment. SLEDD treatments offer the best balance between the advantages and disadvantages of both CRRT and IHD, as they allow a nearly unlimited capacity to tailor the treatment to the needs of the patient while using one single machine.

RATIONALE FOR SLEDD: ADVANTAGES AND DISADVANTAGES

Hemodynamic stability

As already stated, avoiding additional complications should be the first aim of RRT in the ICU. Hemodynamic instability is often a major problem in ICU patients. This instability can be further enhanced by starting RRT, due to changes in circulating volume and plasma osmolarity. In a typical ICU patient with ARF, there is often a conflict between third-space fluid overload, in the form of edema, ascites, and pleural effusion, on the one hand, and intravascular underfilling, on the other, leading to hypotension. During the extracorporeal treatment, excess fluid is removed from the blood compartment. The rate-limiting step for removal of fluid from the body is the transport rate between the extravascular and the intravascular compartments. In many ICU patients, the fluid transport between the intra- and extravascular fluid compartments is hampered by alterations in the permeability of the capillaries by inflammation, and the alterations in plasma colloid or crystalloid osmolarity by hypoalbuminemia and/or electrolyte disturbances. The fluid removal rate is thus often limited, because of inadequate 'refilling' of the vascular bed.

Also, changes in osmolarity can cause hemodynamic instability. During hemodialysis, there is diffusive transport from osmotically active substances down a concentration gradient from the blood to the dialysate. As this transport exceeds the transport of water during regular hemodialysis, this results in a decrease in plasma osmolarity. During hemofiltration, transport of solutes is driven by solute drag, and the ultrafiltered fluid is isotonic. Therefore, there is no change in the blood osmolarity, at least if the substitution fluid has a comparable osmolarity to the blood. Fox and Henderson found a more pronounced increase in heart rate response and a greater decline in peripheral resistance during hemodialysis than during hemofiltration in patients with end-stage renal disease (ESRD).[16]

During hemofiltration, there is often a decrease in body core temperature, as the temperature of the substitution fluid is not completely warmed to body temperature.[17] This cooling will result in vasoconstriction, and thus better preservation of blood pressure. However, this vasoconstriction may also further deteriorate tissue perfusion and cardiac output.

Only limited data actually show that CRRT is really superior to IHD with regard to hemodynamic stability, whereas other, prospective and randomized studies have found no difference. Davenport et al found a stable blood pressure in patients with hepatic failure during CRRT, whereas a small blood pressure drop was noted in patients on IHD.[18] This difference was only present during the first few minutes after the start of RRT. Misset et al[19] did not find a difference in hemodynamic stability between patients on CRRT or on IHD, neither for mean arterial blood pressure, drops in blood pressure, nor for need of vasopressive agents. By applying sodium modeling during IHD, Paganini et al[20] could enhance hemodynamic stability, while increasing the ultrafiltered volume. This once again demonstrates that IHD can be greatly improved for ICU-related ARF when some available modifications are used.[21] Kumar et al[22] found a comparable hemodynamic stability in patients on SLEDD as compared to patients on CRRT.

The implementation of SLEDD allows the tailoring of the treatment to the clinical condition of the patient and the needs of the ICU staff. With one single technique and machine, the treatment can be slow and gentle (if needed), and the intensity of the treatment can be increased (while reducing treatment time) if the patient's condition further improves during the course of the disease.

Adequacy

Some recent studies have pointed to a relationship between delivered dialysis dose in ARF and patient survival, for both IHD and CRRT.[23,24] However, only a few centers measure some form of adequacy parameters in addition to the follow-up of the serum urea or creatinine plasma levels.[3] For water, as well as for solutes, there is a compartmentalization in the body. As outlined above, the rate-limiting step is the equilibration of the solutes between the extravascular compartment(s) and the blood. If the extracorporeal extraction exceeds this equilibration, the blood concentration will go down, and the efficiency of the removal of the toxic solute decreases. If the dialysis is stopped, further equilibration will occur, resulting in an increase of blood levels of the solute in the minutes after cessation of the therapy, a phenomenon called 'rebound'. The magnitude of this rebound increases with the efficiency of the dialysis treatment, and with the resistance for equilibration between the blood and the extravascular compartments. During CRRT, the efficiency is low, and the treatment is continuous, leading to virtually little or no rebound. However, due to the low efficiency of the technique, the treatment has to be performed on a continuous basis to achieve adequacy goals. During short-term, high-efficiency IHD, the reduction in blood concentration of small solutes such as urea is up to 80% and there is usually an important rebound.[25]

Spiegel et al[26] demonstrated that the efficiency not the duration of the therapy was the main determinant of the amount of urea rebound. The overestimation of delivered dose with treatments of the same efficiency but different duration will therefore be the same. However, since treatments with longer duration are mostly less efficient, the difference between estimated and measured adequacy will decrease with longer treatment duration. In CRRT, it takes some time before blood levels of certain markers such as creatinine or urea drop below certain thresholds.

Clark et al have shown that it takes 48–72 hours to obtain stable blood levels of urea during CRRT, because the removal rate is low due to the low efficiency of the technique.[27] In IHD, a saw-tooth pattern in blood urea levels is observed, with levels being part of the time under, and part of time above, the desired blood levels of toxicity markers. During SLEDD, the extraction rate nearly equals the equilibration rate, at least for small solutes such as urea. Marshall et al[28] analyzed urea kinetics during a SLEDD session of 12 hours, with a blood flow of 200 ml/min and a dialysate flow of 100 ml/min, and observed virtually no rebound under these conditions. A single-pool urea kinetic model performed as adequately as a two-pool model, again pointing to the fact that during SLEDD performed under these conditions, there is no urea disequilibrium. Clark et al calculated that with a daily IHD session of 4 hours, it is not possible to maintain a blood urea nitrogen (BUN) below 60 mg/dl in a 90 kg patient.[27] However, this goal can easily be achieved if the duration of the dialysis session is extended. Schlaeper et al[29] compared the efficiency of SLEDD, with a blood flow of 200 ml/min and a dialysate flow of 100 ml/min, to that of CRRT with a dialysate or substitution fluid flow of 15–35 ml/min and a blood flow of 150–200 ml/min. They found a daily Kt/V of 2.4 for SLEDD, whereas for IHD this was only 0.9–1.4. In the setting of chronic hemodialysis, long-term nocturnal dialysis has been associated with excellent phosphorus removal, indicating that during extended, slow dialysis sessions, an almost complete equilibration of phosphorus between the extravascular and the intravascular compartments is achieved. Also in the setting of ICU-related ARF, Tan et al[30] demonstrated a good phosphate control during CRRT, in contrast with IHD. However, the patients in the IHD group received only dialysis 3 times/week with 4-hour sessions.

PRACTICAL ASPECTS OF SLEDD

Practical implementation

Technical requirements
The hardware to perform SLEDD consists of a dialysis monitor and a water treatment system.

As the efficiency in SLEDD can vary from low to high, there is need for some form of online prepared dialysis or substitution fluid to avoid the need for expensive, industrially prepared fluids delivered in bags. There are different ways to obtain this goal (Fig. 15.4). One can opt for a central water supply, with a pipeline distribution system to deliver the treated water on the site where it is needed to feed the dialysis monitor. A second option is a compact water treatment system that is incorporated in the dialysis monitor. A third option is to prepare the water in a central place, and to bring it to the location of the dialysis monitor in a big container, the so-called 'batch method'. Each of these systems has its pros and cons, and it depends on the size of the ICU, and the number of ARF patients to be treated, which system should be preferred. A central water delivery system is expensive, and needs regular maintenance to assure perfect water quality. The pressure on the tap water distribution system should also be sufficient to feed the system. A central delivery system is thus only a useful option in an ICU unit where a great number of ARF patients are treated. In addition, all potential cases of ARF in the hospital should then be centralized in that unit, because the system is not mobile. This is a major drawback, as most contemporary large hospitals have separate medical, coronary and surgical ICUs and burn units. In our opinion, a separate compact water treatment system for each dialysis monitor is a better option. If the hospital or the ICU has a water distribution system that already delivers centrally softened water (less than 0.1 dH and/or less than 1.8 ppm $CaCO_3$), this system will consist of a charcoal cartridge and a reverse osmosis membrane. These systems can be made very compact, and are mostly mounted in the dialysis monitor itself to limit the square meters needed to place the equipment. They allow the preparation of sterile, contaminant-free water at the bedside, starting from tap water. These systems can thus be used for dialysis at any location in the hospital where there is a tap and a drain. In addition, it is also possible to use the system for dialyzing hospitalized CRF patients at the bedside. The combination of a dialysis monitor and a compact water treatment system

A

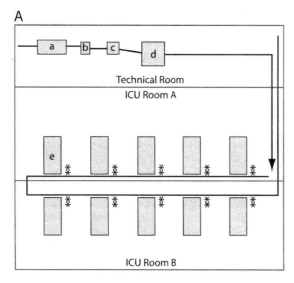

B

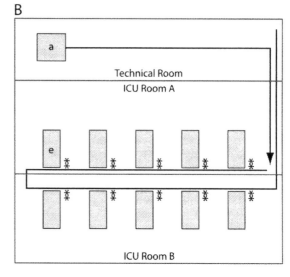

C

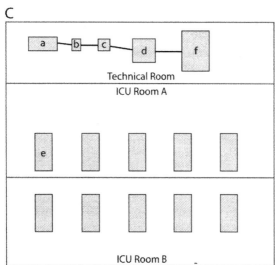

Figure 15.4 Different set-ups for a water treatment system in the intensive care unit (ICU). (A) Central water treatment with pipeline distribution to the dialysis monitor: a = water softener; b = charcoal filter; c = particle filter; d = reverse osmosis unit; e = ICU post. ———— Water pipeline; ‡ = connection for dialysis machine. Note that at every dialysis post, there should also be a drain to collect spent dialysate. (B) Compact water treatment system mounted on the dialysis machine. In this system, there is only need for a water supply (softened tap water) to feed the system and a drain at the bedside of the patient. (C) Batch system: example Genius. The water is prepared at a central place and transported in a large container to the site where the dialysis is performed. There is no need for a tap or a drain at the bedside. f = Preparator for filling and emptying the Genius tank.

is probably the most ideal hardware for most hospitals, as it ensures the lowest cost/utility index.

In the batch system, the water is prepared in a central place and then transported in a big container to the site where the dialysis is performed. In the original format, a small badge of 20–30 L of dialysate was prepared, and transported in an open aluminum container. As the sterility of this fluid could not be guaranteed, the water could only be used for dialysis. Because of the low available volume, the dialysate was often recirculated, which considerably diminished the efficiency of the treatment. This technique has nowadays been abandoned in most ICUs, and should only be accepted in emergency situations where no other

options are available, e.g. for dialysis in disaster areas. However, this old procedure has regained new interest, as a new, actualized format has been proposed over the last years. In the Genius system,[31] the dialysate is prepared in a special device, called the Preparator, which delivers ultrapure dialysate. The dialysate is then pumped into a 75 or 90 L container made of glass, with an incorporated ultraviolet (UV) radiation system that ensures further microbiological purity.[32] The system contains a dialysis monitor, which circulates the dialysate in a single-pass, closed-loop circuit. The fresh dialysate is pumped from the top of the container, whereas the spent dialysate is pumped back into the tank at the bottom. Due to physicochemical differences between fresh and spent dialysate, there is no mixing and there is no recirculation of dialysate.[33]

Whatever water treatment system is used, it is essential that the water delivered is of the highest purity, as it is now accepted that even limited levels of contamination might lead to induction of the inflammatory cascade,[34] which can potentially worsen the systemic inflammatory response that is already present in critically ill patients. It has been argued that the quality of the industrially prepared substitution fluids is superior to that of online prepared fluids. However, the combination of a good water treatment system and a modern dialysis monitor also allows the production of ultrapure water,[35] and in industrially prepared dialysis fluids, contamination can also occur.[36]

Although in principle, all modern dialysis monitors can be used for SLEDD, some special considerations should be taken into account. The monitor should be compact, to fit around the bedside in an often already very crowded ICU environment. The monitor should also be user-friendly, and basic alarms should be easy to understand so that they can be handled by the ICU nurse expeditiously at the bedside. The monitor should be able to deliver the different treatment modalities (hemodialysis, hemodiafiltration, and hemofiltration), and dialysate flow rate and treatment time should be adjustable over a wide range. Despite this flexibility of the monitor, all treatment modalities should, after they have been set up and initiated by the renal nurse, look similar to the ICU nurse in charge.

Most experience with modern dialysis monitors has been described with the Fresenius 2008H machine,[28,29] but also other monitors have been used, such as the Gambro AK Ultra, and the Genius.

An important advantage of the use of 'regular' dialysis monitors over CRRT machines is the accuracy of the ultrafiltration control. CRRT machines mostly use weighing scales or balancing chambers to control the volume of the instilled and ultrafiltered volumes. These weighing scales are prone to decalibration, and their accuracy is limited. In view of the currently advocated high exchange volumes, even errors of 1% can provoke imbalances in fluid status of up to 1 L/24 hours, which is difficult to accept in hemodynamically unstable ICU patients. Dialysis monitors offer more precise ultrafiltration control because they have internal balancing chambers that match incoming and outgoing fluid flow rates very accurately. In the Genius system, ultrafiltration is based on the principle that the dialysate tank is a closed container, and that fluids are not compressible at the low pressures present in the circuit. Therefore, all excess fluid (= ultrafiltration) is allowed to escape through an ultrafiltration line and is collected in a separate receptacle for volumetric control.

Depending upon the desired dialysis modality (hemodialysis, hemodiafiltration or hemofiltration), all different types of membranes can be used for SLEDD. This is in contrast with most CRRT machines, where the membranes are mostly delivered as a package with the tubing system, which of course increases the cost. Although the debate of using complement activating vs low-complement activating and of high-flux vs low-flux membranes is still ongoing,[37] most authors advocate low-complement activating high-flux membranes for SLEDD. High-flux membranes have, at least theoretically, the advantage that there is internal back-filtration, which enhances the convective clearance, and thus the removal of larger solutes such as phosphorus. Also, the larger pore size and the three-dimensional structure provide an increased surface area for adsorption of toxins to the membrane. In addition, most high-flux membranes have an asymmetrical composition, meaning that the permeability is high from the blood side to the dialysate side but low from the dialysate side to the blood side. Because of this property, it is less likely that eventual contaminants present in the dialysate will pass across the membrane to the blood compartment. Low-flux membranes have a much smaller thickness, and therefore a more limited reflection capacity from dialysate to blood side. Therefore, in contrast with what one would imagine intuitively, induction of systemic inflammation by contaminants in the dialysate is less pronounced in high-flux than in low-flux dialysis. It is of note that the Genius system can only work with a high-flux membrane, as there is only a limited transmembranous pressure gradient, so that if a low-flux filter were used, no ultrafiltration would be obtained.

Organizational and nursing aspects

One of the principles of good clinical practice in an open ICU is a smooth cooperation between the different medical disciplines – in this case, the ICU team and the nephrology team. This is extremely important in the dialysis treatment of an ARF patient, most particularly with SLEDD, as this treatment will always require a cooperation between the two teams.

On the medical side, the dialysis treatment prescription should be adapted on a daily basis in consensus between the attending nephrologist and intensivist. Most ideally, the nephrologist will offer knowledge on blood purification therapy and fluid handling, to achieve the treatment goals of the intensivist, who should remain responsible for the overall management of the patient.

On the nursing side, treatment protocols should be prepared that document and define the responsibilities of the different nursing teams. The renal nurse should be in charge of the installation of the equipment, the programming of the desired treatment, and the start and termination of the actual dialysis treatment, including connecting and disconnecting the patient. Once the treatment has started, the ICU nurse should perform hourly monitoring and documentation, and should be able to manage the basic alarms according to simple algorithms. In any case, a renal nurse should be available within an acceptable period of time for advice or assistance. It is essential that, before the SLEDD program is implemented, the renal department provides theoretical and hands-on training of the ICU personnel. In addition, regular update sessions, and short bedside refreshing of important points should be given. The renal department should also be responsible for the maintenance of the machines and the water treatment system. Although, as far as we know, no formal studies have been done on this subject, it is our personal experience that satisfaction with SLEDD is high in both renal and ICU nursing teams for its time-saving and increased efficiency. The ICU nurse is liberated from the hourly fluid balances and bag exchanges, and faces a lower workload. In addition, in view of the reduced treatment time, there is more time left for the actual nursing of the patient, or for medical–technical interventions, which are often a cumbersome task to perform while the patient is connected to a CRRT machine.

Anticoagulation in SLEDD

Anticoagulation and the associated bleeding risk are still the greatest peril of extracorporeal treatments. Fiaccadori et al[38] found a gastrointestinal bleeding rate of 13.4% in a patient population with ARF, with an odds ratio of 2 for patients on CRRT. Ward et al[39] demonstrated that 25% of new episodes of bleeding were attributable to anticoagulation. Martin et al[40] calculated that 3.5–10% of deaths in the ICU were associated with the use

of anticoagulation. Anticoagulation remains an Achilles heel of CRRT, where a continuous struggle is fought between patient bleeding and filter clotting. The major problems are the protracted treatment time, with need for long periods of continuous anticoagulation, and the price of the filter sets, which prohibits frequent change of clotted filters. Reported filter lives vary from a few hours to a few days, depending on the anticoagulation level obtained.[41] Filter clotting not only increases treatment cost and workload (and frustration) of the ICU staff but also limits the efficacy of the treatment. From a theoretical point of view, all anticoagulation strategies that can be implemented in CRRT or IHD can be used for SLEDD. Nevertheless, SLEDD has some important advantages over CRRT with regard to anticoagulation and bleeding risk. In a study of Kumar et al,[22] 31.9% of patients on SLEDD vs only 2.7% on CRRT could be dialyzed without any anticoagulation, and the doses of heparin needed in the remaining patients were far lower in the SLEDD patients.

ACTUAL CLINICAL EXPERIENCE WITH SLEDD

Although it appears that, based on personal contacts with nephrologists in charge of ICU-related ARF patients, SLEDD-like approaches are being used in many centers around the world, the literature on this subject is rather limited. Lonnemann et al used the Genius system, with a blood and dialysate flow rate of 70 ml/min, for 18 hours a day.[32] This resulted in a urea clearance of 65 L/day, and a mean ultrafiltration volume of 120 ml/h without any reported hemodynamic instability. Kumar et al[22] used a Fresenius 2008H machine, with a mean blood flow of 200 ml/min and a dialysate flow of 300 ml/min, for 6–8 hours, on a daily basis. They compared the clearance, hemodynamic stability, and anticoagulation needs of patients on this treatment with those of patients treated by CVVH with a mean blood flow of 170 ml/min and an exchange volume of 2 L/hour. There was no difference in hemodynamic stability or in the need for vasopressive agents. Excellent metabolic control was obtained with both modalities.

CONCLUSIONS

The use of SLEDD has some important advantages that will certainly increase its popularity in the future. SLEDD offers the advantages of IHD (high efficiency, practicality, economy, good ultrafiltration control, and no need for industry-prepared substitution fluids) in combination with the advantages of CRRT (extended treatment and smooth metabolic control) in a modular fashion, using one single type of dialysis machine. Usually, the treatment is started as a 'slow dialysis' with a low blood flow (typically 150 ml/min in double needle) and a low dialysate flow (typically 100–300 ml/min). The ultrafiltration rate is usually also low (max. 350 ml/h). The use of hemodialysis monitors with adapted software allows the implementation of online hemofiltration or hemodiafiltration. Daily evaluation of the patient by a nephrologist and an intensivist is needed, and this collaboration will improve the treatment of the patient. Daily adaptation of dialysis duration, which can range from nearly continuous to regular IHD, is feasible. The blood and dialysate flows, as well as the type of artificial kidney, can be adapted to the needs of the patient. There is an important cost-containment, as the need for expensive 'all-in' sets can be avoided and the 'conventional' membranes and tubings of the chronic dialysis program can be used (better price-setting negotiation and no stock problems). Also, expensive substitution fluid bags are not needed, as dialysate is prepared online. Compared with CRRT, the reduced treatment duration not only reduces the labor costs but also allows more possibilities for diagnostic or therapeutic interventions. Finally, a substantial reduction in need for anticoagulation is realized, and heparin-free dialysis is possible.

For all these reasons, we believe SLEDD offers an important potential for the treatment of ARF in the ICU.

REFERENCES

1. Chertow GM, Christiansen CL, Cleary PD, Munro C, Lazarus JM. Prognostic stratification in critically ill patients with acute renal failure requiring dialysis. Arch Intern Med 1995;155:1505–11.
2. Brivet FG, Kleinknecht DJ, Loirat P, Landais PJ. Acute renal failure in intensive care units – causes, outcome, and prognostic factors of hospital mortality; a prospective, multicenter study. French Study Group on Acute Renal Failure. Crit Care Med 1996;24:192–8.
3. Hyman A, Mendelssohn DC. Current Canadian approaches to dialysis for acute renal failure in the ICU. Am J Nephrol 2002;22:29–34.
4. McCarthy JT. Prognosis of patients with acute renal failure in the intensive-care unit: a tale of two eras. Mayo Clin Proc 1996;71:117–26.
5. Lameire N, Van Biesen W, Vanholder R, Colardijn F. The place of intermittent hemodialysis in the treatment of acute renal failure in the ICU patient. Kidney Int Suppl 1998;66:S110–19.
6. Ronco C, Zanella M, Brendolan A, et al. Answers from the first international course on critical care nephrology questionnaire. Contrib Nephrol 2001;132:196–209.
7. Mehta RL, Letteri JM. Current status of renal replacement therapy for acute renal failure. A survey of US nephrologists. The National Kidney Foundation Council on Dialysis. Am J Nephrol 1999;19:377–82.
8. Paganini EP, Kanagasundaram NS, Larive B, Greene T. Prescription of adequate renal replacement in critically ill patients. Blood Purif 2001;19:238–44.
9. Schiffl H, Lang SM, Fischer R. Daily hemodialysis and the outcome of acute renal failure. N Engl J Med 2002;346:305–10.
10. Bonventre JV. Daily hemodialysis – will treatment each day improve the outcome in patients with acute renal failure? N Engl J Med 2002;346:362–4.
11. Mehta RL, McDonald B, Gabbai FB, et al. A randomized clinical trial of continuous versus intermittent dialysis for acute renal failure. Kidney Int 2001;60:1154–63.
12. Lameire N, Van Biesen W, Vanholder R. Dialysing the patient with acute renal failure in the ICU: the emperor's clothes? Nephrol Dial Transplant 1999;14:2570–3.
13. Dhondt A, Van Biesen W, Vanholder R, Lameire N. Selected practical aspects of intermittent hemodialysis in acute renal failure patients. Contrib Nephrol 2001;132:222–35.
14. Leblanc M, Moreno L, Robinson OP, Tapolyai M, Paganini EP. Bicarbonate dialysate for continuous renal replacement therapy in intensive care unit patients with acute renal failure. Am J Kidney Dis 1995;26:910–17.
15. Leblanc M, Tapolyai M, Paganini EP. What dialysis dose should be provided in acute renal failure? A review. Adv Ren Replace Ther 1995;2:255–64.
16. Fox SD, Henderson LW. Cardiovascular response during hemodialysis and hemofiltration: thermal, membrane, and catecholamine influences. Blood Purif 1993;11:224–36.
17. van der Sande FM, Kooman JP, Konings CJ, Leunissen KM. Thermal effects and blood pressure response during postdilution hemodiafiltration and hemodialysis: the effect of amount of replacement fluid and dialysate temperature. J Am Soc Nephrol 2001;12:1916–20.
18. Davenport A, Will EJ, Davison AM. Effect of renal replacement therapy on patients with combined acute renal and fulminant hepatic failure. Kidney Int Suppl 1993;41:S245–51.
19. Misset B, Timsit JF, Chevret S, et al. A randomized cross-over comparison of the hemodynamic response to intermittent hemodialysis and continuous hemofiltration in ICU patients with acute renal failure. Intensive Care Med 1996;22:742–6.
20. Paganini EP, Sandy D, Moreno L, Kozlowski L, Sakai K. The effect of sodium and ultrafiltration modelling on plasma volume changes and haemodynamic stability in intensive care patients receiving haemodialysis for acute renal failure: a prospective, stratified, randomized, cross-over study. Nephrol Dial Transplant 1996;11 (Suppl 8):32–7.
21. Schortgen F, Soubrier N, Delclaux C, et al. Hemodynamic tolerance of intermittent hemodialysis in critically ill patients: usefulness of practice guidelines. Am J Respir Crit Care Med 2000;62:197–202.
22. Kumar VA, Craig M, Depner TA, Yeun JY. Extended daily dialysis: a new approach to renal replacement for acute renal failure in the intensive care unit. Am J Kidney Dis 2000;36:294–300.
23. Ronco C, Bellomo R, Homel P, et al. Effects of different doses in continuous veno-venous haemofiltration on outcomes of acute renal failure: a prospective randomised trial. Lancet 2000;356:26–30.
24. Tapolyai M, Fedak S, Chaff C, Paganini EP. Delivered dialysis dose may influence ARF outcome in ICU patients. J Am Soc Nephrol 1994;5:530A.

25. Schneditz D, Daugirdas JT. Compartment effects in hemodialysis. Semin Dial 2001;14:271–7.

26. Spiegel DM, Baker PL, Babcock S, Contiguglia R, Klein M. Hemodialysis urea rebound: the effect of increasing dialysis efficiency. Am J Kidney Dis 1995;25:26–9.

27. Clark WR, Mueller BA, Kraus MA, Macias WL. Extracorporeal therapy requirements for patients with acute renal failure. J Am Soc Nephrol 1997;8:804–12.

28. Marshall MR, Golper TA, Shaver MJ, Alam MG, Chatoth DK. Urea kinetics during sustained low-efficiency dialysis in critically ill patients requiring renal replacement therapy. Am J Kidney Dis 2002;39:556–70.

29. Schlaeper C, Amerling R, Manns M, Levin NW. High clearance continuous renal replacement therapy with a modified dialysis machine. Kidney Int Suppl 1999;72:S20–3.

30. Tan HK, Bellomo R, M'Pis DA, Ronco C. Phosphatemic control during acute renal failure: intermittent hemodialysis versus continuous hemodiafiltration. Int J Artif Organs 2001;24:186–91.

31. Fassbinder W. Renaissance of the batch method? Nephrol Dial Transplant 1998;13:3010–12.

32. Lonnemann G, Floege J, Kliem V, Brunkhorst R, Koch KM. Extended daily veno-venous high-flux haemodialysis in patients with acute renal failure and multiple organ dysfunction syndrome using a single path batch dialysis system. Nephrol Dial Transplant 2000;15:1189–93.

33. Dhondt AM, Vanholder RC, De Smet, et al. Studies on dialysate mixing in the Genius single-pass batch system for hemodialysis therapy. Kidney Int 2003;63:1540–7.

34. Schindler R, Lonnemann G, Schaffer J, et al. The effect of ultrafiltered dialysate on the cellular content of interleukin-1 receptor antagonist in patients on chronic hemodialysis. Nephron 1994;68:229–33.

35. Vaslaki L, Karatson A, Voros P, et al. Can sterile and pyrogen-free on-line substitution fluid be routinely delivered? A multicentric study on the microbiological safety of on-line haemodiafiltration. Nephrol Dial Transplant 2000;15 (Suppl 1):74–8.

36. Williams PF, Foggensteiner L. Sterile/allergic peritonitis with icodextrin in CAPD patients. Perit Dial Int 2002;22:89–90.

37. Jaber BL, Cendoroglo M, Balakrishnan VS, et al. Impact of dialyzer membrane selection on cellular responses in acute renal failure: a crossover study. Kidney Int 2000;57:2107–16.

38. Fiaccadori E, Maggiore U, Clima B, et al. Incidence, risk factors, and prognosis of gastrointestinal hemorrhage complicating acute renal failure. Kidney Int 2001;59:1510–19.

39. Ward DM, Mehta RL. Extracorporeal management of acute renal failure patients at high risk of bleeding. Kidney Int Suppl 1993;41:S237–44.

40. Martin PY, Chevrolet JC, Suter P, Favre H. Anticoagulation in patients treated by continuous venovenous hemofiltration: a retrospective study. Am J Kidney Dis 1994;24:806–12.

41. Schetz M. Anticoagulation in continuous renal replacement therapy. Contrib Nephrol 2001;132:283–303.

16

Intensive care management of the patient with chronic renal failure

Robert C Albright Jr and Matthew D Griffin

INTRODUCTION

End-stage renal disease (ESRD) is becoming a common condition. Over 275 000 patients currently receive dialysis care in the United States as of December 31, 2000, whereas over 103 800 patients have functioning renal allografts.[1] Hemodialysis patients have a very high rate of general hospitalization (approximately 2000 admissions per 1000 patient-years at risk), as do renal transplant patients. Although the rates of hospital admission for transplant patients are significantly lower (approximately 800 admissions per 1000 patient-years at risk),[1] this rate still far exceeds the general risk for hospitalization for the general population.[1(p24)] Congestive heart failure and infectious complications are the top reasons for hospitalization admissions among all ESRD patients,[1(p18)] whereas complications resulting from vascular access lead admission rates for patients 67 years old or older in the immediate month following initiation of renal replacement therapy.[1(p18)] The average admission duration for a patient with ESRD on dialysis is approximately 14 days, with an average of two admissions per year.[1] These admissions have high cost implications for our society. The total cost of hospitalization of the ESRD population has increased from over US$3 billion to over US$4.2 billion over the past 5 years.[1(p27)]

Specific rates of intensive care unit (ICU) admission are not available for the ESRD populations in the United States, Europe, or for other regions. In fact, little published data exist in regard to etiology of ICU admissions, rates of ICU admissions, outcomes, or general utility of these activities to our society and the ESRD population as a whole. These issues not withstanding, all practitioners in the ICU environment will deal quite commonly with ESRD patients. This chapter discusses the salient issues with respect to the clinical management of the chronic hemodialysis and renal transplant patient who requires ICU care.

INTENSIVE CARE MANAGEMENT OF THE CHRONIC DIALYSIS PATIENT

Review of clinical issues of dialysis patients treated in ICU settings

Initial evaluation
Often the most important information with respect to initial diagnosis and management of a dialysis patient admitted to a critical care environment is to be obtained from the referring dialysis facility. Crucial historical information, including optimal dry weight, hemodynamic data, medication lists, allergies, access history, anticoagulation regimen and recent laboratory values, and perhaps, most importantly, recent clinical assessments by the dialysis care team are available for dialysis patients, unlike the majority of patients admitted to the ICU. The patient's prior dialysis prescription and advance directives can also be obtained.

Standard attention to ensuring adequate airway, oxygenation, ventilation and circulatory support are mandatory. The dialysis access may be a useful modality for volume and pressor support in an emergency situation. However, these accesses should be treated with the utmost respect, as they serve as the dialysis patient's 'lifeline' for the ongoing dialysis therapy. Dual-lumen central venous dialysis catheters are nearly always loaded to lumen volume with either heparin or sodium citrate. Therefore, these medications must be aspirated prior to introducing infusions through these device. An extremity access may potentially be utilized for resuscitation; however, the fistula or graft should be treated for what it is, essentially an arterial line. Accessing a fistula or graft should only occur with a pressure infusion device, and immediate consultation (as practical) with nephrology and dialysis nursing staff.

Once the dialysis patient is stabilized, several issues deserve comment. Special attention needs to be directed to the patient's access. Blood draws, peripheral arterial or intravenous lines and blood pressure measurements should be done only on the contralateral extremity. Adjustment of all medications for a glomerular filtration rate (GFR) of approximately 10 ml/min should be ensured via communication with pharmacy and the nephrology and critical care teams. Therapeutic drug levels, when available, become even more important tools among the ESRD patients due to difficulties of calculating doses in the setting of rapidly shifting volume status (dialysis). Several medications deserve specific mention. Meperidine compounds should be avoided for analgesia due to rapid accumulation of normeperidine byproducts that lower the seizure threshold.[2] Succinylcholine, a depolarizing paralytic agent utilized for rapid sequence intubations, can often cause significant hyperkalemia, and alternative agents such as etomidate may be more appropriate.[3] Imipenem cilastatin (a broad-spectrum antibiotic) should also be avoided among patients with renal failure due also to propensity for decreased seizure threshold.[4] Nearly all the benzodiazepine agents will exhibit increased duration of clinical effect among the ESRD population; however, no single agent appears to have any specific advantages among these patients. Low molecular weight heparin (LMWH) compounds have dramatically increased half-lives among the dialysis patients.[5] Close monitoring of factor X levels is required when using these agents in the ESRD population. As this monitoring is not yet practical, our medical center has avoided the use of LMWH in dialysis patients.

Nutrition requirements are unique for the dialysis patient. Close attention to nutrition prescription, including appropriate restriction of potassium (<60 mEq/day), sodium (<90 mEq/day), and phosphorus (<800 mg/day), will prevent metabolic complications perhaps leading to increased need for dialysis. Protein requirements for the dialysis patients in the hospital setting are approximately 0.8–1.2 g/kg (ideal body weight or IBW)/day.[6]

Erythropoietin requirements for ESRD patients who are critically ill are usually dramatically increased due to multiple issues. Arguably, erythropoietin is much less effective in this setting and extremely expensive; thus, controversy exists as to its utility.

Cardiac and vascular complications

Among incident hemodialysis patients between the years 1995 and 1999, the 2-year mortality after acute myocardial infarction (MI) was 73%.[1(p172)] In fact, cardiac disease is the major cause of death among patients with ESRD, accounting for 45% of all deaths.[1(p172),7] Furthermore, among patients who suffer acute MI, 1-year survival for those with diabetes as the primary etiology of ESRD is approximately 42%.[1(p172)] One-year survival following cardiac arrest among patients with ESRD treated by chronic dialysis is less than 18% at 1 year.[1(p173)] Interestingly, there appears to be an increased cardiac death rate among ESRD patients on Mondays and Tuesdays (20%) compared with other days of the week (14%).[8]

Caring for these patients is made more challenging by the difficulties in interpretation of cardiac biomarkers. However, recent evidence demonstrates plasma or cardiac troponin T (cTnT) is an important predictor of long-term all-cause mortality and cardiovascular mortality in patients with ESRD.[9,10] Recent guidelines endorsed by both American and European societies of cardiology state that cardiac troponin T and I are the preferred biomarkers for the detection of myocardial injury and diagnosis of MI.[11] Furthermore, although controversy still exists with respect to interpretation of troponins in ESRD, recent literature has supported that troponin T has independent predictive value across the entire spectrum of renal function. Specifically, an elevated troponin T increased the risk of death from MI by 20% with an adjusted odds ratio for death of 2.5 among patients requiring dialysis.[12]

Despite recent reports highlighting the dismal prognosis of ESRD patients with acute coronary syndromes, little is known about how such patients are to be managed.[13] Furthermore, treatment of patients requiring dialysis who suffer acute MIs and are treated in an ICU is complicated by various clinical issues which may challenge the usual standard care for MI. Such modalities as thrombolysis, urgent PTCA (percutaneous coronary transluminal angioplasty), or other adjunctive measures (glycoprotein IIB/IIIA inhibitors) may be contraindicated by bleeding risk, severe hypertension, or limits of care due to perceived quality of life issues. A recently published cohort examined treatment of acute MI among patients with ESRD treated in a cardiac ICU at a tertiary medical center. This study illustrated that standard adjunctive therapy such as ACE (angiotensin-converting enzyme) inhibitors, beta-blockers, aspirin, heparin, and nitrates was suboptimally utilized. Additionally, reperfusion therapy was offered to only 7% of patients with ESRD suffering MI.[14] Whether a more aggressive approach will yield improved outcomes among ESRD patients with acute MI is currently being evaluated in controlled trials.

Congestive heart failure carries an extraordinary risk of mortality as well. Published rates of 50% mortality risk at 2 years following diagnosis are accepted among all ESRD patients, and diabetics have an even greater risk.[1] Maximizing appropriate support measures such as beta blockade, ACE inhibitor/ARBs (angiotensin receptor blockers), digitalis, and appropriate hemoglobin levels, and maintaining optimal volume status among ESRD patients can often be improved, especially in the critical care environment.

Atrial fibrillation has been reported to occur in approximately 9% of dialysis patients.[15,16] While specific etiology of new-onset atrial fibrillation events among dialysis patients has yet to be studied systematically, volume overload, ischemic events, and electrolyte shifts uniquely increase the risk. Medication toxicity, specifically digoxin toxicity, should be ruled out. Therapy for this dysrhythmia should focus on correction of the preceding issues, particularly with respect to provision of dialysis if necessary, along with the standard approach of heart rate control and attention to risks of thromboembolism. The risk of thromboembolism has been reported to vary between 5 and 23%,[15,16] and long-term anticoagulation should be addressed on a case-by-case basis.

Admission for peripheral vascular disease portends a very poor short- and long-term survival. A mortality of 40% has been reported following admission for severe peripheral vascular disease.[1(p172)]

Stroke

Stroke is a common cause of death among all patients on chronic hemodialysis. Recent studies in the hemodialysis patient population have shown a high annual incidence of stroke (12–18 per 1000 patient-years) compared with the general population, and the incidence of brain hemorrhage is two to three times higher than the incidence of infarction.[17,18] These data suggest that hemodialysis treatment is possibly a major trigger of both brain

hemorrhage and infarction, as the majority of events occurred on dialysis days. Cerebrovascular events are a devastating event, with a 50% expected annual mortality noted after admission to an ICU for CVA/TIA (cerebrovascular accident/transient ischemic attack).[1(p172)] Unfortunately, little epidemiologic/outcome data exist with regards to reperfusion strategies in acute stroke among hemodialysis patients.

Infection and sepsis

The most recent US Renal Data Survey System report indicates that, following cardiovascular disease, infection is the second leading cause of death among patients with ESRD. Septicemia accounts for more than 75% of these infectious deaths.[1] The annual percent mortality due to sepsis among ESRD patients is 100- to 300-fold higher for chronic hemodialysis patients and approximately 20-fold higher for renal transplant recipients compared with the general population.[19] In this same study, the mortality rate from sepsis remained approximately 50-fold higher among dialysis patients compared with the general population when multiple variant risk analysis was carried out.[19]

The etiology of sepsis among ESRD patients has yet to be thoroughly stratified. However, evaluation of catheter-based sepsis comparing standard central venous catheterization vs dialysis catheterization did not demonstrate different risks of infection or sepsis between the two groups, according to a recently published small study. This study found no difference in either catheter colonization or catheter-related bacteremia incidents per 1000 days of catheter use between dialysis catheters and central venous catheters. Gram-positive micro-organisms were found to be the predominant causative agents in catheter infections between both groups.[20] This study is in disagreement with prior work, which showed the rate of catheter-related sepsis among dialysis catheters was significantly higher than those of triple-lumen catheters among patients treated in the ICU.[21] However, these studies did not differentiate between short- and long-term dialysis catheters.

Hyperkalemia

Hyperkalemia is a very common issue among dialysis patients and poses a serious mortality risk, with up to 3–5% of deaths among all dialysis patients attributed to hyperkalemia.[22] Unfortunately, the classic electrocardiographic changes of hyperkalemia are particularly insensitive and lack specificity as well among dialysis patients. Concurrent electrolyte and metabolic disturbances strongly influence the degree of electrophysiologic abnormalities. Hypernatremia, hypercalcemia, and alkalemia all increase the cardiac tolerance for hyperkalemia, while the development of hyponatremia, hypocalcemia, and acidemia worsen electrophysiologic effects of hyperkalemia.[22] Unfortunately, no universally applicable threshold correlating potassium level and dysrhythmia exists among dialysis patients.

Following calcium-induced membrane stabilization for life-threatening hyperkalemia, the therapy of choice is urgent dialysis. Serum potassium will usually decline approximately 1 mEq/L/h for the first 3 hours of standard hemodialysis vs 0–1 mEq/L of potassium-containing dialysate; thereafter, a plateau of the serum level develops.[22] Whereas insulin and dextrose therapy has been shown to be efficacious in causing transient shifting of potassium from extra- to intracellular compartments, sodium bicarbonate has been demonstrated to be of very limited benefit among dialysis patients with hyperkalemia.[22] Case reports of colonic mucosal necrosis have been documented among critically ill patients treated with polystyrene sulfonate, a cation exchange resin (Kayexalate), and hence its use in the ICU should be limited.[22]

Gastrointestinal bleeding

Acute gastrointestinal (GI) hemorrhage as a complication of ESRD is well documented in the literature and is considered one of the major causes of morbidity and mortality among patients on dialysis.[23,24] Increased incidence of upper GI bleeding, which often leads to ICU admission, is due to the increased incidence of hemorrhagic complications secondary to anticoagulation of the dialysis procedure, platelet dysfunction, and quantitative abnormalities of the von Willebrand factor. The major causes of upper GI bleeding in patients with ESRD include erosive gastritis, erosive duodenitis, erosive esophagitis, gastroduodenal ulcer, Mallory–Weiss tears, and angiodysplasias.[25] Additionally troublesome is the fact that rebleeding is a much greater problem among patients with ESRD compared to patients without renal failure. Rebleeding occurs more frequently and results in a significantly higher mortality rate among patients on dialysis as compared with the general population of patients treated for upper GI hemorrhage in the ICU (13% vs 2%, respectively, $p <0.05$).[25]

The implication of these data is that it is extremely important to prevent upper GI bleeding among ESRD patients cared for in the ICU. Whether the incidence of 'stress ulceration' is increased among ESRD patients as compared to the general ICU population is unclear. Intuitively, it would appear that, due to the hemostatic abnormalities among ESRD patients, this particular group of patients would be at inordinate risk. Prevention should center on either H_2 blockade or proton pump inhibition. The theoretical risk of aluminum overload precludes the routine use of aluminum sucralfate for patients on chronic dialysis.

Trauma

Little data exist in regard to acute injury or trauma requiring ICU admission among the ESRD population. A recent review of a single center's experience with trauma management among patients with ESRD discovered that the complication and mortality rates among ESRD patients were 50.8% and 13.5%, respectively, as compared with 16.3% and 4.7% among the general trauma population.[23] The increased mortality was attributed to hemorrhagic complications and infectious complications as well as to fluid and acid-based disturbances, which occurred more frequently among the patients with ESRD.[26] Additionally, length of stay among ESRD patients suffering trauma admitted to a Level 1 trauma center is noted to be extended by 55.3%.[27]

Specific dialytic support issues

Dialysis adequacy

Dialysis adequacy of patients requiring hemodialysis in the ICU has recently received well-deserved attention. A link between dialysis adequacy among patients with acute renal failure treated in the ICU and survival is beginning to be shown.[28,29] However, dialysis adequacy of ESRD patients hospitalized in the ICU has not been formally addressed. Multiple factors complicate the adequate delivery of dialysis to an ESRD patient treated in an ICU. Access difficulties are extremely common among patients admitted to the ICU. Clotting and mechanical access complications as well as infectious complications are common. Additionally, utilization of adequate anticoagulation is often contraindicated by the patient's underlying critical illness (coagulopathy, bleeding). Utilization of single-use dialyzers, which are often of lower efficiency, will often require increase in treatment times, which may be impractical in the ICU.

Importantly, hypotension often limits intermittent dialysis therapy as well. Poor access flows in the setting of hypotension or clotting can lead to multiple pump stops and inadequate treatment delivery. An important practical consideration, which may also hinder the adequate delivery of renal replacement among patients admitted to the ICU, is that of limited available time. Often, treatments are shortened in order to allow other required therapeutic and diagnostic procedures to occur. A small retrospective study illustrated these very difficulties. This study found that blood flow rates among hospitalized patients were over 60 ml/min slower and dialysis time was actually shortened by over half an hour. This resulted in a calculated Kt/V value of 1.11 ± 0.1 for hospitalized ESRD patients vs their current outpatient kinetics, which were a Kt/V of 1.38 ± 0.2.[30] An increase in the prescribed treatment duration by 10–15% over the patient's usual outpatient time along with monitoring of dialysis adequacy by weekly performance of urea reduction ratios (with a target of 70%) and/or weekly time averaged concentration of urea of 60 mg/dl has become the standard of care at our institution. Thus far, however, no data definitively linking increased dialysis dose and improved survival among ESRD patients in acute care settings (or ICUs) exist. This obviously deserves attention.

Dialysis modality
Caring for the dialytic needs of a critically ill patient presents many difficulties, as have been delineated above. Occasionally, the clinical situation may dictate a change in modality of renal replacement. Hypotension, access difficulties, or inability to achieve renal replacement goals of azotemia control, fluid balance management, and acid–base and electrolyte balance may require change to continuous renal replacement therapy (CRRT) or a change from peritoneal dialysis to hemodialysis. Challenges arise with respect to access in these circumstances. Placement of temporary dual-lumen central venous access is favored when patients change from intermittent to continuous modalities if their usual dialysis access is either a fistula or graft. Prolonged low-efficiency therapies may be an option, and may allow use of the native extremity access; however, repeated prolonged cannulation of the permanent access can predispose to trauma, bleeding, and difficulties with securing the cannula. Occasionally, the renal replacement needs of peritoneal dialysis patients are unable to be met in the ICU, even with increased frequency of exchanges. This situation requires strong consideration for change in modality to extracorporeal therapies.

INTENSIVE CARE MANAGEMENT OF THE RENAL TRANSPLANT PATIENT

Literature pertaining to the assessment, management, and clinical outcomes of critically ill renal transplant recipients is quite limited. Furthermore, the renal transplant population itself and the pharmacotherapy associated with it have continued to broaden and change during the past two decades. Nevertheless, the presentation of an acutely unwell renal transplant recipient to the ICU represents an opportunity to effectively apply a well-recognized set of diagnostic and therapeutic considerations. Excluding patients admitted to the ICU in the immediate postoperative period, the majority of admissions are for medical disease and the reported hospital mortality is between 10% and 14%.[31,32] Mortality is not well predicted by need for mechanical ventilation, level of renal function, or APACHE II score on admission.[31,32]

As with all acutely ill patients, the first actions taken are likely to have the most impact on patient recovery. In addition, these first management decisions may also significantly influence the prospects for preservation of graft function. Box 16.1 lists some important guiding principles that should be brought to bear when completing the initial evaluation of the critically ill renal transplant recipient. Central to these principles are the need to consider disease entities for which immunosuppression creates a heightened risk[33–41] and the need to generate a modified immunosuppressive strategy that will enhance the patient's likelihood of recovery without unduly jeopardizing the graft. Errors of judgment during the primary work-up may result either from over-reaction (e.g. complete withdrawal of all immunosuppression in a relatively stable patient) or under-reaction (e.g. failure to aggressively pursue diagnostic studies) to the immunosuppressed state. In this regard, it is essential to bear in mind that the symptoms and signs of inflammation that are often used to guide decisions on the early use of diagnostic procedures or empiric treatment may be deceptively subtle or absent in the immunosuppressed patient.[34] The remainder of this section focuses on the pharmacological management of the transplanted patient in the ICU and on the transplant-specific features of individual ICU presentations. Emphasis is placed

---

Box 16.1   Guiding principles for the initial assessment of the critically ill renal transplant recipient

1. Document clearly the primary cause for renal failure, time from transplantation, current immunosuppressive regimen, most recent record of graft function, and most recent immunosuppression trough levels.
2. Document and record all recent additions or changes to the patient's prescription and nonprescription medication schedule.
3. Review potential transplant-related etiologies for the patient's clinical presentation (e.g. opportunistic infection, lymphoma, medication toxicities, corticosteroid withdrawal) and include appropriate diagnostic testing in the primary evaluation.
4. Consider the potential modifying influence of the immunosuppressed state on presenting symptoms and physical signs (e.g. blunted febrile response, lack of peritoneal signs, lack of meningeal signs) and on progression rate of acute illness.
5. Proceed quickly to high-yield diagnostic procedures (e.g. bronchoscopy/BAL, CSF examination, CT/MR imaging).
6. Based on the severity of the clinical presentation, generate and clearly document an immunosuppression management plan that includes:
    (a) overall level of immunosuppression to be employed (e.g. minimal, moderately reduced, unchanged)
    (b) dose, timing, and route of administration of each agent
    (c) timing and frequency of immunosuppression monitoring.
7. While awaiting diagnostic information, begin empiric therapy that takes into account:
    (a) extended differential diagnosis
    (b) baseline level of renal transplant function
    (c) possible interactions with immunosuppressive agents

BAL, bronchoalveolar lavage; CSF, cerebrospinal fluid; CT, computed tomography; MRI, magnetic resonance imaging.

on the primary diagnostic and management decision process.

Immunosuppression management of the acutely ill renal transplant patient

Management of immunosuppression is a central consideration in any transplanted patient admitted to the ICU and requires close attention as part of the primary and ongoing plan of care. Factors that will influence immunosuppression prescription in the critically ill renal transplant recipient include:

- the likelihood of an acute infection at the time of presentation
- the possibility of medication toxicity as a cause or contributing factor to an acute illness
- the routes of drug administration that can be employed during the course of the illness
- the possible interactions with other medications that may be initiated or withdrawn during the illness.

For the patient with an immediately life-threatening infection or neoplasm, it is, undoubtedly, appro-

priate to withdraw all immunosuppression with the exception of a low dose of corticosteroid. As abrupt withdrawal of all immunosuppression may precipitate acute rejection even in a long-standing stable graft, the renal transplant recipient with non-life-threatening infection is best managed by judicious reduction in dose or target through levels of nonsteroid agents. If specific toxicity from one or more immunosuppressive medications is suspected, selective withdrawal with interim increase in corticosteroid or substitution with an alternative agent is indicated. The presence of acute renal impairment may also be an indication for temporary discontinuation of a calcineurin inhibitor.[42,43] In the case of a non-infectious process such as MI, it is important to maintain a stable immunosuppressive regimen with parenteral administration if necessary. Table 16.1 summarizes the features of the commonly used maintenance immunosuppressive agents in renal transplant recipients. Typically, two or three such agents comprise the stable antirejection regimen for a given patient. As indicated, many of these immunosuppressants can be administered via nasogastric tube or intravenously. Maintenance of stable dose intervals and effective monitoring of trough blood levels for cyclosporine A, tacrolimus, and sirolimus are essential to avoid over- or under-immunosuppression as well as the occurrence of specific drug toxicities (see Table 16.1 and Ref 42). Immunosuppression dosage, monitoring, and route of administration should be reviewed daily during the course of a hospital admission for acute illness. With recovery from an infectious process or episode of toxicity, a stepwise reintroduction of baseline immunosuppressive agents can be planned.

Acute respiratory failure

Differential diagnosis
Acute respiratory failure has been reported to be the commonest reason for ICU admission in renal transplant patients.[32] Although infection represents the most frequent etiology, the differential diagnosis is broad and includes a number of non-infectious processes that may mimic an acute pneumonia.[38,39,44]

Infection
During the immediate postoperative period, acute pneumonia is likely to be related to aspiration, nosocomial infection, or pre-existing pulmonary colonization by Gram-positive or Gram-negative bacteria.[34,35] For renal transplant patients presenting from the community, there is a wide variety of potential pathogens, including those commonly associated with community-acquired pneumonia in the general population.[34,39,45] Opportunistic infections that must be considered are:

- Bacteria – *Nocardia* spp. (see Fig. 16.1C for example), *Legionella* spp.
- Mycobacteria – *Mycobacterium tuberculosis*, *Mycobacterium avium-intracellulare*, other atypical mycobacteria
- Fungi – *Pneumocystis carinii*, *Cryptococcus neoformans*, *Aspergillus* spp., *Candida* spp., *Histoplasma capsulatum*, *Coccidioides immitis*, *Blastomyces dermatitidis*, Mucoraceae, others
- Viruses – cytomegalovirus (CMV), influenza A and B, respiratory syncytial virus (RSV), adenovirus, herpes simplex virus (HSV), varicella-zoster (VZV)
- Protozoa – *Toxoplasma gondii*.

Medication toxicity
The monoclonal anti-T-cell antibody OKT3 is used for initial immunosuppression or for treatment of acute rejection. It can cause acute pulmonary edema associated with massive T-cell cytokine release, usually following the first dose.[42] Polyclonal anti-T-cell preparations, including ATGAM and Thymoglobulin, may also be associated with acute respiratory syndromes, although less commonly than OKT3. Intravenous administration of cyclosporine A has also been rarely reported as a cause for acute pulmonary edema. More recently, the immunosuppressive agent sirolimus has been linked with cases of acute interstitial pneumonitis for which no infectious etiology could be identified.[46]

Neoplasia
Post-transplant lymphoproliferative disorder (PTLD) due to B-cell transformation by Epstein–Barr virus (EBV) may progress rapidly in transplant recipients and present acutely as diffuse pulmonary infiltrates or as multifocal pulmonary masses in 5–20% of cases.[36,38] Many other neoplastic processes may also present with more rapidly progressive pulmonary complications (pleural effusion, cavitary lesions, multifocal masses) in renal transplant recipients than in the general population.[37,38]

Thromboembolism and acute pulmonary edema
Pulmonary embolism and acute cardiac failure due to MI or other causes are common following renal transplantation and may present primarily with pulmonary symptoms.[41,47–50] These conditions, which must be considered during the initial evaluation of a transplant patient with acute respiratory failure, are outlined in greater detail in the section on acute cardiovascular syndrome.

Others
Among the uncommon causes of acute respiratory failure in renal transplant recipients are recurrence of vasculitis, fulminant pulmonary calcification, parasitic infestation with *Strongyloides stercoralis*, bronchiolitis obliterans organizing pneumonia (BOOP), and graft versus host disease.

Assessment strategies
Imaging studies may provide important information in narrowing the differential diagnosis and guiding diagnostic procedures. High-resolution computed tomography (CT) of the chest, which can define the anatomic distribution of multifocal processes and accurately detect cavitation or intrathoracic lymph node enlargement, should be considered the primary imaging modality of

Table 16.1 Common maintenance oral immunosuppressive agents in renal transplantation.

Name	Dosing frequency	Therapeutic complications	Notable Interactions	Monitoring strategy	Formulations available	Nasogastric administration	Conversion to Intravenous[a]
Prednisone (Deltasone, Orasone, others)	Once daily	Hypertension, diabetes mellitus, GI bleeding, papilledema, Addisonian crisis	Metabolism increased by enzyme inducers (phenytoin, rifampin)	None	Tablets Liquid Preparations	Yes – liquid preparation	Convert to methylprednisolone (Solumedrol) 10–40 mg daily intravenously[b]
Azathioprine (Imuran)	Once or twice daily	Bone marrow suppression, hepatotoxicity, GI disturbance	Severe pancytopenia with allopurinol	None (dose reduction for leukopenia)	Tablets Intravenous solution	Yes – crushed tablets	Intravenous solution every 24 or 12 hours at 1:1 conversion from oral dose
Mycophenolate mofetil (CellCept)	Twice daily	Bone marrow suppression, GI disturbance	Decreased absorption: antacids cholestyramine	Assay available – trough level (µg/ml) may guide dose adjustment	Capsules Tablets Oral suspension Intravenous solution	Yes – oral suspension *not* opened capsules	Intravenous solution every 12 hours at 1:1 conversion from oral dose
Cyclosporine A (nonmodified: Sandimmune, others) (modified Neoral Gengraf, others)	Twice daily (every 12 hours)	Neurotoxicity, hepatotoxicity, nephrotoxicity, hypertension, hyperkalemia, diabetes mellitus	*Increased levels:* diltiazem, verapamil, ketoconazole, itraconazole, erythromycin, clarithromycin, others *Decreased levels:* rifampin, phenytoin phenobarbital, carbamazepine, others[c]	Trough level (ng/ml) for does adjustment[d]	Capsules Oral solutions Intravenous solution	Yes – oral solutions (maintain patient on non-modified or modified formulation as apropriate)	Intravenous solution every 12 hours at 1:3 conversion from oral dose

Drug	Dosing	Toxicity	Monitoring	Formulations	Can be opened/given	Availability
Tacrolimus (FK506, Prograf)	Twice daily (every 12 hours)	Neurotoxicity, hepatotoxicity, nephrotoxicity, hypertension, hyperkalemia, diabetes mellitus	As for cyclosporine A	Trough level (ng/ml) for dose adjustment[d]	Capsules Intravenous solution	Yes – open capsules	Not recommended for maintenance therapy
Sirolimus (Rapamycin, Rapamune)	Once daily (noon)	Bone marrow suppression, interstitial pneumonitis, hyperlipidemia	As for cyclosporine A	Trough level (ng/ml) for dose adjustment[d]	Tablets (1 mg only) Oral solution	Yes – oral solution	Not available

a For immunosuppression level, equivalent to baseline oral doses.
b Methylprednisolone may increase trough levels of cyclosporine, tacrolimus, and sirolimus.
c See reference 42 for comprehensive lists.
d Trough levels must be drawn prior to dose administration and 12 hours after the previous dose. Depending on time from transplantation and assay used typical maintenance target trough levels are: cyclosporine A, 80–200 ng/ml; tacrolimus, 5–10 ng/ml; and sirolimus, 5–12 ng/ml.

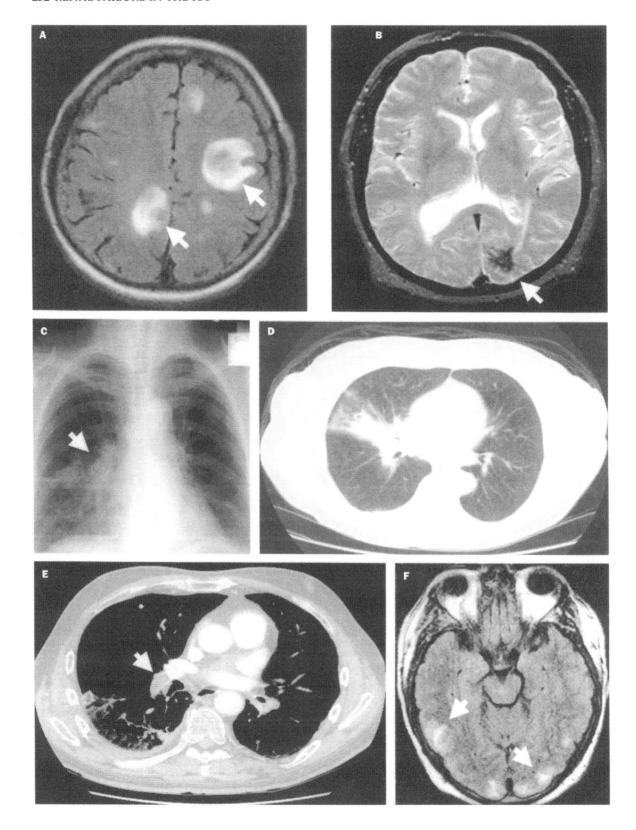

choice in renal transplant recipients with respiratory failure and abnormal chest radiography. Where appropriate, cine-CT angiography, and transthoracic or transesophageal echocardiography can provide specific diagnostic information regarding pulmonary embolism or acute cardiac syndromes.

Bronchoscopy with bronchoalveolar lavage (BAL) is a proven high-yield diagnostic study in renal transplant recipients with acute respiratory illness[51-53] and should be carried out as early as possible. Samples should be submitted for staining, DNA-based analysis, and culture for common community-acquired organisms as well as for opportunistic infections such as *Pneumocystis carinii*, *Legionella* spp., *Nocardia* spp., fungal organisms, mycobacteria, and viruses. Cytological examination of BAL cellular components may also yield evidence of alveolar hemorrhage or of lymphoma. Positive microbiological results are obtained from 60 to 80% of procedures, with multiple organisms isolated in 12-25%.[51-53]

A number of rapid diagnostic tests of blood and urine have become available in recent years that afford an additional opportunity for early diagnosis of opportunistic infections, including legionellosis, histoplasmosis, coccidioidomycosis, cryptococcosis, CMV, and EBV.[33,53] The choice of additional tests to be submitted in the course of the initial evaluation is based on geographic location, history of potential exposures, and clinical features suggestive of specific infections.[33-35,39,45,46,54] Rapid tests, particularly those based on polymerase chain reaction (PCR) technology must, however, be interpreted with caution, as high sensitivity may result in detection of nonpathogenic levels of individual organisms. A quantitative assay or confirmation of infection by another technique is essential to avoid misdiagnosis. Diagnostic tests that rely on the detection of pathogen-specific antibodies (serology) may be inappropriately negative as a result of immunosuppression and should also

be interpreted with caution.[34] Consultation with an infectious disease service during this first diagnostic phase is advisable. If there has been no clear clinical improvement and no diagnostic information has been secured within 48–72 hours of admission, a diagnostic tissue biopsy is required. Depending on the results of imaging studies, this may consist of one or more of the following:

- CT-guided needle biopsy of the lung thoracoscopic lung and/or pleural biopsy
- mediastinoscopy with biopsy of intrathoracic lymph node or mass
- pericardial biopsy
- open lung biopsy
- biopsy of an accessible distant site such as a subcutaneous lymph node or a skin lesion.

Initial therapy

Empiric antimicrobial therapy is indicated in renal transplant recipients presenting with acute respiratory failure unless a clear noninfectious etiology can be rapidly established. The possibility of infection with multiple organisms should be borne in mind.[51-53] Broad-spectrum parenteral antibiotic coverage for Gram-positive and Gram-negative bacteria as well as an agent with activity against atypical agents such as *Mycoplasma* and *Legionella* should be initiated. Opportunistic infections for which initial empiric therapy may be reasonable (depending on disease severity, level of clinical suspicion, use of prophylaxis, and geographic location) include CMV pneumonitis, *Pneumocystis carinii* pneumonia (PCP), fungal pneumonia (*Cryptococcus*, *Aspergillus*, others), nocardial pneumonia, and tuberculosis.[33-35] As indicated in Box 16.1, a plan for immunosuppression adjustment and monitoring must also be generated as part of the initial decision-making. Discontinuation of immunosuppressive agents suspected of being directly responsible for a pulmonary process may be indicated during the primary management plan

Figure 16.1 Imaging studies of acutely ill renal transplant recipients. (A) Neoplasia: post-transplant lymphoproliferative disorder (PTLD) presenting as seizures and altered consciousness is demonstrated as multiple cortical mass lesions on head magnetic resonance imaging (MRI). (B) Opportunistic infection: disseminated aspergillosis presenting as prolonged febrile illness with skin nodules followed by seizures is associated with a single cavitating lesion (arrow) on head MRI. (C) Opportunistic infection: pulmonary nocardiosis presenting as acute cough and dyspnea is detected on chest X-ray as a localized infiltrate and on chest computed tomography (CT) as a right peribronchial mass and wedge-shaped area of consolidation (arrow). Thoracoscopic lung biopsy was required for definitive diagnosis. (D) Acute vascular event: a large occlusive right pulmonary embolism is revealed by CT angiography of the chest in a recent pancreas transplant recipient presenting with acute hypotension, hypoxia, and a new right infiltrate on chest X-ray. (E) Immunosuppressive medication toxicity: leukoencephalopathy due to cyclosporine, presenting as headache followed by seizures, is diagnosed by the presence of multiple T_2-enhancing areas (arrows) in the posterior cerebral vortex on head MRI.

or at a later time if alternative diagnoses have been ruled out.[42,46]

Acute neurologic syndrome

Differential diagnosis

Neurologic abnormalities represent the second most common cause for ICU admission in renal transplant recipients. Presenting features may include altered consciousness, seizures or focal motor or sensory deficits. Onset may be rapid or gradual.[40] As with respiratory failure, infection represents the most frequent etiology but may be mimicked by many other conditions, and a detailed knowledge of prior medical history and medication exposure is essential.[33–35,40,55]

Infection

Infectious agents associated with meningitis and encephalitis in the general community may present with altered or more severe clinical features in immunosuppressed transplant recipients and should be considered in the differential diagnosis for any acute neurologic illness.[40] These include *Neisseria meningitidis*, *Streptococcus pneumoniae*, *Haemophilus influenzae*, *Listeria monocytogenes* and seasonally or geographically restricted viral encephalitides. In addition, underlying medical conditions such as valvular heart disease, diabetes mellitus, artificial joints, and intravascular devices may predispose the transplant recipient to bacteremia and intracranial abscesses. An array of opportunistic infections must also be considered during the initial evaluation:

- Bacteria – *Nocardia* spp.
- Mycobacteria – *Mycobacterium tuberculosis*, atypical mycobacteria
- Fungi – *Cryptococcus neoformans*, *Aspergillus* spp. (see Fig. 16.1B for example), *Candida* spp., *Histoplasma capsulatum*, *Coccidioides immitis*, Mucoraceae, others
- Viruses – HSV, VZV, CMV, EBV, JC virus (progressive multifocal leukoencephalopathy)
- Protozoa – *Toxoplasma gondii*.

Although each of these organisms may be associated more or less commonly with specific presenting features (e.g. focal symptoms or signs with toxoplasmosis and aspergillosis, sinus involvement with mucormycosis) there is substantial clinical overlap and it is essential to proceed rapidly to diagnostic testing.

Medication toxicity

Neurologic side effects occur in up to 25% of patients receiving the calcineurin inhibitors cyclosporine A and tacrolimus (FK506).[40–42] These vary from mild (tremor, headache) to severe (seizures, altered consciousness, cortical blindness, focal motor or sensory loss) and are generally related to blood level of the drug. Acute presentations with severe neurologic changes may occur during first exposure or be precipitated by dose increase, initiation or discontinuation of an interacting medication (see Table 16.1), or a metabolic abnormality such as hypomagnesemia. Two syndromes merit specific consideration in patients receiving these medications. Leukoencephalopathy, presenting with altered consciousness, seizures, and/or focal deficits, is characteristic of calcineurin inhibitor neurotoxicity and is associated with T2-enhancing posterior cerebral lesions in magnetic resonance imaging (MRI) (see Fig. 16.1E). Thrombotic microangiopathy (thrombotic thrombocytopenic purpura) may involve the central nervous system (CNS) and cause seizures or focal deficits. This syndrome is accompanied by evidence of intravascular hemolysis, such as anemia with fragmented erythrocytes, thrombocytopenia, and renal impairment.[56,57]

The anti-T-cell monoclonal antibody OKT3 is also commonly associated with acute neurologic abnormalities, typically within 12–72 hours of the first dose. The most frequent presentation is aseptic meningitis (2% of those receiving OKT3), but acute encephalopathy, psychosis, and acute cerebral edema have also been reported.[40,42] High-dose corticosteroid therapy in the immediate post-transplant period or during treatment for rejection may be associated with acute encephalopathy, often preceded by mood or behavioral disturbance.

Neoplasia

The CNS may be the primary site for EBV-associated PTLD and commonly presents with acute or subacute neurologic abnormalities (see Fig. 16.1A for example).[36,40] As with PTLD at other sites, the distinction between lymphoma and infection is often difficult, and pursuit of an early tissue diagnosis should not be delayed. Overall risk for a number of cancers is increased over time in the renal transplant recipient[37] and metastatic neoplasia may also result in acute neurologic syndromes. Uncommonly, an underlying condition such as von Hippel–Lindau syndrome or tuberous sclerosis may be associated both with renal failure and CNS tumors.

Vascular events and metabolic encephalopathies

Following infection, metabolic encephalopathies and CVAs comprise the second and third most common causes for acute neurologic illness among renal transplant recipients.[40] Patients with renal failure requiring transplantation frequently have a history of additional related or unrelated medical conditions that predispose to encephalopathy, seizures, or stroke. These conditions include diabetes mellitus (hypoglycemic, ketoacidotic, or hyperosmotic coma; cerebrovascular disease), hepatitis B and C (hepatic encephalopathy), depression (medication or other overdose), hypertension (intracerebral hemorrhage, cerebrovascular disease, hypertensive encephalopathy), autosomal dominant polycystic kidney disease (saccular aneurysm/subarachnoid hemorrhage), hypothyroidism (myxedema, thyrotoxicosis), and systemic vasculitis or systemic lupus erythematosus (CNS vasculitis). Uremia due to renal allograft rejection or graft failure for other reasons may also contribute to an acute encephalopathy. Renal transplant artery stenosis may, occasionally, present with acute hypertensive encephalopathy.

Stroke due to atherosclerosis/cerebrovascular embolism is the cause of death in 10–15% of renal transplant recipients.[58] As an acute neurologic presentation, however, it is important to consider this a diagnosis of exclusion in the immunosuppressed patient because potentially reversible conditions such as medication toxicity, PTLD, and a variety of opportunistic infections may present with the rapid development of focal neurologic deficits.

Primary assessment strategy

The broad differential diagnosis for acute neurologic illness in a transplant recipient can be a daunting challenge to the physician assessing such a patient in the ICU. As already emphasized, a detailed past medical history and medication history is essential to understanding the potential for noninfectious causes. A high-resolution imaging study frequently yields important early diagnostic information. Although CT scanning with intravenous contrast may readily detect intracerebral hemorrhage and focal inflammatory or neoplastic lesions, MRI is significantly more sensitive for many of the conditions to which the transplant patients have increased susceptibility and is preferable in this setting.

Unless the initial clinical history or imaging study provide an immediate clear diagnosis, the primary biochemical and hematologic testing should be comprehensive and include assays for liver function, possible drug overdoses, intravascular hemolysis, and metabolic syndromes such as ketoacidosis and hyperosmolality. Blood cultures should be drawn for bacteria and yeast as well as for mycobacteria, viruses and fungi.[33–35] Appropriate serologic and rapid diagnostic testing of blood and/or urine for specific opportunistic infections should be drawn and subsequently interpreted under the guidance of an infectious disease consulting service.[33]

Examination of the cerebrospinal fluid (CSF) is essential if infection and PTLD have not been ruled out within 24 hours or if immediate empiric antimicrobial therapy is planned. In addition to the standard assays (protein and glucose levels, cell count and differential, staining and cultures), an array of testing for opportunistic infection and cytology for detection of lymphoma should be submitted. Rapid tests of CSF for CMV, HSV, EBV, mycobacteria, and individual fungal organisms may provide important diagnostic information within 24–48 hours of admission.

Electroencephalography, although rarely diagnostic, may also allow the differential diagnosis to be narrowed or response to therapy to be monitored in the case of metabolic encephalopathy, HSV encephalitis, or medication toxicity. Transesophageal echocardiography may allow diagnosis of endocarditis or infection of an endovascular device in the patient with evidence of CNS abscesses. CT imaging of the chest and abdomen may reveal evidence of multisystem disease and provide a site for a diagnostic biopsy or another procedure. If no other biopsy site is identified, a biopsy of the brain should be carried out in a transplant recipient with (1) undiagnosed focal intracranial lesions or (2) persistent or worsening encephalopathy despite reversal of potential toxic/metabolic causes and initiation of empiric antimicrobial therapy.

Initial therapy

Immediate discontinuation of potentially neurotoxic immunosuppressive medication is appropriate during the initial diagnostic phase.[40,42] If a severe infection is not suspected, an interim increase in corticosteroid dosage can be used to reduce the risk of acute graft rejection. Seizure control, which may require the use of anticonvulsants that interact significantly with one or more immunosuppressants (see Table 16.1), should be initiated and monitored in consultation with a neurology service. Effective reversal of any meta-bolic abnormalities should be initiated early, including intermittent or continuous dialysis for uremia. In the hypertensive patient, blood pressure control should be aggressively pursued. Unless infection can be rapidly ruled out, empiric antimicrobial therapy should be initiated and comprise broad-spectrum coverage for bacterial agents associated with meningitis. The decision to begin empiric therapy for individual opportunistic infections should be based on disease frequency, severity of illness, geographic risk, or suggestive clinical and/or imaging features. Infectious agents for which this is often appropriate include *Cryptococcus neoformans*, HSV, CMV, VZV, *Toxoplasma gondii*, *Aspergillus* spp., and Mucoraceae.[33–35]

Acute cardiovascular instability

Differential diagnosis
In general, the reasons for acute hypotension, with or without multiorgan failure, are similar in renal transplant recipients to those in other patients, and include infection/sepsis, acute MI, acute pulmonary embolism, hemorrhage/volume depletion, and anaphylaxis. The renal transplant patient has, to varying degrees, an increased risk profile for each of these life-threatening events. In addition, there may be specific etiologies for acute cardiovascular collapse that are peculiar to the immunosuppressed patient or there may be instances in which the symptoms or signs of an underlying organ-specific cause are masked by immunosuppressive medication. The differential diagnosis of acute hypotension in renal transplant recipients is outlined here with these considerations in mind.

Infection/sepsis
The first 4 weeks following transplantation bring together a number of formidable risk factors for bacteremia and sepsis, including pre-existing medical illness, recent surgery, high-level immunosuppression, and indwelling vascular and/or urinary catheters. The incidence and outcomes of bacteremia requiring ICU admission in this early post-transplant period have not been well studied but a high level of suspicion should be maintained for systemic infection in a patient with new onset of fever, weakness, or hypotension. Significant wound infections may be accompanied by only subtle physical signs. The cumulative frequency of urinary infection in renal transplant recipients has been reported at between 35% and 79%.[34,35] Gram-positive and Gram-negative bacteria and *Candida* spp. may be responsible for an episode of acute sepsis, and infection with more than one organism is not uncommon. At later time points following transplant surgery, many patients remain at risk for bacteremia, particularly those with diabetes mellitus, bladder dysfunction, and long-standing intravascular catheters, and those requiring treatment for acute graft rejection. Gastrointestinal infections and infestations such as *Salmonella* spp., *Campylobacter jejuni*, *Listeria monocytogenes*, *Cryptosporidium*, and *Clostridium difficile* toxin may present with cardiovascular collapse due to profound volume depletion and/or accompanying bacteremia. Certain other opportunistic infections may also present as a severe disseminated illness with hemodynamic instability, including legionellosis, fungal infections, tuberculosis, and disseminated VZV infection.[33–35]

Acute cardiac failure
Ischemic heart disease is at least twice as frequent in renal transplant recipients as in the general population and higher still in those with diabetes mellitus.[41,58,59] Cardiovascular disease is currently the single greatest cause of mortality following renal transplantation.[41,58,59] Acute MI is, therefore, a common occurrence among transplant patients and carries a 1-year mortality of approximately 25%.[58] As with many other acute illnesses, the classical symptoms of myocardial ischemia may be altered in the immunosuppressed patient and the diagnosis must not be overlooked in a transplant recipient admitted to the ICU with hypotension. Hypertensive cardiomyopathy and dilated cardiomyopathy are frequent pre-existing conditions in many patients receiving renal transplants but typically remain stable or improve following transplantation. Less commonly, a cardiomyopathy due to viral infection may result in rapid onset of cardiac failure in a transplant recipient without prior severe myocardial disease. Pericarditis and pericardial effusion may also present with acute cardiac failure and, in the transplant recipient, may be due to opportunistic infection (particularly viral, mycobacterial, and fungal agents), or to PTLD.[60] In the case of a patient presenting with recurrent unexplained episodes of pulmonary edema, a stenosis of the transplant artery or of the iliac artery proximal to the transplant anastomosis should be suspected.[61]

Acute pulmonary embolus

Pulmonary embolism should be ruled out early in any transplant recipient presenting with unexplained hypoxia or cardiovascular instability. Thromboembolic events, including deep venous thrombosis (DVT), have been reported in 5–18% of patients following renal transplantation and pulmonary embolism in 0.5–3%, with a mortality of up to 30%.[47–50,62] Polycystic kidney disease, factor V Leiden heterozygosity, and pancreas transplantation are associated with additional increased risk of thromboembolism.[50,62]

Acute hemorrhage

Hypovolemia due to acute hemorrhage may occur at any time post-transplant. The use of high-dose corticosteroid therapy during the first 6 months may be associated with a higher risk of bleeding from GI lesions during this period. Common etiologies for acute upper or lower GI hemorrhage that must be borne in mind in renal transplant recipients include peptic ulcer disease, variceal bleeding due to underlying liver disease, ischemic colitis, lymphoma (PTLD), and infection with CMV.

Medication toxicity

Cardiovascular collapse due to immunosuppressive medication is not a frequent occurrence but should be considered following administration of monoclonal or polyclonal anti-T-cell preparation (OKT3, ATGAM, Thymoglobulin) or in patients receiving pooled human immunoglobulins for the first time. Anaphylaxis due to other specific medications is no more or less common in the transplant population than in other patient groups. However, the frequency of polypharmacy among renal transplant recipients emphasizes the need to thoroughly document all new exposures in the patient admitted because of acute hypotension.

Primary assessment and management strategy

The primary evaluation of the renal transplant patient with acute cardiovascular instability is fundamentally no different from that of nontransplanted patients. Hemodynamic monitoring and echocardiography may provide an early distinction between cardiogenic and noncardiogenic causes. Timely diagnosis and aggressive management of MI (including thrombolysis or angioplasty) is highly appropriate in renal transplant recipients and there is evidence that recent improvement in in-hospital mortality for this patient population has paralleled that of non-ESRD patients.[41] Pulmonary embolus should be rapidly ruled out where appropriate by a high-sensitivity test such as cine-CT angiography. Consideration of possible etiologies should be extended to include *Candida* sepsis, other disseminated opportunistic infections, complicated lymphoma, and recently administered antibody therapies. In the case of upper or lower GI bleeding, brushings and biopsies should be liberally taken during endoscopy to detect CMV or HSV. Even in the absence of striking symptoms and signs, the presence of an acute pulmonary or intraabdominal process should be considered early and actively pursued by CT scan if doubt remains (see relevant sections for additional discussion). Empiric antibiotic therapy with broad-spectrum coverage for Gram-positive and Gram-negative bacteria is appropriate if a noninfectious cause cannot be quickly confirmed. Additional empiric antimicrobial therapy for *Legionella* spp., *Listeria monocytogenes*, *Candida* spp., other fungal infections, CMV, and VZV may be indicated for patients with suggestive clinical presentations or documented exposure.[33–35] Early consultation with an infectious disease service is advisable in the case of an immunosuppressed patient with suspected disseminated infection.

Acute renal failure

Differential diagnosis

The investigation of acute renal transplant dysfunction typically revolves around the detection of graft rejection. In the current era of transplantation, however, acute rejection is rarely associated with severe systemic manifestations. In the case of the critically ill renal transplant recipient, reduced graft function is unlikely to be due to rejection and should be evaluated and managed in the context of the presenting illness.[63] Important causes of acute renal transplant failure with systemic illness are outlined in the following paragraphs.

Ischemic nephropathy

As with the native kidney, the transplanted kidney is susceptible to ischemic nephropathy in the context of bacteremia/sepsis, hypoperfusion following acute cardiovascular event, hypertensive crisis, trauma, dehydration, or exposure to nephrotoxic agents. The concomitant use of a calcineurin inhibitor results in higher sensitivity to ischemic nephropathy and may also delay recovery from an episode of acute renal failure. The presence of chronic renal allograft rejection or transplant artery stenosis may also predispose to renal failure during the course of a systemic illness.

Medication toxicity

Acute encephalopathy due to cyclosporine A or tacrolimus is associated with high blood level of these drugs and, for this reason, is commonly accompanied by reduced renal function.[40,42] Recovery of neurological and renal function typically occurs within days of reducing or discontinuing calcineurin inhibitor therapy.[40] Both cyclosporine A and tacrolimus may also precipitate a thrombotic microangiopathy with predominant renal features (hemolytic uremic syndrome (HUS)).[56,57] In this case, evidence of intravascular hemolysis may require discontinuation of the causative drug. Drug-induced interstitial nephritis may also occur in the renal transplant patient and should be considered in the differential diagnosis of acute renal transplant failure during treatment of an acute infection or other illness.

Neoplasia

Post-transplant lymphoproliferative disorder not infrequently involves the organ transplant itself and a graft recipient with acute illness due to PTLD may develop renal failure as a result of parenchymal invasion of the transplant by lymphomatous cells.[36]

Allograft-related infection

The combination of cardiovascular collapse with acute renal transplant dysfunction may result not only from ischemic nephropathy but also from graft pyelonephritis, from infection of a peritransplant fluid collection (lymphocele), or from ureteral stenosis with pyonephrosis. In addition to the Gram-negative bacteria commonly responsible for urinary infection, the presence of a Gram-positive bacterial or candidal infection should be considered when initiating empiric antimicrobial therapy. Opportunistic infection with CMV or a tissue-invasive fungus may also directly involve the renal transplant and result in renal impairment.

Primary assessment and management strategy

Renal transplant dysfunction in the context of an acute systemic illness can be initially evaluated with urinalysis; urine microscopy, eosinophil count and culture; blood testing for evidence of intravascular hemolysis; measurement of trough cyclosporine A or tacrolimus level; and imaging by ultrasound with Doppler study of the graft vasculature.[64] Nephrotoxic medication (including calcineurin inhibitor therapy) should be withdrawn or avoided and the use of intravenous radiologic contrast minimized where possible. The indications for and prescription of intermittent or continuous hemodialysis in the renal transplant recipient do not currently differ from those for nontransplanted patients.[63] Graft and patient outcomes for renal transplant recipients requiring dialysis during an ICU admission have not been well studied. Renal allograft biopsy should be considered under the following circumstances:

- persistent unexplained renal failure despite successful treatment of known underlying illnesses
- laboratory or imaging study suggestive but not diagnostic of a treatable renal parenchymal process
- lack of tissue diagnosis of suspected lymphoma or other systemic process that may involve the transplant
- new onset of graft dysfunction during recovery from an acute illness.

Additional interventions that may be indicated under specific circumstances include ultrasound or CT-guided aspiration of peritransplant fluid collection and percutaneous nephrostomy of an acutely obstructed renal transplant.

Acute abdominal syndromes

Differential diagnosis

Acute abdominal emergencies requiring surgical intervention are relatively common in renal transplant recipients (5.7% in one series[65]) and may occur both early and late post-transplant.[66] The presenting symptoms for intra-abdominal conditions that require urgent surgery are notoriously vague in patients receiving immunosuppressive medication and a delay in intervention of greater than 24 hours is associated with substantially increased mortality.[67] The possibility of acute perforation of a viscus must always be considered in the differential diagnosis of an acutely ill transplant recipient with abdominal pain, even in the absence of abdominal guarding and rigidity. The causes of bowel perforation for which transplant patients have specific susceptibility as a result of pre-existing disease or immunosuppression are diverticulosis, intestinal lymphoma, CMV colitis, pseudomembranous colitis, and ischemic colitis.[65-68] The frequency of bowel perforation among renal transplant recipients is reported to be between 0.5% and 2%.[66,67] Many other intra-abdominal processes may be responsible for acute illness in the renal transplant patient, including acute cholecystitis, acute intestinal ischemia, mechanical bowel obstruction, acute appendicitis, acute pancreatitis, complicated peptic ulcer disease, ruptured abdominal aortic aneurysm, and volvulus. For these conditions the risk following renal transplantation is not clearly increased. However, in each case, the effect of immunosuppression on characteristic symptoms and signs may delay presentation or diagnosis until an advanced stage. Less commonly, opportunistic infections other than CMV may cause bowel perforation or intra-abdominal abscess. These include atypical mycobacteria, *Nocardia* spp., and *Candida* spp. As discussed in the following section, the presence of a pancreas transplant is associated with a number of additional intra-abdominal conditions.

Primary assessment and management strategy

The primary goal of evaluating a transplant recipient with an acute abdominal syndrome should be to prevent a delay in surgical intervention if such is indicated. The presence of hemodynamic instability and/or metabolic acidosis in a patient with vague abdominal symptoms or signs raises the possibility of a significant intra-abdominal catastrophe and the strategy of intermittent physical examination and plain radiography can prove costly. A CT scan of the abdomen and pelvis (with intravenous contrast if possible) should be considered the primary imaging study of choice and early surgical consultation obtained if there is evidence of an intra-abdominal process. Colonoscopy can be of specific diagnostic value for CMV colitis, pseudomembranous colitis, and colonic PTLD, but should not be performed until a bowel perforation has been ruled out. Ultrasound- or CT-guided aspiration of a localized intra-abdominal fluid collection can also be of diagnostic value for an abscess or perforated viscus. Empiric antimicrobial therapy with broad coverage for Gram-positive, Gram-negative, and anaerobic micro-organisms is appropriate if an acute abdominal emergency is suspected. If there remains doubt about a perforation following radiologic imaging, an exploratory laparotomy is preferable to proceeding with endoscopy or to a strategy of continued observation.

The pancreas transplant recipient – special considerations in the ICU

Pancreas transplantation may be carried out in combination with kidney transplantation or as a single organ graft for diabetic patients without advanced renal impairment. Pancreas exocrine secretions may be directed to the urinary bladder ('bladder-drained') or to the small intestine ('enteric drained').[69,70] Immunosuppressive management and many of the risks for acute illness are similar in pancreas and kidney transplant recipients. A number of specific points should, however, be borne in mind when assessing critical illness in a patient who has received a pancreas transplant:

1. Underlying atherosclerosis, microvascular disease, and autonomic dysfunction are extremely common as a result of prior complicated diabetes mellitus.
2. Risk for thromboembolism is higher following pancreas transplantation compared to kidney transplantation (see Fig. 16.1D for example).
3. PTLD and CMV infection are significantly more common following pancreas transplantation compared to kidney transplantation.
4. Intra-abdominal complications peculiar to pancreas transplantation are not uncommon and include graft pancreatitis, leakage of exocrine contents into the peritoneal cavity (with or without infection), graft thrombosis, and intra-abdominal abscess.
5. For patients with bladder-drained pancreas transplants, in whom chronic exocrine secretion into the urine occurs, profound dehydration and acidosis may occur in the setting of an acute GI illness or other source of fluid loss.[69-72]

The modifying effect of immunosuppression on abdominal symptoms and signs cannot be overemphasized in the case of the acutely unwell pancreas transplant recipient and a CT scan of the abdomen and pelvis (with intravenous contrast if possible) should be considered early in the evaluation. The presence of leakage from a bladder-drained pancreas graft may be demonstrated by a cystogram or a CT cystogram.

CONCLUSIONS

The population of patients with ESRD is expected to reach over 600 000 in the United States by 2010[1] and will, undoubtedly, require increasing amounts of healthcare resources, including those of the ICU. Despite the complexity that is often involved in their care, the assessment and management of an acutely unwell dialysis or renal transplant patient is a rewarding and, at times, inspiring experience. These individuals and their families have overcome (often repeatedly) great adversity and frequently teach us the value of applying an organized, multidisciplinary plan of care. The temptation to adopt a passive approach to diagnosis and therapy because of a perceived poor prognosis should be resisted unless this is clearly the patient's wish. Indeed, a failure to consider active management for acute illness means only that the expectation of high mortality rates becomes a 'self-fulfilling prophecy'. Cardiovascular disease deserves specific attention in this regard, with current information indicating that standard medical management is often not offered to the ESRD patient. Clinical studies are needed to begin to assess the outcomes of specific therapies for this population in the critical care environment, but we strongly advocate the application of therapies that have proven benefit in the general population for acutely ill ESRD patients if at all possible.

ACKNOWLEDGMENTS

The authors wish to acknowledge the dedication and support of colleagues and coworkers from the Mayo Clinic Dialysis and Kidney/Pancreas Transplant Programs and Critical Care Services. Our thanks also to Mr Michael DeBernardi for helpful review of the manuscript and to Ms Kathy Mandery for manuscript preparation.

REFERENCES

1. US Renal Data System. USRDS 2002 annual data report: atlas of end-stage renal disease in the US. Bethesda, MD: National Institutes of Health, National Institute of Diabetes and Digestive and Kidney Diseases; 2002:18.
2. Davies G, Kingswood C, Street M. Pharmacodynamics of opioids in renal dysfunction. Clin Pharmacokinet 1996;31:410–22.
3. Bishop M, Hornbein TF. Prolonged effect of succinylcholine after neostigmine and pyridostigmine administration in patients with renal failure. Anesthesiology 1983;58:384–6.
4. Gibson TP, Demetriades JL, Bland JA. Imipenem/cilastatin: Pharmacokinetic profile in renal insufficiency. Am J Med 1985;78 (Suppl A)54–61.
5. Weitz JI. Low molecular weight heparins. N Engl J Med 1997;337: 688–98.
6. KDOQI Nutrition Workgroup. Management of protein and energy intake. Am J Kidney Dis 2000;35,6(Suppl 2):540–1.
7. Herzog CA, Ma JV, Collings AJ. Poor long-term survival after acute myocardial infarction among patients on long-term dialysis. N Engl J Med 199;339:779–805.
8. Blyer AJ, Russell GB, Satko SG. Sudden and cardiac death rates in hemodialysis patients. Kidney Int 1999;55:1553–9.
9. Dierkes J, Domrose U, Westphal S, et al. Cardiac troponin T predicts mortality in patients with end-stage renal disease. Circulation 2000;102:1964–9.
10. Ooi DS, Zimmerman D, Gram J, et al. Cardiac troponin T predicts long-term outcomes in hemodialysis patients. Clin Chem 2001; 47:412–17.
11. Joint European Society of Cardiology/American College of Cardiology Committee. Myocardial infarction defined: a consensus document of the Joint European Society of Cardiology/American College of Cardiology Committee for the redefinition of myocardial infarction. J Am Coll Cardiol 2000;36:959–69.
12. Aviles RJ, Askari AT, Lindhal B, et al. Troponin T levels in patients with acute coronary syndromes with or without renal dysfunction. N Engl J Med 2002;346(26):2047–52.
13. Herzog CA. Acute myocardial infarction in patients with end-stage renal disease. Kidney Int Suppl 1999;71:S130–3.
14. Wright RS, Reeder GS, Herzog CA, et al. Acute myocardial infarction and renal dysfunction: a high risk combination. Ann Intern Med 2002;137:563–70.
15. Ansari N, Maurs T, Femfeld DA. Symptomatic atrial arrhythmias in hemodialysis patients. Renal Failure 2001;23(1):71–6.
16. Vasaquez E, Sanchez-Perales C, Borrego F, et al. Influence of atrial fibrillation on the morbido-mortality of patients on hemodialysis. Am Heart J 2000;140:886–90.
17. Iseki K, Fukiyama K. Predictors of stroke in patients receiving chronic hemodialysis. Kidney Int 1996;50:1672–5.
18. Kawamura M, Fujimoto F, Hisanaga S, et al. Incidence, outcome, and risk factors of cerebrovascular events in patients undergoing maintenance hemodialysis. Am J Kidney Dis 1998;31:991–6.
19. Sarnak MJ, Jaber BL. Mortality caused by sepsis in patients with end-stage renal disease compared with the general population. Kidney Int 2000;58:1758–64.
20. Souweine B, Traore O, Aublet-Cuvelier B, et al. Dialysis and central venous catheter infections in critically ill patients: results of a prospective study. Crit Care Med 1999;27:2394–8.
21. Eyer S, Brummitt C, Crossley K, et al. Catheter-related sepsis: prospective randomized study of three methods of long-term catheter maintenance. Crit Care Med 1990;18:1073–9.
22. Ahmed J, Weisberg LS. Hyperkalemia in dialysis patients. Semin Dial 2001;14(5):348–56.
23. Chalasani N, Cotsonis G, Wilcox CM. Upper gastrointestinal bleeding in patients with chronic renal failure: role of vascular ectasis. Am J Gastroenterol 1996;91:2329–32.
24. Alvarez L, Puleo J, Balint JA. Investigation of gastrointestinal bleeding in patients with end-stage renal disease. Am J Gastroenterol 1993;88:30–3.
25. Tsai CJ, Hwang JC. Investigation of upper gastrointestinal hemorrhage in chronic renal failure. J Clin Gastroenterol 1996;22:2–5.
26. Blake AM, Toker SI, Dickerman R, Dunn EL. Trauma management in the end-stage renal disease patient. Am Surgeon 2002; 68(5):425–9.
27. Lorelli DR, Kralovich AA, Seguin C. The impact of pre-existing end-stage renal disease on survival in acutely injured trauma patients. Am Surg 2001;67(7):693–6.
28. Schiffert H, Lang SM, Fisher R. Daily hemodialysis and the outcome of acute renal failure. N Engl J Med 2002;346(5):305–10.
29. Ronco C, Bellomo R, La Greca GL. Effects of different doses in continuous veno-venous hemofiltration on outcomes of acute renal failure: a perspective randomized trial. Lancet 2001; 356(9223):26–30.
30. Obialo CI, Hernandes B, Carter D. Delivered dialysis dose is

suboptimal in hospitalized patients. Am J Nephrol 1998; 18:525–30.

31. Sadaghdar H, Lakshmipathi C, Bowles SA, et al. Outcome of renal transplant recipients in the ICU. Chest 1995;107:1402–5.

32. Kogan A, Singer P, Cohen J, et al. Readmission to an intensive care unit following liver and kidney transplantation: a 50 month study. Transplant Proc 1999;31:1892–3.

33. Patel R, Paya CV. Infections in solid-organ transplant recipients. Clin Microbiol Rev 1997;10:86–124.

34. Rubin RH. Infectious complications of renal transplantation. Kidney Int 1993;44:221–36.

35. Sia IG, Paya CV. Infectious complications following renal transplantation. Surg Clin N Am 1998;78:95–112.

36. Paya CV, Fung JJ, Nalesnik MA, et al. Epstein–Barr virus-induced posttransplant lymphoproliferative disorders. Transplantation 1999;68:1517–25.

37. Penn I. Cancers in renal transplant recipients. Adv Ren Replace Ther 2000;7:147–56.

38. Rosenow EC, Wilson WR, Cockerill FR III. Pulmonary disease in the immunocompromised host. (1) Mayo Clin Proc 1985;60: 473–87.

39. Rosenow EC, Wilson WR, Cockerill FR III. Pulmonary disease in the immunocompromised host (2). Mayo Clin Proc 1985;60: 610–31.

40. Jeffrey JA, Raps EC. Critical neurological illness in the immunocompromised patient. Neurol Clin 1995;13:659–77.

41. Kasiske BL. Ischemic heart disease after renal transplantation. Kidney Int 2002;61:356–69.

42. Kahan BD, Ponticelli C. Established immunosuppressive drugs: clinical and toxic effects. In: Kahan BD, Ponticelli C, eds. Principles and practice of renal transplantation. London: Martin Dunitz; 2000:349–414.

43. Bennett WM, Burdmann EA, Ahdoh TF, et al. Nephrotoxicity of immunosuppressive drugs. Nephrol Dial Transplant 1994; 9(Suppl 4):141–5.

44. Edelstein CL, Jacobs JC, Moosa MR. Pulmonary complications in 110 consecutive renal transplant recipients. S Afr Med J 1995; 85:160–3.

45. Anderson DJ, Jordan MC. Viral pneumonia in recipients of solid organ transplants. Semin Respir Infect 1990;5:38–49.

46. Morelon E, Stern M, Israël-Biet D, et al. Characteristics of sirolimus-associated interstitial pneumonitis in renal transplant patients. Transplantation 2001;72:787–90.

47. Humar A, Johnson EM, Gillingham KJ, et al. Venous thromboembolic complications after kidney and kidney–pancreas transplantation: a multivariate analysis. Transplantation 1998;65:229–34.

48. Allen RDM, Michie CA, Murie JA, et al. Deep venous thrombosis after renal transplantation. Surg Gynecol Obstetr 1987;164: 137–42.

49. Gruber SA, Pescovitz RL, Simmons RL, et al. Thromboembolic complications after renal transplantations: results from the randomized trial of cyclosporine v azathioprine-antilymphocyte globulin. Transplant Proc 1987;19:1815–16.

50. Tveit DP, Hypolite I, Bucci J, et al. Risk factors for hospitalization resulting from pulmonary embolism after renal transplantation in the United States. J Nephrol 2001;14:361–8.

51. Reichenberger F, Dickenmann M, Binet I, et al. Diagnostic yield of bronchoalveolar lavage following renal transplantation. Transplant Infect Dis 2001;3:2–7.

52. Sternberg RI, Baughman RP, Dohn MN, et al. Utility of bronchoalveolar lavage in assessing pneumonia in immunosuppressed renal transplant recipients. Am J Med 1993;95:358–64.

53. Johnson PC, Hogg KM, Sarosi GA. The rapid diagnosis of pulmonary infections in solid organ transplant recipients. Semin Respir Infect 1990;5:2–9.

54. John GT, Shankar V, Abraham AM, et al. Risk factors for posttransplant tuberculosis. Kidney Int 2001;60:1148–53.

55. Sakhuja V, Sud K, Kalra OP, et al. Central nervous system complications in renal transplant recipients in a tropical environment. J Neurol Sci 2001;183:89–93.

56. Singh N, Gayowski T, Marino IR. Hemolytic uremic syndrome in solid-organ transplant recipients. Transpl Int 1996;9:68–75.

57. Young BA, Marsh CL, Alpers CE. Cyclosporine-associated thrombotic microangiopathy/hemolytic uremic syndrome following kidney and kidney–pancreas transplantation. Am J Kidney Dis 1996;28:561–71.

58. Aakhus S, Dahl K, Widerøe TE. Cardiovascular morbidity and risk factors in renal transplant patients. Nephrol Dial Transplant 1999;14:648–54.

59. Herzog CA, Ma JZ, Collins AJ. Long-term survival of renal transplant recipients in the United States after acute myocardial infarction. Am J Kidney Dis 2000;36:145–52.

60. Sever MS, Steinmuller DR, Hayes JM, et al. Pericarditis following renal transplantation. Transplantation 1991;51:1229–32.

61. Butterworth PC, Bolia A, Nicholson ML. Recurrent pulmonary oedema caused by iliac artery stenosis in a renal transplant recipient. Nephron 1998;79:119–20.

62. Wüthrich RP, Cicvara-Muzar S, Booy C, et al. Heterozygosity for the factor V Leiden (G1691A) mutation predisposes renal transplant recipients to thrombotic complications and graft loss. Transplantation 2001;72:549–50.

63. Ronco C, Bellomo R. Acute renal failure in patients with kidney transplant: continuous versus intermittent renal replacement therapy. Renal Failure 1996;18:461–70.

64. O'Neill WC, Baumgarten DA. Ultrasonography in renal transplantation. Am J Kidney Dis 2002;39:663–78.

65. Gutiérrez de la Barrera M, Gonzalez R, Zúñiga J, et al. Acute abdomen requiring emergency surgery in renal allograft recipients during a single center cohort follow-up. Transplant Proc 1996;28:3333–4.

66. Pirenne J, Lledo-Garcia E, Benedetti E, et al. Colon perforation after renal transplantation: a single-institution review. Clin Transplant 1997;11:88–93.

67. Stelzner M, Vlahakos DV, Milford EL, et al. Colonic perforation after renal transplantation. J Am Coll Surg 1997;184:63–9.

68. Soravia C, Baldi A, Kartheuser A, et al. Acute colonic complications after kidney transplantation. Acta Chir Belg 1995;95:157–61.

69. Sollinger HW, Odorico JS, Knechtle SJ, et al. Experience with 500 simultaneous pancreas–kidney transplants. Ann Surg 1998; 228:284–96.

70. Auchincloss H, Shaffer D. Pancreas transplantation. In: Ginns LC, Cosimi AB, Morris PJ, eds. Transplantation, Oxford: Blackwell Science; 1999:395–421.

71. Stratta RJ. Mortality after vascularized pancreas transplantation. Surgery 1998;124:823–30.

72. Troppman C, Gruesner AC, Dunn DL, et al. Surgical complications requiring early relaparotomy after pancreas transplantation. Ann Surg 1998;227:255–68.

III

Consultative nephrology in the intensive care unit

17

Clinical pharmacology and therapeutics

Gary R Matzke and Gilles Clermont

CRITICAL ILLNESS AND ACUTE ORGAN SYSTEM FAILURE

Progress in emergency response systems and resuscitation techniques has resulted in a significant improvement in the immediate survival of victims of severe trauma, burns, and infection. However, many early survivors develop a syndrome of progressive and sequential dysfunction of multiple organ systems that may result in prolonged morbidity or death.[1] *Multiple organ dysfunction syndrome* (MODS) accounts for most of the late-onset deaths in critically ill patients.[2,3] Large US epidemiologic studies indicate that physiologic changes, organ failure rates, and survival are similar among patients with infectious and noninfectious causes of MODS.[4,5] Furthermore, organ failure, both in terms of the number of organs failing[6] and the degree of organ dysfunction,[6,7] is the strongest predictor of death. It is estimated that 750 000 cases of sepsis, accompanied by organ dysfunction warranting hospitalization, occur in the USA each year at an annual cost exceeding $16 billion.[8]

Organ dysfunction impairs the metabolism and/or elimination of a large number of pharmacotherapeutic agents used in the treatment of critically ill patients. A prospective study of the incidence of organ dysfunction suggested that 8.8% and 40.2% of patients admitted to an intensive care unit (ICU) will develop hepatic or renal dysfunction, respectively.[9] These data support the importance of recognizing MODS early and the prompt initiation of individualized pharmacotherapeutic regimens.

ACUTE RENAL FAILURE, CHRONIC KIDNEY DISEASE, AND CLINICAL OUTCOME

The incidence of acute renal failure (ARF) on admission to an intensive care unit varies between 5.4% and 25% of patients, depending on how ARF is defined. Renal replacement therapy may be required in 5% of all patients admitted to an ICU, and one-third of these will have baseline renal function impairment.[10] Critically ill patients with ARF are generally sicker, with higher mean APACHE III scores, greater hemodynamic instability, longer ICU length of stay, and higher ICU and hospital mortality than patients without ARF. Recent data suggest that ICU and hospital mortality was roughly 4-fold higher in patients with ARF.[11] Critically ill patients with chronic kidney disease (CKD) have poorer outcomes than patients with normal renal function, as illustrated by the inclusion of CKD as a significant predictor of hospital mortality in APACHE mortality prediction tools.[12,13] However, patients with CKD who have a similar severity of illness, on admission, to those with ARF have a better outcome; mortality in CKD is half of that of patients with ARF, but still double that of patients without renal dysfunction (Fig. 17.1).[10,11] Increased mortality associated with ARF may therefore not be caused by loss of organ function only, since in this case the prognosis of ARF and CKD patients would be comparable. The difference in prognosis is thus probably related to the clinical circumstances that lead to renal dysfunction.

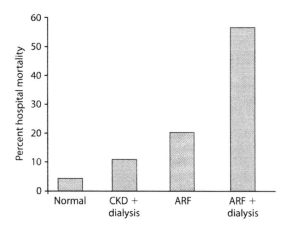

Figure 17.1 Prognostic importance of chronic kidney disease (CKD) and acute renal failure (ARF) in critically ill patients. Hospital mortality is increased in patients with chronically dialysed CKD admitted to the ICU compared to patients who never develop renal dysfunction during their ICU stay. ARF considerably increases the risk of death, in proportion to the intensity of ARF, with a mortality of almost 60% in those patients requiring dialysis. (Adapted from Clermont et al[11] with permission.)

QUANTITATION OF RENAL AND HEPATIC FUNCTION/INJURY

Accurate assessment of renal and hepatic function in critically ill patients is important since the development of multisystem organ failure has been definitively associated with poor prognosis. Furthermore, serial estimates or measurements of renal function are routinely recommended to guide adjustment of drug dosage regimens for individual patients to optimize clinical response and minimize adverse consequences. Although the degree of hepatic injury has been associated with alterations in the distribution and elimination of many drugs,[14–16] no clinically useful noninvasive index of liver function has been developed to guide drug dosage regimen adjustment.[17,18] At the present time, there is no good hepatic counterpart to creatinine clearance (CL_{CR}) or glomerular filtration rate (GFR) estimation or measurements which are sensitive, accurate indices of renal function.

Measurement of renal function

The calculation of CL_{CR} from a timed urine collection with creatinine measurement in serum and urine has been the standard clinical index of renal function. Urine is difficult to accurately collect in

the ICU setting and the fact that many commonly utilized medications interfere with creatinine measurement, especially if colorimetric assay methods such as the Jaffé method are utilized,[19–21] limits the utility of this readily available approach.

Several alternatives to CL_{CR} measurement have been proposed, including:

- the administration of radioactive (^{125}I iothalamate, ^{51}Cr-EDTA, or ^{99m}Tc-DTPA) or nonradioactive (iohexol, iothalamate and inulin) markers of GFR
- the estimation of CL_{CR} or GFR in patients with stable or unstable renal function
- measurement of aminoglycoside (AG) clearance in those receiving one of the agents in this class for therapeutic purposes.[22]

The measurement of GFR, although scientifically sound, is clinically impractical because intravenous (IV) or subcutaneous (SQ) administration of the marker and the collection of multiple timed blood and urine collections makes the test extremely expensive ($500–1500 per measurement) and difficult to perform.

Estimation of CL_{CR} or GFR, however, requires only routinely collected laboratory and demographic data and thus is inexpensive and clinically feasible. The Cockroft and Gault method for CL_{CR}[23] and the Levey method for GFR[24,25] have been demonstrated to correlate well with CL_{CR} and GFR measurements which utilized timed urine collections in individuals with stable renal function:[24,26]

Cockroft and Gault
Men: $CL_{CR} = (140 - Age) \, IBW/(S_{CR} \times 72)$
Women: $CL_{CR} \times 0.85$

Levey et al.
GFR $= 186 \times (S_{CR})^{-1.154} \times [Age]^{-0.203} \times$
$[0.742$ if female$] \times [1.210$ if African-American$]$
('four-variable' (abbreviated) equation in Levey[25]

where IBW = ideal body weight and S_{CR} = serum creatinine.

These methods, however, lose their predictive performance in certain patient populations, e.g. those with liver disease[27–29] as well as critically ill patients with unstable renal function.[19,30,31] Although several methods for CL_{CR} estimation in patients with unstable renal function have been proposed,[21] their ability to estimate CL_{CR} has not been rigorously assessed and at the present time their use cannot be recommended.

The final option, measurement of AG clearance has been shown by Zarowitz et al[22] to be highly correlated with GFR (inulin clearance) in a small population of critically ill patients. This observation extends the data from numerous controlled studies, which indicate a significant relationship between gentamicin or tobramycin clearance and measured CL_{CR} or GFR.[32] This approach may thus be a practical method for serial determinations of renal function in those critically ill patients with documented or suspected infection.

Measurement of hepatic function

Clinically available 'liver function tests' (i.e. serum albumin, bilirubin, alanine aminotransferase, aspartate aminotransferase, etc.) reflect the presence of liver injury but, unlike CL_{CR} or GFR, they do not provide a continuous index of hepatic function or a useful tool for drug therapy individualization. This should not be a surprising finding since 'liver function' is a complex compilation of individual pathways of drug metabolism which may be impacted by liver blood flow, the degree of protein binding of the drug, and the type of liver injury.[14–16]

Although there is no single clinical test of liver function that correlates well with drug clearance, some investigators have proposed indices which utilize discontinuous clinical observations plus laboratory values to predict patient survival and secondarily to prioritize allocation of organs for liver transplantation and categorize the degree of liver dysfunction. The most widely accepted of those methods is Pugh's modification of Child's classification scheme.[33] Recently, Kamath and colleagues have developed a new scoring system (Model for End-Stage Liver Disease [MELD]) and tested it in multiple independent patient groups.[34,35] These scoring systems may be useful to follow an individual patient's course or for comparison of drug disposition between those with mild vs severe organ dysfunction. However, they lack the sensitivity necessary to quantitatively project drug dosage requirements for acutely ill patients.

Three alternatives to measuring endogenous markers of liver function have been proposed:

1. administration of probes for the assessment of hepatic blood flow, e.g. indocyanine green, lidocaine, or galactose[36,37]
2. ingestion of model substrates for the phenotypic determination of the activity of multiple cytochrome P450 (CYP) isozymes or Phase II enzymatic processes, i.e. the 'cocktail approach'[38,39]
3. to ascertain the patient's genotype for those metabolic pathways which are polymorphic.

In some academic research environments, these techniques are currently being evaluated in healthy volunteers, patients with stable liver disease, as well as critically ill patients.

The major limitation of these specific approaches is the multiplicity of processes that may be involved in the hepatic and extrahepatic metabolism of many drugs. Additional limitations include the influence of concomitant drugs on analytical determinations; the effect of concomitant medications or procedures on enzyme activity (induction or inhibition); the invasiveness of the approach that may require the administration of investigational drugs; and, finally, the need for confidentiality of the genetic data that may be generated. At this time, the clinical application of these new techniques for the quantification of liver function is limited.

ALTERED DRUG DISPOSITION AND METABOLISM IN CRITICALLY ILL PATIENTS

Renal insufficiency

Effect on drug absorption
The absorption of a drug from the gastrointestinal (GI) tract may be altered due to renal disease or the result of drug interactions with concomitant medications. Systemic availability of some drugs is increased in CKD patients as a result of a decrease in metabolism during the drug's first pass through the GI tract and liver.[40,41] The systemic availability of four β-blockers, dextropropoxyphene, and dihydrocodeine is increased; however, clinical consequences have been demonstrated only with dextropropoxyphene and dihydrocodeine. The lack of association between the increased systemic availability of the β-blockers and clinical consequences may be a result of an alteration in the responsiveness of patients with renal disease to these agents, as has been reported with propranolol in the elderly.[42]

Effect on drug distribution
The volume of distribution of several drugs is significantly increased in patients with severe

CKD.[32,41,43] Increases may be the result of fluid overload, decreased protein binding, altered tissue binding, or may be an artifact due to the use of an inappropriate calculation method.

The three most commonly used volume of distribution terms are volume of the central compartment (V_c), volume of the terminal phase (V_β), and volume of distribution at steady state (V_{ss}). The V_c, which approximates extracellular fluid volume (approx. 0.2–0.25 L/kg total body weight or TBW) or blood volume (0.05–0.08 L/kg TBW) for many drugs, may be increased in CKD and especially in those with oliguric ARF, which is often accompanied by fluid overload. V_{ss}, will often be similar in magnitude to V_β. In situations in which V_β is much larger than V_{ss}, V_β may reflect the elimination rate more than the distribution volume. Because V_{ss} has the advantage of being independent of drug elimination, it may be the most appropriate volume term to use when one desires to ascertain the influence of renal insufficiency on drug distribution volume.[44]

Effect on drug metabolism

In rat models of CKD, protein expression of several CYP enzymes, including CYP3A1 and CYP3A2 (corresponding to human CYP3A4), is reduced in the liver by as much as 75%.[45] This change appears to be the result of reduced mRNA expression, which indicates transcriptionally mediated down-regulation.[46] Subsequently, enzyme-selective breath test analysis has indicated that CKD has a differential effect on enzyme activity, with CYP2C11 and CYP3A2 being significantly reduced (by 35%), while CYP1A2 activity was unchanged.[47]

Clinical data to support this premise include observations of reduced nonrenal clearance (CL_{NR}) for several drugs in patients with severe CKD.[41,48] These data should be interpreted cautiously because concurrent drug intake, age, smoking habit, and alcohol intake were not often controlled. Furthermore, the possibility of pharmacogenetic variation must be considered. Prediction of the effect of CKD on the metabolism of a particular drug is thus difficult; e.g. nifedipine, nitrendipine, and nisoldipine are all apparently metabolized in vivo by CYP3A4, yet the metabolism of nifedipine is increased,[49] the metabolism of nitrendipine is decreased,[50] and the metabolism of nisoldipine is unaffected by renal failure.[51] Preliminary data suggest a differential effect of CKD on other CYP enzymes: CYP2C19 is reduced, whereas CYP2D6 is not affected.[52] This differential effect on individual enzymes may help to explain some of the conflicting reports of drug metabolism alterations in the presence of severe CKD. The reductions in CL_{NR} for those with CKD are generally proportional to the reductions in GFR. Critically ill patients with ARF, however, may have a higher residual nonrenal clearance of some drugs than patients with CKD who have a similar CL_{CR}.[53–55] This may occur because of less exposure to or accumulation of uremic waste products that may alter hepatic function. A CL_{NR} value in a patient with ARF that is higher than anticipated based on data from CKD patients would result in lower than expected, possibly subtherapeutic, serum concentrations.

Effect on renal excretion

Renal clearance (CL_R) is the composite of GFR, tubular secretion (Cl_{sec}), and reabsorption (Cl_{reabs}):

$$CL_R = (GFR \times f_u) + CL_{sec} - CL_{reabs}$$

where f_u is the fraction of the drug unbound to plasma proteins. Drug elimination by GFR occurs by a diffusion process, but Cl_{sec} and CL_{reabs} are bidirectional processes that involve carrier-mediated renal transport systems. The anionic and cationic secretory pathways are responsible for the transport of a number of acidic and basic drugs, respectively. Other important renal transport systems include the nucleoside and p-glycoprotein transporters, which are involved in the renal tubular excretion of dideoxynucleosides (e.g. zidovudine, dideoxyinosine) and digoxin, respectively.[56] An acute or chronic progressive reduction in GFR thus results in a decrease in CL_R; for drugs that are extensively renally secreted $(CL_R > 300 \text{ ml/min})$, the loss of filtration clearance (up to 120 ml/min) will have less of an impact than for those drugs which are primarily dependent on GFR.

Hepatic insufficiency

Effect on drug absorption

The impact of liver disease on drug absorption/bioavailability has not been well characterized, but is typically offset by a decrease in metabolism and/or an increase in drug distribution. Orally administered drugs may undergo gut wall metabolism as they are absorbed, as well as metabolism in the liver before they reach the systemic circulation. Increased portal pressure has been associated with intestinal edema and reduced absorption of nutrients.[57] The administration of osmotically active substances such as lactulose decreases GI transit time and may also impair absorption.[58] Finally, the decreased availability of bile salts and acids may compromise the absorption of lipophyllic compounds.

Effect on drug distribution

Chronic liver disease affects drug distribution in a number of ways. First, volume of distribution is typically increased because of an increase in total body water, clinically evidenced by the presence of ascites, pleural effusions and peripheral edema.[59] Secondly, hypoalbuminemia results in decreased protein binding for drugs. Thirdly, the accumulation of endogenous compounds such as bilirubin, which has a high affinity for binding sites on albumin, may displace acidic molecules from their binding sites.[60,61] The last two mechanisms result in an effective redistribution that increases the apparent volume of distribution. Consequently, half-life can be increased independent of a reduction in the intrinsic elimination capacity of the liver. The pharmacodynamic consequences of decreased drug binding are difficult to quantify in practice, but are likely to be more important for extensively bound drugs and for patients with higher Child–Pugh scores, marked hypoalbuminemia and hyperbilirubinemia, and significant fluid overload.[62]

Effect on drug metabolism

Liver disease can affect drug disposition mechanisms, blood flow, and intrinsic clearance differentially, and hepatic reserve may vary substantially in different hepatic conditions; thus the relationship between liver insufficiency and drug metabolism is intricate.[63] For example, bilirubin elimination must fall by 90% before hyperbilirubinemia develops, while disturbances in the urea cycle (clinically manifested by hyperammonemia) may be detectable when liver function falls to below 60% capacity.[64] Co-administration of drugs sharing disposition pathways further complicates our understanding. When hepatocytes have a high affinity for a particular substance such that hepatic clearance is large relative to liver blood flow, the elimination of this substance is classified as blood flow rate dependent.[65,66] Conditions where hepatic blood flow may be impaired include cirrhosis, portal hypertension, liver resection surgery, severe decreases in actual or effective intravascular volume, as well as vasopressor therapy. Several enzyme systems contribute to this activity, including the cytochrome P450 system (CYP), as well as

a variety of esterases, hydrolases, dehydrogenases, and reductases. Only the CYP system has been extensively studied in the context of chronic liver disease.[67] Because drugs are metabolized by different CYP isozymes, which may be differentially affected in liver disease, the impact of liver disease on the metabolism of a given drug will depend on which CYP is responsible for its metabolism. Conjugative pathways, such as glucuronidation, are typically maintained until quite late in the clinical course of liver disease,[68] so that the metabolism of some drugs frequently used in the ICU, such as lorazepam and morphine, is relatively well preserved.

Acute liver disease

The pathophysiology of acute liver disease (ALD) is quite different from chronic liver disease and there may be a wide range in the severity of the acute affliction. Although portal hypertension is not a major feature of ALD, oral drug absorption is markedly affected by ileus, nausea, and vomiting. Unless ALD is severe and leads to fulminant failure, there is typically minimal fluid accumulation and probably modest impact on volume of distribution, although hypoalbuminemia can be quite marked. Reduction in liver blood flow is associated with extensive organ damage and is probably only seen in severe ALD. Viral hepatitis has minimal impact on the metabolism of warfarin and phenytoin, while the metabolism of meperidine, diazepam, and lorazepam are significantly affected.[69–71] This appears to be secondary to a differential impact on CYP isoenzyme activity. This effect has not been well documented in other forms of ALD. Patients with fulminant hepatic failure typically present with extensive organ damage and extreme alterations in metabolism, often warranting liver transplantation.[72] The use of extracorporeal liver-assist devices remains investigational and their impact on drug disposition, as opposed to hemodialysis for renal failure, has not been well documented.[73]

Dosing guidelines

Because liver function is difficult to quantify and because different aspects of liver function may deteriorate at different rates, guidelines for drug dosing are generally vague, although some general principles apply (Table 17.1).[74–93] Because hepatic reserve is usually considerable, drug dosage reductions are rarely recommended in mild liver disease or for drugs given acutely, especially if given intravenously. A small (<25%)

Table 17.1	Guidelines for dosing of commonly used drugs in liver dysfunction.		
Elimination mechanism	**Drug**	**Dosing modification**	**References**
Flow-limited	Lidocaine	Decrease by 50%	234
	Metoprolol	Consider decrease	75
	Propranolol	Decrease in severe disease	76
	Labetalol	Decrease oral dose	77
	Verapamil	Decrease by 50%	78
	Morphine	Decrease in severe disease	79, 80
	Midazolam	Decrease	81
	Flumazenil	Consider decrease	82
	Omeprazole	None	83
Enzyme-limited	Cefoperazone	Decrease	84
	Clindamycin	Decrease in severe disease	85
	Metronidazole	Decrease	86
	Nafcillin	Decrease in severe disease	87
	Phenytoin	Decrease in severe disease	88
	Phenobarbital	Decrease in severe disease	74
	Procainamide	Consider decrease	89
	Atracurium	Decrease dose for infusion	90

reduction of drug dosage should be considered for those drugs given orally, where the route of metabolism is predominantly hepatic. In severe liver disease, when drugs are administered chronically, and when there is associated renal dysfunction, reduction of drug dosages of 50% or more may be necessary.[94]

Multisystem organ failure

The onset of MODS is associated with macroscopic organ dysfunction, leading to hypotension, reduced tissue blood flow and a reprioritization of metabolism associated with a marked dysregulation of the inflammatory response. Tumor necrosis factor (TNF) and interleukin-6 (IL-6), for example, have been shown to profoundly modify the acute-phase response in the liver, reprioritizing synthetic pathways and down-regulating the CYP system.[95,96] In addition, MODS is a dynamic process and its impact on drug absorption and disposition varies over time. It is the confluence of these factors that mandates clinicians to be especially vigilant in proper dosing of drugs in patients with MODS.

STRATEGIES FOR DRUG THERAPY INDIVIDUALIZATION

Knowledge of basic pharmacokinetic principles combined with the drug disposition properties of a particular compound and the type and degree of pathophysiologic alterations associated with critical illness makes it possible for the clinician to design an individualized therapeutic regimen. This section provides a practical approach for drug dosage individualization for critically ill patients as well as those receiving continuous renal replacement therapy or hemodialysis.

The design of individualized therapeutic regimens for critically ill patients requires an assessment of the functional capacity of the major organ systems and is dependent on the availability of an accurate characterization of the relationship between the pharmacokinetic parameters of a given drug and organ function. Secondary references such as the *American Hospital Formulary Service (AHFS) Drug Information,*[97] and text books[98] are excellent sources of information about a drug's pharmacokinetic characteristics in subjects with normal renal and hepatic function. However, they often do not provide the explicit relationships of the kinetic parameters of interest (total body clearance and distribution volume) with a continuous index of organ function such as CL_{CR} or GFR. Ideally, one should be able to identify relationships between total body clearance (CL_T), elimination rate constant (Ke) or distribution volume (V_D) with an index of renal (CL_{CR} or GFR) or hepatic function (Child–Pugh score). These relationships, along with the patient's CL_{CR}, will enable prediction of the patient's kinetic parameters and the subsequent formulation of a therapeutic regimen to attain the desired therapeutic outcome. The clinical measurement or estimation of GFR or CL_{CR} remains the primary guiding factor for drug dosage regimen design in critically ill patients.[41] The estimation of CL_{CR} for adults and children is most accurate for individuals of average muscle mass for their age, weight, and height. The creatinine clearance of emaciated and obese adult patients is difficult to predict.

The importance of an alteration in renal function on drug disposition depends on two factors: the fraction of drug normally eliminated by the kidney unchanged and the degree of renal insufficiency. If the relationships of CL_T or Ke with CL_{CR} are not known, then one can estimate the kinetic parameters of the patient provided the fraction of the drug that is eliminated renally unchanged (f_e) in subjects with normal renal function is known. This approach assumes that the change in CL_T or Ke is proportional to CL_{CR}, that renal disease does not alter the drug's metabolism, that the metabolites if formed are inactive and nontoxic, that the drug obeys first-order (linear) kinetic principles, and that it is adequately described by a one-compartment model. If these assumptions are true, then the kinetic parameter/dosage adjustment factor (Q) can be calculated as:

$$Q = 1 - [f_e(1 - KF)]$$

and the estimated total body clearance can be calculated as

$$CL_{PT} = CL_{normT} \times Q$$

where CL_{normT} is the value in patients with normal renal function and KF is the ratio of the patient's CL_{CR} to an assumed normal value of 120 ml/min.

The best method for dosage regimen adjustment is dependent on the desired goal; i.e. the maintenance of a similar peak (C_{max}), trough (C_{min}), or average steady-state drug concentration (C_{ave}). If there is a significant relationship between C_{max} and

clinical response[99] (e.g. aminoglycosides) or toxicity[100] (e.g. quinidine, phenobarbital, and phenytoin), then attainment of the specific target values is critical. In this case, the dose and dosing interval may both need to be changed. If, however, no specific target values for C_{max} or C_{min} concentrations have been reported (e.g. antihypertensive agents and benzodiazepines), then attaining the same C_{ave} may be appropriate (see Fig. 17.2).

The desired C_{ave} profile, can be achieved by decreasing the dose ($D_{PT} = D_{NORM} \times Q$) or prolonging the dosing interval (τ) ($\tau_{PT} = \tau_{NORM}/Q$). If the size of the dose is reduced while the dosing interval remains unchanged, the C_{max} will be lower and the C_{min} higher. Alternatively, if the dosing interval is increased, the C_{max} and C_{min} in the patient will be similar to those with normal renal function. This dosage adjustment method is often utilized because it results in a reduction in nursing and pharmacy time, as well as in the supplies associated with frequent drug administration (Fig. 17.2).

Continuous renal replacement therapy

There are marked differences with regard to drug removal between intermittent hemodialysis and

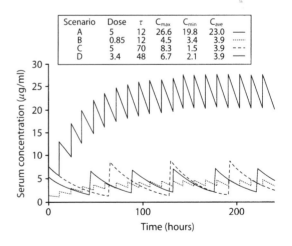

Scenario	Dose	τ	C_{max}	C_{min}	C_{ave}	
A	5	12	26.6	19.8	23.0	——
B	0.85	12	4.5	3.4	3.9	·······
C	5	70	8.3	1.5	3.9	- - -
D	3.4	48	6.7	2.1	3.9	——

Figure 17.2 Without a change in dosage regimen this patient would achieve excessive steady-state serum concentrations (Scenario A). Although the average steady-state concentrations (C_{ave}) are identical, the concentration–time profile will be markedly different if one changes the dose and maintains the dosing interval (τ) constant (Scenario B), vs changing the dosing interval (τ) and maintaining the dose constant (Scenario C) or changing both (Scenario D). (Used with permission from Frye and Matzke[101].)

the three primary types of continuous renal replacement therapy (CRRT):

- continuous arteriovenous or venovenous hemofiltration (CAVH/CVVH)
- continuous arteriovenous or venovenous hemodialysis (CAVHD/CVVHD)
- continuous arteriovenous or venovenous hemodiafiltration (CAVHDF/CVVHDF).

CAVH/CVVH primarily removes drugs via convection/ultrafiltration (the passive transport of drugs at the concentration which they exist in plasma water into the ultrafiltrate). The clearance of a drug is thus a function of the permeability of the hemofilter, which is called the sieving coefficient (SC) and the rate of ultrafiltrate formation (UFR). The SC of a drug can be simply calculated as the concentration in the ultrafiltrate (C_{uf}) divided by the concentration in the plasma entering the hemofilter (C_a):

$$SC = C_{uf}/C_a.$$

Although the SC is most precisely characterized as:

$$SC = (2C_{uf})/[(C_a/1 - \theta) + (C_v/1 - \theta)]$$

where C_v is the concentration in the plasma effluent and θ is 0.0107 times the total protein concentration in plasma, this approach is rarely utilized.[101] The SC is often approximated by the fraction unbound to plasma proteins (f_u), because plasma concentrations of the drug of interest may not be readily available. Thus, the clearance by CAVH/CVVH can be estimated as:

$$CL_{CVVH} = UFR \times f_u.$$

Clearance of a drug by CAVHDF/CVVHDF can be estimated, providing the blood flow rate is greater than 100 ml/min and dialysate flow rate (DFR) is between 8 and 33 ml/min as:

$$CL_{CVVHDF} = (UFR + DFR) \times (f_u \text{ or } SC).$$

If UFR is negligible (<3 ml/min) as is often the case with CAVHD/CVVHD, CL_{CVVHD} can be estimated as the product of DFR and f_u or SC. In the clinical setting, the CL_{CVVHDF} or CL_{CVVHD} is calculated as the product of the combined ultrafiltrate and dialysate flow rate and ratio of the concentration of the drug in this fluid to the plasma concentration.

An algorithmic approach for drug dosage adjustment in patients undergoing CRRT has been proposed.[102] Individualization of therapy for a patient receiving CRRT therapy is dependent on the patient's residual renal function and the clearance of the drug by the mode of CRRT they are receiving. The patient's residual drug clearance can be predicted based on their CL_{CR} and the relationship between CL_T or Ke of the drug with CL_{CR}. The CRRT clearance can be ascertained from the literature or estimated as described above. The CRRT clearance, SC, and recommend initial dosage regimens of selected drugs which are frequently utilized in ICU patients receiving CAVH/CVVH are listed in Table 17.2.[54,103–127] Values observed in patients receiving CAVVHD/CVVHD or CAVHDF/CVVHDF are listed in Table 17.3.[103,108,109,112,113,120,125,128–142]

Hemodialysis

The impact of intermittent acute hemodialysis on a patient's drug therapy is dependent on the characteristics of the drug and the dialysis conditions. Drug-related factors include the molecular weight, protein binding, and volume of distribution.[41] The dialysis prescription factors include the composition of the dialyzer, the surface area, and blood and dialysate flow rates. Over 150 dialyzers composed of cellulose-based, semisynthetic or synthetic materials (e.g. polysulfone, polymethylmethacrylate, or polyamide) are currently available in the USA. The semisynthetic and synthetic dialyzers used in high-flux hemodialysis (HFD) have the largest ultrafiltration rates and pore sizes and more closely mimic the filtration characteristics of the human kidney. This allows the passage of most solutes, including drugs that have a molecular weight of 15 000 or less.[143] High-molecular-weight drugs such as vancomycin are significantly cleared by this mode of dialysis and the clearance of many smaller drugs has also been reported to be significantly increased (Table 17.4).[140,144–180] The net result is that the patient receiving high-flux dialysis will require larger doses to maintain the desired concentrations.

The impact of hemodialysis on drug therapy is not answerable by simple 'yes-no' reference materials. Quantification of the impact of hemodialysis is necessary for the clinician who needs to design a dosing regimen for an individual patient. The effect of hemodialysis on drug disposition can be calculated in several ways.[41] The difference between the half-life during dialysis ($t_{1/2,onHD}$), and

Table 17.2 Pharmacokinetics and clearance of drugs in patients receiving CVVH/CAVH.

Drug	Hemofilter	UFR (ml/h)	$t_{1/2}$ (h)*	CL_T (ml/min)*	SC*	CL_{CVVH} (ml/min)*	Dosage recommendation
Acyclovir	PS-A	150	88	0.39	NR	NR	5 mg/kg q 12 h
Amikacin	PS	600	29.7	10.5	0.93	10.1	IND
	PS	1152	11.4	39	NR	16.4	
Amrinone	PS	245–576	–	40.8	0.8–1.4	2.4–14.4	None provided
Atracurium	PA	1140	–	502.5	NR	8.25	None provided
Ceftazidime	AN69[a]	500–1000	–	–	0.97	7.5–15.6	500 mg q 12 h
	PMMA	500–1000	–	–	0.8	6.7–12.9	
	PS	500–1000	–	–	0.97	7.6–15.5	
Ceftriaxone	AN69	500–1000	–	–	0.48	4–7.7 h	300 mg q 12 h
	PMMA	500–1000	–	–	0.86	7.1–11.9 h	
	PS	500–1000	–	–	0.82	6.9–11.3 h	
	PA	1200–1800	10.8	39.3	0.69	16.6	1000 mg q 24 h
Cefuroxime	PS	850	7.9	32	NR	11	0.75–1.0 g q 24 h
Ciprofloxacin	AN69[a]	1000	18.5	84.4	0.72	12.4	400 mg q 24 h
Fluconazole	AN69[a]	1167	37.7	25.3	0.96	17.5	400–800 mg q 24 h
Gentamicin	PS	140–393	34.6	11.6	NR	3.47	IND
	PS	322.3	65.4	NR	NR	1.5–12.5	
Imipenem	PS	1000	2.9	108.3	0.8	13.3	500 mg q 6–8 h
	PS	1000	3	64.4	0.8	13.3	
	PS	72–828	2.2	103	1.16	6.6	
Cilastatin	PS	72–828	13.8	29	0.77	4	
Levofloxacin	AN69	1155	26.9	42.3	0.62	11.5	250 mg q 24 h
Meropenem	PA	1500–1800	6.37	76	0.63	16.7	0.5–1.0 g q 12 h
	PAN	6000–9000	8.7	52	1.17	22	
	PS	2760	2.3	143.7	1.09	49.7	
	PAN	100–2000	5.9	64.7	0.95	24.9	
Phenytoin	PS	165	–	–	0.37	1.02	IND
Piperacillin (PIP)	NR	1560	5.9	42	–	NR	PIP: 4 g q 12 h
Tazobactam (TAZO)	NR	1560	8.1	74	–	NR	PIP/TAZO:2.25– 3.375 g q 8 h
Ticarcillin	PS	NR	4.60	29.7	0.83	12.3	2 g q 8–12 h
Clavulanic acid	PS	NR	2.45	128.5	1.69	25.2	
Tobramycin	PS	140–393	34.6	11.7	–	3.5	IND
Vancomycin	PA	1000	36.5	21.9	0.7	23.3	750–1250 mg q 24 h
	AN69[a]	500–1000	–	–	0.7	5.6–11.7	
	PMMA	500–1000	–	–	0.86	6.9–14.4	
	PS	500–1000	–	–	0.68	5.6–11.4	
	PA	1231	4.1	185	0.73–0.79	152.6	
	PS	NR	45	13.8	0.5–0.94	6.3	
	PS	1000–2000	18.4	28.5	0.8	6.7–13.3	

CL_{CVVH} = CVVH clearance; CL_T = total body clearance; SC = sieving coefficient; $t_{1/2}$ = half-life; UFR = ultrafiltration rate; V_d = volume of distribution; NR = not reported; – = data not determined; IND = dosage individualization required; [a] = Amicon diafilter 20; * = Data are mean or range.

Table 17.3 Pharmacokinetics and clearance of drugs in patients receiving CAVHD/CVVHD.

Drug	Hemofilter	DFR (L/h)	UFR (ml/h)	$t_{1/2}$ (h)*	CL_T (ml/min)*	SC*	CL_{CVVHD} (ml/min)*	Dosage recommendation
Acyclovir	AN69	0.9–1.0	65–115	30	1.2	NR	NR	5 mg/kg q 12 h
Ceftazidime	AN69[a]	1.0–2.0	448	14.7	24.8	0.86	13.1–15.2	1 g q 24 h
	AN69	1.0–2.0	30–180	–	–	0.97	13.5–21.6	0.5–1 g q 12 h
	PMMA	1.0–2.0	30–180	–	–	0.80	16.6–27.5	
	PS	1.0–2.0	30–180	11.9	31.3	0.97	14.5–24.2	
Ceftriaxone	AN69	1.0–2.0	30–180	–	–	0.48	11.7–13.2 h	250 mg q 12 h
	PMMA	1.0–2.0	30–180	–	–	0.86	19.8–30.5 h	300 mg q 12 h
	PS	1.0–2.0	30–180	–	–	0.82	21.8–29.6 h	
Cefuroxime	AN69[a]	1.0–2.0	448	12.6	22.3	0.9	14–16.2	750 mg q 12 h
Ciprofloxacin	AN69[a]	1.0–2.0	434	6.4	264.3	0.76	16.2–19.9	300 mg q 12 h
	AN69	1	NR	9.4	203	0.70	37	
	AN69	0.8–1	1044	8.3	146	0.63	21	
Fluconazole	AN69[a]	1	–	33.8	21.6	1.04	25	400–800 mg q 12 h
	AN69	1	1158	23.8	37.9	0.88	30.5	
Ganciclovir	AN69[a]	1	–	18.9	32.6	0.84	12.9	2.5 mg/kg q 24 h
Gentamicin	AN69[a]	1	420	27	20.5	–	5.2	IND
Imipenem	AN69[b]	1.0–3.0	500	1.9, 1.7	134	1.05	16–30	500 mg q 6–8 h
	PS	1.5	NR	3.5	183	NR	11.6	
Cilastatin	AN69[b]	1	500	14.9, 9.2	13, 21	0.68	10	
Levofloxacin	AN69	1	1110	18.6	51.2	0.60	21.7	250 mg q 24 h
Meropenem	PAN	2	NR	4.3	141.3	1.02	20	1000 mg q 8–12 h
	PAN	1.6	NR	4.5	54.6	1.06	30.4	
	PAN	1–1.5	NR	4.4	78.7	0.92	38.9	
Mezlocillin	AN69 & PS	1.0–2.0	0–200	1.1–8.8	31–253	NR	11–44.9	2–4 g q 24 h
Sulbactam	AN69 & PS	1.0–2.0	0–200	4.3–6.4	32–54	NR	10.1–22.8	0.5 g q 24 h
Piperacillin (PIP)	AN69	1.50	80–200	4.3	47	0.84	22	PIP: 4 g q 12 h
Tazobactam (TAZO)	AN69	1.50	80–200	5.6	29.5	0.64	17	PIP/TAZO 3.375 g q 8–12 h
Teicoplanin	AN69[b]	1	258–650	99	9.2	NR	3.6	LD: 800 mg 400 mg q 24 h × 2, then q 48–72 h
Vancomycin	AN69[a]	1.0–2.0	570	24.7	31	0.66	12.1–16.6	7.5 mg/kg q 12 h
	AN69[a]	0.5	474	13.9	38.9	NR	4.2	
	AN69[a]	1	162	56.3	17.1	NR	8.1	
	AN69	1.0–2.0	30–180	–	–	0.7	10–13.4	
	PMMA	1.0–2.0	30–180	–	–	0.86	14.7–27.0	1.0–1.5 g q 24 h
	PS	1.0–2.0	30–180	27.2	35.7	0.68	11.4–22.1: 22.3	0.85–1.35 g q 24 h

CL_{CVVH} = CVVH clearance; CL_T = total body clearance; SC = sieving coefficient; $t_{1/2}$ = half-life; UFR = ultrafiltration rate; V_d = volume of distribution; NR = not reported; – = data not determined; IND = dosage individualization required; LD = loading dose; * = data are mean or range; [a] = Amicon diafilter 20; [b] = Amicon diafilter 30.

Table 17.4   Hemodialysis clearance and fraction removed by hemodialysis.

Drug	Dialyzer utilized	Type of dialyzer*	Calculated % removed in # of hours		CL_D (ml/min)*	Dosage recommendation
Acyclovir	UNK	UNK	45	in 3 hours	113	5–10 mg/kg q 24 h
	UNK	UNK	51	in 4–5 hours	UNK	LD: 6 mg/kg MD: 3 mg/kg q 12 h
Amikacin	Multiple	CU,CA,RC,PA	20–90	in 4 hours	32–125	LD: 5–7.5 mg/kg MD: IND q 48 h
Ampicillin	CDAK 3500	CA	35–40	in 4 hours	30–60	1000 mg q 12 h
Sulbactam	C-DAK 3500	CA	45	in 4 hours	87.1	0.75–1.5 g q 24–48 h
Aztreonam	GAMBRO LUNDIA	CU	38	in 4 hours	43	LD: 1 g MD: 05 g q 12 h
Cefazolin	BAXTER CT 190	CTA	NR		30.9	15–20 mg/kg q 48–72 h
	TERUMO T175/220	C	NR		20.0	
	BAXTER CA170/210	CA	NR		15.1	
	FRESENIUS F80	POLY	50	in 3–4 hours	38	1 g q 48–72 h
Cefmetazole	BAXTER CA170/210	CA	60	in 3 hours	86.1	2 g q 48–72 h
Ceftazidime	BAXTER CF 2308	CU	41.3	in 4 hours	60	1 g q 48 h
	FRESENIUS F-60	POLY	77.3	in 4 hours	155	1 g q 24 h
Cefepime	BAXTER CA210/170	CA	68	in 3 hours	158	1–2 g q 48–72 h
	FRESENIUS F-60	POLY	72	in 3.5 hours	126.8	
Ceftriaxone	BELLCO BL611	H	21	in 4 hours	24	0.5–1 g q 24 h
	FRESENIUS E2	CU	22	in 4 hours	31.6	
	FRESENIUS F40	POLY	24	in 4 hours	41.9	
Ceftizoxime	GAMBRO LUNDIA	C	NR		44.8	1 g q 48 h
Clavulanic acid	BELLCO BL 612-M	CU	65	in 4 hours	92.8	100 mg q 12–24 h
Ticarcillin	BAXTER UF II	CU	NR		46.0	3 g q 12 h
Fluconazole	UNK	UNK	40–50	in 4 hours	NR	0.2–0.8 g q 48 h
	UNK	UNK	38	in 3 hours	NR	
Ganciclovir	GAMBRO LUNDIA IC 3L	CU	62.5	in 4 hours	48.3	LD: 5 mg/kg MD: 0.5 mg/kg q 48–72 h
Gentamicin	Multiple	CA,CU,CR	40–50	in 4 hours	27–58	LD: 1.7 mg/kg MD: 0.8 mg/kg q 48–72 h or IND
	FRESENIUS F-80	POLY	50–60	in 3 hours	116	LD: 2 mg/kg MD: 1 mg/kg q 48–72 h or IND
Imipenem/ cilistatin	GAMBRO LUNDIA 1m2	CU	55–63	in 4 hours	84/41	0.25–0.5 g q 12 h
Meropenem	GAMBRO GFE 11,15,18	CU	NR		19	0.5 g q 24 h
	UNK	CU	51	in 4 hours	22	1 g q 48–72 h
Metronidazole	Multiple	CA,CU,RC	44.9	in 4 hours	70–125	0.5–1.0 g q 8 h
Mezlocillin	Multiple	CU,C	62	in 6 hours	24–67	2–4 g q 8 h
Ofloxacin	GAMBRO IC 3N	CU	21.5	in 4 hours	59.2	200 mg q 24–48 h
Phenobarbital	UNK	UNK	NR		60.5	30 mg q 6–8 h
Piperacillin (PIP)	BAXTER CF 1511	CU	42	in 4 hours	78.2	4 g q 12 h
	BAXTER CA210	CA	31	in 3 hours	69.4	
Sulfamethoxazole	TERUMO TE-10	CU	57	in 4 hours	42	See Trimethoprim
Tazobactam (TAZO)	BAXTER CA210	CA	39	in 3 hours	94.6	PIP/TAZO 2.25 g q8h

Table 17.4 *Continued.*

Drug	Dialyzer utilized	Type of dialyzer*	Calculated % removed in # of hours		CL_D (ml/min)*	Dosage recommendation
Teicoplanin	FRESENIUS F8	POLY	9	in 4 hours	3.9	6 mg/kg q 72 h
	FRESENIUS F60	POLY	20	in 4 hours	NR	
	FRESENIUS F60	POLY	19.3	in 3–4 hours	39.7	LD: 800 mg MD: 400 mg day 2, 3, 5, 12, 19 & IND
Tobramycin	CDAK 3500	CA,CU	NR		30–55	LD: 1.7 mg/kg MD: 0.8–1.0 mg/kg q 48–72 h or IND
Trimethoprim	TERUMO TE-10	CU	44	in 4 hours	38	5 mg/kg q 48–72 h
Vancomycin	BAXTER CA-210	C	12.8	in 4 hours	NR	15 mg/kg, q 7 days
	FRESENIUS F-80	POLY	45.7	in 4 hours	130.7	LD: 15–25 mg/kg, MD: 5 mg/kg q 48–72 h
	BAXTER CT-190	CTA	25.2	in 4 hours	100.7	
	Hospal, Filtral 16	PA	NR		54.4	

UNK = unknown; NR = not reported; C = cellulose; CA = cellulose acetate; CTA = cellulose triacetate; CU = cuprophane; CR = cuprammonium rayon; H = hemophan; PMMA = polymethylmethocralate; PA = polyacryonitrile; POLY = polysulfone; IV = in vitro data; RC = regenerated cellulose; LD = loading dose; MD = maintenance does; * = mean or range; IND = individualize.

the half-life of the drug when the patient is off dialysis provides only a crude guide to the impact of dialysis. The $t_{1/2,onHD}$ may not be interpretable in ARF patients because declining plasma drug concentrations during dialysis represent elimination by the patient, which may be considerable, as well as by dialysis. Furthermore, if significant rebound in drug concentrations after dialysis has been reported, the removal of drug by the dialysis procedure may be perceived to be artificially high, depending on when, after dialysis, the post-dialysis concentration is collected.[126,153,155]

A more accurate means of assessing the effect of hemodialysis is to calculate the dialyzer clearance (CL_D) of the drug.[41] The clearance from blood (CL^b_D) can be calculated as

$$CL^b_D = Q_b [(A_b - V_b)/A_b]$$

where Q_b is blood flow through the dialyzer, A_b is the concentration of drug in blood going into the dialyzer, and V_b is the concentration of drug in the blood leaving the dialyzer. Because drug concentrations are generally determined in plasma, the previous equation is usually modified to allow calculation of plasma clearance by the dialyzer

$$CL^p_D = Q_p [(A_p - V_p)/A_p]$$

where p represents plasma and Q_p is plasma flow, which equals Q_b (1 − hematocrit). Finally, the recovery clearance approach can be utilized for the determination of dialyzer clearance:

$$CL^r_D = R/AUC_{0-t}$$

where R is the total amount of drug recovered unchanged in the dialysate and AUC_{0-t} is the area under the predialyzer plasma concentration–time curve during hemodialysis.[41]

Drug dosage regimen individualization can be accomplished by using values of CL_D, volume of distribution, or half-life during dialysis from the literature.[32,41,43,100] Because clearance terms are additive, the total clearance during dialysis can be calculated as the sum of the patient's residual total body clearance (CL_{PT}) and CL_D. The half-life during the period between dialysis treatments can then be calculated using an estimate of the drug's distribution volume (V_D).

Once the key pharmacokinetic parameters have been estimated, they may be used to simulate the plasma concentration–time profile of the drug for the individual patient and ascertain how much drug to administer and when. This approach to drug therapy individualization can be accomplished in a stepwise fashion assuming first-order elimination of the drug and a one-compartment model. The CL_D and fraction of drug removed during hemodialysis for several drugs commonly administered to ICU patients are listed in Table 17.4 along with initial dosage recommendations.

EMERGING CHALLENGES IN CRITICAL ILLNESS PHARMACOTHERAPY

Management of anemia

Recent studies suggest that, although transfusion of red blood cells to maintain hematocrit may be harmful to patients,[181] there is probably a threshold below which outcome is so adversely affected by anemia associated with acute illness that transfusions should be considered.[182–185] Transfusions have been proposed as part of early goal-directed therapy in patients with severe sepsis, an intervention strategy that appears to be highly beneficial.[186] Because of the recent concerns with infectious agents and the ongoing potential problems with transfusion reactions, alternatives to blood products to maintain hematocrit have been sought with vigor. Recombinant human erythropoietin may become widely used in the ICU setting, where temporary marrow dysfunction is a very common problem associated with the postoperative state or organ dysfunction.[187] Few trials have explored the role of erythropoietin in reducing the need for red cell transfusion in the critically ill and the guidelines for potential use remain unclear.[183,188] The introduction of this potentially expensive modality should be directed by careful pharmacoeconomic assessment that includes potential long-term complications related to transfusion therapy.

Management of sedation and pain in the intensive care unit

Recent efforts to document and standardize sedation practice have led to several evidence-based guidelines regarding the drugs of choice and optimal method of delivery in critically ill patients.[189–191] The use of appropriate drug regimens and routes of administration (e.g. epidural or patient-controlled analgesia) relate predominantly to proper education and dissemination of existing

guidelines. Newer and more expensive drugs, such as propofol, will find appropriate therapeutic niches, but should be considered as adjcts, and not substitutions, to the more widely recommended regimens. Rigorous pharmacoeconomic assessment should be completed before the acceptance of these agents on hospital formularies.[192,193] It is paramount that the use of drugs with proven safety profiles and minimal hemodynamic compromise is optimized (predominantly benzodiazepines and opiates); for example, daily interruption of infusions of sedative drugs has been associated with decreased duration of mechanical ventilation.

Neuromuscular paralysis

An improved understanding of the long-term implications of neuromuscular paralysis[194] and the development of improved techniques in the delivery of mechanical ventilation have redefined the role of neuromuscular paralysis in the ICU.[195–197] Because of the possibility of prolonged weakness and its devastating consequences, despite adequate monitoring, and the difficulty in titrating sedation in paralyzed patients, neuromuscular blockade should be restricted to situations where mechanical ventilation cannot be provided safely and adequately otherwise.[198] Adequately sedated patients may tolerate ventilation modalities such as inverse ratio ventilation and high-frequency ventilation without continuous administration of paralytic agents. There are therefore no recommended indications for neuromuscular paralysis, although the experienced clinician will recognize their utility in a limited number of patients.[199]

Antibiotic resistance

The rapid emergence of multidrug-resistant strains of ICU pathogens, their documented role in the pathogenesis of infection, and the increase in the size of a vulnerable population of immunoincompetent patients have resulted in the initiation of major institutional efforts to contain the spread of organisms such as vancomycin-resistant *enterococcus faecium*, vancomycin-insensitive or resistant strains of staphylococci, and multidrug-resistant Gram-negative bacteria.[200–203] Successful strategies to contain this spread will depend heavily on antibiotic cycling, controlled use of broad-spectrum agents, and simpler, but time-honored physical modalities.[204] Furthermore, institutional strategies are intrinsically limited in their potential success, since many of these organisms are now prevalent in the community. Broader interventions targeting nursing homes, other community-based healthcare delivery arenas, and regional hospital systems are likely to be required to enhance the effectiveness of interventions designed to contain the spread of highly resistant organisms.[205–207]

PHARMACOECONOMICS OF PHARMACOTHERAPEUTIC INTERVENTIONS IN THE INTENSIVE CARE UNIT

The cost of care of critically ill patients is impacted because of the aging population, more people being admitted to the ICU, and the high costs of designer drugs and new generations of antibiotics. Decisions to include emerging therapies on hospital formularies are increasingly driven by attempts to quantify the 'added-value' of these therapies over existing alternatives and over other drugs also competing for acceptance in the marketplace of ICU therapies. Methods for the valuation of effects and costs of interventions are undergoing intense development. Recently, the Panel on Cost-Effectiveness in Health and Medicine (PCEHM) formulated recommendations that constitute a useful template for comparative evaluation of pharmacotherapeutic agents.[208,209] The medical literature often reports societally based economic analyses of emerging or existing therapies. Such evaluations should indeed be conducted. However, payers, pharmacies, and end-users will typically have specific interests that diverge from this societal perspective. Accordingly, published pharmacoeconomic assessments may or may not have direct relevance for healthcare providers and payers, depending on the cost and level of compensation of this therapy in a given environment.

Measuring effect

A new therapy, when evaluated as part of a randomized trial, is typically compared to a placebo or standard of care.[210] Thus, one really measures incremental benefit or detriment of the new therapy. Effect can be measured a number of ways, including lives saved, avoidance of adverse effects, the need for expensive treatment modalities, or the achievement of a specific endpoint thought to have societal or human value, such as avoidance of tracheal intubation and mechanical ventilation.

Endpoints that are specific for a given intervention in a critically ill patient may not allow fair comparisons of efficacy with interventions in other patient populations competing for healthcare dollars. Therefore, a common metric to measure effect is required to conduct such comparisons.[211] Although a life saved appears to be a fairly universal unit of effect, some attempt should be made at further describing the quality of life during this time. For example, it would be inappropriate to believe that an intervention allowing patients to live 3 more months with life support in the ICU but without other health benefits is indeed beneficial. Several scales have been described to quantify quality or utility of life.[208,212,213] These scales attribute, on a scale of 0 (dead or worst possible quality of life) to 1 (perfect quality of life), some value to quality of life. Muliplying survival by quality of life yields quality-adjusted life years (QALYs). The PCEHM has recommended the use of the QALY as the most desirable measure of effect. QALYs can be compared across interventions in different venues of health care and elsewhere.[214]

Measuring cost

When comparing interventions in health care, several components of costs can be evaluated in addition to direct medical costs. Recent guidelines of the PCEHM recommend including indirect costs such as lost wages and intangible costs such as valuation of suffering whenever possible.[208,209] Furthermore, attempts should be made to evaluate costs for as long a period as differences in clinical effects persist, possibly a life time.[215] The perspective of analysis will dictate which costs are included. Although, the PCEHM also recommends adapting a societal perspective when reporting costs, healthcare providers or pharmacists may clearly have a very different perspective on the valuation of costs. Institutional or corporate decisions and policies (such as the inclusion of an expensive drug on formulary) are typically based on a nonsocietal perspective, and may not necessarily follow a utilitarian principle. This creates a difficult situation in the current economic context. There is a clear temptation for payers and providers to neglect incremental effects between two drugs in favor of a more immediate cost-saving strategy and thus reduce pharmacoeconomic assessment to a cost-minimization exercise. This tacitly assumes equal effect between drug A and drug B.

Comparing cost-effectiveness

Dividing incremental costs by incremental effects yields a cost-effectiveness ratio, the recommended metric to express cost-effectiveness across a large breath of curative or preventive health interventions.[214] A decade ago, Laupacis et al published guidelines on adoption and utilization of emerging technologies.[216] These authors suggest that therapies can be classified into five grades of recommendation. A grade A intervention is more effective and cheaper than standard therapy. Grades B through D are more effective and more costly; grade B technology costs less than $20 000/QALY, grade C $20 000–$100 000/QALY, and a grade D more than $100 000/QALY. A grade E intervention is more expensive and harmful, and thus should never be adopted. Since evaluating incremental costs and effectiveness is associated with uncertainties, results of cost-effectiveness analyses are typically presented as a best-estimate cost-effectiveness ratio with 95% confidence intervals or ellipse of confidence (Fig. 17.3).[217]

Differences in perspectives can then be more completely illustrated. For example, a drug administered to neonates costs $1000, but results in one additional life saved this year out of the 1000 neonates treated. The hospital pharmacy perspective is that this drug is hardly cost-effective ($1 000 000/life saved). Society, on the other hand, considers that this neonate will have 80 years of good health and evaluates a cost-effectiveness of $12 500/QALY. From a societal perspective drug A therefore represents a highly desirable intervention. Mechanisms to resolve those divergences will require multilateral efforts that will include rethinking reimbursement strategies and possibly rescaling what is currently considered societally acceptable and affordable.

IMPROVING PHARMACOTHERAPY IN THE INTENSIVE CARE UNIT

Medication errors

The landmark report of the Institute of Medicine attributed between 44 000 and 98 000 deaths annually to medical errors.[218–220] A significant proportion of these medical errors are related to the administration of drugs to patients. Medication-related errors may contribute to as many as 7000 deaths annually. Recent reports suggest rates between 3.13 and 6.5 adverse drug events per 1000 orders, with the rate of significant errors to be 1.81

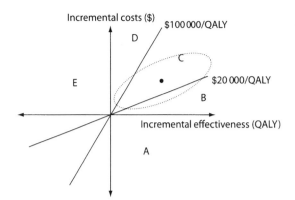

Figure 17.3 The cost-effectiveness plane. Incremental costs (cost of new therapy − costs of established standard) are typically depicted on the y-axis, while incremental effectiveness, quantified in quality-adjusted life years (QALYs), is depicted on the x-axis. The best estimate of the cost-effectiveness ratio of a new therapy is represented by a point in the x–y plane. The uncertainty around this estimate may be represented in several ways: a 95% confidence ellipse around the best estimate is an intuitive way of representing this uncertainty. The cost-effectiveness plane is divided in zones representing the spectrum (A–E) between more-effective/less-costly therapies (zone A) and less-effective/more-costly (zone E) therapies. Standard thresholds of acceptability ($20 000/QALY and $100 000/QALY lines) have been published. See the text for more details.

per 1000 orders, or 20% of all adverse drug events.[221,222] Moreover, medication errors are underreported and many are preventable.[223]

The Leapfrog Group, a coalition of more than 100 public and private organizations that provide healthcare benefits, has promulgated three major initiatives to enhance the safety and quality of care of critically ill patients (www.leapfroggroup.org). The first of these initiatives is computerized physician entry of medication orders, a practice that could reduce serious medication errors by as much as 86%. It is to be expected that a growing number of payers, private and public, will require computerized physician order entry. The other two initiatives include the presence of dedicated intensive care specialists and the regionalization of surgery in high-volume, high-expertise centers.[224]

The pharmacist in the intensive care unit

A growing number of ICUs include a muldisciplinary team during patient rounds. Improved communication and positive attitudes have been linked to improved outcomes.[225] Given the substantial number of preventable medication errors, the participation of a dedicated pharmacist on ICU rounds would appear to be a positive contribution to patient safety and ultimately promote positive outcomes.[226] Pharmacists positively contribute to the implementation of practice guidelines.[227] Data now suggest that a rounding clinical pharmacist decreases the number of adverse events,[228] contributes to decreased antibiotic resistance,[229] may yield substantial cost saving,[230,231] and therefore would be a cost-effective member of the ICU team.[232,233] We have also observed that clinical pharmacists play an active role in teaching medical trainees and assuring therapeutic continuity as house staff and staff physicians rotate through the ICU.

REFERENCES

1. Baue AE. Multiple, progressive, or sequential systems failure. A syndrome of the 1970's. Arch Surg 1975;110:779–81.
2. Faist E, Baue AE, Dittmer H, Heberer G. Multiple organ failure in polytrauma patients. J Trauma 1983;23:775–87.
3. Sauaia A, Moore FA, Moore EE, et al. Epidemiology of trauma deaths: a reassessment. J Trauma 1995;38:185–93.
4. Brazier J, Roberts J, Deverill M. The estimation of a preference-based measure of health from the SF-36. J Health Economics 2002; 21:271–92.
5. Sands KE, Bates DW, Lanken PN, et al. Epidemiology of sepsis syndrome in 8 academic medical centers. Academic Medical Center Consortium Sepsis Project Working Group. JAMA 1977; 278:234–40.
6. Vincent JL, Moreno R, Takala J, et al. The SOFA (Sepsis-related Organ Failure Assessment) score to describe organ dysfunction/failure. On behalf of the Working Group on Sepsis-related Problems of the European Society of Intensive Care Medicine. Intensive Care Med 1996;22:707–10.
7. Wheeler A, Carmichael L, Christman B. Renal function abnormalities in sepsis. J Respir Crit Care Med 1995;151:A317.
8. Angus DC, Linde-Zwirble WT, Lidicker J, et al. Epidemiology of severe sepsis in the United States: analysis of incidence, outcome, and associated costs of care. Crit Care Med 2001;29:1303–10.
9. Vincent JL, deMendonca A, Cantraine F, et al. Use of SOFA score to assess the incidence of organ dysfunction/failure in intensive care units: results of a multicenter, prospective study. Crit Care Med 1998;26:1793–800.
10. Metnitz PG, Krenn CG, Steltzer H, et al. Effect of acute renal failure requiring renal replacement therapy on outcome in critically ill patients. Crit Care Med 2002;30:2051–8.
11. Clermont G, Acker CG, Angus DC, et al. Renal failure in the ICU: comparison of the impact of acute renal failure and end-stage renal disease on ICU outcomes. Kidney Int 2002;62:986–96.
12. Knaus WA, Draper EA, Wagner DP, Zimmerman JE. APACHE II: a severity of disease classification system. Crit Care Med 1985; 13:818–29.
13. Knaus WA, Wagner DP, Draper EA, et al. The APACHE III prognostic system. Rick prediction of hospital mortality for critically ill hospitalized adults. Chest 1991;100:1619–36.
14. Kubisty CA, Arns PA, Wedlund PJ, Branch RA. Adjustment of medications in liver failure. In: Chernow B, ed. The pharmacologic approach to the critically ill patient. Baltimore: Williams and Wilkins; 1994:95–113.

15. McKindley DS, Hanes S, Boucher BA. Hepatic drug metabolism in critical illness. Pharmacotherapy 1998;18(4):759–78.
16. Brouwer KLR, Dukes GE, Powell JR. Influence of liver function on drug disposition. In: Evans WE, Schentag JJ, Jusko WJ, eds. Applied pharmacokinetics: principles of therapeutic drug monitoring. Vancouver: Applied Therapeutics; 1992:1–59.
17. Bass N, Williams R. Guide to drug dosage in hepatic disease. Clin Pharmacokinet 1988;15:396–420.
18. Williams RL. Drug administration in hepatic disease. N Engl J Med 1983;309(26):1616–22.
19. Robert S, Zarowitz BJ. Is there a reliable index of glomerular filtration rate in critically ill patients? DICP 1991;25:169–78.
20. Ducharme MP, Smythe M, Strohs G. Drug-induced alterations in serum creatinine concentrations. Ann Pharmacother 1993;27: 622–33.
21. Comstock TJ. Quantification of renal function. In: Dipiro JT, Talbert RL, Yee GC, et al, eds. Pharmacotherapy: a pathophysiologic approach. New York: McGraw-Hill; 2002:753–69.
22. Zarowitz BJ, Robert S, Peterson EL. Prediction of glomerular filtration rate using aminoglycoside clearance in critically ill medical patients. Ann Pharmacother 1992;26:1205–10.
23. Cockroft DW, Gault MH. Prediction of creatinine clearance from serum creatinine. Nephron 1976;16:31–41.
24. Levey AS, Bosch JP, Lewis JB. A more accurate method to estimate glomerular filtration rate from serum creatinine: a new prediction equation. Ann Intern Med 1999;130:461–70.
25. Levey AS, Greene T, Kusek JW, Beck GJ. A simplified equation to predict glomerular filtration rate from serum creatinine. J Am Soc Nephrol 2000;11:A0828.
26. Luke DR, Halstenson CE, Opsahl JA. Validity of creatinine clearance estimates in the assessment of renal function. Clin Pharmacol Ther 1990;48:503–8.
27. Orlando R, Floreani M, Padrini R, Palatini P. Evaluation of measured and calculated creatinine clearances as glomerular filtration markers in different stages of liver cirrhosis. Clin Nephrol 1999; 51:341–7.
28. Caregaro L, Menon F, Angeli P. Limitations of serum creatinine level and creatinine clearance as filtration markers in cirrhosis. Arch Intern Med 1994;154:201–5.
29. DeSanto NG, Anastasio P, Loguercio C. Creatinine clearance: an inadequate marker of renal filtration in patients with early posthepatitic cirrhosis (Child A) without fluid retention and muscle wasting. Nephron 1995;70:421–4.
30. Pesola GR, Akhavan I, Madu A, Shah NK, Carlon GC. Prediction equation estimates of creatinine clearance in the intensive care unit. Intensive Care Med 1993;19:39–43.
31. Martin C, Alaya M, Bras J, Saux P, Gouin F. Assessment of creatinine clearance in intensive care patients. Crit Care Med 1990; 18:1224–6.
32. St.Peter WL, Redic-Kill KA, Halstenson CE. Clinical pharmacokinetics of antibiotics in patients with impaired renal function. Clin Pharmacokinet 1992;22(3):169–210.
33. Pugh RNH. Transection of the oesophagus for bleeding oesophageal varices. Br J Surg 1973;60:646.
34. Kamath PS, Wiesner RH, Malinchoc M, et al. A model to predict survival in patients with end-stage liver disease. Hepatology 2001;33:464–70.
35. Wiesner RH, McDiarmid SV, Kamath PS, et al. MELD and PELD: application of survival models to liver allocation. Liver Transpl 2001;7(7):567–80.
36. Nagel RA, Dirix LY, Hayllar KM, et al. Use of quantitative liver function tests – caffeine clearance and galactose elimination capacity – after orthotopic liver transplantation. J Hepatol 1990; 10:149–57.
37. Hu OYP, Tang HS, Chang CL. Novel galactose single point method as a measure of residual liver function: example of

cefoperazone kinetics in patients with liver cirrhosis. J Clin Pharmacol 1995;35:250–8.

38. Frye RF, Matzke GR, Adedoyin A, Porter JA, Branch RA. Validation of the five-drug 'Pittsburgh cocktail' approach for assessment of selective regulation of drug-metabolizing enzymes. Clin Pharmacol Ther 1997;62:365–76.

39. Streetman DS, Bleakley JF, Kim JS, et al. Combined phenotypic assessment of CYP1A2, CYP2C19, CYP2D6, CYP3A, N-acetyltransferase-2, and xanthine oxidase with the 'Cooperstown cocktail'. Clin Pharmacol Ther 2000;68:375–83.

40. Dressman JB, Bass P, Ritschel WA, et al. Gastrointestinal parameters that influence oral medications. J Pharm Sci 1993;82(9):857–72.

41. Matzke GR, Comstock TJ. Influence of renal function and dialysis on drug disposition. In: Burton ME, Shaw LM, Schentag JJ, Evans WE, eds. Applied pharmacokinetics and pharmacodynamics: principles of therapeutic drug monitoring. Philadelphia: Lippincott Williams & Wilkins; 2006:188–212.

42. Vestal RE, Wood AJ, Shand DG. Reduced β-receptor sensitivity in the elderly. Clin Pharm Ther 1979;26:181–6.

43. St Peter WL, Halstenson CE. Pharmacologic approach in patients with renal failure. In: Chernow B, ed. The pharmacologic approach to the critically ill patient. Baltimore: Williams and Wilkins; 1994:41–79.

44. Koup J. Disease states and drug pharmacokinetics. J Clin Pharmacol 1989;29:674–9.

45. Elston AC, Bayliss MK, Park GR. Effect of renal failure on drug metabolism by the liver. Br J Anaesth 1993;71:282–90.

46. Leblond F, Guevin C, Demers C. Downregulation of hepatic cytochrome P450 in chronic renal failure. J Am Soc Nephrol 2001; 12:326–32.

47. Leblond FA, Giroux L, Villeneuve JP, Pichette V. Decreased in vivo metabolism of drugs in chronic renal failure. Drug Metab Dispos 2000;28:1317–20.

48. Kim YG, Shin JG, Shin SG, et al. Decreased acetylation of isoniazid in chronic renal failure. Clin Pharmacol Ther 1993;54(6):612–20.

49. van Bortel L, Bohm R, Mooij J, Schiffers P, Rahn KH. Total and free steady-state plasma levels and pharmacokinetics of nifedipine in patients with terminal renal failure. Eur J Clin Pharmacol 1989;37(2):185–9.

50. Aronoff GR. Pharmacokinetics of nitrendipine in patients with renal failure: comparison to normal subjects. J Cardiovasc Pharmacol 1984;6(Suppl 7):S974–6.

51. Van Harten J, Burggraaf J, van Brummelen P. Influence of renal function on the pharmacokinetics and cardiovascular effects of nisoldipine after single and multiple dosing. Clin Pharmacokinet 1989;16:55–64.

52. Frye RF, Matzke GR, Alexander ACM. Effect of renal insufficiency on CYP activity. Clin Pharmacol Ther 1996;59:155.

53. Macias WL, Mueller BA, Scarim SK. Vancomycin pharmacokinetics in acute renal failure: preservation of non-renal clearance. Clin Pharmacol Ther 1991;50:688–94.

54. Mueller BA, Scarim SK, Macias WL. Comparison of imipenem pharmacokinetics in patients with acute or chronic renal failure treated with continuous hemofiltration. Am J Kidney Dis 1993; 21(2):172–9.

55. Heinemeyer G, Link J, Weber W. Clearance of ceftriaxone in critical care patients with acute renal failure. Intensive Care Med 1990;16:448–53.

56. Bendayan R. Renal drug transport – a review. Pharmacotherapy 1996;16:971–85.

57. Blaschke TF, Rubin PC. Hepatic first-pass metabolism in liver disease. Clin Pharmacokinet 1979;4(6):423–32.

58. Holgate AM, Read NW. Relationship between small bowel transit time and absorption of a solid meal. Influence of metoclopramide, magnesium sulfate, and lactulose. Dig Dis Sci 1983; 28(9):812–19.

59. Kiszka-Kanowitz M, Henriksen JH, Moller S, Bendtsen F. Blood volume distribution in patients with cirrhosis: aspects of the dual-head gamma-camera technique. J Hepatol 2001;35(5):605–12.

60. Petersen CE, Ha CE, Harohalli K, Feix JB, Bhagavan NV. A dynamic model for bilirubin binding to human serum albumin. J Biol Chem 2000;275(28):20985–95.

61. Thiessen JJ, Sellers EM, Denbeigh P, Dolman L. Plasma protein binding of diazepam and tolbutamide in chronic alcoholics. J Clin Pharmacol 1976;16(7):345–51.

62. Huet PM, Villeneuve JP. Determinants of drug disposition in patients with cirrhosis. Hepatology 1983;3(6):913–18.

63. Roos FJ, Zysset T, Reichen J. Differential effect of biliary and micronodular cirrhosis on oxidative drug metabolism. In vivo-in vitro correlations of dextromethorphan metabolism in rat models. Biochem Pharmacol 1991;41(10):1513–19.

64. Goldberg DM, Brown D. Advances in the application of biochemical tests to diseases of the liver and biliary tract: their role in diagnosis, prognosis, and the elucidation of pathogenetic mechanisms. Clin Biochem 1987;20(2):127–48.

65. Bjorkman S, Redke F. Clearance of fentanyl, alfentanil, methohexitone, thiopentone and ketamine in relation to estimated hepatic blood flow in several animal species: application to prediction of clearance in man. [erratum appears in J Pharm Pharmacol 2000;52(12):203–4.]. J Pharm Pharmacol 2000;52(9):1065–74.

66. Keiding S. Hepatic clearance and liver blood flow. J Hepatol 1987; 4(3):393–8.

67. Bastien MC, Leblond F, Pichette V, Villeneuve JP. Differential alteration of cytochrome P450 isoenzymes in two experimental models of cirrhosis. Can J Physiol Pharmacol 2000;78(11):912–19.

68. Poupon RY, Raizman A, Brumault JC, Infante R, Darnis F. [Hepatic biotransformation and conjugation of dehydrocholic acid in patients with cirrhosis (author's transl)]. [French]. Gastroenterol Clin Biole 1979;3(12):879–84.

69. Williams RL, Schary WL, Blaschke TF, et al. Influence of acute viral hepatitis on disposition and pharmacologic effect of warfarin. Clin Pharmacol Ther 1976;20(1):90–7.

70. Blaschke TF, Meffin PJ, Melmon KL, Rowland M. Influence of acute viral hepatitis on phenytoin kinetics and protein binding. Clin Pharmacol Ther 1975;17(6):685–91.

71. Wilkinson GR. The effects of liver disease and aging on the disposition of diazepam, chlordiazepoxide, oxazepam and lorazepam in man. Acta Psychiatr Scand Suppl 1978;274:56–74.

72. Hoofnagle JH, Carithers RL Jr, Shapiro C, Ascher N. Fulminant hepatic failure: summary of a workshop. Hepatology 1995;21(1):240–52.

73. Pascher A, Sauer IM, Hammer C, Gerlach JC, Neuhaus P. Extracorporeal liver perfusion as hepatic assist in acute liver failure: a review of world experience. Xenotransplantation 2002;9(5):309–24.

74. Alvin J, McHorse T, Hoyumpa A, Bush MT, Schenker S. The effect of liver disease in man on the disposition of phenobarbital. J Pharmacol Exp Ther 1975;192(1):224–35.

75. Regardh CG, Jordo L, Ervik M, et al. Pharmacokinetics of metoprolol in patients with hepatic cirrhosis. Clin Pharmacokinet 1981;6:375–88.

76. Wood AJ, Kornhauser DM, Wilkinson GR, Shand DG, Branch RA. The influence of cirrhosis on steady-state blood concentrations of unbound propranolol after oral administration. Clin Pharmacokinet 1978;3:478–87.

77. Homeida M, Jackson L, Roberts CJ. Decreased first-pass metabolism of labetalol in chronic liver disease. Br Med J 1978;2:1048–50.

78. Woodcock BG, Rietbrock I, Vohringer HF, Rietbrock N. Verapamil disposition in liver disease and intensive-care patients: kinetics, clearance, and apparent blood flow relationships. Clin Pharmacol Ther 1981;29:27–34.

79. Patwardhan RV, Johnson RF, Hoyumpa A Jr, et al. Normal metabolism of morphine in cirrhosis. Gastroenterology 1981;81:1006–11.

80. Hasselstrom J, Eriksson S, Persson A, et al. The metabolism and bioavailability of morphine in patients with severe liver cirrhosis. Br J Clin Pharmacol 1990;29:289–97.

81. MacGilchrist AJ, Birnie GG, Cook A, et al. Pharmacokinetics and pharmacodynamics of intravenous midazolam in patients with severe alcoholic cirrhosis. Gut 1986;27:190–5.

82. Janssen U, Walker S, Maier K, von Gaisberg U, Klotz U. Flumazenil disposition and elimination in cirrhosis. Clin Pharm Ther 1989;46:317–23.

83. Andersson T, Olsson R, Regardh CG, Skanberg I. Pharmacokinetics of [^{14}C]omeprazole in patients with liver cirrhosis. Clin Pharm 1993;24:71–8.

84. Boscia JA, Korzeniowski OM, Snepar R, et al. Cefoperazone pharmacokinetics in normal subjects and patients with cirrhosis. Antimicrob Agents Chemother 1983;23:385–9.

85. Eng RH, Gorski S, Person A, Mangura C, Chmel H. Clindamycin elimination in patients with liver disease. J Antimicrob Chemother 1981;8:277–81.

86. Farrell G, Baird-Lambert J, Cvejic M, Buchanan N. Disposition and metabolism of metronidazole in patients with liver failure. Hepatology 1984;4(4):722–6.

87. Marshall JP, Salk WB, Elam RO, Wilkinson GR, Schenker S. Disposition of nafcillin in patients with cirrhosis and extrahepatic biliary obstruction. Gastroenterology 1977;73:1388–92.

88. Olsen GD, Bennett WM, Porter GA. Morphine and phenytoin binding to plasma proteins in renal and hepatic failure. Clin Pharmacol Ther 1975;17(6):677–84.

89. du SP, Erill S. Metabolism of procainamide and p-aminobenzoic acid in patients with chronic liver disease. Clin Pharm Ther 1977;22:588–95.

90. Parker CJ, Hunter JM. Pharmacokinetics of atracurium and laudanosine in patients with hepatic cirrhosis. Br J Anaesth 1989;62:177–83.

91. Bass NM, Williams RL. Guide to drug dosage in hepatic disease. Clin Pharmacokin 1988;15(6):396–420.

92. Hayes PC. Liver disease and drug disposition. BJA: Br J Anaesth 1992;68(5):459–61.

93. Westphal JF, Brogard JM. Drug administration in chronic liver disease. Drug Saf 1997;17(1):47–73.

94. Sonne J. Drug metabolism in liver disease: implications for therapeutic drug monitoring. Ther Drug Monit 1996;18(4):397–401.

95. Zheng H, Webber S, Schuetz E, et al. Cytochrome P4503A5 and TNF-a genotypes are associated with tacrolimus dosing in pediatric heart transplant patients. Hum Immunol 2002;63:S15.

96. Siewert E, Bort R, Kluge R, et al. Hepatic cytochrome P450 down-regulation during aseptic inflammation in the mouse is interleukin 6 dependent. Hepatology 2000;32:49–55.

97. McEvoy GK, Litvak K, Welsh OH. American Hospital Formulary Service, drug information. Bethesda: American Society of Hospital Pharmacists; 2001.

98. Thummel KE, Shen DD. Design and optimization of dosage regimens: pharmacokinetic data. In: Haradman JG, Limbird LE, Goodman GA, eds. The pharmacological basis of therapeutics. New York: McGraw-Hill; 2001:1917–2024.

99. Craig WA. Pharmacokinetic/pharmacodynamic parameters: rationale for antibacterial dosing of mice and men. Clin Infect Dis 1998;26:1–12.

100. Murphy JE. Clinical pharmacokinetics pocket reference, 2nd edn. Bethesda: American Society of Hospital Pharmacists; 2001.

101. Frye RF, Matzke GRM. Drug therapy individualization for patients with renal insufficiency. In: Dipiro JT, Talbert RL, Yee GC, et al, eds. Pharmacotherapy: A pathophysiologic approach. New York: McGraw Hill; 2002:939–52.

102. Joy MS, Matzke GR, Armstrong DK, Marx MA, Zarowitz BJ. A primer on continuous renal replacement therapy for critically ill patients. Ann Pharmacother 1998;32(3):362–75.

103. Bleyzac N, Barou P, Massenavette B, et al. Assessment of acyclovir intraindividual pharmacokinetic variability during continuous hemofiltration, continuous hemodiafiltration, and continuous hemodialysis. Ther Drug Monit 1999;21(5):520–5.

104. Armendariz E, Chelluri L, Ptachcinski R. Pharmacokinetics of amikacin during continuous veno-venous hemofiltration [see comments]. Crit Care Med 1990;18(6):675–6.

105. Robert R, Rochard E, Malin F, Bouquet S. Amikacin pharmacokinetics during continuous veno-venous hemofiltration [letter; comment]. Crit Care Med 1991;19(4):588–9.

106. Lawless S, Restaino I, Azin S, Corddry D. Effect of continuous arteriovenous haemofiltration on pharmacokinetics of amrinone. Clin Pharmacokin 1993;25(1):80–2.

107. Shearer ES, O'Sullivan EP, Hunter JM. Clearance of atracurium and laudanosine in the urine and by continuous venovenous haemofiltration [see comments]. BJA: Br J Anaesth 1991;67(5):569–73.

108. Matzke GR, Frye RF, Joy MS, Palevsky PM. Determinants of ceftazidime clearance by continuous venovenous hemofiltration and continuous venovenous hemodialysis. Antimicrob Agents Chemother 2000;44(6):1639–44.

109. Matzke GR, Frye RF, Joy MS, Palevsky PM. Determinants of ceftriaxone clearance by continuous venovenous hemofiltration and hemodialysis. Pharmacotherapy 2000;20(6):635–43.

110. Kroh UF, Lennartz H, Edwards DJ, Stoeckel K. Pharmacokinetics of ceftriaxone in patients undergoing continuous veno-venous hemofiltration. J Clin Pharmacol 1996;36:1114–19.

111. Weiss LG, Cars O, Danielson BG, Grahnen A, Wikstrom B. Pharmacokinetics of intravenous cefuroxime during intermittent and continuous arteriovenous hemofiltration. Clin Nephrol 1988;30(5):282–6.

112. Malone RS, Fish DN, Abraham E, Teitelbaum I. Pharmacokinetics of levofloxacin and ciprofloxacin during continuous renal replacement therapy in critically ill patients. Antimicrob Agents Chemother 2001;45(10):2949–54.

113. Muhl E, Martens T, Iven H, Rob P, Bruch HP. Influence of continuous veno-venous haemodiafiltration and continuous venovenous haemofiltration on the pharmacokinetics of fluconazole. Eur J Clin Pharmacol 2000;56(9–10):671–8.

114. Zarowitz BJ, Anandan JV, Dumler F, Jayashankar J, Levin N. Continuous arteriovenous hemofiltration of aminoglycoside antibiotics in critically ill patients. J Clin Pharmacol 1986;26(8):686–9.

115. Lehman ME, Kolb KW. Gentamicin elimination in a patient undergoing continuous ultrafiltration. Clin Pharm 1985;4(3):327–30.

116. Keller E, Fecht H, Bohler J, Schollmeyer P. Single-dose kinetics of imipenem/cilastatin during continuous arteriovenous haemofiltration in intensive care patients. Nephrol Dial Transplant 1989;4(7):640–5.

117. Ververs TFT, van Dijk A, Vinks AA, et al. Pharmacokinetics and dosing regimen of meropenem in critically ill patients receiving continuous venovenous hemofiltration. Crit Care Med 2000;28(10):3412–16.

118. Quale JM, O'Halloran JJ, DeVincenzo N, Barth RH. Removal of vancomycin by high-flux hemodialysis membranes. Antimicrob Agents Chemother 1992;36(7):1424–6.

119. Zoer J, Schrander-van der Meer AM, van Dorp WT. Dosage recommendation of vancomycin during haemodialysis with highly permeable membranes. Pharm World Sci 1997;19(4):191–6.

120. Torras J, Cao C, Rivas MC, et al. Pharmacokinetics of vancomycin in patients undergoing hemodialysis with polyacrylonitrile. Clin Nephrol 1991;36(1):35–41.

121. Lau AH, Kronfol NO. Effect of continuous hemofiltration on phenytoin elimination. Ther Drug Monit 1994;16(1):53–7.
122. van der Werf TS, Mulder PO, Zijlstra JG, Uges DR, Stegeman CA. Pharmacokinetics of piperacillin and tazobactam in critically ill patients with renal failure, treated with continuous veno-venous hemofiltration (CVVH). Intensive Care Med 1997;23(8):873–7.
123. Lindsay CA, Bawdon R, Quigley R. Clearance of ticarcillin-clavulanic acid by continuous venovenous hemofiltration in three critically ill children, two with and one without concomitant extracorporeal membrane oxygenation. Pharmacotherapy 1996;16(3):458–62.
124. Thomson AH, Grant AC, Rodger RS, Hughes RL. Gentamicin and vancomycin removal by continuous venovenous hemofiltration. DICP 1991;25(2):127–9.
125. Joy MS, Matzke GR, Frye RF, Palevsky PM. Determinants of vancomycin clearance by continuous venovenous hemofiltration and continuous venovenous hemodialysis. Am J Kidney Dis 1998;31(6):1019–27.
126. Matzke GR, O'Connell MB, Collins AJ, Keshaviah PR. Disposition of vancomycin during hemofiltration. Clin Pharmacol Ther 1986;40(4):425–30.
127. Macias WL, Mueller BA, Scarim SK. Vancomycin pharmacokinetics in acute renal failure: preservation of nonrenal clearance [see comments]. Clin Pharmacol Ther 1991;50(6):688–94.
128. Davies SP, Lacey LF, Kox WJ, Brown EA. Pharmacokinetics of cefuroxime and ceftazidime in patients with acute renal failure treated by continuous arteriovenous haemodialysis. Nephrol Dial Transplant 1991;6(12):971–6.
129. Lambrecht L, Gunderson B, St Peter WL, Swan SK. Antibiotic removal on continuous veno-venous hemodialysis. Pharmacother 2000;20:347.
130. Davies SP, Azadian BS, Kox WJ, Brown EA. Pharmacokinetics of ciprofloxacin and vancomycin in patients with acute renal failure treated by continuous haemodialysis. Nephrol Dial Transplant 1992;7(8):848–54.
131. Wallis SC, Mullany DV, Lipman J, Rickard CM, Daley PJ. Pharmacokinetics of ciprofloxacin in ICU patients on continuous veno-venous haemodiafiltration. Intensive Care Med 2001;27(4):665–72.
132. Nicolau DP, Crowe H, Nightingale CH, Quintiliani R. Effect of continuous arteriovenous hemodiafiltration on the pharmacokinetics of fluconazole. Pharmacotherapy 1994;14(4):502–5.
133. Boulieu R, Bastien O, Bleyzac N. Pharmacokinetics of ganciclovir in heart transplant patients undergoing continuous venovenous hemodialysis. Ther Drug Monit 1993;15(2):105–7.
134. Ernest D, Cutler DJ. Gentamicin clearance during continuous arteriovenous hemodiafiltration. Crit Care Med 1992;20(5):586–9.
135. Vos MC, Vincent HH, Yzerman EP. Clearance of imipenem/cilastatin in acute renal failure patients treated by continuous hemodiafiltration (CAVHD). Intensive Care Med 1992;18(5):282–5.
136. Schoumacher R, Chevalier RL, Gomez RA, et al. Enhanced clearance of vancomycin by hemodialysis in a child. Pediat Nephrol 1989;3(1):83–5.
137. Bastani B. Invivo comparison of three different hemodialysis membranes for vancomycin clearance; cuprophan, cellulose acetate, and polyacrylonitrile. Dial Transplant 1988;17:527.
138. Rohde B, Werner U, Hickstein H, Ehmcke H, Drewelow B. Pharmacokinetics of mezlocillin and sulbactam under continuous veno-venous hemodialysis (CVVHD) in intensive care patients with acute renal failure. Eur J Clin Pharmacol 1997;53(2):111–15.
139. Mueller SC, Majcher-Peszynska J, Hickstein H, et al. Pharmacokinetics of piperacillin-tazobactam in anuric intensive care patients during continuous venovenous hemodialysis. Antimicrob Agents Chemother 2002;46(5):1557–60.
140. Wolter K, Claus M, Wagner K, Fritschka E. Teicoplanin pharmacokinetics and dosage recommendations in chronic hemodialysis patients and in patients undergoing continuous veno-venous hemodialysis. Clin Nephrol 1994;42(6):389–97.
141. Santre C, Leroy O, Simon M, et al. Pharmacokinetics of vancomycin during continuous hemodiafiltration. Intensive Care Med 1993;19(6):347–50.
142. Reetze-Bonorden P, Bohler J, Kohler C, Schollmeyer P, Keller E. Elimination of vancomycin in patients on continuous arteriovenous hemodialysis. Contrib Nephrol 1991;93:135–9.
143. Konstantin P. Newer membranes: cuprophan versus polysulfone versus polyacrylonitrile. In: Bosch JP, ed. Contemporary issues in nephrology. Hemodialysis: high efficiency treatments. New York: Churchill Livingstone; 1993:63–78.
144. Krasny HC, Liao SH, de Miranda P, et al. Influence of hemodialysis on acyclovir pharmacokinetics in patients with chronic renal failure. Am J Med 1982;73(1A):202–4.
145. Almond MK, Fan S, Dhillon S, Pollock AM, Raftery MJ. Avoiding acyclovir neurotoxicity in patients with chronic renal failure undergoing haemodialysis. Nephron 1995;69(4):428–32.
146. Lanao JM, Dominguez-Gil A, Tabernero JM, Macias JF. Influence of type of dialyzer on the pharmacokinetics of amikacin. Int J Clin Pharmacol Ther Toxicol 1983;21(4):197–202.
147. Armstrong DK, Hodgman T, Visconti JA, et al. Hemodialysis of amikacin in critically ill patients. Crit Care Med 1988;16(5):517–20.
148. Davies BE, Boon R, Horton R, Reubi FC, Descoeudres CE. Pharmacokinetics of amoxycillin and clavulanic acid in haemodialysis patients following intravenous administration of Augmentin. Br J Clin Pharmacol 1988;26(4):385–90.
149. Blum RA, Kohli RK, Harrison NJ, Schentag JJ. Pharmacokinetics of ampicillin (2.0 grams) and sulbactam (1.0 gram) coadministered to subjects with normal and abnormal renal function and with end-stage renal disease on hemodialysis. Antimicrob Agents Chemother 1989;33(9):1470–6.
150. Gerig JS, Bolton ND, Swabb EA, Scheld WM, Bolton WK. Effect of hemodialysis and peritoneal dialysis on aztreonam pharmacokinetics. Kidney Int 1984;26(3):308–18.
151. Sowinski KM, Mueller BA, Grabe DW, et al. Cefazolin dialytic clearance by high-efficiency and high-flux hemodialyzers. [erratum appears in Am J Kidney Dis 2001;37(5):1111]. Am J Kidney Dis [online] 2001;37(4):766–76.
152. Fogel MA, Nussbaum PB, Feintzeig ID, et al. Cefazolin in chronic hemodialysis patients: a safe, effective alternative to vancomycin. Am J Kidney Dis 1998;32(3):401–9.
153. Halstenson CE, Guay DR, Opsahl JA, et al. Disposition of cefmetazole in healthy volunteers and patients with impaired renal function. Antimicrob Agents Chemother 1990;34(4):519–23.
154. Toffelmire EB, Reymond J, Brouard R, et al. Dialysis clearance in high flux hemodialysis with reuse using ceftazidime as the model drug. Clin Pharmacol Ther 1989;45(2):160.
155. Barbhaiya RH, Knupp CA, Forgue ST, et al. Pharmacokinetics of cefepime in subjects with renal insufficiency. Clin Pharmacol Ther 1990;48(3):268–76.
156. Schmaldienst S, Traunmuller F, Burgmann H, et al. Multiple-dose pharmacokinetics of cefepime in long-term hemodialysis with high-flux membranes. Eur J Clin Pharmacol 2000;56(1):61–4.
157. Gabutti L, Taminelli-Beltraminelli L, Marone C. Clearance of ceftriaxone during haemodialysis using cuprophane, haemophane and polysulfone dialysers. Eur J Clin Pharmacol 1997;53(2):123–6.
158. Cutler RE, Blair AD, Burgess ED, Parks D. Pharmacokinetics of ceftizoxime. J Antimicrob Chemother 1982;10(Suppl C):91–7.

159. Parry MF, Neu HC. Pharmacokinetics of ticarcillin in patients with abnormal renal function. J Infect Dis 1976;133(1):46–9.

160. Toon S, Ross CE, Gokal R, Rowland M. An assessment of the effects of impaired renal function and haemodialysis on the pharmacokinetics of fluconazole. Br J Clin Pharmacol 1990; 29(2):221–6.

161. Berl T, Wilner KD, Gardner M, et al. Pharmacokinetics of fluconazole in renal failure. J Am Soc Nephrol 1995;6(2):242–7.

162. Swan SK, Munar MY, Wigger MA, Bennett WM. Pharmacokinetics of ganciclovir in a patient undergoing hemodialysis. Am J Kidney Dis 1991;17(1):69–72.

163. Matzke GR, Halstenson CE, Keane WF. Hemodialysis elimination rates and clearance of gentamicin and tobramycin. Antimicrob Agents Chemother 1984;25(1):128–30.

164. Agarwal R, Cronin RE. Heterogeneity in gentamicin clearance between high-efficiency hemodialyzers. Am J Kidney Dis 1994; 23(1):47–51.

165. Amin NB, Padhi ID, Touchette MA, et al. Characterization of gentamicin pharmacokinetics in patients hemodialyzed with high-flux polysulfone membranes. Am J Kidney Dis 1999; 34(2):222–7.

166. Verpooten GA, Verbist L, Buntinx AP, et al. The pharmacokinetics of imipenem (thienamycin-formamidine) and the renal dehydropeptidase inhibitor cilastatin sodium in normal subjects and patients with renal failure. Br J Clin Pharmacol 1984;18(2): 183–93.

167. Christensson BA, Nilsson-Ehle I, Hutchison M, et al. Pharmacokinetics of meropenem in subjects with various degrees of renal impairment. Antimicrob Agents Chemother 1992;36(7):1532–7.

168. Leroy A, Fillastre JP, Borsa-Lebas F, Etienne I, Humbert G. Pharmacokinetics of meropenem (ICI 194,660) and its metabolite (ICI 213,689) in healthy subjects and in patients with renal impairment. Antimicrob Agents Chemother 1992;36(12):2794–8.

169. Somogyi A, Kong C, Sabto J, et al. Disposition and removal of metronidazole in patients undergoing haemodialysis. Eur J Clin Pharmacol 1983;25(5):683–7.

170. Lau AH, Chang CW, Sabatini S. Hemodialysis clearance of metronidazole and its metabolites. Antimicrob Agents Chemother 1986;29(2):235–8.

171. Brogard JM, Comte F, Spach MO, Lavillaureix J. Pharmacokinetics of mezlocillin in patients with kidney impairment: special reference to hemodialysis and dosage adjustments in relation to renal function. Chemotherapy 1982;28(5):318–26.

172. Thorsteinsson SB, Steingrimsson O, Asmundsson P, Bergan T. Pharmacokinetics of mezlocillin during haemodialysis. Scand J Infect Dis Suppl 1981;29:59–63.

173. Janicke DM, Mangione A, Schultz RW, Jusko WJ. Mezlocillin disposition in chronic hemodialysis patients. Antimicrob Agents Chemother 1981;20(5):590–4.

174. Kampf D, Borner K, Pustelnik A. Multiple dose kinetics of ofloxacin and ofloxacin metabolites in haemodialysis patients. Eur J Clin Pharmacol 1992;42(1):95–9.

175. Streete JM, Berry DJ, Jones JA, Groggin MJ. Clearance of phenylethylmalonamide during haemodialysis of a patient with renal failure. Ther Drug Monit 1990;12(3):281–3.

176. Heim-Duthoy KL, Halstenson CE, Abraham PA, Matzke GR. The effect of hemodialysis on piperacillin pharmacokinetics. Int J Clin Pharmacol Ther Toxicol 1986;24(12):680–4.

177. Johnson CA, Halstenson CE, Kelloway JS, et al. Single-dose pharmacokinetics of piperacillin and tazobactam in patients with renal disease. Clin Pharmacol Ther 1992;51(1):32–41.

178. Nissenson AR, Wilson C, Holazo A. Pharmacokinetics of intravenous trimethoprim-sulfamethoxazole during hemodialysis. Am J Nephrol 1987;7(4):270–4.

179. Thalhammer F, Rosenkranz AR, Burgmann H, et al. Single-dose pharmacokinetics of teicoplanin during hemodialysis therapy using high-flux polysulfone membranes. Wien Klin Wochenschr 1997;109(10):362–5.

180. Halstenson CE, Berkseth RO, Mann HJ, Matzke GR. Aminoglycoside redistribution phenomenon after hemodialysis: netilmicin and tobramycin. Int J Clin Pharmacol Ther Toxicol 1987;25(1):50–5.

181. Hebert PC, Wells G, Blajchman MA, et al. A multicenter, randomized, controlled clinical trial of transfusion requirements in critical care. Transfusion Requirements in Critical Care Investigators, Canadian Critical Care Trials Group. N Engl J Med 1999; 340:409–17.

182. Ely EW, Bernard GR. Transfusions in critically ill patients. N Engl J Med 1999;340:467–8.

183. Corwin HL, Gettinger A, Rodriguez RM, et al. Efficacy of recombinant human erythropoietin in the critically ill patient: a randomized, double-blind, placebo-controlled trial. Crit Care Med 1999;27(11):2346–50.

184. Goodnough LT, Bach RG. Anemia, transfusion, and mortality. N Engl J Med 2001;345:1272–4.

185. Wu WC, Rathore SS, Wang Y, Radford MJ, Krumholz HM. Blood transfusion in elderly patients with acute myocardial infarction. N Engl J Med 2001;345:1230–6.

186. Rivers E, Nguyen B, Havstad S, et al. Early goal-directed therapy in the treatment of severe sepsis and septic shock. N Engl J Med 2001;345:1368–77.

187. Rodriguez RM, Corwin HL, Gettinger A, et al. Nutritional deficiencies and blunted erythropoietin response as causes of the anemia of critical illness. J Crit Care 2001;16(1):36–41.

188. Corwin HL. Anemia in the critically ill: the role of erythropoietin. Semin Hematol 2001;38(3:Suppl 7):Suppl 32.

189. Mascia MF, Koch M, Medicis JJ. Pharmacoeconomic impact of rational use guidelines on the provision of analgesia, sedation, and neuromuscular blockade in critical care. Crit Care Med 2000;28:2300–6.

190. Ostermann ME, Keenan SP, Seiferling RA, Sibbald WJ. Sedation in the intensive care unit: a systematic review. JAMA 2000; 283:1451–9.

191. Kress JP, Pohlman AS, O'Connor MF, Hall JB. Daily interruption of sedative infusions in critically ill patients undergoing mechanical ventilation. N Engl J Med 2000;342:1471–7.

192. McCollam JS, O'Neil MG, Norcross ED, Byrne TK, Reeves ST. Continuous infusions of lorazepam, midazolam, and propofol for sedation of the critically ill surgery trauma patient: a prospective, randomized comparison. Crit Care Med 1999; 27(11):2454–8.

193. Miller LJ, Wiles-Pfeifler R. Propofol for the long-term sedation of a critically ill patient. Am J Crit Care 1998;7(1):73–6.

194. Davis NA, Rodgers JE, Gonzalez ER, Fowler AA. Prolonged weakness after cisatracurium infusion: a case report. Crit Care Med 1998;26:1290–2.

195. Topulos GP. Neuromuscular blockage in adult intensive care. New Horiz 1993;1:447–62.

196. May JR, Rutkowski AF. The role of nondepolarizing neuromuscular blocking agents in mechanically ventilated patients. J Med Assoc Ga 1994;83:473–6.

197. Hoyt JW. The shifting sands of mechanical ventilation. Crit Care Med 1998;26:1162–3.

198. Hansen-Flaschen JH, Brazinsky S, Basile C, Lanken PN. Use of sedating drugs and neuromuscular blocking agents in patients requiring mechanical ventilation for respiratory failure. A national survey. JAMA 1991;266(20):2870–5.

199. Eriksson LI. Ventilation and neuromuscular blocking drugs. Acta Anaesth Scand Suppl 1994;102:11–15.

200. Mayhall CG. The epidemiology and control of VRE: still struggling to come of age [letter; comment]. Infect Control Hosp Epidemiol 1999;20(10):650–2.

201. Miller NC, Rudoy RC. Vancomycin intermediate-resistant *Staphylococcus aureus* (VISA). Orthopaed Nurs 2000;19(6):45–8.

202. Linares J. The VISA/GISA problem: therapeutic implications. Clin Microbiol Infect 2001;7:Suppl 15.

203. Poole K. Multidrug resistance in Gram-negative bacteria. Curr Opin Microbiol 2001;4(5):500–8.

204. CDC VRE guidelines still relevant. Hospital Peer Rev 1998; 23(2):25–7.

205. Padiglione AA, Grabsch E, Wolfe R, Gibson K, Grayson ML. The prevalence of fecal colonization with VRE among residents of long-term-care facilities in Melbourne, Australia. Infect Control Hosp Epidemiol 2001;22(9):576–8.

206. Carrico RM, Niner S. Multidrug resistant organisms – VRE and MRSA: practical home care tips. Home Healthcare Nurse 2002; 20(1):23–8.

207. Zansky S, Wallace B, Schoonmaker-Bopp D, et al. From the Centers for Disease Control and Prevention. Outbreak of multi-drug resistant Salmonella Newport – United States, January–April 2002. JAMA 2002;288(8):951–3.

208. Gold MR, Siegel JE, Russell LB, Weinstein MC. Cost-effectiveness in health and medicine. New York: Oxford University Press; 1996.

209. Weinstein MC, Siegel JE, Gold MR, Kamlet MS, Russell LB. Recommendations of the Panel on Cost-effectiveness in Health and Medicine. JAMA 1996;276:1253–8.

210. [The Helsinki Accords of the World Medical Association: guidelines for physicians concerning biomedical experiments on humans] Klinicheskaia Meditsina 2000;78(9):13–14.

211. Angus DC, Rubenfeld GD, Roberts MS, et al. Understanding costs and cost-effectiveness in critical care: report from the Second American Thoracic Society Workshop on Outcomes Research. Am J Respir Crit Care Med 2002;165(4):540–50.

212. Black NA, Jenkinson C, Hayes JA, et al. Review of outcome measures used in adult critical care. Crit Care Med 2001; 29:2119–24.

213. Torrance GW, Feeny DH, Furlong WJ, et al. Multiattribute utility function for a comprehensive health status classification system. Health Utilities Index Mark 2. Med Care 1996;34:702–22.

214. Chapman RH, Stone PW, Sandberg EA, Bell C, Neumann PJ. A comprehensive league table of cost-utility ratios and a sub-table of 'panel-worthy' studies. Med Decis Making 2000;20:451–67.

215. van Hout BA, Angus DC. How should we measure the economic consequences of critical illness? In: Angus DC, Carlet J, eds. Surviving intensive care. Vincent J-L (series ed) Update in Intensive Care and Emergency Medicine No. 39. Berlin: Springer-Verlag, 2003:221–34.

216. Laupacis A, Feeny D, Detsky AS, Tugwell PX. How attractive does a new technology have to be to warrant adoption and utilization? Tentative guidelines for using clinical and economic evaluations. Can Med Assoc J 1992;146:473–81.

217. van Hout BA, Al MJ, Gordon GS, Rutten FF. Costs, effects and C/E ratios alongside a clinical trial. Health Econ 1994;3:309–19.

218. Kohn LT, Corrigan JM, Donaldson MS. To err is human: building a safer health system. Washington, DC: Institute of Medicine; 2000.

219. Leape LL. Institute of Medicine medical error figures are not exaggerated. JAMA 2000;284:95–7.

220. McDonald CJ, Weiner M, Hui SL. Deaths due to medical errors are exaggerated in Institute of Medicine report. JAMA 2000; 284:93–4.

221. Bates DW, Cullen DJ, Laird N, et al. Incidence of adverse drug events and potential adverse drug events. Implications for prevention. ADE Prevention Study Group. JAMA 1995;274:29–34.

222. Lesar TS, Briceland L, Stein DS. Factors related to errors in medication prescribing. JAMA 1997;277:312–17.

223. Cullen DJ, Sweitzer BJ, Bates DW, et al. Preventable adverse drug events in hospitalized patients: a comparative study of intensive care and general care units. Crit Care Med 1997;25:1289–97.

224. Milstein A, Galvin RS, Delbanco SF, Salber P, Buck CR Jr. Improving the safety of health care: the leapfrog initiative. Eff Clin Pract 2000;3:313–16.

225. Sexton JB, Thomas EJ, Helmreich RL. Error, stress and teamwork in medicine and aviation: cross sectional surveys. BMJ 2000;320:745–9.

226. Bond CA, Raehl CL, Franke T. Clinical pharmacy services and hospital mortality rates [see comments]. Pharmacotherapy 1999; 19(5):556–64.

227. Devlin JW, Holbrook AM, Fuller HD. The effect of ICU sedation guidelines and pharmacist interventions on clinical outcomes and drug cost. Ann Pharmacother 1997;31(6):689–95.

228. Leape LL, Cullen DJ, Clapp MD, et al. Pharmacist participation on physician rounds and adverse drug events in the intensive care unit. JAMA 1999;282:267–70.

229. Ibrahim KH, Gunderson B, Rotschafer JC. Intensive care unit antimicrobial resistance and the role of the pharmacist. Crit Care Med 2001;29:N108–13.

230. Chuang LC, Sutton JD, Henderson GT. Impact of a clinical pharmacist on cost saving and cost avoidance in drug therapy in an intensive care unit. Hosp Pharm 1994;29:215–18.

231. Krupicka MI, Bratton SL, Sonnenthal K, Goldstein B. Impact of a pediatric clinical pharmacist in the pediatric intensive care unit. Crit Care Med 2002;30:919–21.

232. Ellinoy BR. Critical care pharmacist: an essential intensivist [letter; comment]. Crit Care Med 2001;29(5):1092–3.

233. Papadopoulos J, Rebuck JA, Lober C, et al. The critical care pharmacist: an essential intensive care practitioner. Pharmacotherapy 2002;22(11):1484–8.

234. Thomson PD, Melmon KL, Richardson JA, et al. Lidocaine pharmacokinetics in advanced heart failure, liver disease, and renal failure in humans. Ann Intern Med 1973;78(4):499–508.

18

Clinical toxicology

Marc Ghannoum and Martine Leblanc

INTRODUCTION

Drug poisoning, either deliberate or accidental, accounts for a significant portion of healthcare resources. According to statistics published by the American Association of Poison Control Centers (AAPCC), there are annually about 2 million cases of overdose in the USA;[1-13] adding the undeclared cases and the ones who die before receiving medical care, the actual number is probably over 5 million. About 85% are accidental, 10% are deliberate, and 5% are consequent to therapeutic errors. Furthermore, poisonings represent about 10–15% of total intensive care unit (ICU) admissions.[14]

American data have shown reduced morbidity and mortality in poisoned patients over the last 15 years (fatalities account for less than 0.1% of reported intoxications). Better understanding of pharmacokinetics, structured studies, new consensus guidelines, optimization of supportive care, and evolving extracorporeal therapies (ECTs) have permitted improved care for intoxicated patients.

EVALUATION OF THE INTOXICATED PATIENT

Clinical history

Although often difficult to obtain because of altered mental status or lack or cooperation, history-taking is essential for subsequent care and should always be sought. Of primordial importance are the nature of the implied poison, quantity, method of administration, delay since exposure, and symptoms on admission. Past medical history should include history of renal disease, heart disease, drug abuse, and seizure disorder. If these are unobtainable, collateral information and identification of empty bottles can be helpful.

Physical examination

Examination may provide several useful hints on the type of substance ingested. Although a general physical examination is certainly advisable, time is often a limiting factor. Evaluation of vital signs and toxidromes (cluster of specific signs after ingestion of a distinct poison) can orient the physician to the incriminating substance (Table 18.1). Breath examination can also be rewarding (Table 18.2). Finally, as in every case of impaired sensorium, every patient should have a thorough neurologic examination with attention to trauma and focal signs.

Laboratory and drug levels

Anion gap
A positive anion gap with or without an associated osmolar gap can provide important clues to the ingested substance while waiting for a toxicology screen. It can be calculated by the following:

$$\text{Anion gap} = Na^+ - (Cl^- + HCO_3^-)$$

The value must be corrected for hypoalbuminemia (by adding 2.5 mEq/L for every 10 g/L of albumin deficit). Normal value is between 8 and 12 mEq/L. The differential diagnosis of an abnormal anion gap is summarized in Box 18.1.

Table 18.1 Vital signs and toxidromes with different substances.

Substance	Example	BP	P	RR	Temp	Early mental status	Pupils	Bowel sounds	Sweat	Other specific signs
Sympaticomimetics	Cocaine	↑	↑	↑	↑	↑	↑	↑	↑	Seizures (horizontal and vertical nystagmus for PCP)
Anticholinergics	Antihistaminics	↑	↑	↑	↑	↑	↑	↓	↓	Flushed skin, urinary retention (hypotension, seizure, QT prolongation and lethargy for tricyclic antidepressants)
Cholinergics	Organophosphates	V	↓	↓	↓	↓	↓	↑	↑	Salivation, lacrimation, urination, bronchorrhea, paralysis
Opiates	Morphine	↓	↓	↓	↓ / N	↓	↓	↓	↓ / N	Pulmonary edema
Opiate withdrawal		↑	↑	–	–	↑	↑	↑	↑	Hyperactivity, piloerection
Sedatives	Benzodiazepines	↓	↓	↓	↓	↓	↓	↓	↓	
Sedative withdrawal		↑	↑	↑	↑	↑	↑	V	↑	Seizure, tinnitus
SSRIs	Aspirin	V	↑	↑	↑	V	–	V	↑	↑ Anion gap, tinnitus, pulmonary edema
Serotonin	Paroxetine	↑↓	↑	V	↑	↑	↑	–	↑	Myoclonus, muscle rigidity
Neuroleptic malignant	Haloperidol	V	↑	V	↑	↓	–	–	↑	Muscle rigidity, tremor
Methemoglobin		↓	↑	↑	V	↓	–	–	–	Blue skin
CO		V	V	↑	↓	↓	–	–	–	Red skin, seizures
Iron		↓	↑	↑	–	V	–	↑	–	Gastrointestinal bleeding

↑ = increase; ↓ = decrease; BP = blood pressure; P = pulse; RR = respiratory rate; V = variable; CO = carbon monoxide; PCP = phencyclidine; SSRIs, selective serotonin reuptake inhibitors; Temp = temperature.

Table 18.2 Breath associated with the ingestion of different substances.

Breath odor	Substance
Bitter almonds	Cyanide
Garlic	Arsenic, organophosphates, thallium
Rotten eggs	Sulfuric group
Mint	Methyl salicylate
Fruity	Ketoacidosis, alcohols
Glue-like	Toluene
Moth balls	Naphthalene
Pears	Chloral hydrate
Gasoline	Hydrocarbons
Ammoniac	Hepatic insufficiency

Osmolar gap

An osmolar gap is the difference between measured osmolality (OSMm, performed by freezing point depression) and calculated osmolality (OSMc). It can be calculated as:

$$OSMm - OSMc = OSMm - (2 \times Na^+ + glucose + urea)$$

where glucose and blood urea nitrogen (BUN) are in mmol/L. Normal values are 10–15 mOsm/kgH$_2$O. An osmolar gap (above that level) represents the addition of exogenous osmols, most frequently methanol, ethylene glycol, isopropanol, ethanol, and also propylene glycol.[15]

Drug levels

Although drug levels are clearly helpful to point out which drugs were ingested, drug levels must be interpreted with extreme caution in the toxicologic

<table>
<tr><td>

Box 18.1   Differential diagnosis of an elevated anion gap

Elevated anion gap = MUDPILE CAT:
   Methanol, Uremia, Diabetes, Paraldehyde,
   Iron/Isoniazid, Lactates, Ethylene glycol, CO, ASA
   (Acetylsalicylic acid), Toluene
Decreased anion gap:
   Lithium, Boric acid
</td></tr>
</table>

setting.[16–18] Positive qualitative or quantitative tests do not necessarily signify that there is clinical toxicity, and a negative result does not exclude serious poisoning (absorption may not have been complete yet). Furthermore, many drugs do not have a readily available assay or are very expensive. As results take a long time to obtain, supportive measures should never be delayed. Drug levels are particularly helpful if:[18]

- levels help to guide specific therapy for drugs,[19] such as salicylates, lithium, CO, digoxin, theophylline, ethylene glycol, iron, and methanol.
- levels correlate fairly well with short-term risk in the asymptomatic patient, as in the case of acetaminophen[16]
- severe symptoms when no other indicator of disease exists.

For salicylates and acetaminophen, nomograms have been recommended to ascertain clinical risk according to blood levels. However, they are not recommended in chronic overdoses, delayed absorption preparation, and with concomitant hepatic or renal failure.

Finally, urine and hair analysis can detect drugs long after exposure (days or even months as compared to hours for blood). These may be useful for cocaine abuse, anabolic steroids, or mercury exposition.[19] Saliva samples correlate well with blood concentrations and may eventually become useful, considering how practical they are to collect.[20]

Complementary investigation
Since overdoses are frequently accompanied by metabolic disturbances, extended laboratory analyses should be performed, including electrolytes, complete blood count, creatine kinase, glucose, urea, creatinine, blood gas, albumin, urinalysis and hepatic enzymes. Other investigations include electrocardiogram (ECG), which may help to assess the toxicity of tricyclic antidepressants, and chest X-ray

for aspiration. Abdominal series can detect radiopaque drugs (iron, enteric salicylates) but often delays unnecessarily treatment.

STABILIZATION

Supportive therapy is the mainstay for all overdoses, and is solely sufficient in the large majority of cases. Although every poisoning must be handled on an individual basis, the initial approach is always the same.

Cardiorespiratory stabilization

As in every emergency setting, priority is given to ABC (airways, breathing, and circulation). Intubation may be required for respiratory tract protection or hypoventilation. In general, poisoned patients are considered to be hypovolemic, and most need some kind of volume replacement. Hypotensive patients often benefit from inotropic support, after adequate fluid optimization. Sinus tachycardia is the most frequent arrhythmia encountered and usually does not need to be treated. More serious rhythm abnormalities can be corrected by standard resuscitation procedures.

The coma cocktail

Since assessment of a comatose patient can be difficult, administration of an empiric therapy has been recommended to reverse certain coma-inducing substances, although much controversy remains about its indications.

- Oxygen – administration of 100% oxygen to all patients seems adequate and safe as a first step.
- Dextrose – hypertonic dextrose (50 ml of 50% dextrose) was once given indiscriminately to all intoxicated patients. Although current literature continues to support this,[21] some authors now suggest dextrose only in cases of documented hypoglycemia, given the widespread availability of reagents for rapid testing, and the potential risk of deteriorating neurologic insult.[22]
- Thiamine – a 100 mg intravenous (IV) dose can be given to most comatose patients with acceptable safety. There is still some debate as to whether thiamine should be given before dextrose to prevent precipitation of Wernicke's

encephalopathy. Current opinion does not support this hypothesis.

- Naloxone – can reverse opiate intoxication and may be given to most patients. However, caution should be given to the fact that it may precipitate withdrawal symptoms and that the half-life of naloxone is often shorter than the opiate itself; hence, the need to repeat doses or to begin an infusion.
- Flumazenil – administration of flumazenil has been proposed to antagonize benzodiazepine toxicity. However, there have been data on the proconvulsing effect of flumazenil in tricyclic antidepressant overdose; furthermore, toxicity with benzodiazepines is only very rarely fatal. Therefore, flumazenil should not be blindly used in the comatose patient unless monotoxicity with benzodiazepines has been documented and if head trauma and seizure history have been excluded.[22,23] Again, continuous infusion may be necessary considering its short half-life.

Other supportive measures

Seizures often accompany overdoses. They should initially be treated with benzodiazepines; diazepam is perhaps the ideal choice because it can be given intravenously, endotracheally, orally, or rectally.[24] Phenytoin may also be used (as well as for its antiarrhythmic effects) but is not always effective in toxic seizures. Drug-induced hyperthermia must be treated aggressively: first, clothing should be removed and IV fluids administered. Cooling blankets and ice packs can then be added (with caution) until the body temperature reaches 38–39°C.[25] Finally, consultation with a certified poison center can guide evaluation and management, especially for unusual substances or atypical presentations.

Admission to the intensive care unit

Of patients declared through AAPCC, 25% receive management in an hospital, whereas 3% require admission to an ICU.[1-13] Of these, It is acknowledged that 50% were unnecessary. Although the initial clinical picture for a given patient may look grim, mortality was only about 2% for patients admitted in an ICU, in one study.[14] Instead, admission in the ICU should be reserved for cases:[26]

- requiring intubation
- with hemodynamic instability requiring intravenous arrhythmics or vasopressors

- needing treatment for convulsions
- requiring ECT, such as hemodialysis or hemoperfusion
- with tricyclic overdose and tachyarrhythmia (>100 bpm), any significant change on the ECG (including QRS >0.1 s), anticholinergic signs, or neurological symptoms
- for massive overdoses of known substances causing delaying toxicity, such as *Amanita* mushrooms and enteric-coated products.[27]

GASTROINTESTINAL DECONTAMINATION

Methods to limit gastrointestinal (GI) absorption have always been one of the most debated subjects in toxicology; controversy originates from the absence of prospective trials clearly showing improved outcome with decontamination, and lack of efficacy of methods blindly accepted for decades. Recently, the American Academy of Clinical Toxicology and the European Association of Poison Centers and Clinical Toxicologists have reviewed relevant data and published jointly some specific recommendations on different modalities to help decision-making.

In general, the sooner the decontamination, the better: 1 hour is the general cut-off for efficacy for most decontamination techniques, an interesting point since the average time of ingestion to presentation is about 2 hours.[28] Accepted contraindications for GI decontamination include an unprotected airway (absent gag/loss of consciousness); in these situations, endotracheal intubation may permit decontamination. Furthermore, decontamination methods should not be given in the presence of GI tract pathology: ileus for whole bowel irrigation (WBI), significant hemorrhage, or esophageal rupture. They should never be used for ingestion of corrosives, hydrocarbons or strong acids or bases because of risk of mucosal injury and aspiration pneumonia. However, when used adequately, all decontamination techniques have a high index of safety.[28,29] As for the agent used, current opinion favors single-dose activated charcoal, except for specific circumstances.

Ipecac

A single dose of 20 ml of ipecac causes emesis in nearly 90% of patients, but its efficacy at reducing absorption is debatable. As seen from the AAPCC report (Table 18.3), ipecac is used less frequently (from 7% in 1989 to less then 1% of overdoses in 2001), probably because it delays administration and efficacy of charcoal.[1-13,30] There are no more indications for its use,[31] except perhaps for infants intoxicated at home. Nevertheless, if tried, it should be administered no more than 60 minutes after ingestion.[32]

Gastric lavage

A once very popular technique, gastric lavage consists of inserting a tube into the stomach to wash out and retrieve its content. For maximum efficacy, it must be done via the largest tolerable orogastric tube (minimum 36F), but even then, substance removal is unpredictable.[33] There remains some concern that lavage may push unabsorbed drug into the small bowel and increase absorption. Lavage should be reserved for very selected cases, i.e. after a potentially life-threatening ingestion,[33] ingestion of substances not bound to charcoal, or with medications such as aspirin that can delay gastric emptying.[34]

Activated charcoal

Known to be an effective agent for over 150 years, activated charcoal (AC) can adsorb particles through its enormous surface area. It works for most drugs but is not effective for alcohols,

organophosphates, cyanide, acids, bases, and metal salts (lithium, iron). It is most efficacious for patients arriving within 1 hour of ingestion[35] and is probably at least better than lavage. Ideally, the ratio of AC:toxin should be 10:1, but since the quantity of toxin ingested is often unknown, the dose of administered AC is usually 1–2 g/kg. Single-dose AC can be given without a laxative, as it does not cause constipation. AC may bind antidotes given orally, but it does not limit their use clinically.[36]

Cathartics

Cathartics (sorbitol and magnesium sulfate being the most popular) promote substance evacuation from the GI tract. With repeated use, they can produce electrolyte disturbances. Their efficacy is very questionable and they should never be used alone. Some physicians recommend adding cathartics to charcoal to improve its palatability. According to the most recent position statement, cathartics are not recommended as a method of gut decontamination.[37]

Whole bowel irrigation

Whole bowel irrigation exerts its effect by cleansing the bowel of an ingested substance. The agent of choice in this method is polyethylene glycol (GoLYTELY®), which is given by a nasogastric

Table 18.3	AAPCC report on the use of absorption prevention (in percent) in poisonings from 1989 to 2001.						
Year	Human exposures	Ipecac	Single-dose charcoal	Cathartic	Lavage	Other emetics	WBI
1989	1581540	7.0%	NA	5.4%	2.6%	0.24%	NA
1990	1713462	6.1%	NA	5.5%	2.9%	0.24%	NA
1991	1837939	5.2%	NA	5.9%	3.2%	0.23%	NA
1992	1864188	4.3%	NA	5.9%	3.3%	0.23%	NA
1993	1751476	3.7%	6.5%	5.2%	3.4%	0.27%	0.071%
1994	1926438	2.7%	6.5%	5.1%	3.5%	0.27%	0.073%
1995	2023089	2.3%	6.9%	5.3%	3.6%	0.30%	0.084%
1996	2155952	1.8%	6.6%	4.8%	3.0%	0.29%	0.089%
1997	2192088	1.5%	6.5%	4.5%	2.4%	0.29%	0.091%
1998	2241082	1.2%	6.3%	3.8%	2.0%	0.28%	0.089%
1999	2201156	1.0%	6.2%	3.1%	1.7%	0.30%	0.094%
2000	2168248	0.8%	6.2%	2.7%	1.5%	0.31%	0.111%
2001	2267979	0.7%	6.2%	2.5%	1.3%	0.33%	0.110%

NA = not available; WBI = whole bowel irrigation.

tube. It can decrease bioavailability of agents that are not bound by AC (iron, lithium) and be useful for concealed packs of sealed drugs.[38,39] Some authors have used WBI up to 16 hours after ingestion of sustained-release medications.[40] Unfortunately, large doses are necessary (2 L/h continuously, for a total of 4–6 doses), which makes compliance questionable.

Others

Sometimes, endoscopy, or even laparoscopy, become necessary to recuperate pills. Resins such as sodium polystyrene sulfonate may also show some efficacy in reducing absorption of lithium and iron.

ANTIDOTES

Antidotes have a folkloric appeal because they can potentially reverse life-threatening symptoms quickly. Although toxicologic research is advancing in this area, present knowledge is unfortunately incomplete to offer this solution in most cases. Antidotes work by three general mechanisms: either by displacing poison from its target site (naloxone), inhibiting formation of toxic metabolites (fomepizole, N-acetylcysteine), or acting as an antibody (Digibind, antivenom). The latter are perhaps the most efficacious (up to 90% efficacy in digitalis overdose in 1 study[41]) and can sometimes obviate other costly and complicated treatment such as ECT. Unfortunately, antidotes are often costly to develop and to administer. Besides the coma cocktail described earlier, there are a number of specific antidotes (Table 18.4). Doses can be obtained from the complete review from Trujillo et al.[42]

ELIMINATION ENHANCEMENT

For serious poisonings, especially when decontamination is no longer useful (after 1–2 hours), it is necessary to consider methods to promote poison elimination.

Forced diuresis

Although once universally used in lithium and salicylate overdoses, forced diuresis is no longer recommended because of its lack of efficacy and risk of circulatory overload. Salicylates elimination, notably, is more enhanced with simple alkaline diuresis than forced saline diuresis.[43]

Multiple doses of activated charcoal

Multiple doses of activated charcoal (MDAC), in addition to binding unabsorbed drug from the GI tract, can enhance back-diffusion of substances from the blood through the intestinal lumen (intestinal dialysis); MDAC can also interrupt enterohepatic recirculation of some drugs. MDAC efficacy (in some cases, showing comparable clearances to ECTs) was demonstrated for theophylline, phenobarbital, carbamazepine, quinine, and dapsone, while it remains controversial for salicylates;[44,45] in such cases, MDAC should be considered,[46] although there is no proof of improved mortality or morbidity.[44] Generally, a first dose of 50–100 g of AC will be administered, followed by 12.5–25 g every hour with a cathartic (to avoid obstruction) until acceptable drug levels are obtained. Premedication with an intravenous antiemetic might be necessary in some patients. They should be continued until evidence of clinical or laboratory improvement (even after initiation of ECT).

pH alteration

Substances that are weak acids, with a dissociation constant (pKa) lower than serum pH, can become preferentially ionized after systemic alkalinization. This charged state does not easily cross cellular membranes; hence the appeal of pH alteration to reduce cellular toxicity. By the same mechanism, alkalinization will favor the formation of ionized drug in the tubular lumen, a state which is not freely reabsorbable, thereby increasing its elimination via urine.

Examples of drugs that can be eliminated successfully by this mechanism are salicylic acid (pK_a 3.0), phenobarbital ($pK_a = 7.2$) and chlorpropamide ($pK_a = 4.8$). For aspirin, alkalinization is particularly effective, and a urinary pH of 7–8 is recommended. Since tricyclic antidepressants are weak bases, alkalinization does not favor their elimination. However, administration of bicarbonate is nevertheless effective because it favors protein binding, decreasing the free (and toxic) fraction. It may also prevent blockade of sodium channels, which is one of the mechanisms of toxicity attributed to

Table 18.4 Summary of available specific antidotes for various poisons.

Poison	Antidote
ACEI	Angiotensin II
Acetaminophen	N-acetylcysteine
Anticholinergics	Physostigmine (except with tricyclic overdose)
Arsenic, copper, mercury, gold, iron, radium, uranium, selenium	Dimercaprol (BAL)
Benzodiazepines	Flumazenil
Beta-blockers	Isoproterenol, glucagon
Calcium channel blockers	Calcium, glucagons
Carbon monoxide	O_2 100%, hyperbaric chamber
Cyanates	100% O_2, amyl nitrite, sodium nitrite, sodium thiosulfate, hydroxycobalamin
Digitalis	Digoxin-specific antibody fragments
Drug-induced dystonic reaction	Diphenyhydramine
Drug-induced parkinsonism	Biperiden
Fluoride	Calcium
Heparin	Protamine sulfate
Insulin, sulfonylureas	Octreotide, glucagon, dextrose
Iron, aluminum	Deferoxamine
Isoniazid	Pyridoxine
Lead, nickel, cobalt, zinc, selenium	Calcium disodium edentate (EDTA)
Methanol, ethylene glycol	Ethanol, fomepizole
Methemoglobinemia	Methylene blue
Methotrexate	Folinic acid
Neuroleptic malignant syndrome	Dantrolene
Nondepolarizing neuromuscular agents	Neostigmine
Opiates	Naloxone
Organophosphates (muscarinic)	Atropine
Organophosphates (nicotinic)	Pralidoxime (2-PAM)
Serotonin syndrome	Cyproheptadine (Periactin)
Thallium	Prussian blue
Tricyclic antidepressants	Bicarbonate
Warfarin	Vitamin K, fresh frozen plasma (FFP)

ACEI = angiotensin-converting enzyme inhibitor; BAL = British antilewisite; EDTA = ethylene diaminetetraacetic acid.

tricyclics. Administration of bicarbonate in alcohol and isoniazid poisoning corrects acidosis but does not enhance elimination: 1–2 mEq/kg of bicarbonate every 3–4 hours is a reasonable amount (avoiding the delivery of excessive amounts of sodium). Acidification of urine has been recommended in overdoses of amphetamines, phencyclidine, and quinine, but this procedure can carry considerable risk, especially in the presence of concomitant metabolic acidosis.

Extracorporeal removal therapies

Elimination enhancement by ECT has become an area of growing interest with emerging procedures. In some cases, use of these techniques may provide excellent drug clearance as compared to endogenous clearance, even in presence of intact renal and hepatic function. Despite the promise of ECT, however, very few reports have shown improved outcome compared to supportive measures. Benefits of ECT should be weighted against potential risks of the procedure, pharmacokinetics of the drug, time to initiate therapy, and valuable alternatives to ECT.[47,48] Indications of ECT are summarized in Box 18.2.[49,50]

Toxins have different characteristics, which render them more or less amenable to different types of ECT, the following being the most important:

- *Volume of distribution (V_d)* – although a drug may be entirely cleared from the plasma (= high plasma clearance), this may only represent a minor percentage of total body stores. The smaller the volume of distribution, the more a drug is confined to plasma. A spectacular example is chloroquine: because of its enormous V_d, total body clearance with hemoperfusion (HP) is only 2 L/h.[51]
- *Tissue-to-plasma transfer* – once the drug is cleared from plasma, there can be a significant delay for redistribution from the tissue pool (where a drug exerts its toxic effects) into the intravascular compartment. This is the presumed reason why ECT does not significantly remove organophosphates.[52]
- *Protein binding* – usually, free drug is easier to clear by ECT than drug bound to plasma proteins. However, in overdose, high drug concentration can saturate binding sites, permitting clearance by hemodialysis (HD). Valproic acid[53] and salicylates are such examples.

Box 18.2   General indications for extracorporeal removal therapy (ECT)

Absolute (all must be present)
Exposure to toxic drug
Drug properties that make ECT clearance possible (e.g. low V_d)
Severe overdose suggested by either biochemistry (toxic levels), exposure (absorption of sustained-release drugs), or clinical status (coma, cardiovascular compromise or hypoventilation)

Relative
Deteriorating condition despite maximal supportive therapy
No alternative equally effective treatment (e.g. antidotes)
Inadequate endogenous elimination mechanisms (renal or hepatic failure)

V_d = volume of distribution.

- *Molecular weight* – to be cleared, a molecule must be able to pass through the pores of the artificial membrane. In general, molecules under 2000 Da can be removed by diffusion (during HD), whereas middle molecules (as large as 40 000 Da) can pass through porous membranes with convection (during hemofiltration or HF). Table 18.5 shows examples of drugs for which ECT is not likely to be effective.

Hemodialysis
During HD, molecules transfer from plasma to a dialysate solution (and vice versa) down a concentration gradient through a semipermeable membrane. This allows removal of poisons and correction of associated metabolic abnormalities. Hemodialysis is especially effective to accelerate elimination of substances of low molecular weight, hydrosoluble, poorly bound to plasma proteins and with a low V_d: lithium and alcohols are such ideal molecules.

Generally, high-flux dialyzers are preferred in cases of poisonings because they can improve clearances of some toxins better than standard membranes and, occasionally, better than modalities previously deemed more efficacious; this is the case for carbamazepine and phenobarbital.[54–56] Venovenous access is usually provided by dual-lumen catheters inserted in the internal jugular, subclavicular vein, or femoral vein. The former two need X-ray placement confirmation of the catheter (hence delay), whereas the latter carries higher blood recirculation (loss of efficiency). Some centers use two separate single-lumen catheters inserted in two different central veins to avoid recirculation, but this entails increased complications. Finally, blood flow should be maximized to 400 ml/min whenever possible. Volume removal

---

Table 18.5   Drugs for which extracorporeal removal therapies (ECTs) are not effective.

Drug	Reason why ECT not used
Acetaminophen, narcotics	Efficient antidote
Benzodiazepines	Low mortality even if excessive amounts
Paraquat (late presentation)	Will not improve outcome
Tricyclic antidepressants	Very high V_d
Vitamin C	Not toxic

V_d = volume of distribution.

(or ultrafiltration) is rarely necessary because poisoned patients are generally hypovolemic and subject to hypotension, unless there is lung edema or oliguric renal failure. Care must be given to the prescription of the dialysate bath, since intoxicated patients do not have the same metabolic parameters as chronic renal failure patients (in particular, they may not be hyperkalemic, hyperphosphatemic, or acidotic). The bath should then be readjusted accordingly. Finally, ethanol can also be added to the acid concentrate of dialysate during methanol overdose to offset its removal by hemodialysis.[57]

The extracorporeal circuit should ideally be fully anticoagulated (in order to maximize efficiency) unless the patient is at major risk for bleeding. In such a case, tight heparinization or saline flushes are practical alternatives. Duration of the dialysis session will depend on desired clinical or biochemical surrogates, but is at least 4–6 hours in most cases. Drugs that have a large V_d can be redistributed after hemodialysis, producing a rebound effect, often requiring another session.

Hemofiltration

For HF, blood is passed through a hemofilter in which water and particles are removed by convective forces or solvent drag (as opposed to diffusive forces in conventional HD) and replaced by a physiologic solution containing electrolytes and alkali. Hemofiltration is usually applied in a continuous setting but can also be intermittent. Hemofiltration can remove molecules up to 40 000 Da and is therefore well suited for substances such as aminoglycosides or vancomycin.[58–60]

Hemoperfusion

The principle of HP is based on the passage of blood through a cartridge (instead of a hemofilter) containing a substance with nonspecific adsorptive properties. These substances usually contain activated charcoal, as nonionic resins (XAD-4, polystyrene) are infrequently used today. Resins bind to lipid-soluble drugs , whereas charcoal may bind to a greater variety of substances. Charcoal is coated with a membrane to improve biocompatibility. The advantage of HP is its capacity to extract substances of variable molecular weight (100–40 000 Da), which are liposoluble and\or bound to plasma proteins (since charcoal competes with proteins for binding). However, certain toxins, such as alcohols, saturate the filter very quickly and their elimination is better suited by HD. Furthermore, the HP circuit does not offer dialysis and, therefore, if there are significant acid–base or electrolyte abnormalities, it will be necessary to resort to HD or to combine both types of treatments. HP may also be performed continuously, with good results.[61]

As observed in the AAPCC report (Table 18.6), HD is gaining favor over HP; this may be due to the lesser availability of HP and to the emergence

Table 18.6   AAPCC report on the use of extracorporeal removal therapies (ECTs) for poisoning from 1989 to 2001.

Year	Human exposures	Hemodialysis	Hemoperfusion	Other ECT
1989	1581540	418	191	63
1990	1713462	584	148	97
1991	1837939	692	162	117
1992	1864188	640	164	139
1993	1751476	646	64	80
1994	1926438	743	82	49
1995	2023089	772	59	53
1996	2155952	839	61	35
1997	2192088	927	55	33
1998	2241082	978	48	26
1999	2201156	1049	33	25
2000	2168248	1207	43	39
2001	2267979	1280	45	26

of high-performance dialyzers.[1–13] Paraquat and theophylline overdoses were perhaps the best indications of HP; unfortunately, in the first case, patients often present when it is too late for therapy to be effective and, in the second case, HD remains effective and life-saving. For these reasons, the future of HP is uncertain.

Complications related to HP are mainly thrombocytopenia and leukopenia, both of which may be reduced using a polymer membrane-coated resin. Hypocalcemia, hypoglycemia, and hypothermia may also be seen. Cartridges are prone to coagulation; to avoid this, blood flows should be maintained to at least 200 ml/min and heparinization maintained. The filter must be changed on a regular basis because saturation occurs approximately 2–3 hours after onset of treatment. As in dialysis, rebound following treatment can also be observed in hemoperfusion.

Continuous therapies: venovenous hemodialysis, hemoperfusion, hemofiltration, and hemodiafiltration

Drugs removed by these modalities have lower hourly clearances than intermittent therapies but can be maintained for much longer periods (>24 hours as compared to 4–6 hours). Procainamide, for example, has better daily clearance by continuous hemodiafiltration than intermittent HD clearance.[62] In general, continuous therapies are preferred:

- for hemodynamically unstable patients
- given their continuous nature, they allow better mobilization of intratissular accumulation of the toxin (in chronic overdoses especially where most of drug burden is not in plasma), thus preventing rebound[63]
- more readily available than hemodialysis in some centers, especially in the ICU setting.

Peritoneal dialysis

Unfortunately, drug clearance with peritoneal dialysis (PD) is insufficient to be considered for poisonings. In lithium and barbiturates for example, clearance is only 10 ml/min. Perhaps PD can be restricted to patients already receiving this form of renal replacement in the presence of a mild, non-threatening intoxication, or as adjunct to other effective treatment.[50]

Plasmapheresis

In plasmapheresis (PP), plasma (and all its solutes) is separated from blood and replaced by either 5% albumin or fresh frozen plasma. Usually, removal of 1–3 L in one or two sessions is sufficient for overdoses, although most experience is limited to anecdotal reports. It is more difficult to perform than HD, does not correct metabolic problems, and exposes the patient to blood products. Plasmapheresis should be considered in cases of serious poisonings with substances of low V_d, very tightly bound to proteins, of molecular weight up to 3 000 000 Da (digoxin–fab complexes), or for toxin-related hemolysis.[64,65] Plasmapheresis is presently recognized and accepted therapy for *Amanita* mushroom poisoning.[64–66]

Exchange transfusion

In exchange transfusion (ET), blood is removed from the patient and completely replaced by whole blood. This technique has the advantage of clearing drug that is tightly bound to erythrocytes. Today, it is almost only reserved for infants, in very special circumstances. There are some anecdotal reports for quinine,[67] and theophylline poisoning,[68–70] whereas it is controversial for methotrexate.[71] The risk and benefit profiles for ET need to be further assessed.

Combination therapy

Intuitively, it seems interesting to combine different approaches to optimize decontamination. Hemodialysis and hemoperfusion (by placing the dialyzer first and the cartridge second) can both be done serially and have been used successfully in many cases.[72] This could permit correction of electrolyte abnormalities with HD, while taking advantage of the better clearance with HP (and perhaps delaying saturation of the cartridge). PP (to clear drug-bound toxin) and HP (to clear low- and middle-weight toxins) can also be combined.[73] Another example is to combine ECT with an antidote. While digoxin is not easily cleared by HD, plasmapheresis can clear fab–digoxin complex successfully, in cases of renal failure.[74] Mercury/dimercaptosuccinic acid with continuous therapy[75] and iron/deferoxamine with hemodialysis are other examples.

Others

Albumin dialysis using molecular absorbent recirculating system (MARS) has been recommended in acetaminophen overdose, not for specific removal of the drug but for replacement of hepatic function.[76] Other liver replacement strategies have been described with limited experience.[77] Cardiopulmonary bypass and intra-aortic balloon counterpulsation have also been suggested to compensate temporarily for ineffective cardiac and pulmonary functions until recovery of overdose occurs.[78] Although these areas are promising avenues for the future, at present there are not enough data to support their current use considering their high rate of complications.

Table 18.7 is a summary of preferable ECT according to specific drug properties. Table 18.8 shows a summary of common drug overdoses, their characteristics, and ideal method of removal.

SPECIFIC INTOXICATIONS

Salicylates

Salicylates are one of the most commonly abused drugs. Symptoms of toxicity (observed with as little as 200 mg/kg) include nausea, tinnitus and dizziness, which can progress to fever, hypoglycemia, seizures, and coma. Noncardiogenic edema and high anion gap metabolic acidosis accompanied with respiratory alkalosis (by direct stimulation of respiratory centers) are classic findings. Levels do not adequately reflect clinical risk because toxicity is dependent on salicylate central nervous system (CNS) concentration and on the type of poisoning (worse when chronic) rather than plasma levels. However, it is generally accepted that adverse outcomes are associated with concentrations above 2.5 mmol/L and possibly death if above 6.5 mmol/L.

Management of salicylate poisoning should begin with activated charcoal decontamination. Repeated doses may increase elimination. Salicylates are weak acids (pK_a = 3.0); when ionized, they do not diffuse through cellular membranes (while they freely do when unionized). Intracerebral accumulation of salicylates is therefore dependent on blood pH; the lower the pH, the more the cellular toxicity. Thus, alkalinization (target plasma pH = 7.50–7.55) becomes an essential component of therapy. Urinary alkalinization (by elevating urinary pH from 5 to 7.5) is also a critical step to salicylate elimination and should be performed without delay, even before initiating ECT.[79] Hypoglycemia and hypokalemia often accompany salicylate poisoning and glucose and potassium, respectively, should be replenished accordingly.

Elimination of salicylates can be accelerated by ECT. Hemodialysis is the chosen method because it also corrects associated metabolic changes. In cases of hemodynamic instability, continuous hemodialfiltration has been used successfully.[80] Accepted indications of hemodialysis are the following:[49,81]

- salicylate levels above 7 mmol/L in acute toxicity, or above 2.2 mmol/L in chronic poisoning

Table 18.7 Preferred extracorporeal therapy according to certain drug characteristics.	
Characteristics of drug	**Choice of technique**
Low molecular weight (<2000 Da)	HD
Higher molecular weight	PF/HP/HF
Thrombocytopenia	HD
Water soluble	HD
Renal, metabolic disturbance	HD
Low V_d	HD
Low protein binding	HD
Not adsorbable with charcoal (alcohols, lithium, heavy metals)	HD
Lipid soluble	HP
High protein binding	PF/HP
Molecules very tightly bound to serum proteins, or within large complexes	PF
High V_d	Continuous therapies
Hypotension	Continuous therapies
High tissue binding with slow transfer	Continuous therapies

V_d = volume of distribution; HD = hemodialysis; HF = hemofiltration; HP = hemoperfusion; PF = plasmapheresis.

Table 18.8 Summary of common drug overdoses.

Drug	MW	V_d (L/kg)	Plasma protein binding	Method of removal[a]	Evidence[b]	Comments
Acetaminophen	151	1	10%		3	
Amanita toxin	919	0.3	2%	PP >HD, HP	2	Not likely effective after 12 hours
Aminoglycosides	>500	0.3	2%	HF >HD	2	
Amitriptyline	277	10	96%		4	
Bromide	35	0.7	0%	HD	1	
Cannabis	314	10	99%		4	
Carbamazepine	236	1.4	75%	HP, HD, HF	2	HD perhaps better with new dialyzers
Calcium channel blockers					4	Verapamil is an exception
Chloral hydrate	165	0.8	75%	HD	2	
Chloroquine	158	150	60%		4	HP ineffective
Cocaine	303	1.5	10%		3	
Colchicine	399	4	50%		4	
Digoxin	781	8	25%	PF, HF	2	Only indicated for Fab–dig complex in renal failure
Ethylene glycol	62	0.6	0%	HD	1	
Heroin	369	25	40%		4	
Isopropanol	46	0.6	0%	HD	1	
K+	39	0.6	0%	HD	1	
Lithium	7	1	0%	HD	1	Consider slow procedures
Lorazepam	321	1	93%		3	
Metformin	166	7	1%	HD	2	Highly bound to tissue proteins but removed quickly by hemodialysis
Methanol	32	0.6	0%	HD	1	
Methotrexate	454	0.8	50%	HP, HF, HP + HD	2	Consider slow procedures
Morphine	285	3.5	35%		4	
Organophosphates	300				4	Very slow tissue-to-plasma transfer
Paraquat	186	1	6%	HP >HD	2	Slow procedure perhaps better
Phenobarbital	232	0.9	50%	HP >HD, HF	2	HD perhaps better with new dialyzers
Phenytoin	252	0.6	90%	HP	2	HD perhaps better with new dialyzers
Procainamide	272	1.5	10%	HDF	2	Slow procedure perhaps better
Propylene glycol	76	0.6	0%	HD	1	
Quinine	783	1.5	80%	HP, PF, ET	2	
Salicylates	138	0.2	90%	HD	1	Protein binding lower in overdose
Theophylline	180	0.5	50%	HP >HD	1	
Thyroxine	777	0.2	99.9%	PP	2	
Valproic acid	144	0.2	90%	HP	2	Protein binding lower in overdose
Vancomycin	1500	0.7	55%	HF	1	

ET = exchange transfusion; HD = hemodialysis; HP = hemoperfusion; HF = hemofiltration; HDF = hemodiafiltration; PF = plasma filtration; PP = plasmapheresis.

[a] Most of these values were taken from reports using low-efficiency dialyzers with suboptimal dialysis parameters.

[b] (1) Proven and accepted as efficient; (2) may be efficient clinically but controversial; (3) removable by extracorporeal therapy (ECT) but not clinically indicated; (4) not removable by ECT in sufficient quantity.

For other abbreviations, see text.

- presence of renal failure
- clinical deterioration despite optimal therapy
- persistent acidemia
- serious end-organ complications (coma, pulmonary edema, etc.).

Ethylene glycol and methanol

Ethylene glycol (EG) intoxications are most often the result of voluntary or involuntary ingestion of antifreeze, while methanol can be found in numerous commercial fuels and undistilled alcohol. Early presentation for both intoxications can be confused with ethanol abuse. Unfortunately, if not treated rapidly, patients may have progressive neurologic dysfunction (seizures, coma), renal failure, and cardiopulmonary disease. Patients taking methanol can develop blindness.

Specific diagnosis can often be time-consuming. Clues to the diagnosis are metabolic acidosis with elevated anion gap and accompanying osmolar gap. Ethylene glycol also has findings of hypocalcemia, oxalate crystals in urine, and renal failure by crystal precipitation.

Besides supportive measures, decontamination should include gastric lavage if within 1 hour of ingestion (charcoal is not effective). These compounds are not toxic per se, but their metabolites are (mainly glycolic acid and oxalic acid for EG and formic acid for methanol through the action of alcohol dehydrogenase). Therefore, goals should be oriented towards delaying breakdown of the offending drug, accelerating elimination of the drug and its metabolites, and treating the acidosis, by HD or by exogenous administration of bicarbonate. Ethanol blocks the action of alcohol dehydrogenase with better affinity than toxic alcohols; fomepizole (4-methylpyrazole, 4-MP) is another potent inhibitor of alcohol dehydrogenase and is an accepted therapy for both types of overdose.[82–84] It has fewer side effects and is easier to administer than ethanol and can sometimes avoid the need for HD in the case of EG. It is unclear if this compensates for its much higher cost. Here are the indications of ethanol or 4-MP use:

- metabolic acidosis
- presence of urinary oxalate crystals
- symptomatic overdose
- osmolar gap over 15 mOsm/kgH$_2$O
- EG levels above 3 mmol/L or methanol levels above 6 mmol/L.

For EG overdose, thiamine (100 mg IV) and pyridoxine (100 mg IV) transform glyoxalate into a nontoxic metabolite. For methanol, in symptomatic patients, leucovorin (1 mg/kg IV, max = 50 mg), followed by folic acid 1 to 2 mg/kg IV every 4 hours for 6 doses (or more during HD), can facilitate transformation of formic acid to carbon dioxide. Since toxic alcohols are soluble in water, low molecular weight, unbound to plasma proteins, and have a low V_d, they are the ideal drugs for dialysis. The indications to proceed to HD are the following:

- symptoms of toxicity and\or deterioration within the first hours following admission
- in the presence of refractory acidosis or severe electrolyte abnormalities
- EG levels above 8 mmol/L or methanol levels above 15 mmol/L
- renal failure
- presence of visual signs in methanol toxicity.

Asymptomatic patients (with no metabolic acidosis) and tolerable levels do not need HD. If HD is required, ethanol infusion must be increased to maintain desired ethanol levels or ethanol can be added to the dialysate.[59] HD will be continued until obtaining EG levels lower than 3 mmol/L, methanol levels under 6 mmol/L, osmolar gap lower than 3 mOsm/L and disappearance of acidosis. Ethanol or 4-MP should be continued until the toxic alcohol becomes undetectable.[85]

Lithium

Lithium currently remains a first-line therapy for bipolar disorders. It is usually available as a carbonate salt. GI absorption is fast, with peak concentrations 4 hours after ingestion. Lithium is not metabolized and its elimination is almost exclusively renal. Lithium has a narrow therapeutic window (0.8–1.2 mEq/L).

Clinical presentation of lithium poisoning is variable; it depends partially on the level but also on the type of poisoning (acute or chronic). GI symptoms occur frequently early. Thereafter, nervous system conditions may include confusion, tremors, hyperreflexia, delirium, convulsions, and coma. Renal effects include concentration capacity defects, a reflection of chronic use. ECG changes can sometimes be seen (T-wave flattening, prolonged QT, appearance of a U wave).

Gastric lavage should be initiated if indicated (charcoal does not adsorb lithium). Kayexalate (sodium polystyrene sulfonate) may bind absorbed or unabsorbed lithium in the bowel,[86,87] but is insufficient as monotherapy. Intestinal irrigation with polyethylene glycol may be as beneficial.[88] To improve elimination, forced saline diuresis or diuretic therapy were formerly recommended, but are no longer used. It is preferable to maintain adequate hydration with saline to induce diuresis. As for salicylates, lithium is ideally removed by HD. It is recommended when:

- there is massive documented ingestion
- levels are above 3.5 mEq/L in acute poisoning
- patients are symptomatic in subacute or chronic poisonings (levels do not correlate well with tissue accumulation in such cases).

However, because of the intracellular accumulation and of delay in tissue redistribution, HD is often complicated by rebound. As a consequence, it is sometimes necessary to prolong HD or to repeat sessions, particularly during chronic poisonings in which the tissular accumulation is more extensive. To avoid rebound, continuous renal replacement therapies have been used successfully.[89] Dialysis should be continued until levels are under 1 mEq/L.

Theophylline

The popularity of theophylline has been increasing again recently in treatment for asthma and chronic obstructive pulmonary disease (COPD). It has a narrow therapeutic window (from 55 to 111 μmol/L). Symptoms of toxicity appear in most patients with levels from 111 to 167 μmol/L and are almost universal when above 167 μmol/L. Symptomatology may be mild (nausea, abdominal pain, agitation), severe (supraventricular arrhythmias, seizures, hypotension), or fatal (ventricular arrhythmias, status epilepticus, shock). About 90% of theophylline overdoses are due to chronic exposures[90] and 10% are lethal. Again, there is correlation between the serum peak levels and degree of toxicity in acute but not chronic intoxications.

Administration of MDAC is recommended, even after complete absorption of theophylline. WBI may be considered for sustained-release preparations. If the patient vomits, antiemetics and ranitidine are useful (not cimetidine, which slows down theophylline metabolism). For arrhythmias, verapamil, adenosine, lidocaine as well as selective β-blockers have been successfully tried, whereas convulsions are best controlled with IV diazepam. Serum potassium and phosphate are often low because of transcellular shifts; they should be monitored closely and corrected if necessary.

Theophylline poisoning is amenable to ECT. Hemoperfusion is the best method of removal. It can eliminate significantly more drug than hemodialysis, because of added removal of intraerythrocyte drug.[49] However, new high-performance membranes offer excellent clearances and, therefore, HD remains a perfectly valid alternative. Combined HD with HP is also feasible, with perhaps the best results.[91,92] Continuous techniques,[93] exchange transfusion or plasmapheresis may also be effective (although experience is very limited) but probably less than HP or HD and are complicated to use.[49,59] Criteria for ECR are the following:[49,91]

- acute poisoning with levels >555 μmol/L
- refractory arrhythmias and/or convulsions
- chronic poisoning with levels >330 μmol/L
- chronic poisoning with levels >220 μmol/L in patients presenting with lung, cardiac, or hepatic disease, or over 60 years old
- patients who do not tolerate activated charcoal.

Treatment should be maintained until symptoms disappear or levels are below 280 μmol/L.[93]

REFERENCES

1. Litovitz TL, Klein-Schwartz W, Rodgers GC Jr, et al. 2001 Annual report of the American Association of Poison Control Centers Toxic Exposure Surveillance System. Am J Emerg Med 2002; 20(5):391–452.
2. Litovitz TL, Klein-Schwartz W, White S, et al. 2000 Annual report of the American Association of Poison Control Centers Toxic Exposure Surveillance System. Am J Emerg Med 2001;19(5): 337–95.
3. Litovitz TL, Klein-Schwartz W, White S, et al. 1999 Annual report of the American Association of Poison Control Centers Toxic Exposure Surveillance System. Am J Emerg Med 2000;18(5): 517–74.
4. Litovitz TL, Klein-Schwartz W, Caravati EM, et al. 1998 Annual report of the American Association of Poison Control Centers Toxic Exposure Surveillance System. Am J Emerg Med 1999; 17(5):435–87.
5. Litovitz TL, Klein-Schwartz W, Dyer KS, et al. 1997 Annual report of the American Association of Poison Control Centers Toxic Exposure Surveillance System. Am J Emerg Med 1998;16(5): 443–97.
6. Litovitz TL, Smilkstein M, Felberg L, et al. 1996 Annual report of the American Association of Poison Control Centers Toxic Exposure Surveillance System. Am J Emerg Med 1997;15(5):447–500.
7. Litovitz TL, Felberg L, White S, Klein-Schwartz W. 1995 Annual report of the American Association of Poison Control Centers Toxic Exposure Surveillance System. Am J Emerg Med 1996; 14(5):487–537.
8. Litovitz TL, Felberg L, Soloway RA, Ford M, Geller R. 1994 Annual report of the American Association of Poison Control

Centers Toxic Exposure Surveillance System. Am J Emerg Med 1995;13(5):551–97.

9. Litovitz TL, Clark LR, Soloway RA. 1993 Annual report of the American Association of Poison Control Centers Toxic Exposure Surveillance System. Am J Emerg Med 1994;12(5):546–84.

10. Litovitz TL, Holm KC, Clancy C, et al. 1992 Annual report of the American Association of Poison Control Centers Toxic Exposure Surveillance System. Am J Emerg Med 1993;11(5):494–555.

11. Litovitz TL, Holm KC, Bailey KM, Schmitz BF. 1991 Annual report of the American Association of Poison Control Centers National Data Collection System. Am J Emerg Med 1992;10(5): 452–505.

12. Litovitz TL, Bailey KM, Schmitz BF, Holm KC, Klein-Schwartz W. 1990 Annual report of the American Association of Poison Control Centers National Data Collection System. Am J Emerg Med 1991;9(5):461–509.

13. Litovitz TL, Schmitz BF, Bailey KM. 1989 Annual report of the American Association of Poison Control Centers National Data Collection System. Am J Emerg Med 1990;8(5):394–442.

14. Henderson A, Wright M, Pond SM. Experience with 732 acute overdose patients admitted to an intensive care unit over six years. Med J Aust 1993;158(1):28–30.

15. Parker MG, Fraser GL, Watson DM, Riker RR. Removal of propylene glycol and correction of increased osmolar gap by hemodialysis in a patient on high dose lorazepam infusion therapy. Intensive Care Med 2002;28(1):81–4.

16. Dawson AH, Whyte IM. Therapeutic drug monitoring in drug overdose. Br J Clin Pharmacol 1999;48(3):278–83.

17. Hammett-Stabler CA, Pesce AJ, Cannon DJ. Urine drug screening in the medical setting. Clin Chim Acta 2002;315(1–2):125–35.

18. Warner A. Setting standards of practice in therapeutic drug monitoring and clinical toxicology: a North American view. Ther Drug Monit 2000;22(1):93–7.

19. Goulle JP, Lacroix C. Toxicological analysis in the dawn of the third millenium. Ann Biol Clin 2001;59(5):605–12.

20. Kintz P, Samyn N. Use of alternative specimens: drugs of abuse in saliva and doping agents in hair. Ther Drug Monit 2002;24(2): 239–46.

21. Hoffman RS, Goldfrank LR. The poisoned patient with altered consciousness. Controversies in the use of a 'coma cocktail'. JAMA 1995;274(7):562–9.

22. Doyon S, Roberts JR. Reappraisal of the 'coma cocktail'. Dextrose, flumazenil, naloxone, and thiamine. Emerg Med Clin North Am 1994;12(2):301–16.

23. Weinbroum AA, Flaishon R, Sorkine P, Szold O, Rudick V. A risk-benefit assessment of flumazenil in the management of benzodiazepine overdose. Drug Saf 1997;17(3):181–96.

24. Kulig K. Initial management of ingestions of toxic substances. N Engl J Med 1992;18;326(25):1677–81.

25. Chan TC, Evans SD, Clark RF. Drug-induced hyperthermia. Crit Care Clin 1997;13(4):785–808.

26. Brett AS, Rothschild N, Gray R, Perry M. Predicting the clinical course in intentional drug overdose: implications for use of the intensive care unit. Arch Int Med 1987;147:133–7.

27. Bosse GM, Matyunas NJ. Delayed toxidromes. J Emerg Med 1999;17(4):679–90.

28. Pond SM, Lewis-Driver DJ, Williams GM, Green AC, Stevenson NW. Gastric emptying in acute overdose: a prospective randomised controlled trial. Med J Aust 1995;163(7):345–9.

29. Bond GR. The role of activated charcoal and gastric emptying in gastrointestinal decontamination: a state-of-the-art review. Ann Emerg Med 2002;39(3):273–86.

30. Goldfrank LR. Managing the patient with an unknown overdose. In: Goldfrank LR, Flomenbaum NE, Lewin NA, et al, eds.

Goldfrank's toxicologic emergencies, 6th edn. Stamford, Conn.: Appleton and Lange; 1998:515–40.

31. Harris CR, Kingston R. Gastrointestinal decontamination. Which method is best? Postgrad Med 1992;92(2):116–22,125,128.

32. Krenzelok EP, McGuigan M, Lheur P. Position statement: ipecac syrup. American Academy of Clinical Toxicology; European Association of Poisons Centres and Clinical Toxicologists. J Toxicol Clin Toxicol 1997;35(7):699–709.

33. Vale JA. Position statement: gastric lavage. American Academy of Clinical Toxicology; European Association of Poisons Centres and Clinical Toxicologists. J Toxicol Clin Toxicol 1997;35(7):711–19.

34. Bateman DN. Gastric decontamination – a view for the millennium. J Accid Emerg Med 1999;16(2):84–6.

35. Chyka PA, Seger D. Position statement: single-dose activated charcoal. American Academy of Clinical Toxicology; European Association of Poisons Centres and Clinical Toxicologists. J Toxicol Clin Toxicol 1997;35(7):721–41.

36. Perrone J, Hoffman RS, Goldfrank LR. Special considerations in gastrointestinal decontamination. Emerg Med Clin North Am 1994;12(2):285–99.

37. Barceloux D, McGuigan M, Hartigan-Go K. Position statement: cathartics. American Academy of Clinical Toxicology; European Association of Poisons Centres and Clinical Toxicologists. J Toxicol Clin Toxicol 1997;35(7):743–52.

38. Sporer KA. Whole-bowel irrigation in the management of ingested poisoning. West J Med 1993;159(5):601.

39. Tenenbein M. Position statement: whole bowel irrigation. American Academy of Clinical Toxicology; European Association of Poisons Centres and Clinical Toxicologists. J Toxicol Clin Toxicol 1997; 35(7):753–62.

40. Tenenbein M. Recent advancements in pediatric toxicology. Pediatr Clin North Am 1999;46(6):1179–88.

41. Antman EM, Wenger TL, Butler VP Jr, Haber E, Smith TW. Treatment of 150 cases of life-threatening digitalis intoxication with digoxin-specific Fab antibody fragments. Final report of a multicenter study. Circulation 1990;81(6):1744–52.

42. Trujillo MH, Guerrero J, Fragachan C, Fernandez MA. Pharmacologic antidotes in critical care medicine: a practical guide for drug administration. Crit Care Med 1998;26(2):377–91.

43. Prescott LF, Balali-Mood M, Critchley JA, Johnstone AF, Proudfoot AT. Diuresis or urinary alkalinisation for salicylate poisoning? Br Med J 1982;285(6352):1383–6.

44. Bradberry SM, Vale JA. Multiple-dose activated charcoal: a review of relevant clinical studies. J Toxicol Clin Toxicol 1995; 33(5):407–16.

45. Johnson D, Eppler J, Giesbrecht E, et al. Effect of multiple-dose activated charcoal on the clearance of high-dose intravenous aspirin in a porcine model. Ann Emerg Med 1995;26(5):569–74.

46. Vale JA, Krenzelok EP, Barecloux GD. Position statement and practice guidelines on the use of multi-dose activated charcoal in the treatment of acute poisoning. American Academy of Clinical Toxicology; European Association of Poisons Centres and Clinical Toxicologists. J Toxicol Clin Toxicol 1999;37(6):731–51.

47. Webb D. Charcoal haemoperfusion in drug intoxication. Br J Hosp Med 1993;49(7):493–6.

48. Garella S. Extracorporeal techniques in the treatment of exogenous intoxications. Kidney Int 1988;33:735–54.

49. Garella S, Lorch JA. Hemodialysis and hemoperfusion for poisoning. American Kidney Foundation Nephrology Letter 1993; 10:1–19.

50. Winchester JF, Kitiyakara C. Use of dialysis and hemoperfusion in treatment of poisoning. In: Daugirdas JT, Blake PG, Ing TS, eds. Handbook of dialysis, 3rd edn. Philadelphia, PA: Lippincott, Williams and Wilkins, 2001:263–77.

51. Kawasaki C, Nishi R, Uekihara S, Hayano S, Otagiri M. Charcoal hemoperfusion in the treatment of phenytoin overdose. Am J Kidney Dis 2000;35(2):323–6.

52. Martinez-Chuecos J, del Carmen Jurado M, Paz Gimenez M, Martinez D, Menendez M. Experience with hemoperfusion for organophosphate poisoning. Crit Care Med 1992;20(11):1538–43.

53. Hicks LK, McFarlane PA. Valproic acid overdose and haemodialysis. Nephrol Dial Transplant 2001;16(7):1483–6.

54. Tapolyai M, Campbell M, Dailey K, Udvari-Nagy S. Hemodialysis is as effective as hemoperfusion for drug removal in carbamazepine poisoning. Nephron 2002;90(2):213–5.

55. Palmer BF. Effectiveness of hemodialysis in the extracorporeal therapy of phenobarbital overdose. Am J Kidney Dis 2000; 36(3):640–3.

56. Peces R, Alvarez R. Effectiveness of hemodialysis with high-flux polysulfone membrane in the treatment of life-threatening methanol intoxication. Nephron 2002;90(2):216–18.

57. Dorval M, Pichette V, Cardinal J, et al. The use of an ethanol- and phosphate-enriched dialysate to maintain stable serum ethanol levels during haemodialysis for methanol intoxication. Nephrol Dial Transplant 1999;14(7):1774–7.

58. Golper TA. Drug removal during continuous hemofiltration or hemodialysis. Contrib Nephrol 1991;93:110–16.

59. Pond SM. Extracorporeal techniques in the treatment of poisoned patients. Med J Aust 1991;154(9):617–22.

60. Akil IO, Mir S. Hemodiafiltration for vancomycin overdose in a patient with end-stage renal failure. Pediatr Nephrol 2001;16(12): 1019–21.

61. Lin JL, Lim PS. Continuous arteriovenous hemoperfusion in acute poisoning. Blood Purif 1994;12(2):121–7.

62. Leblanc M, Pichette V, Madore F, et al. N-Acetylprocainamide intoxication with torsades de pointes treated by high dialysate flow rate CAVHD. Crit Care Med 1995;23:589–93.

63. Riegel W. Use of continuous renal replacement therapy for detoxification? Int J Artif Organs 1996;19(2):111–12.

64. Jander S, Bischoff J, Woodcock BG. Plasmapheresis in the treatment of Amanita phalloides poisoning: II. A review and recommendations. Ther Apher 2000;4(4):308–12.

65. Kale-Pradhan PB, Woo MH. A review of the effects of plasmapheresis on drug clearance. Pharmacotherapy 1997;17(4):684–95.

66. St Nenov D, Sv Nenov K. Therapeutic apheresis in exogenous poisoning and in myeloma. Nephrol Dial Transplant 2001;16 (Suppl 6):101–2.

67. Burrows AW, Hambleton G, Hardman MJ, Wilson BD. Quinine intoxication in a child treated by exchange transfusion. Arch Dis Child 1972;47(252):304–5.

68. Shannon MW, Wernovsky G, Morris C. Exchange transfusion in the treatment of severe theophylline intoxication. Vet Hum Tox 1991;33:354.

69. Henry GC, Wax PM, Howland MA, Hoffman RS, Goldfrank LR. Exchange transfusion for the treatment of a theophylline overdose in a premature neonate. Vet Hum Toxicol 1991;33:354.

70. Shannon M, Wernovsky G, Morris C. Exchange transfusion in the treatment of severe theophylline poisoning. Pediatrics 1992;89(1): 145–7.

71. Benezet S, Chatelut E, Bagheri H, et al. Inefficacy of exchange-transfusion in case of a methotrexate poisoning. Bull Cancer 1997; 84(8):788–90.

72. Fiedler R, Baumann F, Deschler B, Osten B. Haemoperfusion combined with haemodialysis in ifosfamide intoxication. Nephrol Dial Transplant 2001;16(5):1088–9.

73. Splendiani G, Zazzaro D, Di Pietrantonio P, Delfino L. Continuous renal replacement therapy and charcoal plasmaperfusion in treatment of amanita mushroom poisoning. Artif Organs 2000; 24(4):305–8.

74. Rabetoy GM, Price CA, Findlay JW, Sailstad JM. Treatment of digoxin intoxication in a renal failure patient with digoxin-specific antibody fragments and plasmapheresis. Am J Nephrol 1990;10(6):518–21.

75. Pai P, Thomas S, Hoenich N, et al. Treatment of a case of severe mercuric salt overdose with DMPS (dimercapo-1-propane sulphonate) and continuous haemofiltration. Nephrol Dial Transplant 2000;15(11):1889–90.

76. McIntyre CW, Fluck RJ, Freeman JG, Lambie SH. Use of albumin dialysis in the treatment of hepatic and renal dysfunction due to paracetamol intoxication. Nephrol Dial Transplant 2002;17(2): 316–7.

77. Stockmann HB, Hiemstra CA, Marquet RL, IJzermans JN. Extracorporeal perfusion for the treatment of acute liver failure. Ann Surg 2000;231(4):460–70.

78. Larkin GL, Graeber GM, Hollingsed MJ. Experimental amitriptyline poisoning: treatment of severe cardiovascular toxicity with cardiopulmonary bypass. Ann Emerg Med 1994;23(3):480–6.

79. Higgins RM, Connolly JO, Hendry BM. Alkalinization and hemodialysis in severe salicylate poisoning: comparison of elimination techniques in the same patient. Clin Nephrol 1998;50(3): 178–83.

80. Wrathall G, Sinclair R, Moore A, Pogson D. Three case reports of the use of haemodiafiltration in the treatment of salicylate overdose. Hum Exp Toxicol 2001;20(9):491–5.

81. Richlie DG, Anderson RJ. Contemporary management of salicylate poisoning: when should hemodialysis and hemoperfusion be used? Semin Dial 1996;9(3):257–64.

82. Brent J, McMartin K, Phillips S, et al. Fomepizole for the treatment of ethylene glycol poisoning. Methylpyrazole for Toxic Alcohols Study Group. N Engl J Med 1999;340(11):832–8.

83. Brent J, McMartin K, Phillips S, Aaron C, Kulig K. Fomepizole for the treatment of methanol poisoning. N Engl J Med 2001;344(6): 424–9.

84. Barceloux DG, Krenzelok EP, Olson K, Watson W. American Academy of Clinical Toxicology Practice Guidelines on the Treatment of Ethylene Glycol Poisoning. Ad Hoc Committee. J Toxicol Clin Toxicol 1999;37(5):537–60.

85. Jones A. Recent advances in the management of poisoning. Ther Drug Monit 2002;24(1):150–5.

86. Ghannoum M, Ayoub P, Lavergne V, Fortin MC, Roy L. Lithium intoxication treated with sodium polystyrene sulfonate, report of 4 cases. Unpublished data.

87. Roberge RJ, Martin TG, Schneider SM. Use of sodium polystyrene sulfonate in a lithium overdose. Ann Emerg Med 1993;22(12): 1911–15.

88. Smith SW, Ling LJ, Halstenson CE. Whole-bowel irrigation as a treatment for acute lithium overdose. Ann Emerg Med 1991; 20(5):536–9.

89. Leblanc M, Raymond M, Bonnardeaux A, et al. Lithium poisoning treated by high-performance continuous arteriovenous and venovenous hemodiafiltration. Am J Kidney Dis 1996;27(3): 365–72.

90. Sessler CN. Theophylline toxicity: clinical features of 116 consecutive cases. Am J Med 1990;88(6):567–76.

91. Benowitz NL, Toffelmire EB. The use of hemodialysis and hemoperfusion in the treatment of theophylline intoxication. Semin Dial 1993;6(4):243–52.

92. Hootkins R Sr, Lerman MJ, Thompson JR. Sequential and simultaneous 'in series' hemodialysis and hemoperfusion in the management of theophylline intoxication. J Am Soc Nephrol 1990;1(6):923–6.

93. Okada S, Teramoto S, Matsuoka R. Recovery from theophylline toxicity by continuous hemodialysis with filtration. Ann Intern Med 2000;133(11):922.

19

Other nonazotemic/nonrenal renal replacement therapy indications

Miet Schetz

INTRODUCTION

Continuous renal replacement therapy (CRRT) is often regarded as one of the more important advances in intensive care medicine in recent years. The use of CRRT in critically ill patients with acute renal failure (ARF) combined with cardiovascular instability, severe fluid overload, cerebral edema, or hypercatabolism is widely accepted.[1] CRRT is also used in some nonrenal indications and these are less well established. These nonrenal indications are based on the presumed elimination of inflammatory mediators (systemic inflammatory response syndrome (SIRS) and sepsis, acute respiratory distress syndrome (ARDS), cardiopulmonary bypass (CPB)), on the removal of fluid (ARDS, CPB, congestive heart failure (CHF)), or on the elimination of nonuremic endogenous toxic solutes (inborn errors of metabolism, lactic acidosis, crush injury, tumor lysis syndrome). This chapter reviews the available evidence for each of these nonrenal indications. The use of CRRT in intoxications will not be discussed.

SEPSIS AND SIRS

Severe sepsis and septic shock continue to be a major cause of morbidity and mortality in critically ill patients.[2] The sepsis syndrome begins with the recognition of microbial products by phagocytic leukocytes and other immune cells that are activated and release toxic cytokines and other mediators. These mediators activate various plasma cascade systems and attract further immune cells, resulting in the release of secondary mediators and amplification of the host response. This innate host response has developed to protect the organism: at a local level it serves to contain, kill and remove foreign material. However, a generalized host response is probably maladaptive and harms the host. In sepsis an 'inflammatory imbalance' exists with either excessive inflammation resulting in multiple organ dysfunction, probably through widespread endothelial damage, or excessive anti-inflammation resulting in immunosuppression. The mediators released in sepsis include pro-inflammatory cytokines (e.g. tumor necrosis factor-α (TNF-α) and interleukins (IL-1, IL-6 and IL-8)), anti-inflammatory cytokines (e.g. IL-10, soluble TNF receptors, IL-1ra), release products of the coagulation, complement and contact system, arachidonic acid metabolites, reactive oxygen species, and nitric oxide.[3,4] Already more than 15 years ago, hemofiltration was suggested to be beneficial for septic patients, an effect that was hypothesized to be related to the extracorporeal removal of these inflammatory mediators.[5]

Rationale for the use of hemofiltration in sepsis

Inflammation and anti-inflammation are both harmful and protective and this hampers their modulation by treatment. In addition, the complexity of the host response, with important redundancy, synergy, antagonism and feedback regulation, makes the development of pharmacologic interventions extremely difficult.[6–8] The simultaneous removal of several mediators with most pronounced effect on those with the highest concentration, thus dampening the pro-inflammatory as well as the anti-inflammatory effect, could make hemofiltration an interesting alternative for the treatment of sepsis. However,

CRRT is a rather invasive treatment, requiring the introduction of a large catheter and continuous anticoagulation. In addition, the indiscriminate removal of circulating substances may induce imbalances or deficiencies. And finally, it represents an important cost and workload. It is thus obvious that we need scientific evidence before this treatment can be widely advocated in septic patients without renal failure.

Are inflammatory mediators removed by continuous renal replacement therapy?

Theoretically, CRRT can affect the plasma level of inflammatory mediators by elimination in the ultrafiltrate (*convection*), by elimination in the dialysate (*diffusion*), by adsorption to the membrane (*adsorption*), or by eliminating substances that influence their production. Most of the inflammatory mediators are in the small to middle molecular weight range (Table 19.1) and are therefore amenable to convective removal from the circulation. Diffusion, a size-dependent process, is less suitable for removal of these larger solutes. Convective removal depends on both the filtration rate (Q_f) and the sieving coefficient (ratio of ultrafiltrate to plasma concentration). The reported sieving coefficients of inflammatory mediators[9-22] (summarized in Table 19.1) vary considerably, which may have several explanations:

1. the use of membranes with different cut-off
2. the timing of the sampling, since the sieving coefficient may increase over time after adsorption has reached saturation[9] or may decrease over time due to polarization of proteins on the surface[10,11]
3. Q_f also may affect the sieving coefficient, higher filtration rates inducing more protein polarization[10,11]
4. the use of different assays.

The reported sieving coefficients are generally not very high. Molecular weight does not appear to be the sole determinant of sieving, probably because of differences in three-dimensional structure and

Table 19.1   The molecular weight and sieving coefficient of sepsis mediators.

Mediator	MW (Da)	S	Reference
Endotoxin fragments	100 000		
TNF-α (trimer)	51 000	0–0.3	9–19
TNF sR I	33 000	0.09	18
TNF sR II	30 000	0.01	17,18
IL-1β	17 000	0.04–0.86	10,11
IL-1ra	22 000	0.28–0.45	17,18
IL-6	26 000	0.02–0.86	10–12,15
IL-6 sR	65 000		
IL-8	8000	0.1–0.8	10–12,20
IL-10	14 000	0–1.15	10,12,16,21
IFN-γ	20 000		
TGF-β		0.59	21
C3a/C5a	11 000	0.2–0.77	19
Procalcitonin	13 000	0.04–0.1	22
Endothelin	2500	0.19–0.3	40
Bradykinin	1000		
Arachidonic acid			
Metabolites	600	0.5–0.9	15,40

TNF = tumor necrosis factor; IL = interleukin; IFN = interferon; TGF = transforming growth factor; MW = molecular weight (daltons); S = sieving coefficient.

charge. In addition, many inflammatory cytokines are bound to aspecific binding proteins (e.g. α_2-macroglobulin[23]) or to specific binding substances (e.g. soluble receptors for TNF and IL-6[24,25]) or remain cell-associated,[26] thus hampering their passage through the membrane.

Adsorption is an alternative pathway of extracorporeal elimination of mediators and recent evidence suggests that it might even be the predominant elimination route of cytokines,[16,27] which would plead for the use of filters with high surface area. However, adsorption reaches saturation after a few hours[16,18,28] and might even be followed by release of mediators.[18,29] In order to obtain a maximal effect, frequent filter changes will thus be required. It is interesting to note that Kellum et al found higher adsorptive TNF removal with hemofiltration than with hemodialysis, suggesting that convective transport with exposure of the filtrate to the inner structure of the membrane increases the adsorptive area.[27] Adsorption depends on both membrane and mediator characteristics, which explains the diverging results in different trials. In particular, the AN69 membrane appears to have a high adsorptive capacity, and adsorption of both complement components and cytokines has been described.[9,12,16,18,27,30–33] Two recent in-vitro investigations did not find adsorption of TNF, IL-1, IL-6, IL-8, or IL-10 to cellulose acetate or to polyamide.[10,11]

Whether the convective or adsorptive removal with CRRT will influence the plasma level of inflammatory mediators not only depends on the extent of their elimination but also on their kinetic behavior. Most mediators have a short half-life, pointing to a high endogenous clearance. Their persistent presence in the circulation should therefore be attributed to an ongoing production rather than a slow elimination. Compared with the high endogenous clearance, the contribution of the extracorporeal clearance, especially when 'renal' operational characteristics are used, will be negligible and can therefore not be expected to influence plasma levels.[34]

Since the plasma levels of inflammatory mediators may vary considerably over time[35,36] and are influenced by many clinical conditions and therapeutic interventions,[37,38] uncontrolled observations can neither prove nor exclude a significant impact of the extracorporeal treatment. Unfortunately, few trials in this field have a prospective controlled design. Most of the experimental trials do not find an effect on TNF levels.[15,29,39,40] Also the levels of arachidonic acid metabolites do not seem to be affected.[15,29,40] Bellomo et al found a lower endothelin level in the filtered animals, somewhat unexpectedly in view of the significant increase of the blood pressure.[40] Yekebas et al, on the other hand, noted that hemofiltration attenuated the increase of TNF levels after the induction of septic pancreatitis. However, extracorporeal treatment also attenuated the hyporesponsiveness of lipopolysaccharide (LPS)-stimulated polymorphonuclear neutrophils (PMNs), resulting in higher TNF levels in the later phase.[21] A few small randomized trials have compared hemofiltration with standard treatment in patients with inflammatory syndromes without ARF. No significant differences were found with regard to the levels of C3a, C5a, IL-6, IL-8, IL-10, or TNF,[41–44] with the exception of Braun et al who report a somewhat more pronounced decrease of TNF in the filtered group.[41] Wakabayashi et al also found lower IL-6 and IL-8 levels during hemofiltration than during a control period between two treatments.[45] Two clinical trials using high-volume hemofiltration (HVHF) also show a significant effect on some mediators. Journois et al compared zero-balanced HVHF (total $Q_f = 5$ L/m^2) with no treatment during CPB in children undergoing elective surgery for congenital heart disease. They found lower C3a, TNF, and IL-10 levels immediately after the procedure and lower IL-1 and IL-6 levels 24 hours later, suggesting that cytokine-inducing substances were eliminated during HVHF.[46] Cole et al report on 11 patients with septic shock and multiple organ failure who were treated with HVHF in a cross-over design, comparing a Q_f of 6 L/h with 1 L/h, each for 8 hours with a washout period between the treatments. The higher Q_f resulted in significantly lower plasma levels of C3a and C5a.[47]

In conclusion, although both convection and adsorption of inflammatory mediators have clearly been shown, there is limited evidence for a significant effect of this extracorporeal removal on the plasma level of these substances, and certainly not with the operational characteristics that are currently used. The mediator network in sepsis is extremely complex and incompletely elucidated and it is not clear which mediators have to be eliminated to what extent. The answer to this question might even differ according to the underlying pathology or the phase of the disease process. Since the ultimate goal of hemofiltration in sepsis and inflammation is to improve organ dysfunction and survival, focusing on the clinical effect of hemofiltration is probably more important than looking at mediator elimination.

Continuous renal replacement therapy in animal models of sepsis

Many experimental studies have been performed to test the hypothesis that hemofiltration improves the outcome of sepsis (summarized in Table 19.2);[14,21,29,39,40,48–57] such studies use different hypo- or hyperdynamic sepsis models with variable clinical relevance. CRRT is always isovolemic, is mostly started early after the induction of sepsis and, with a few exceptions, only the (very) short-term effect of the procedure is evaluated. Different membranes are used and, probably very important, filtration rates vary considerably between 10 and 200 ml/kg/h (HVHF). Short-term survival is either not assessed or improved. Those studies that evaluate the effect of zero-balanced hemofiltration on respiratory parameters found either no effect or an improvement in oxygenation (especially with HVHF) and/or lung mechanics. Most, but not all, studies find an improvement of hemodynamic parameters, with an increase of mean arterial pressure (MAP) and systemic vascular resistance (SVR) being the most consistent finding, whereas an improved cardiac output (CO) is less frequently observed. Early treatment appears to be more effective than late.[56] The most striking hemodynamic effect is seen with HVHF,[39,51,53] although even here the results are not always consistent.[57] This would suggest the convective removal of a myocardial depressant substance. The presence of such a substance in the filtrate[49,58] and its decrease in the circulation during CRRT[49,56] has indeed been demonstrated. Bellomo et al, on the other hand, showed that 'medium volume HF' resulted in an immediate (after 15 minutes) increase of blood pressure, which would argue against an important contribution of convective removal.[40] Yekebas et al, in an elegant study with the use of different Q_f and filter duration, demonstrated that both high filtration rates and frequent filter changes have a beneficial hemodynamic effect, suggesting that both convection and adsorption may contribute.[21] Another way to increase convective removal is to increase the membrane pore size. Lee et al compared two membranes with 50 kDa and 100 kDa pore size and found an improved survival with the large pore membrane.[59] Kline et al found an improved systolic function and myocardial efficiency with a large-pore polysulfone membrane (unfortunately, no treatment group with standard pore size filter was included in this experiment).[60] Some investigators have looked beyond the cardiopulmonary effect and evaluated aspects of immune function. DiScipio and Burchard, in a nonlethal model of intra-abdominal infection, demonstrated that continuous arteriovenous hemofiltration (CAVH) attenuates polymorphonuclear phagocytosis during the first 48 h.[55] Whether this represents an advantage remains to be proven. Other aspects of PMN function, such as oxidative burst or chemotaxis, were not assessed. Yekebas et al, on the other hand, found that continuous venovenous hemofiltration (CVVH) in animals with septic pancreatitis resulted in decreased C-reactive protein (CRP) and white blood cell (WBC) count, improved in-vitro cytokine release by endotoxin-stimulated PMN, improved monocyte major histocompatibility complex (MHC) II antigen expression and improved oxidative burst and phagocytosis by PMN. These effects too were accentuated by high filtration rates and frequent filter changes, suggesting a contribution of both convection and adsorption.[21]

Clinical data on continuous renal replacement therapy in sepsis or inflammatory syndromes

A large number of uncontrolled clinical observations report an improvement of hemodynamic parameters during CRRT.[16,17,19,61–63] An improvement in oxygenation can mostly be attributed to a negative fluid balance.[62,64–67] Only a few randomized trials with limited patient numbers compare 'prophylactic' CRRT with no extracorporeal treatment in patients with (mostly post-traumatic) SIRS without ARF. The most striking effect is an increase of SVR and MAP and an attenuation of the hyperdynamic circulation.[42,45,68,69] Only limited filtration rates (300–1000 ml/h) were used in these studies. Cole et al performed a prospective randomized trial, comparing CVVH with Q_f of 2 L/h with conservative treatment in patients with early SIRS without ARF. They could not establish a difference in the mean cumulative multiple organ dysfunction score (MODS) or in the duration of vasopressor requirement.[44] However, a cross-over design between CVVH with Q_f of 6 L/h and 1 L/h in septic patients with ARF showed a significant reduction of the norepinephrine requirements with the higher filtration rates.[47] Other clinical studies also suggest a beneficial effect of HVHF.

Oudemans-van Straaten et al performed a prospective cohort analysis of 306 patients, treated with HVHF (mean Q_f 3.8 L/h in runs of 100 L, median 2 runs). Indications for HVHF were circulatory shock and pulmonary edema with or without ARF. In a subgroup of patients with therapy-resistant low cardiac output syndrome, CO and MAP increased during HVHF. In a subgroup of patients with high cardiac output, SVR increased despite decreasing norepinephrine doses. The arterial oxygenation improved most clearly in the patients with low PaO_2/FiO_2 ratio. None of these effects was related to the fluid balance (all uncontrolled observations!). The standardized mortality ratio (observed/predicted mortality) was low; however, it was not different from that of the whole intensive care unit (ICU) population in this closed unit.[70] Another uncontrolled study was performed with short-term HVHF ($Q_f = 35$ L/4 h) in 20 patients with severe refractory hypodynamic septic shock ($n = 11$). Hemodynamic responders ($n = 11$), defined by increase of CO, mixed venous oxygen saturation (SvO_2) and pH and decrease of epinephrine dose, had a significantly better survival (82% vs 0%). In addition, they appeared to have a longer time interval from ICU admission to HVHF and a higher body weight, pointing to the importance of treatment timing and dose. However, this still remains an uncontrolled observation.[71] Ronco et al performed a prospective randomized trial comparing three different hemofiltration doses (20–35–45 ml/kg/h) in 425 patients with ARF.[72] A subgroup analysis of 52 patients with sepsis shows a lower mortality in the group treated with 45 ml/kg/h (53%) vs the other two groups (82% in the 35 ml/kg/h group and 75% in the 20 ml/kg/h group), although the numbers are probably too small to reach statistical significance.[73]

In summary, a limited number of clinical studies suggest hemodynamic stabilization during CVVH, especially with HVHF, in septic patients. The few studies suggesting an improved survival are either uncontrolled[70,71] or include a very small patient number.[73] The mechanism of the hemodynamic effect is not clear. It can point to the removal of inflammatory mediators with cardiovascular activity or to the removal of other vasoactive substances. Whether a decrease of norepinephrine requirement is a valid outcome parameter is debatable. It indeed points to an improvement of cardiovascular failure. However, a recent prospective, multicenter, observational study on the pattern of organ dysfunction in septic patients showed that an improvement of the cardiovascular score over time, in contrast to an improvement of other failing organs, was not associated with a better outcome.[74] In addition, other interventions known to increase

blood pressure were not always associated with better outcome. A recent large prospective randomized trial with a nitric oxide synthase inhibitor was stopped early because of an increased mortality in patients receiving the drug.[75] Hemodynamic parameters can therefore not be a valid outcome parameter to analyze the effect of this powerful procedure with many possible (unmeasured) effects.

A few authors also evaluated the effect of CVVH on the immune system. Lonnemann et al report an improvement of the in-vitro LPS-induced TNF production during CRRT in septic patients, pointing to an improved immune function.[76] Hoffmann, on the other hand, demonstrated that ultrafiltrate of septic patients stimulates the TNF release by monocytes and suppresses the IL-2 and IL-6 production by lymphocytes.[77] Mariano et al demonstrated that CVVH reduces the priming activity of the serum of septic patients on neutrophil chemiluminescence, a finding they attribute to the removal of IL-8.[20]

Conclusion

Administration of appropriate antibiotics together with the removal of the septic source and hemodynamic stabilization remain the mainstay in the treatment of sepsis. Although the evidence for a clinically important extracorporeal elimination of inflammatory mediators is not very strong, hemofiltration appears to have some effect in patients with sepsis and other inflammatory syndromes. The mechanism of this effect, however, remains unclear. Studies looking at mediator elimination suggest that adsorption is the most important clearance mechanism. This would imply that we should give preference to membranes with high adsorptive capacity and high surface area, combined with frequent filter changes. Studies looking at the hemodynamic effect suggest that high filtration rates are important, whereas immune function seems to benefit from a combination of high filtration rates and frequent filter changes. However, HVHF remains a cumbersome and riskful procedure that should be restricted to the setting of clinical trials until such a trial, performed prospectively and randomized, has proven a beneficial effect on the survival of septic patients.

Besides hemofiltration, other extracorporeal blood purification techniques for sepsis are under investigation. Examples are plasmapheresis,[78,79] coupled plasma filtration and adsorption[80,81] and

Table 19.2 Overview of experimental trials on the use of hemofiltration in sepsis.

Main author	Animal (weight)	Model	Sepsis	Timing	Duration	Technique	Membrane	Q_f (ml/kg/h)	Hemodynamics	Respiratory	Survival
Gomez 1990[48]	Dogs (20–35 kg)	E.coli bolus+ infusion/5 h	Hyperdynamic	4 h	2–3 h	CAVH (pumped)	PA	14–50	Improved (EsEmax)	No effect	NA
Stein 1990–91[49,50]	Pigs (28–32 kg)	Endotoxin infusion to PAP × 2	Hypodynamic	15 min after PAP	3.5 h	CVVH	PS	20	Slight improvement	Improved mechanics No effect on oxygenation	Trend to improvement
Grootendorst 1992[51]	Pigs (36–39 kg)	Endotoxin 'bolus'	Hypodynamic	30 min	3.5 h	CVVH	PS	170	Improved (MAP, CO, RVEF)	Improved pO$_2$	NA
Lee 1993[52]	Piglets (5–10 kg)	Live Staphylococcus aureus	?	0 h	6 h	CAVH	PS	50–200	No consistent effect	No effect	Improved
Grootendorst 1994[53]	Pigs (33–39 kg)	Clamping AMS	Hypodynamic	30 min before	3 h	CVVH	Cu	160–180	Improved (MAP,CO, LVSW)	NA	60% vs 0% (24 h)
Heideman 1994[14]	Rats (0.4 kg)	Endotoxin 'bolus'	Hypodynamic	Before LPS	4 h	CAVH	PS	25–40	No effect	NA	Improved
Freeman 1995[54]	Dogs (7–13 kg)	Infected clot intraperitoneal	Hypodynamic	1 h	6 h		PS	60	No effect	NA	Trend to decrease
DiScipio 1997[55]	Pigs (15–20 kg)	Cecal ligation and puncture	?	1.5 h	72 h	CAVH	PS	8–10	No effect	No effect	NA
Ishihara 1999[29]	Pigs (30–45 kg)	Endotoxin infusion/24 h	?	0.5 h	24 h	CVVH	PA	22–30	NA	No effect	NA
Mink 1999[56]	Dogs (20–30 kg)	Pneumonia	Hypodynamic	2 h vs 5 h	3 h	CAVH	?	33	Improved if early (MAP and SW)	No effect	NA
Rogiers 1999[39]	Dogs (±28 kg)	Endotoxin 'bolus'	Hyperdynamic	1 h	3.5 h	CVVH	PA	100 or 200	Improved (more if 200)	No effect	NA

Bellomo 2000[40]	Dogs (19–22 kg)	Endotoxin 'bolus'	Hypodynamic	Before LPS 3 h	CVVH	AN69	87	Improved (MAP, SVR, not CO)	NA	NA
Yekebas 2001[21]	Pigs (21–30 kg)	Septic pancreatitis	Hyperdynamic	When SVR 70%	60 h	CVVH	AN69	20 or 100	Improved (MAP, SVR, CO)	NA	67% vs 0% (24 h)
Ullrich 2001[57]	Pigs (25–30 kg)	Endotoxin infusion/2 h	Hypodynamic	3 h	4 h	CVVH	PS	150–180	No effect	Improved oxygenation and mechanics	NA

AMS = arteria mesenterica superior; PAP = pulmonary artery pressure; SVR = systemic vascular resistance; CAVH = continuous arteriovenous hemofiltration; CVVH = continuous venovenous hemofiltration; PA = polyamide; PS = polysulfone; Cu = cuprophane; AN69 = polyacrylonitrile; MAP = mean arterial pressure; SW = stroke work; CO = cardiac output; NA = not assessed; LPS = lipopolysaccharide; RVEF = right ventricular ejection fraction; LVSW = left ventricular stroke work.

polymyxin B immobilized fibers.[82,83] A further discussion of these treatments is beyond the scope of this chapter.

ACUTE RESPIRATORY DISTRESS SYNDROME

Three mechanisms could explain a beneficial effect of CRRT on ARDS:

1. CRRT-induced hypothermia *reduces CO_2 production*. The decreased ventilatory requirement in turn reduces the risk of ventilator-induced lung injury.
2. *Elimination of inflammatory mediators* is discussed in the previous section. Variable effects on oxygenation and lung mechanics have been reported with zero-balanced hemofiltration in animal models of sepsis or other inflammatory syndromes (see Table 19.2).[29,39,49–52,55–57] In a small randomized trial in patients with ARDS, Cosentino et al found an even better oxygenation in the control group than in the (zero-balanced) hemofiltered group.[84]
3. In most clinical studies the beneficial effect of hemofiltration on gas exchange can be attributed to *fluid removal*.[62,64–67] Fluid management in ARDS and sepsis remains, however, controversial.[85] In observational studies negative fluid balances have indeed been associated with improved outcome.[86,87] However, this could also be an expression of the greater capillary leak and fluid requirement in sicker patients. Theoretically, a reduction of the hydrostatic pressure in the pulmonary circulation will reduce the pressure gradient, driving the formation of edema.

Humphrey and co-workers indeed showed that a reduction in pulmonary capillary wedge pressure (PCWP) is associated with an improved survival in ARDS patients. However, what they actually showed was a better survival in the patients who responded to diuretics, dialysis, or ultrafiltration with a lowering of PCWP, compared with (probably sicker) patients in whom the same treatment had no effect on the wedge pressure.[88] Laggner et al compared the effect of ultrafiltration on the extravascular lung water (EVLW) of patients with cardiogenic pulmonary edema and ARDS and showed a decrease of the shunt fraction in both groups. However, the reduction of EVLW was less pronounced in ARDS patients in whom hemofiltration also induced a decrease of cardiac output

and O_2 delivery.[89] Ultrafiltration in ARDS patients should therefore only be performed under close hemodynamic monitoring.

CARDIOPULMONARY BYPASS

Cardiac surgery provokes a vigorous inflammatory response due to the surgical trauma, blood loss or transfusion, hypothermia, CPB, nonpulsatile flow, ischemia reperfusion, and endotoxemia.[90] In addition, during CPB, hemodilution is required in order to reduce the amount of transfused blood and to improve viscosity during hypothermia. Both the inflammatory response and hemodilution result in accumulation of extravascular water, organ dysfunction (especially pulmonary and myocardial dysfunction), and coagulopathy. This problem is most pronounced in children because of the often greater complexity of the operative procedure, requiring longer periods of extracorporeal circulation, the small blood volume compared to the bypass circuit, and the limited capacity for water removal in neonates.

In an attempt to reduce this 'postperfusion syndrome', filtration techniques have been applied during and after CPB. When, during rewarming on CPB, a proportion of the blood passes through a filter and both the patient and the circuit content are hemoconcentrated, the procedure is called conventional ultrafiltration (CUF). It was initially introduced to treat patients with chronic renal failure, preoperative fluid overload, extreme hemodilution, and prolonged CPB.[91–96] Modified ultrafiltration (MUF), applied shortly after CPB during 10–15 minutes, allows for greater efficiency of filtration because there is no requirement to maintaining the reservoir level.[97–99] In adults the effects of these filtration techniques on hemodynamics, oxygenation, blood loss, and transfusion requirement remain controversial, often short-lasting and with limited clinical benefit.[100–104] In pediatric cardiac surgery (especially modified), ultrafiltration has shown beneficial effects on postoperative weight gain,[97] blood loss, and/or transfusion requirement,[97,105–108] on oxygenation or duration of mechanical ventilation,[105,107,108] on pulmonary compliance,[109] on blood pressure,[97,105,107] on myocardial contractility,[110,111] on myocardial diastolic function,[110] on myocardial edema,[110,111] and on pulmonary vascular resistance.[111–113] Experimental data also suggest a beneficial effect of MUF on the cerebral metabolic recovery after deep hypothermic circulatory arrest.[114] In this animal study MUF appeared more effective than transfusion, which led the authors to the conclusion that MUF acts by other mechanisms than increased O_2 delivery. However, a subsequent animal study showed that a higher perfusate hematocrit was more effective than MUF in improving neurologic recovery.[115] The deleterious effects of autologous transfusion on tissue oxygenation might be a possible explanation for this discrepancy.[116]

Whether the beneficial effects of ultrafiltration are attributed solely to removal of excess water and the concomitant increase of the coagulation factors, hematocrit, and colloid oncotic pressure, or whether removal of inflammatory mediators also contributes, remains a matter of debate. Controlled clinical studies have indeed shown inconsistent effects of ultrafiltration on cytokine levels,[99,105,110,117–119] which is not unexpected in view of the limited duration, the limited volumes removed, and the hemoconcentration. If removal of mediators does indeed contribute substantially to the observed effect, an increase of Q_f with partial substitution of the filtered volume may be required to maximize the effect. Ming et al found lower cytokine levels with the use of 'balanced ultrafiltration'.[120] Journois et al performed a randomized trial in which they compared MUF with (very) high-volume (5000 ml/m²) zero-balanced hemofiltration during CPB followed by MUF in children undergoing surgical correction of congenital heart disease under hypothermic CPB. After HVHF, the hemofiltered group had lower levels of C3a and TNF. However after 24 hours the difference in TNF was more pronounced and also the levels of IL-1, IL-6, and IL-8 were lower. The author concludes, therefore, that HVHF removes cytokine-inducing substances. The dampened inflammatory response is manifested clinically as a lower body temperature, less blood loss, lower neutrophil count, and less oxidative damage to the lungs.[46] The use of zero-balanced HVHF in an animal experiment with deep hypothermic circulator arrest also resulted in improved oxygenation, lung compliance, cardiac output, and pulmonary vascular resistance.[121] Hiramatsu et al used 'dilutional' hemofiltration during CPB combined with MUF and found, compared with CUF, a lower endothelin level and pulmonary vascular resistance in children after the Fontan procedure.[113]

In conclusion, most of the observed beneficial effects of CUF and MUF can be attributed to the removal of excess water. Whether modulation of the inflammatory response is possible with simple ultrafiltration is questionable. On the other

hand, limited evidence in children suggests that the use of HVHF during CPB might have an anti-inflammatory effect.

CONGESTIVE HEART FAILURE

Congestive heart failure, a leading cause of morbidity and mortality in Western countries, is characterized by the hyperstimulation of vasoconstrictive and sodium-retaining neurohumoral systems (renin–angiotensin–aldosterone system (RAAS), adrenergic system, arginine–vasopressin system). This neurohormonal activation induces structural and conformational changes in the heart, resulting from altered loading conditions and/or the direct action of these biologically active molecules.[122] Modern treatment of CHF is based on the correction of this overstimulation and consists of angiotensin-converting enzyme (ACE) inhibitors, aldosterone antagonists, beta-blockers, and diuretics.[123] In advanced stages of CHF (NYHA class III and IV), patients become refractory to conservative measures and pharmacologic interventions. Advanced CHF significantly affects the quality of life and imposes a major burden on healthcare resources. In these patients symptoms can be relieved by the removal of fluid and sodium with simple ultrafiltration, as was already suggested more than 25 years ago.[124,125]

Patients with CHF under standard pharmacotherapy appear to have a lower than normal blood volume.[126] Hemodynamic stability during ultrafiltration can therefore only be preserved through an adequate plasma refilling that, fortunately, appears to be more rapid in patients with expanded interstitial space.[127,128] Marenzi et al found efficient plasma refilling during ultrafiltration of 500 ml/h in patients with refractory CHF.[129] The endpoint of the ultrafiltration treatment is usually an increase of the hematocrit by 10% of baseline. Overly aggressive ultrafiltration with hypovolemia-induced hypotension can be avoided by the use of blood volume monitors.[130] Special care should be taken in patients on ACE inhibitors, because these drugs may interfere with the defense mechanisms toward hypovolemia (activation of RAAS). In addition, the hypotension that is sometimes seen after the start of CRRT appears to be, at least partially, mediated by bradykinin, the breakdown of which is prevented by ACE inhibition.[131] On the other hand, ACE inhibitors are important to counteract the body's response to ultrafiltration-induced dehydration, explaining the more sustained effect of ultrafiltration in patients on ACE inhibition.[132]

A typical response to ultrafiltration in heart failure consists of an improvement of the clinical and functional condition, with reduction of the radiologic signs of lung congestion, relief of respiratory distress, improved oxygenation and pulmonary compliance, decreased filling pressures with preserved or even increased CO, increased exercise performance, decreased peripheral edema and ascites, increased diuresis, and restored responsiveness to diuretics.[129,133–141] Most of these effects are easily explained by a reduction of interstitial fluid volume. Two mechanisms have been suggested to explain the decreased filling pressures with preserved CO: (1) the heart is operating on the horizontal part of the ventricular function curve or (2) removal of the constraining effect of the overhydrated lungs reduces the absolute filling pressures, but not the transmural or the effective filling pressures, and improves the diastolic properties of the heart.[129,133,136,137] Another insufficiently explained observation is the decrease of neuroendocrine factors after ultrafiltration in overhydrated patients,[135,136,138,142] whereas ultrafiltration normally induces an increase of plasma renin activity and catecholamines.[143,144] Proposed explanations are an improved cardiac performance with lowered sympathetic drive (however, decreased neurohumoral stimulation is also seen when CO remains unchanged) or regression of organ congestion, which results in improved clearance of norepinephrine. The reduced release or enhanced clearance of salt- and water-retaining hormones may explain the restored diuresis and diuretic responsiveness. Alternative explanations are an increase of renal perfusion pressure or restored sensitivity to atrial natriuretic factor.

Compared with an additional bolus of furosemide, and despite a similar fluid removal, ultrafiltration appears to result in a better and more sustained effect.[139] The greater sodium removal with ultrafiltration might be responsible for the different neurohumoral response and, consequently, a more favorable water and salt balance post ultrafiltration. The direct stimulating effect of loop diuretics on renin secretion via the macula densa may also contribute to the more rapid fluid reaccumulation with furosemide.[145,146] Additional research will be needed in order to determine whether the observed neuroendocrine effect has a beneficial effect on survival of patients with refractory CHF.

LACTIC ACIDOSIS

Hyperlactatemia is common in critically ill patients, especially in those with sepsis. This hyperlactatemia may or may not be accompanied by acidosis, depending on the balance of other ions.[147] Although hypoperfusion and hypoxia play a dominant role in lactate production in ischemic states (shock lactate), current evidence suggests that elevated lactate levels may also result from an increased glycolytic flux stimulated by catecholamines and inflammatory mediators (stress lactate).[148] In addition to increased production, decreased hepatic clearance also contributes to hyperlactatemia.[149] Whether lactic acidosis and/or hyperlactatemia are in themselves harmful and should be corrected remains a matter of debate.[150,151] A few case reports have suggested that CRRT, by extracorporeal elimination of lactate, may contribute to this correction.[152–154] Hemofiltration with sodium bicarbonate in the substitution fluid will correct acidosis as long as the HCO_3^- is eliminated via the lungs. The remaining Na increases the strong ion difference, resulting in a decreased dissociation of water and an increased pH.[147] The effect of CRRT on the lactate level depends on the contribution of the extracorporeal clearance to the total body clearance. In patients with normal lactate level and stable hemodynamic and respiratory status, the contribution of continuous bicarbonate hemodiafiltration to the total body clearance of lactate (normally 1500–4500 mmol/day) only represents 0.5–3.2%.[155] These authors conclude that the reported reduction in lactate level during hemofiltration probably reflects an improvement in acid–base and metabolic status, leading to enhanced lactate metabolism.[156] It is, however, not inconceivable that in patients with increased lactate level and reduced endogenous clearance due to liver dysfunction, the contribution of extracorporeal elimination might become clinically important, especially if extracorporeal clearance is substantial (high-volume hemofiltration or dialysis).

CRUSH INJURY

Rhabdomyolysis, a syndrome of skeletal muscle breakdown with leakage of muscle contents, is caused by a variety of mechanisms affecting myocytes and muscle membranes.[157] Severe rhabdomyolysis results in ARF through three main pathways: tubular obstruction by myoglobin precipitation with Tamm–Horsfall proteins or urate crystal formation at low urine pH, heme protein-induced lipid peroxidation of proximal tubular cells, and renal vasoconstriction due to hypovolemia (caused by massive uptake of water by the damaged muscles) and release of vasoactive mediators.[158] Early volume replacement, with or without urinary alkalinization, represents the single most important treatment to prevent the development of ARF.[159] Absolute indications for renal replacement therapy are established ARF with hyperkalemia, uncorrectable acidosis, or fluid overload. Some authors have suggested that the extracorporeal removal of myoglobin with 'prophylactic' CRRT could alter the course of myoglobinuric ARF. The molecular weight of myoglobin is 17 000 Da, which excludes important diffusive removal but is indeed compatible with convective removal.[160] The presence of myoglobin in the ultrafiltrate has been demonstrated in case reports and small case series.[161–165] The reported sieving coefficient varies between 0.15[166] and 0.6.[165] Whether this extracorporeal removal affects the plasma level is, however, not clear from these uncontrolled observations. Other authors found a rapid fall in myoglobin levels, regardless of renal function or the method of blood purification, suggesting important extrarenal disposition of myoglobin with limited contribution of the renal replacement therapy.[167,168] The need for continuous anticoagulation may also represent an important disadvantage of CRRT in these (mostly) traumatized patients.

TUMOR LYSIS SYNDROME

Tumor lysis syndrome (TLS) is an oncologic emergency, which is mostly precipitated by chemotherapy- or radiation-induced rapid lysis of malignant cells. The syndrome consists of hyperuricemia, hyperkalemia, hyperphosphatemia, and hypocalcemia and results from the rapid release of intracellular contents into the circulation. The pathogenesis of ARF in this setting is incompletely elucidated. Several mechanisms may play a role: uric acid nephropathy, hyperphosphatemia/hypocalcemia-induced nephrocalcinosis, xanthine nephropathy, adenosine-induced vasoconstriction, and/or volume depletion. Risk factors for TLS are large tumor burden and/or rapidly dividing tumors, high lactate dehydrogenase levels, pre-existing renal disease and/or volume depletion, acidic urine, and young age. The key to the management of TLS lies in prevention: intensive hydration, urinary alkalinization (decreases urate crystal

formation but favors calcium phosphate precipitation), allopurinol, and/or urate oxidase.[169–171] In patients with established ARF, early extracorporeal treatment will be required in order to prevent dangerous accumulation of uric acid, potassium, and phosphorus. Both uric acid and phosphate are small molecules that require high diffusive clearance. Compared with intermittent dialysis, CRRT are better tolerated, may prevent rebound hyperkalemia, and improve the control of hyperphosphatemia.[172–174] However, relatively high extracorporeal clearances are required to obtain optimal metabolic control.[175] Whether propylactic use of CRRT (initiated before the start of chemotherapy in high-risk patients) is useful, as suggested by a few case reports,[176,177] remains to be proven.

INBORN ERRORS OF METABOLISM

Inborn errors of metabolism (e.g. ornithine transcarbamylase deficiency, maple syrup urine disease) cause emergency situations with unconsciousness, convulsions, hyperpnea and hyperpyrexia due to hyperammonemia and/or high levels of branched-chain amino acids and their α-keto acid derivatives. These toxic metabolites have to be eliminated immediately after diagnosis to avoid irreversible brain damage. Endogenous incorporation into protein synthesis by nutritional support and removal by extracorporeal techniques are the two treatment options. Although the best clearance rates are achieved with intermittent hemodialysis, this treatment is often not tolerated by these critically ill (and mostly very small) patients. Several case reports suggest that CVVH, and especially continuous venovenous hemodialysis (CVVHD), is rapidly effective in clearing the low molecular weight toxic metabolites, allowing the patients to recover their neurologic status.[178–187] An experimental study confirmed the superiority of diffusive solute removal in this setting.[188] Hemofiltration-induced hypothermia may also contribute to the beneficial effect by lowering the enzymatic rate of production of the toxins.[189]

HYPOTHERMIA

Mild cases of hypothermia (core temperature >32°C) can be treated with active external rewarming procedures. Severe hypothermia (core temperature $<28°C$) is often associated with cardiac arrest, and rapid core rewarming with CPB is therefore the method of choice.[190] CPB requires expertise, is very invasive, and the equipment is not always available in smaller hospitals. In moderate or severe hypothermia without cardiac arrest, CRRT, now commonly performed in general hospitals, can be used safely and effectively for core rewarming, as illustrated by several case reports and case series.[191-197] In an experimental model of moderate hypothermia, CVVH with warming of the replacement fluid has been shown to be more effective than standard methods (warmed humidified gases, warmed intravenous fluid, external warm-water blankets and warm gastric lavage).[198] If combined with hyperinfusion of heated crystalloids, CRRT allows correction of the artificially induced fluid overload. Since hypothermia itself induces a prolongation of the clotting times,[199] and platelet dysfunction,[200] the extracorporeal rewarming can probably be started without anticoagulation.

REFERENCES

1. Schetz MRC. Classical and alternative indications for continuous renal replacement therapy. Kidney Int Suppl 1988;66:S129–32.
2. Angus D, Wax RS. Epidemiology of sepsis: an update. Crit Care Med 2001;29(Suppl):S109–16.
3. Pinsky MR. Sepsis: a pro- and anti-inflammatory disequilibrium syndrome. Contrib Nephrol 2001;132:354–66.
4. Vincent JL, De Backer D. Pathophysiology of septic shock. Advn Sepsis 2001;1:87–92.
5. Gotloib L, Barzilay E, Shustak A, et al. Hemofiltration in septic ARDS. The artificial kidney as an artificial endocrine lung. Resuscitation 1986;13:123–32.
6. Dubois MJ, Vincent JL. Clinically-oriented therapies in sepsis: a review. J Endotoxin Res 2000;6:463–9.
7. van der Poll T. Immunotherapy of sepsis. Lancet Infect Dis 2001;1:165–74.
8. Glauser MP. Pathophysiologic basis of sepsis: considerations for future strategies of intervention. Crit Care Med 2000;28(9 Suppl): S4–8.
9. Van Bommel EF, Hesse CJ, Jutte NH, et al. Cytokine kinetics (TNF-α, IL-1β, IL-6) during continuous hemofiltration: a laboratory and clinical study. Contrib Nephrol 1995;116:62–75.
10. Uchino S, Bellomo R, Goldsmith D, et al. Super high flux hemofiltration: a new technique for cytokine removal. Intensive Care Med 2002;28:651–5.
11. Uchino S, Bellomo R, Goldsmith D, et al. Cytokine removal with a large pore cellulose triacetate filter: an ex vivo study. Int J Artif Organs 2002;25:27–32.
12. Bouman CS, van Olden RW, Stoutenbeek CP. Cytokine filtration and adsorption during pre- and postdilution hemofiltration in four different membranes. Blood Purif 1998;16:261–8.
13. Bellomo R, Tipping P, Boyce N. Continuous veno-venous hemofiltration with dialysis removes cytokines from the circulation of septic patients. Crit Care Med 1993;21:522–6.
14. Heidemann SM, Ofenstein JP, Sarnaik AP. Efficacy of continuous arteriovenous hemofiltration in endotoxic shock. Circ Shock 1994;44:183–7.
15. Bottoms G, Fessler J, Murphey E, et al. Efficacy of convective removal of plasma mediators of endotoxic shock by continuous veno-venous hemofiltration. Shock 1996;5:149–54.
16. De Vriese AS, Colardyn FA, Philippe JJ, et al. Cytokine removal during continuous hemofiltration in septic patients. J Am Soc Nephrol 1999;10:846–53.
17. Heering P, Morgera S, Schmitz FJ, et al. Cytokine removal and cardiovascular hemodyanmics in septic patients with continuous hemofiltration. Intensive Care Med 1997;23:288–96.
18. Van Bommel EFH, Hesse CJ, Jutte NHPM, et al. Impact of continuous hemofiltration on cytokines and cytokine inhibitors in oliguric patients suffering from systemic inflammatory response syndrome. Ren Fail 1997;19:443–54.
19. Hoffmann JN, Hartl WH, Deppisch R, et al. Effect of hemofiltration on hemodynamics and systemic concentrations of anaphylatoxins and cytokines in human sepsis. Intensive Care Med 1996;22:1360–7.
20. Mariano F, Tetta C, Guida G, Triolo G, Camussi G. Hemofiltration reduces the serum priming activity on neutrophil chemiluminescence in septic patients. Kidney Int 2001;60:1598–605.
21. Yekebas EF, Eisenberger CF, Ohnesorge H, et al. Attenuation of sepsis-related immunoparalysis by continuous veno-venous hemofiltration in experimental porcine pancreatitis. Crit Care Med 2001;29:1423–30.
22. Meisner M, Huttemann E, Lohs T, Kasakov L, Reinhart K. Plasma concentrations and clearance of procalcitonin during continuous veno-venous hemofiltration in septic patients. Shock 2001; 15:171–5.
23. LaMarre J, Wollenberg GK, Gonias SL, Hayes MA. Cytokine binding and clearance properties of proteinase-activated alpha 2–macroglobulins. Lab Invest 1991;65:3–14.
24. Van Zee KJ, Kohno T, Fisher E, et al. Tumor necrosis factor soluble receptors circulate during experimental and clinical inflammation and can protect against excessive tumor necrosis factor alpha in vitro and in vivo. Proc Natl Acad Sci 1992;89:4845–9.
25. Fernandez-Botran R. Soluble cytokine receptors: basic immunology and clinical applications. Crit Rev Clin Lab Sci 1999;36:165–224.
26. Munoz C, Misset B, Fitting C, et al. Dissociation between plasma and monocyte-associated cytokines during sepsis. Eur J Immunol 1991;21:2177–84.
27. Kellum JA, Johnson JP, Kramer D, et al. Diffusive vs. convective therapy: effects on mediators of inflammation in patient with severe systemic inflammatory response. Crit Care Med 1998;26:1995–2000.
28. Ronco C, Tetta C, Lupi A, et al. Removal of platelet-activating factor in experimental continuous arteriovenous hemofiltration. Crit Care Med 1995;23:99–107.
29. Ishihara S, Ward JA, Tasaki O, et al. Effects of long-term hemofiltration on circulating mediators and superoxide production during continuous endotoxin administration. J Traum Infect Crit Care 1999;46:894–9.
30. Cheung AF, Chenoweth DE, Otsuka D, Henderson LW. Compartmental distribution of complement activation products in artificial kidneys. Kidney Int 1986;30:74–80.
31. Barrera P, Janssen EM, Demacker PNM, Wetzels JFM, Van der Meer JWM. Removal of interleukin-1β and tumor necrosis factor from human plasma by in vitro dialysis with polyacrylonitrile membranes. Lymphokine Cytokine Res 1992;11:99–104.
32. Lonnemann G, Schindler R, Dinarello CA, Koch KM. Removal of circulating cytokines by hemodialysis membranes in vitro. In: Faist E, Meakins J, Schildberg FW eds. Host defense dysfunction in shock and sepsis. Berlin: Springer-Verlag; 1992;613–23.
33. Gasche Y, Pascual M, Suter PM, et al. Complement depletion during haemofiltration with polyacrylonitrile membranes. Nephrol Dial Transplant 1996;11:117–19.

34. Schetz M, Ferdinande P, Van den Berghe G, Verwaest C, Lauwers P. Removal of pro-inflammatory cytokines with renal replacement therapy: sense or nonsense? Intensive Care Med 1995;21:169–76.

35. Marecaux, G, Pinsky MR, Dupont E, Kahn RJ, Vincent JL. Blood lactate levels are better prognostic indicators than TNF and IL-6 levels in patients with septic shock. Intensive Care Med 1996;22:404–8.

36. Damas P, Canivet JL, de Groote D, et al. Sepsis and serum cytokine concentrations. Crit Care Med 1997;25:405–12.

37. Alkharfy KM, Kedllum JA, Matzke GR. Unintended immunomodulation: Part II. Effects of pharmacological agents on cytokine biosynthesis. Shock 2000;13:346–60.

38. Alkharfy KM, Kedllum JA, Matzke GR. Unintended immunomodulation: Part I. Effects of common clinical conditions on cytokine biosynthesis. Shock 2000;13:333–45.

39. Rogiers P, Zhang H, Smail N, Pauwels D, Vincent JL. Continuous venovenous hemofiltration improves cardiac performance by mechanisms other than tumor necrosis factor-alpha attenuation during endotoxic shock. Crit Care Med 1999;27:1848–55.

40. Bellomo R, Kellum J, Gandhi CR, Pinsky MR, Ondulik B. The effect of intensive plasma water exchange by hemofiltration on hemodynamics and soluble mediators in canine endotoxemia. Am J Respir Crit Care Med 2000;161:1429–36.

41. Braun N, Rosenfeld S, Giolai M, et al. Effect of continuous hemodiafiltration on IL-6, TNF-α, C3a, and TCC in patients with SIRS/septic shock using two different membranes. Contrib Nephrol 1995;116:89–98.

42. Sander A, Armbruster W, Sander B, et al. Hemofiltration increases IL-6 clearance in early systemic inflammatory response syndrome but does not alter IL-6 and TNF alpha plasma concentrations. Intensive Care Med 1997;23:878–84.

43. Sanchez-Izquierdo Riera JA, Perez Vela JL, Lozano Quintana MJ, et al. Cytokines clearance during venovenous hemofiltration in the trauma patient. Am J Kidney Dis 1997;30:483–8.

44. Cole L, Bellomo R, Hart G, et al. A phase II randomized, controlled trial of continuous hemofiltration in sepsis. Crit Care Med 2002;30:100–6.

45. Wakabayashi Y, Kamijou Y, Soma K, Ohwada T. Removal of circulating cytokines by continuous hemofiltration in patients with systemic inflammatory response syndrome or multiple organ dysfunction syndrome. Br J Surg 1996;83:393–4.

46. Journois D, Israel Biet D, Pouard P, et al. High-volume, zero-balanced hemofiltration to reduce delayed inflammatory response to cardiopulmonary bypass in children. Anesthesiology 1996;85:965–76.

47. Cole L, Bellomo R, Journois D, et al. High-volume haemofiltration in human septic shock. Intensive Care Med 2001;27:978–86.

48. Gomez A, Wang R, Unruh H, et al. Hemofiltration reverses left ventricular dysfunction during sepsis in dogs. Anesthesiology 1990;73:671–85.

49. Stein B, Pfenninger E, Grunert A, Schmitz JE, Hudde M. Influence of continuous haemofiltration on haemodynamics and central blood volume in experimental endotoxic shock. Intensive Care Med 1990;16:494–9.

50. Stein B, Pfenninger E, Grunert A, et al. The consequences of continuous haemofiltration on lung mechanics and extravascular lung water in a porcine endotoxic shock model. Intensive Care Med 1991;17:293–8.

51. Grootendorst AF, van Bommel EFH, van der Hoven B, van Leengoed LAMG, van Osta ALM. High volume hemofiltration improves right ventricular function in endotoxin-induced shock in the pig. Intensive Care Med 1992;18:235–40.

52. Lee PA, Matson JR, Pryor RW, Hinshaw LB. Continuous arteriovenous hemofiltration therapy for *Staphylococcus aureus*-induced septicemia in immature swine? Crit Care Med 1993;21:914–24.

53. Grootendorst AF, van Bommel EFH, van Leengoed LAMG, et al. High volume hemofiltration improves hemodynamics and survival of pigs exposed to gut ischemia and reperfusion. Shock 1994;2:72–8.

54. Freeman BD, Yatsiv I, Natanson C, et al. Continuous arteriovenous hemofiltration does not improve survival in a canine model of septic shock. J Am Coll Surg 1995;180:286–92.

55. DiScipio AW, Burchard KW. Continuous arteriovenous hemofiltration attenuates polymorphonuclear leukocyte phagocytosis in porcine intra-abdominal sepsis. Am J Surg 1997;173:174–80.

56. Mink SN, Li X, Bose D, et al. Early but not delayed continuous arteriovenous hemofiltration improves cardiovascular function in sepsis in dogs. Intensive Care Med 1999;25:733–43.

57. Ullrich R, Roeder G, Lorber C, et al. Continuous venovenous hemofiltration improves arterial oxygenation in endotoxin-induced lung injury in pigs. Anesthesiology 2001;95:428–36.

58. Grootendorst AF, Van Bommel EFH, Leengoed LAMG, et al. Infusion of ultrafiltrate from endotoxemic pigs depresses myocardial performance in normal pigs. J Crit Care 1993;8:161–9.

59. Lee PA, Pryor RW, Matson JR. Effects of filter pore size on efficacy of continuous arteriovenous hemofiltration (CAVH) therapy in improving morbidity and mortality in an immature swine model of *Staphylococcus aureus* (*S. aureus*)-induced sepsis. Blood Purif 1998;16:113.

60. Kline JA, Gordon BE, Williams C, et al. Large-pore hemodialysis in acute endotoxin shock. Crit Care Med 1999;27:588–96.

61. Meloni C, Morosetti M, Turani F, et al. Cardiac function and oxygen balance in septic patients during continuous hemofiltration. Blood Purif 1998;16:140–6.

62. Koperna T, Vogl SE, Poschl GP, et al. Cytokine patterns in patients who undergo hemofiltration for treatment of multiple organ failure. World J Surg 1998;22:443–8.

63. Klouche K, Cavadore P, Portales P, et al. Continuous veno-venous hemofiltration improves hemodynamics in septic shock with acute renal failure without modifying TNFalpha and IL6 plasma concentrations. J Nephrol 2002;15:150–7.

64. DiCarlo J, Dudley TE, Sherbotie JR, Kaplan BS, Costarino AT. Continuous arteriovenous hemofiltration/dialysis improves pulmonary gas exchange in children with multiple organ system failure. Crit Care Med 1990;18:822–6.

65. Garzia F, Todor R, Scalea T. Continuous arteriovenous hemofiltration countercurrent dialysis (CAVH-D) in acute respiratory failure (ARDS). J Trauma 1991;31:1277–85.

66. Laggner AN, Druml W, Lenz K, Schneeweiss BS, Grimm G. Influence of ultrafiltration/hemofiltration on extravascular lung water. Contrib Nephrol 1991;93:65–70.

67. Bagshaw ONT, Anaes FRC, Hutchinson A. Continuous arteriovenous hemofiltration and respiratory function in multiple organ system failre. Intensive Care Med 1992;18:334–8.

68. Riegel W, Ziegenfuss T, Rose S, Bauer M, Marzi I. Influence of venovenous hemofiltration on posttraumatic inflammation and hemodynamics. Contrib Nephrol 1995;116:56–61.

69. S-Izquierdo Riera JA, Alted E, Lozano MJ, et al. Influence of continuous hemofiltration on the hemodynamics of trauma patients. Surgery 1997;122:902–8.

70. Oudemans-van Straaten HM, Bosman RJ, van der Spoel JI, Zandstra DF. Outcome of critically ill patients treated with intermittent high-volume haemofiltration: a prospective cohort analysis. Intensive Care Med 1999;25:814–21.

71. Honore PM, Jamez J, Wauthier M, et al. Prospective evaluation of short-term, high-volume isovolemic hemofiltration on the hemodynamic course and outcome in patients with intractable circulatory failure resulting from septic shock. Crit Care Med 2000;28:3581–7.

72. Ronco C, Bellomo R, Homel P, et al. Effects of different doses in continuous veno-venous haemofiltration on outcomes of acute renal failure: a prospective randomised trial. Lancet 2000;356:26–30.

73. Reiter K, Bellomo R, Ronco C. High volume hemofiltration in sepsis. In: Vincent JL, ed. 2002 yearbook of intensive care and emergency medicine. Berlin: Springer-Verlag 2002:129–41.

74. Russell JA, Singer J, Bernard G, et al. Changing pattern of organ dysfunction in early human sepsis is related to mortality. Crit Care Med 2000;28:3405–11.

75. Grover R, Lopez A, Lorente J. Multicenter, randomized, placebo-controlled, double blind study of the nitric oxide synthase inhibitor 546C99: effect on survival in patients with septic shock. Crit Care Med 1999;27:A33.

76. Lonnemann G, Bechstein M, Linnenweber S, Burg M, Koch KM. Tumor necrosis factor-alpha during continuous high-flux hemodialysis in sepsis with acute renal failure. Kidney Int Suppl 1999;72:S84–7.

77. Hoffmann JN, Hartl WH, Deppisch R, et al. Hemofiltration in human sepsis: evidence for elimination of immunomodulatory substances. Kidney Int 1995;48:1563–70.

78. Reeves JH, Butt WW, Shann F, et al. Continuous plasmafiltration in sepsis syndrome. Plasmafiltration in Sepsis Study Group. Crit Care Med 1999;27:2096–104.

79. Schmidt J, Mann S, Mohr VD, et al. Plasmapheresis combined with continuous venovenous hemofiltration in surgical patients with sepsis. Intensive Care Med 2000;26:532–7.

80. Tetta C, Gianotti L, Cavaillon JM, et al. Coupled plasma filtration-adsorption in a rabbit model of endotoxic shock. Crit Care Med 2000;28:1526–33.

81. Ronco C, Brendolan A, Lonnemann G, et al. A pilot study of coupled plasma filtration with adsorption in septic shock. Crit Care Med 2002;30:1250–5.

82. Nemoto H, Nakamoto H, Okada H, et al. Newly developed immobilized polymyxin B fibers improve the survival of patients with sepsis. Blood Purif 2001;19:361–9.

83. Teramoto K, Nakamoto Y, Kunitomo T, et al. Removal of endotoxin in blood by polymyxin B immobilized polystyrene-derivative fiber. Ther Apher 2002;6:103–8.

84. Cosentino F, Paganini E, Lockrem J, Stoller J, Wiedemann H. Continuous arteriovenous hemofiltration in the adult respiratory distress syndrome. A randomized trial. Contrib Nephrol 1991;93:94–7.

85. Schuller D, Mitchell JP, Calandrino FS, Schuster DP. Fluid balance during pulmonary edema. Is fluid gain a marker or a cause of poor outcome? Chest 1991;100:1068–75.

86. Simmons RS, Berdine GG, Seidenfeld JJ, et al. Fluid balance and the adult respiratory distress syndrome. Am Rev Respir Dis 1987;135:924–9.

87. Alsous F, Khamiees M, DeGirolamo A, Amoateng Adjepong Y, Manthous CA. Negative fluid balance predicts survival in patients with septic shock: a retrospective pilot study. Chest 2000;117:1749–54.

88. Humphrey H, Hall J, Sznajder I, Silverstein M, Wood L. Improved survival in ARDS patients associated with a reduction in pulmonary capillary wedge pressure. Chest 1990;97:1176–80.

89. Laggner AN, Druml W, Lenz K, Schneeweiss B, Grimm G. Influence of ultrafiltration/hemofiltration on extravascular lung water. Contrib Nephrol 1991;93:65–70.

90. Laffey JG, Boylan JF, Cheng DCH. The systemic inflammatory response to cardiac surgery: implications for the anesthesiologist. Anesthesiology 2002;97:215–52.

91. Intonti F, Alquati P, Schiavello R, Alessandrini F. Ultrafiltration during open-heart surgery in chronic renal failure. Scand J Thorac Cardiovasc Surg 1981;15:217–20.

92. Hakim M, Wheeldon D, Bethune DW, et al. Haemodialysis and haemofiltration on cardiopulmonary bypass. Thorax 1985;40:101–6.

93. Magilligan DJ, Oyama C. Ultrafiltration during cardiopulmonary bypass: laboratory evaluation and initial clinical experience. Ann Thorac Surg 1984;37:33–9.

94. Magilligan DJ. Indications for ultrafiltration in the cardiac surgical patient. J Thorac Cardiovasc Surg 1985;89:183–9.

95. Boldt J, Kling D, von Bormann B, Scheld HH, Hempelmann G. Extravascular lung water and hemofiltration during complicated cardiac surgery. Thorac Cardiovasc Surg 1987;35:161–5.

96. Solem JO, Stahl E, Kugelberg J, Steen S. Hemoconcentration by ultrafiltration during open-heart surgery. Scand J Thorac Cardiovasc Surg 1988;22:271–4.

97. Naik SK, Knight A, Elliott M. A prospective randomized study of a modified technique of ultrafiltration during pediatric open-heart surgery. Circulation 1991;84(5 Suppl):III422–31.

98. Elliott MJ. Ultrafiltration and modified ultrafiltration in pediatric open heart operations. Ann Thorac Surg 1993;56:1518–22.

99. Wang MJ, Chiu IS, Hsu CM, et al. Efficacy of ultrafiltration in removing inflammatory mediators during pediatric cardiac operations. Ann Thorac Surg 1996;61:651–6.

100. Tassani P, Richter JA, Eising GP, et al. Influence of combined zero-balanced and modified ultrafiltration on the systemic inflammatory response during coronary artery bypass grafting. J Cardiothorac Vasc Anesth 1999;13:285–91.

101. Boga M, Islamoglu, Badak I, et al. The effects of modified hemofiltration on inflammatory mediators and cardiac performance in coronary artery bypass grafting. Perfusion 2000;15:143–50.

102. Grunenfelder J, Zund G, Schoeberlein A, et al. Modified ultrafiltration lowers adhesion molecule and cytokine levels after cardiopulmonary bypass without clinical relevance in adults. Eur J Cardiothorac Surg 2000;17:77–83.

103. Leyh RG, Bartels C, Joubert-Hubner E, Bechtel JF, Sievers HH. Influence of modified ultrafiltration on coagulation, fibrinolysis and blood loss in adult cardiac surgery. Eur J Cardiothorac Surg 2001;19:145–51.

104. Battista-Luciani G, Menon T, Vecchi B, Auriemma S, Mazzucco A. Modified ultrafiltration reduces morbidity after adult cardiac operations: a prospective, randomized clinical trial. Circulation 2001;104(12 Suppl 1):I253–9.

105. Journois D, Pouard P, Greeley WJ, et al. Hemofiltration during cardiopulmonary bypass in pediatric cardiac surgery. Effects on hemostasis, cytokines, and complement components. Anesthesiology 1994;81:1181–9.

106. Koutlas TC, Gaynor JW, Nicolson SC, et al. Modified ultrafiltration reduces postoperative morbidity after cavopulmonary connection. Ann Thorac Surg 1997;64:37–42.

107. Bando K, Turrentine MW, Vijay P, et al. Effect of modified ultrafiltration in high-risk patients undergoing operations for congenital heart disease. Ann Thorac Surg 1998;66:821–7.

108. Hennein HA, Kiziltepe U, Barst S, et al. Venovenous modified ultrafiltration after cardiopulmonary bypass in children: a prospective randomized study. J Thorac Cardiovasc Surg 1999;117:496–505.

109. Keenan HT, Thiagarajan R, Stephens KE, et al. Pulmonary function after modified venovenous ultrafiltration in infants: a prospective, randomized trial. J Thorac Cardiovasc Surg 2000;119:501–5.

110. Davies MJ, Nguyen K, Gaynor JW, Elliott MJ. Modified ultrafiltration improves left ventricular systolic function in infants after cardiopulmonary bypass. J Thorac Cardiovasc Surg 1998;115:361–9.

111. Rivera ES, Kimball TR, Bailey WW, et al. Effect of veno-venous ultrafiltration on myocardial performance immediately after cardiac surgery in children. A prospective randomized study. J Am Coll Cardiol 1998;32:766–72.

112. Bando K, Vijay P, Turrentine MW, et al. Dilutional and modified ultrafiltration reduces pulmonary hypertension after operations for congenital heart disease: a prospective randomized study. J Thorac Cardiovasc Surg 1998;115:517–25.

113. Hiramatsu T, Imai Y, Kurosawa H, et al. Effects of dilutional and modified ultrafiltration in plasma endothelin-1 and pulmonary vascular resistance after the Fontan procedure. Ann Thorac Surg 2002;73:861–5.

114. Skaryak LA, Kirshbom PM, DiBernardo LR, et al. Modified ultrafiltration improves cerebral metabolic recovery after circulatory arrest. J Thorac Cardiovasc Surg 1995;109:744–51.

115. Shin'oka T, Shum-Tim D, Laussen PC, et al. Effects of oncotic pressure and hematocrit on outcome after hypothermic circulatory arrest. Ann Thorac Surg 1998;65:155–64.

116. Marik PE, Sibbald WJ. Effect of stored-blood transfusion on oxygen delivery in patients with sepsis. JAMA 1993;269:3024–9.

117. Millar AB, Armstrong L, van der Linden J, et al. Cytokine production and hemofiltration in children undergoing cardiopulmonary bypass. Ann Thorac Surg 1993;56:1499–502.

118. Saatvedt K, Lindberg H, Geiran OR, et al. Ultrafiltration after cardiopulmonary bypass in children: effects on hemodynamics, cytokines and complement. Cardiovasc Res 1996;31:596–602.

119. Pearl JM, Manning PB, McNamara JL, Saucier MM, Thomas DW. Effect of modified ultrafiltration on plasma thromboxane B2, leukotriene B4, and endothelin-1 in infants undergoing cardiopulmonary bypass. Ann Thorac Surg 1999;68:1369–75.

120. Ming ZD, Wei W, Hong C, Wei Z, Xiang DW. Balanced ultrafiltration, modified ultrafiltration, and balanced ultrafiltration with modified ultrafiltration in pediatric cardiopulmonary bypass. J Extra Corpor Technol 2001;33:223–6.

121. Nagashima M, Shin'oka T, Nollert G, et al. High-volume continuous hemofiltration during cardiopulmonary bypass attenuates pulmonary dysfunction in neonatal lambs after deep hypothermic circulatory arrest. Circulation 1998;98(19 Suppl):II378–84.

122. Greenberg B. Treatment of heart failure: state of the art and prospectives. J Cardiovasc Pharmacol 2001;38(Suppl 2)S59–63.

123. Gomberg-Maitland M, Baran DA, Fuster V. Treatment of congestive heart failure: guidelines for the primary care physician and the heart failure specialist. Arch Intern Med 2001;161:342–52.

124. Silverstein ME, Ford CA, Lysaght MJ, Henderson LW. Treatment of severe fluid overload by ultrafiltration. N Engl J Med 1974;291:747–51.

125. Asaba H, Bergstrom J, Furst P, Shaldon S, Wiklund S. Treatment of diuretic-resistant fluid retention with ultrafiltration. Acta Med Scand 1978;204:145–9.

126. Feigenbaum MS, Welsch MA, Mitchell M, et al. Contracted plasma and blood volume in chronic heart failure. J Am Coll Cardiol 2000;35:51–5.

127. Koomans HA, Geers AB, Mees EJD. Plasma volume recovery after ultrafiltration in patients with chronic renal failure. Kidney Int 1984;26:848–54.

128. de Vries JP, Kouw PM, van der Meer NJ, et al. Non-invasive monitoring of blood volume during hemodialysis: its relation with post-dialytic dry weight. Kidney Int 1993;44:851–4.

129. Marenzi G, Lauri G, Grazi M, et al. Circulatory response to fluid overload removal by extracorporeal ultrafiltration in refractory congestive heart failure. J Am Coll Cardiol 2001;38:963–8.

130. Ronco C, Bellomo R, Ricci Z. Hemodynamic response to fluid withdrawal in overhydrated patients treated with intermittent ultrafiltration and slow continuous ultrafiltration: role of blood volume monitoring. Cardiology 2001;96:196–201.

131. Stoves J, Goode NP, Visvanathan R, et al. The bradykinin response and early hypotension at the introduction of continuous renal replacement therapy in the intensive care unit. Artif Organs 2001;25:1009–13.

132. Agostini PG, Marenzi G, Guazzi M, Guazzi MD. Influence of ACE inhibition on fluid metabolism in chronic heart failure and its pathophysiological relevance. J Cardiovasc Pharmacol Ther 1996;1:279–86.

133. Rimondini AA, Cipolla CM, Bella PD, et al. Hemofiltration as short-term treatment for refractory heart failure. Am J Med 1987;83:43–8.

134. L'Abbate A, Emdin M, Piacenti M, et al. Ultrafiltration: a rational treatment for heart failure. Cardiology 1989;76:384–90.

135. Cipola MC, Grazi S, Rimondini A, et al. Changes in circulating norepinephrine with hemofiltration in advanced congestive heart failure. Am J Cardiol 1990;66:987–94.

136. Agostoni PG, Marenzi GC, Pepi M, et al. Isolated ultrafiltration in moderate congestive heart failure. J Am Coll Cardiol 1993;21:424–31.

137. Pepi M, Marenzi GC, Agostoni PG, et al. Sustained cardiac diastolic changes elicited by ultrafiltration in patients with moderate congestive heart failure: pathophysiological correlates. Br Heart J 1993;70:135–40.

138. Marenzi G, Grazi S, Giraldi F, et al. Interrelation of humoral factors, hemodynamics, and fluid and salt metabolism in congestive heart failure: effects of extracorporeal ultrafiltration. Am J Med 1993;94:49–56.

139. Agostino P, Marenzi G, Lauri G, et al. Sustained improvement in functional capacity after removal of body fluid with isolated ultrafiltration in chronic cardiac insufficiency. Am J Med 1994;96:191–9.

140. Marenzi GC, Lauri G, Guazzi M, Perego GB, Agostoni PG. Ultrafiltration in moderate heart failure. Exercise oxygen uptake as a predictor of the clinical benefits. Chest 1995;108:94–8.

141. Canaud B, Leray-Moragues H, Garred LJ, et al. Slow isolated ultrafiltration for the treatment of congestive heart failure. Am J Kidney Dis 1996;28(Suppl 3):S67–73.

142. Guazzi MD, Agostoni P, Perego B, et al. Apparent paradox of neurohumoral axis inhibition after body fluid volume depletion in patients with chronic congestive heart failure and water retention. Br Heart J 1994;72:534–9.

143. Zucchelli P, Catizone L, Esposti ED, et al. Influence of ultrafiltration on plasma renin activity and adrenergic system. Nephron 1978;21:317–24.

144. Baldamus CA, Ernst W, Lysaght MJ, Shaldon S, Koch KM. Hemodynamics in hemofiltration. Int J Artif Organs 1983;6:27–31.

145. Martinez-Maldonado M, Gely R, Tapia E, Benabe JE. Role of macula densa in diuretics-induced renin release. Hypertension 1990;16:261–8.

146. Ellison DH. Diuretic therapy and resistance in congestive heart failure. Cardiology 2001;96:132–43.

147. Kellum JA. Recent advances in acid–base physiology applied to critical care. In: Vincent JL, ed. 1998 yearbook of intensive care and emergency medicine. Berlin: Springer-Verlag; 1998:577–87.

148. Gore DC, Jahoor F. Lactic acidosis during sepsis is related to increased pyruvate production, not deficits in oxygen availability. Ann Surg 1996;224:97–102.

149. Levraut J, Ciebiera JP, Chave S, et al. Mild hyperlactatemia in stable septic patients is due to impaired lactate clearance rather than overproduction. Am J Respir Crit Care Med 1998;157:1021–6.

150. Veech RL. The untoward effects of the anions of dialysis fluid. Kidney Int 1988;34:587–97.

151. Kellum JA, Song M, Subramanian S. Acidemia: good, bad or inconsequential. In: Vincent JL, ed. 2002 yearbook of intensive care and emergency medicine. Berlin: Springer-Verlag; 2002:510–16.

152. Barton IK, Streather CP, Hilton PJ, Bradley RD. Successful treatment of severe lactic acidosis by haemofiltration using a bicarbonate-based replacement fluid. Nephrol Dial Transplant 1991;6:668–70.

153. Kirschbaum B, Galishoff M, Reines HD. Lactic acidosis treated with continuous hemodiafiltration and regional citrate anticoagulation. Crit Care Med 1992;20:349–53.

154. Forni G, Darling K, Evans M, Hilton PJ, Treacher DF. Lactate intolerance with continuous venovenous haemofiltration: the role of bicarbonate-buffered haemofiltration. Clin Intensive Care 1998;9:40–2.

155. Levraut J, Ciebiera JP, Jambou P, et al. Effect of continuous venovenous hemofiltration with dialysis on lactate clearance in critically ill patients. Crit Care Med 1997;25:58–62.

156. Poole RC, Halestrap AP. Transport of lactate and other monocarboxylates across mammalian plasma membranes. Am J Physiol 1993;264:C761–82.

157. Warren JD, Blumbergs PC, Thompson PD. Rhabdomyolysis: a review. Muscle Nerve 2002;25:332–47.

158. Holt SG, Moore KP. Pathogenesis and treatment of renal dysfunction in rhabdomyolysis. Intensive Care Med 2001;27:803–11.

159. Better OS, Stein JH. Early management of shock and prophylaxis of acute renal failure in traumatic rhabdomyolysis. N Engl J Med 1990;322:825–9.

160. Maduell F, Navarro V, Cruz C, et al. Osteocalcin and myoglobin removal in on-line hemodiafiltration versus low- and high-flux hemodialysis. Am J Kidney Dis 2002;40:582–9.

161. Winterberg B, Ramme K, Tenschert W, et al. Hemofiltration in myoglobinuric acute renal failure. Int J Artif Organs 1990;13:113–16.

162. Berns JS, Cohen RM, Rudnick MR. Removal of myoglobin by CAVH-D in traumatic rhabdomyolysis. Am J Nephrol 1991;11:73–5.

163. Bellomo R, Daskalakis M, Parkin G, Boyce N. Myoglobin clearance during acute continuous hemodiafiltration [Letter]. Intensive Care Med 1991;17:509.

164. Bastani B, Frenchie D. Significant myoglobin removal during continuous veno-venous haemofiltration using F80 membrane [Letter]. Nephrol Dial Transplant 1997;12:2035–6.

165. Amyot SL, Leblanc M, Thibeault Y, Geadah D, Cardinal J. Myoglobin clearance and removal during continuous venovenous hemofiltration. Intensive Care Med 1999;25:1169–72.

166. Nicolau DP, Feng YJ, Wu AH, Bernstein SP, Nightingale CH. Evaluation of myoglobin clearance during continuous hemofiltration in a swine model of acute renal failure. Int J Artif Organs 1996;19:578–81.

167. Wakabayashi Y, Kikuno T, Ohwada T, Kikawada R. Rapid fall in blood myoglobin in massive rhabdomyolysis and acute renal failure. Intensive Care Med 1994;20:109–12.

168. Shigemoto T, Rinka H, Matsuo Y, et al. Blood purification for crush syndrome. Ren Fail 1997;19:711–19.

169 Sallan S. Management of acute tumor lysis syndrome. Semin Oncol 2001;28(2 Suppl 5):9–12.

170. Jeha S. Tumor lysis syndrome. Semin Hematol 2001;38(4 Suppl 10):4–8.

171. Altman A. Acute tumor lysis syndrome. Semin Oncol 2001;28(2 Suppl 5):3–8.

172. Sakarcan A, Quigley R. Hyperphosphatemia in tumour lysis syndrome: the role of dialysis and continuous veno-venous hemofiltration. Pediatr Nephrol 1994;8:351–3.

173. Schelling JR, Ghandour FZ, Strickland TJ, Sedor JR. Management of tumor lysis syndrome with standard continuous arteriovenous hemodialysis: case report and a review of the literature. Ren Fail 1998;20:635–44.

174. Agha-Razii M, Amyot SL, Pichette V, et al. Continuous venovenous hemodiafiltration for the treatment of spontaneous tumor lysis syndrome complicated by acute renal failure and severe hyperuricemia. Clin Nephrol 2000;54:59–63.

175. Pichette V, Leblanc M, Bonnardeaux A, et al. High dialysate flow rate continuous arteriovenous hemodialysis: a new approach for the treatment of acute renal failure and tumour lysis syndrome. Am J Kidney Dis 1994;23:591–6.

176. Heney D, Essex-Cater A, Brocklebank JT, Bailey CC, Lewis IJ. Continuous arteriovenous haemofiltration in the treatment of tumour lysis syndrome. Pediatr Nephrol 1990;4:245–7.

177. Saccente SL, Kohaut EC, Berkow RL. Prevention of tumor lysis syndrome during veno-venous hemofiltration. Pediatr Nephrol 1995;9:569–73.

178. Sperl W, Geiger R, Maurer H, Guggenbichler IP. Continuous arteriovenous hemofiltration in hyperammonemia of newborn babies. Lancet 1990;336:1192–3.

179. Thompson GN, Butt WW, Shann FA, et al. Continuous venovenous hemofiltration in the management of acute decompensation in inborn errors of metabolism. J Pediatr 1991;118:879–84.

180. Falk M, Knight JF, Roy LP, et al. Continuous venovenous hemofiltration in the acute treatment of inborn errors of metabolism. Pediatr Nephrol 1995;9:569–73.

181. Falk MC, Knight JF, Roy Lo, et al. Continuous venovenous haemofiltration in the acute treatment of inborn errors of metabolism. Pediatr Nephrol 1994;8(3):330–3.

182. Schaefer F, Straube E, Oh J, Mehls O, Mayatepek E. Dialysis in neonates with inborn errors of metabolism. Nephrol Dial Transplant 1999;14:910–18.

183. Summar M, Pietsch J, Deshpande J, Schulman G. Effective hemodialysis and hemofiltration driven by an extracorporeal membrane oxygenation pump in infants with hyperammonemia. J Pediatr 1996;128:379–82.

184. Wong KY, Wong SN, Lam SY, Tam S, Tsoi NS. Ammonia clearance by peritoneal dialysis and continuous arteriovenous hemodiafiltration. Pediatr Nephrol 1998;12:589–91.

185. Chen CY, Chen YC, Fang JT, Huang CC. Continuous arteriovenous hemodiafiltration in the acute treatment of hyperammonaemia due to ornithine transcarbamylase deficiency. Ren Fail 2000;22:823–36.

186. Jouvet P, Jugie M, Rabier D, et al. Combined nutritional support and continuous extracorporeal removal therapy in the severe acute phase of maple syrup urine disease. Intensive Care Med 2001;27(11):1798–806.

187. Picca S, Dionisi-Vici C, Abeni D, et al. Extracorporeal dialysis in neonatal hyperammonemia: modalities and prognostic indicators. Pediatr Nephrol 2001;16:862–7.

188. Gouyon JB, Semama D, Prévot A, Desgres J. Removal of branched-chain amino acids and alpha-ketoisocaproate by haemofiltration and haemodiafiltration. J Inher Metab Dis 1996;19:610–20.

189. Whitelaw A, Bridges S, Leaf A, Evans D. Emergency treatment of neonatal hyperammonaemic coma with mild systemic hypothermia. Lancet 2001;358:36–8.

190. Danzl DF, Pozos RS. Accidental hypothermia. N Engl J Med 1994;331:1756–60.

191. Gentilello LM, Cobean RA, Offner PJ, Soderberg RW, Jurkovich GJ. Continuous arteriovenous rewarming: rapid reversal of hypothermia in critically ill patients. J Trauma 1992;32:316–27.

192. Hekmat K, Abel M, Zimmermann R, Ruskowski H. Diabetisches Koma mit tiefer Hypothermie. Erfolgreiche Reanimation mittels Hamofiltration. [Diabetic coma with deep hypothermia. Successful resuscitation with hemofiltration]. Anaesthesist 1994;43:750–2.

193. Brodersen HP, Meurer T, Bolzenius K, Konz KH, Larbig D. Hemofiltration in very severe hypothermia with favorable outcome. Clin Nephrol 1996;45:413–15.

194. van der Maten J, Schrijver G. Severe accidental hypothermia: rewarming with CVVHD. Neth J Med 1996;49:160–3.

195. Garlow L, Kokiko J, Pino-Marina R. Hypothermia in a 62-year-old man: use of the continuous arteriovenous rewarming technique. J Emerg Nurs 1996;22:477–80.

196. Spooner K, Hassani A. Extracorporeal rewarming in a severely hypothermic patient using venovenous haemofiltration in the accident and emergency department. J Accid Emerg Med 2000;17:422–4.

197. Heise D, Rathgeber J, Burchardi H. Schwere, akzidentelle Hypothermie: Aktive Wiedererwarmung durch einen einfachen extrakorporalen veno-venosen Warmekreislauf. [Severe, accidental hypothermia: active rewarming with a simple extracorporeal veno-venous warming-circuit]. Anaesthesist 1996;45:1093–6.

198. Seigler RS, Golding E, Blackhurst DW. Continuous venovenous rewarming: results from a juvenile animal model. Crit Care Med 1998;26:2016–20.

199. Rohrer MJ, Natale AM. Effect of hypothermia on the coagulation cascade. Crit Care Med 1992;20:1402–5.

200. Michelson AD, Barnard MR, Khuri SF, et al. The effects of aspirin and hypothermia on platelet function in vivo. Br J Haematol 1999;104:64–8.

20

Acid–base disorders

Kyle J Gunnerson, Ramesh Venkataraman, and John A Kellum

CLASSIFICATION OF ACID–BASE DISORDERS

Identification

Acid–base homeostasis is defined by the pH of blood plasma and by the conditions of the acid–base pairs that determine it. Normally, arterial plasma pH is maintained between 7.35 and 7.45. Because blood plasma is an aqueous solution containing both volatile (carbon dioxide) and fixed acids, its pH will be determined by the net effects of all these components on the dissociation of water.[1-3] The determinants of blood pH can be grouped into two broad categories, respiratory and metabolic. Respiratory acid–base disorders are disorders of carbon dioxide (CO_2) tension, whereas metabolic acid–base disorders comprise all other conditions affecting the pH. This later category includes disorders of both weak acids (often referred to as buffers, although the term is imprecise) and strong acids and bases (including both organic and inorganic acids). The terms *acidemia* or *alkalemia* represent only blood hydrogen concentration and therefore the pH. The terms *acidosis* and *alkalosis* refer to the actual physiologic (or pathophysiologic) process.[4] Acid–base disorders can be recognized by any of the following conditions:

1. an alteration in the pH of the arterial blood (pH <7.35 signifying an acidemia, whereas a pH >7.45 signifies an alkalemia)
2. an arterial partial pressure of CO_2 ($PaCO_2$) outside the normal range (35–45 mmHg).
3. a plasma bicarbonate (HCO_3^-) concentration outside the normal range (22–26 mEq/L)
4. an arterial standard base excess (SBE) ≥5 or ≤−5 mEq/L.

Base excess (BE) is the quantity of metabolic acidosis or alkalosis defined as the amount of acid or base that must be added to a sample of whole blood in vitro in order to restore the pH of the sample to 7.40 while the pCO_2 is held at 40 mmHg.[5] While this calculation is quite accurate in vitro, inaccuracy exists when applied in vivo in that BE changes with changes in pCO_2.[6,7] This effect is understood to be due to equilibration across the entire extracellular fluid space (whole blood + interstitial fluid). When the BE equation is modified to account for an 'average' content of hemoglobin across this entire space, a value of 5 g/dl is used instead and this defines the standard BE (i.e. the SBE). It should be pointed out that this value does not represent the true content of hemoglobin suspended in the volume of whole blood together with interstitial fluid, but rather an empiric estimate which improves the accuracy of the BE. It can be argued that the entire extracellular fluid space is involved in acid–base balance since this fluid flows through blood vessels and lymphatics, mixing constantly.[8] Thus, the value of SBE is that it quantifies the change in metabolic acid–base status in vivo. It is of interest that BE is only accurate in vivo when it assumes a constant hemoglobin concentration.[8]

Regrettably, while the above criteria are useful in identifying an acid–base disorder, the absence of all four criteria cannot exclude a mixed acid–base disorder, alkalosis + acidosis, which is completely matched. Fortunately, such conditions are quite rare. Assessment of the anion gap (see below) may also be useful in detecting these mixed disorders. Since cellular metabolism is acid-producing, any process that limits CO_2 excretion from the lungs will rapidly induce respiratory acidosis, whereas any process that limits fixed acid excretion from the kidneys will induce metabolic acidosis, albeit more slowly. Similarly, independent excess endogenous or exogenous acid flux into the bloodstream will also induce metabolic acidosis.

Etiology of acid–base disorders

Changes in the pH of water-containing solutions occur as a result of alterations in one or more of the primary determinants of water dissociation. In blood plasma, water dissociation is determined by changes in pCO_2, strong ions, or weak acids.[1-3] Strong ions are those ions that are completely (or almost completely) ionized at physiologic pH, such as Na^+, Cl^-, K^+, Mg^{2+}, Ca^{2+}, and lactate. Abnormal ions such as ketones and sulfate are also strong ions. Importantly, HCO_3^- is not a strong ion, nor is H^+, because these ions do not remain ionized (they form uncharged molecules: CO_2 and H_2O). The net charge of strong cations and strong anions is known as the strong ion difference (SID).[2] When cations are greater than anions, SID is positive and when anions are greater than cations SID is negative. In a normal healthy adult, the SID is somewhere around 40–42 mEq/L.[2] In other words, as SID becomes more positive, H^+, a 'weak' cation decreases (and pH increases) in order to maintain electrical neutrality (Fig. 20.1). The weak acids are those nonvolatile acids which, unlike strong ions, exist in both ionized (A^-) or protonated (AH) forms. The sum of A^- and AH is known as A_{TOT}. Blood pH is determined by pCO_2, SID, and A_{TOT}. Respiratory abnormalities involve derangements in pCO_2 homeostasis, whereas metabolic abnormalities involve SID or, less commonly, A_{TOT}. A graphical representation is shown in Figure 20.2.

Clinical significance of acid–base disorders

Severe derangements in acid–base variables and/or plasma pH can be life-threatening. Respiratory depression and altered sensorium can occur as a consequence of either severe alkalemia or acidemia. Severe alkalemia may induce seizures and severe acidosis can cause or contribute to circulatory shock.[3] Although acid–base disorders appear to be associated with poor outcome in many clinical subsets, it remains unclear whether these alterations are themselves causally related to the outcome or merely markers of adverse pathophysiologic states.[9-11] It has been noted that severe alterations in arterial pH may occur without long-term clinical consequences (e.g. exercise-induced

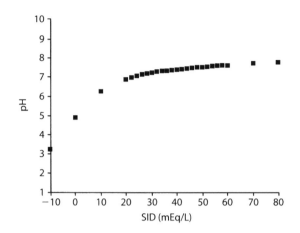

Figure 20.1 Plot of pH vs strong ion difference (SID). For this plot, A_{TOT} and pCO_2 were held constant at 18 mEq/L and 40 mmHg, respectively, and a water dissociation constant for blood of 4.4×10^{-14} Eq/L is assumed. Note how steep the pH curve becomes at SID <20 mEq/L. (Adapted from Kellum[37] with permission.)

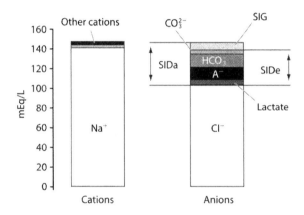

Figure 20.2 Charge balance in blood plasma. 'Other cations' include Ca^{2+} and Mg^{2+}. The strong ion difference (SID) is always positive (in plasma) and SID − SIDe (effective) must always equal zero. Any difference between SIDe and apparent (SIDa) is the strong ion gap (SIG) and must represent unmeasured anions. (Adapted from Kellum[37] with permission.)

lactic acidosis and permissive hypercapnia). Furthermore, the available evidence does not suggest that correcting acid–base derangements improves clinical outcomes.[12] However, there is evidence that acidosis and alkalosis produce adverse clinical effects and most clinicians believe that treating provides (at least symptomatic) benefit.[3] There are adverse consequences to therapy, however (discussed below), and therefore caution is advised.

Diagnosing acid–base disorders

There are four broad categories of acid–base disorders:

1. metabolic acidosis
2. metabolic alkalosis
3. respiratory acidosis (acute and chronic)
4. respiratory alkalosis (acute and chronic).

Acid–base disorders are further divided into simple (or pure), denoting a single process, and complex (or mixed), denoting a condition where two or three processes are occurring simultaneously. Simple acid–base disorders result in predictable patterns, both in terms of carbonic acid equilibrium and physiologic compensation. Table 20.1 outlines the observed changes in pCO_2, bicarbonate, and arterial SBE seen with simple acid–base disorders.[13] When measured acid–base variables fall outside of the parameters described in Table 20.1, complex acid–base disorders exist. Table 20.1 also describes the expected compensatory changes that follow simple acid–base derangements. When normal compensation does not occur, a complex acid–base disorder also exists. It is possible, though rare, that a mixed disorder might occur such that opposing processes (alkalosis and acidosis) are completely balanced, giving the impression of normal acid–base balance.[13]

Acid–base disorders can be suspected from the plasma electrolytes but require arterial blood gas measurement to confirm or help exclude. The first step is to determine the primary process by the following formulae:

1. If arterial pH is <7.35 and pCO_2 <40 mmHg, there is a metabolic acidosis
2. If arterial pH is <7.35 and pCO_2 >40 mmHg, there is a respiratory acidosis
3. If arterial pH is >7.45 and pCO_2 <40 mmHg, there is a respiratory alkalosis
4. If arterial pH is >7.45 and pCO_2 >40 mmHg, there is a metabolic alkalosis
5. If any other pattern exists, there is a complex (mixed) disorder.

Classification of a complex acid–base disorder is accomplished first by examining the pH. If the pH is <7.35, at least one type of acidosis is present, and if the pH is >7.45, at least one type of alkalosis is present. The values of compensatory changes shown in Table 20.1 should be used to determine if a complex disorder is present.[13] Examples:

1. A simple metabolic acidosis will manifest as a SBE <−3 mEq/L, a plasma bicarbonate concentration <22 mmol/L. In addition, the pCO_2 will equal 1.5 × bicarbonate + 8 (alternatively the expected pCO_2 can be found by the simple formula $pCO_2 = 40 + SBE$); either formula has a range of ± 2. If the arterial pCO_2 is outside this range, a secondary respiratory acid–base disorder is present (respiratory alkalosis if pCO_2 is lower than expected and respiratory acidosis if pCO_2 is higher than expected).
2. A simple chronic respiratory acidosis will manifest as a pH <7.35, a pCO_2 >45 mmHg. The plasma bicarbonate concentration should be equal to $pCO_2 − 40/3] + 24$ and the SBE should equal 0.4 × ($pCO_2 − 40$ – the ranges are again ± 2).

Table 20.1 Observational acid–base patterns.			
Disorder	**HCO_3^- (mEq/L)**	**pCO_2 (mmHg)**	**SBE (mEq/L)**
Metabolic acidosis	<22	= (1.5 × HCO_3^-) + 8 = 40 + SBE	<−3
Metabolic alkalosis	>26	= (0.7 × HCO_3^-) + 21 = 40 + (0.6 × SBE)	>+3
Acute respiratory acidosis	= [(pCO_2 − 40)/10] + 24	>45	= 0
Chronic respiratory acidosis	= [(pCO_2 − 40)/3] + 24	>45	= 0.4 × (pCO_2 − 40)
Acute respiratory alkalosis	= 24 − [(40 − pCO_2)/5]	<35	= 0
Chronic respiratory alkalosis	= 24 − [(40 − pCO_2)/2]	<35	= 0.4 × (pCO_2 − 40)

Source: compiled from various sources. The changes in standard base excess (SBE) were taken from Schlichtig et al.[13]

METABOLIC ACIDOSIS

Classification and emergency management of metabolic acidosis

Except when it is a part of a complex (mixed) disorder, metabolic acidosis is manifest by acidemia (arterial pH <7.35), hypobicarbonatemia (HCO_3^- <22 mmol/L), hypocarbia (pCO_2 <40 mmHg), and a reduced SBE (<−3 mEq/L). Metabolic acidosis may induce a variety of adverse clinical effects (Table 20.2), some of which can be life-threatening. When alterations in mental status or respiratory function occur, control of the patient's airway is advisable. Metabolic acidosis may contribute to hypotension, and resuscitation with volume and/or vasoactive medications may be necessary. Caution must be exercised when treating acidosis with sodium bicarbonate, particularly if ventilation is compromised. The increase in pCO_2 can worsen the acidemia and hypercarbia (transiently) and can precipitate acute respiratory failure.[12]

Metabolic acidosis can be subdivided into two broad categories: increased anion gap (AG) and normal AG (hyperchloremic) acidosis. The AG is determined by the formula:

$$AG = (Na^+ + K^+) - (Cl^- + HCO_3^-).$$

The normal range for the AG is 8–12 mEq/L and reflects the unaccounted for negatively charged

---

Table 20.2 Potential clinical effects of metabolic acid–base disorders.

Metabolic acidosis	Metabolic alkalosis
Cardiovascular	**Cardiovascular**
Decreased inotropy	Increased inotropy (Ca^{2+} entry)
Arterial vasodilatation	Digoxin toxicity
Venous vasoconstriction	Alters coronary blood flow[a]
Conduction defects	
Oxygen delivery	**Oxygen delivery**
Decreased 2,3-DPG (late)	Increased 2,3-DPG (delayed)
Decreased oxy-Hb binding	Increased oxy-Hb affinity
Metabolic effect	**Metabolic effect**
Protein wasting	Hypokalemia
Bone demineralization	Hypocalcemia
Insulin resistance	Hypophosphatemia
Catecholamine, PTH, and aldosterone stimulation	Impaired enzyme function
Neuromuscular	**Neuromuscular**
Respiratory depression	Neuromuscular excitability
Decreased sensorium	Encephalopathy
	Seizures
	Respiratory depression
Electrolytes	
Hyperkalemia	
Hypercalcemia	
Hyperuricemia	
Gastrointestinal effect	
Emesis	

[a]Animal studies have shown both increased and decreased coronary artery blood flow.

2,3-DPG = 2,3-diphosphoglycerate; oxy-Hb = oxyhemoglobin; PTH = parathyroid hormone.

species present in the blood under normal (e.g. proteins, phosphates) and pathophysiologic (e.g. lactic acid, ketones, sulfates) conditions. However, if the patient's albumin and phosphate concentrations are low, their AG will be reduced.[14] One should be aware of a falsely normal AG in a patient with hypoalbuminemia of hypophosphatemia; see Figure 20.3. The normal AG is made up predominantly by albumin and phosphate and can be estimated from the following equation:

$$AG = 2(\text{albumin g/dl}) + 0.5(\text{phosphate mg/dl}).^{14}$$

For international units:

$$AG = 0.2(\text{albumin g/L}) + 1.5(\text{phosphate mmol/L})$$

Clues to the existence of a balanced complex disorder include the emergence of imbalance on repeated measurements or the presence of an abnormal anion gap.[3]

Step 1
Once a metabolic acidosis is identified, the first step should be to calculate the AG as described above. An increased AG metabolic acidosis is due to acids whose anions are not normally measured by routine electrolyte determinations (e.g. lactate, ketones, toxins) whereas normal AG acidoses are due to abnormalities in chloride homeostasis – see Table 20.3. In the case of an increased AG, the change in SBE (and if there is no respiratory disorder, the change in bicarbonate concentration) (except isopropanol) should be equal to the increase in the AG from its normal value. If the change in SBE is larger than the change in the AG, a concomitant normal anion gap (hyperchloremic) acidosis is also present.

If the AG is increased, the putative anion should be sought and, when possible, its concentration compared to the change in the AG. Strong ions such as lactate produce a 1:1 increment in the AG for each mEq/L increase in their concentration. When the increase in AG is larger than the increase in strong ions, other acids must be present.[15]

Step 2
If a normal AG (hyperchloremic) metabolic acidosis is present, its cause can be determined by examining the urine SID. If the kidneys are functioning normally in a metabolic acidosis, the urine SID should be negative as the kidney excretes strong anions in excess of strong cations (see Table 20.3).[16] Renal tubular defects are then manifest by a failure to excrete the chloride load and a resulting positive urine SID.[16]

Step 3
If a patient has an increased AG metabolic acidosis, looking for an osmolar gap might also help determine the etiology. Osmolar gap is the difference between the measured serum osmolarity and calculated serum osmolarity:

$$(2 \times Na) + \text{Glucose}/18 + \text{BUN}/2.8$$

where BUN is the blood urea nitrogen. A gap of more than 10 mmol/dl is indicative of the presence of a toxin in the blood that increases its osmolarity. Alcohols (ethanol, methanol, and ethylene glycol toxicity) typically cause AG metabolic acidosis varying with osmolar gaps.[17] The evaluation of the urine sediment, specifically for calcium oxalate, can be useful in diagnosing ethylene glycol ingestions.

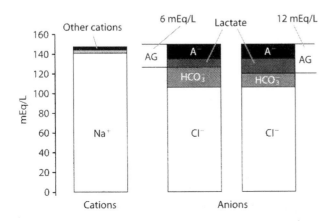

Figure 20.3 A⁻ represents weak acids, mostly albumin and phosphates. Note how an elevated lactate contributes to a widened anion gap (AG). One can also appreciate how hypoalbuminemia could falsely represent a 'normal' anion gap (AG) even if lactate is elevated. (Adapted from Kellum[37] with permission.)

Table 20.3 Differential diagnosis of metabolic acidosis: decreased strong ion difference (SID).	
A Increased anion gap	
Endogenous acids	**Toxic ingestions**
Renal failure	Ethylene glycol
Lactic acid	Paraldehyde
Ketosis (diabetic, starvation, alcohol)	Methanol
Nonketotic hyperosmolar hyperglycemia	Toluene
Unknown (sepsis, hepatic failure)	Salicylate
	Elemental iron
B Normal anion gap	
Renal tubular acidosis	**Nonrenal**
Urine SID (Na + K − Cl) >0	Urine SID (Na + K − Cl) <0
Distal (type I)	*Gastrointestinal*
Urine pH >5.5	Diarrhea
	Small bowel/pancreatic drainage
Proximal (type II)	*Iatrogenic*
Urine pH <5.5 and low serum K^+	Saline
	Parenteral nutrition
Aldosterone deficiency (type IV)	
Urine pH <5.5 and high serum K^+	

Step 4

The next step in characterizing a metabolic acidosis is to determine if a respiratory disorder is also present. The expected arterial pCO_2 in response to a metabolic acidosis can be determined either using the bicarbonate concentration or the SBE. Measured pCO_2 >2 mmHg more than expected indicates a concomitant respiratory acidosis, whereas measured pCO_2 <2 mmHg less than expected indicates a respiratory alkalosis.[13]

- $pCO_2 = 1.5 \times HCO_3^- + 8$
- $pCO_2 = 40 + SBE$

Causes of metabolic acidosis

Metabolic acidosis results from a decrease in the SID or an increase in A_{TOT} or both. When the SID is decreased (or A_{TOT} is increased) as a result of anions other than Cl^-, the AG increases. This may occur as a result of either endogenous or exo-

genous acids or both. The classical metabolic acidosis of renal failure is an early hyperchloremic acidosis, usually with an SBE not in excess of −10, followed by a gradual increase in the AG as the accumulation of sulfate, phosphate and other organic acids occurs.[18] Although some of these substances are strong ions (e.g. sulfate), peak concentrations are relatively low and therefore even in untreated end-stage renal disease, AG rarely exceeds 5 mEq/L over predicted.

Ketones from diabetic ketoacidosis induce an increased AG metabolic acidosis that may be profound. Starvation ketosis may also cause acidosis but it is usually quite mild.[19] Lactic acidosis is perhaps the most common cause of an increased AG metabolic acidosis. Lactic acidosis and patients with shock often represent inadequate resuscitation, whereas lactic acidosis occurring in well-perfused patients generally represents increased glucose metabolism, decreased lactate utilization, oxidative stress, or acute lung injury.[20–23]

Unknown anions can be responsible for the large AGs occasionally seen in patients with sepsis, liver failure, and nonketotic hyperosmolar hyperglycemia.[19,24,25] Several toxins, including methanol, ethylene glycol, paraldehyde, and toluene, induce an increased AG metabolic acidosis.[17] The presence of an osmolar gap (see above) along with an AG acidosis suggests intoxication by one of these alcohols. Salicylate toxicity classically induces a mixed picture of increased AG metabolic acidosis and respiratory alkalosis.[26]

Metabolic acidoses associated with a normal AG are due to abnormalities in Cl^- homeostasis. This may occur either by abnormalities of Cl^- handling by the kidneys or the intestinal tract or due to chloride poisoning.[3] In a renal tubular acidosis (RTA), the kidney fails to excrete Cl^- in excess of Na^+ and K^+. These disorders can be further differentiated on the basis of urine pH and plasma K^+ concentration (see Table 20.3).[16] *Type I* (distal) RTA can be caused by inherited disease, drugs (amphotericin B, lithium, toluene), nephrocalcinosis, idiopathic hypercalciuria, hypervitaminosis D, hyperthyroidism, hyperparathyroidism, autoimmune disorders, hypergammaglobulinemia, or interstitial nephropathies. *Type II* (proximal) RTA can be due to Wilson's disease, drugs (heavy metals, carbonic anhydrase inhibitors), hyperparathyroidism, amyloid, nephritic syndrome, renal transplant, myeloma, hypervitaminosis D, vitamin D deficiency, chronic active hepatitis, outdated tetracycline, or scleroderma. *Type IV* RTA is an imprecise category that includes all other forms of RTA: it can be due to selective aldosterone deficiency, usually associated with interstitial disease, especially lead or diabetes. Drugs, especially nonsteroidal anti-inflammatory agents and cyclosporine, have also been reported to cause type IV RTA.

Diarrhea or small bowel/pancreatic drainage impairs electrolyte reabsorption from the gastrointestinal tract such that Na^+ is lost in excess of Cl^-. The result is a decrease in the SID and a hyperchloremic metabolic acidosis.[3] Chloride poisoning occurs when large volumes of nonphysiologic solutions such as saline are given intravenously. HCl infusion will also produce the same effect, albeit more rapidly.[27–29]

Clinical management of metabolic acidosis

Many metabolic acidoses are self-limiting and do not require specific therapy. For example, exercise (or seizure)-induced lactic acidosis resolves quickly when muscles are rested and should not be treated except perhaps by transiently increasing ventilation. The physiologic response to metabolic acidosis is to increase ventilation and reduce pCO_2. This is generally the safest way to treat acute metabolic acidosis. It is usually best to identify and treat the underlying cause of metabolic acidosis whenever possible. Tissue hypoperfusion should always be excluded in patients with lactic acidosis.

In general, treatment of acute metabolic acidosis with sodium bicarbonate has not been shown to be beneficial and may be harmful.[12] However, there is insufficient evidence in severe or symptomatic patients and many clinicians use sodium bicarbonate in such conditions. Use of sodium bicarbonate by infusion rather than bolus injection induces less arterial hypotension and intracranial hypertension, and thus may be safer.[30] Chronic metabolic acidoses (e.g. chronic renal failure) require therapy to increase the SID. Oral sodium bicarbonate therapy is most commonly used.[31,32]

Use of nonbicarbonate buffers such as TRIS have occasionally been used for severe metabolic acidosis, though published reports are limited.[33] Severe metabolic acidosis may require treatment with continuous renal replacement therapy. The combination of hypokalemia and acidosis is particularly dangerous. These patients have profound total body K^+ depletion. K^+ must be administered before the pH is corrected (whether by decreasing pCO_2, or alkali therapy), since serum K^+ will fall further as the pH is increased.

Specific therapy is required for toxic ingestions (e.g. methanol, ethylene glycol), as these conditions can prove fatal without therapy.[17] Patients with proximal or type IV RTA rarely develop life-threatening acidosis, whereas patients with distal RTA may. In addition, distal RTA may be associated with hypokalemia, sometimes severe.[31,32]

Metabolic acidosis is associated with worse outcome in a variety of patient subsets (trauma, sepsis, respiratory failure).[9,11,34] However, there is little evidence that treating acidosis improves outcome.[12] Most clinicians believe that severe acidosis should be treated and avoidance of iatrogenic acidosis (chloride poisoning), where possible, seems appropriate.[35]

METABOLIC ALKALOSIS

Except when part of a complex (mixed) disorder, metabolic alkalosis is manifest by alkalemia (arterial pH >7.45), hyperbicarbonatemia (HCO_3^-

>26 mmol/L), hypercarbia (pCO_2 >40 mmHg), and an increased SBE (>3 mEq/L). Severe metabolic alkalosis in an intact ventilatory system requires the plasma bicarbonate concentration to be >45 mmol/L.[36]

Diagnosis and classification of metabolic alkalosis

Metabolic alkalosis can be subdivided into two broad categories: chloride-responsive and chloride-unresponsive metabolic alkalosis. A careful history and physical examination will reveal most causes of metabolic alkalosis. Most cases of acute metabolic alkalosis are due to losses from the gastrointestinal (GI) tract (vomiting or gastric drainage), to volume contraction, or to the administration of nonchloride-containing sodium salts (e.g. acetate, citrate, lactate). Chronic metabolic alkalosis is unusual and is usually the result of mineralocorticoid excess or chronic diuretic use. The urine Cl^- concentration can be used to help narrow the differential diagnosis. In so-called chloride-responsive metabolic alkalosis, the urine Cl^- concentration is usually <10 mmol/L. Urinary Cl^- losses in excess of Na^+ losses result in an increase in the plasma SID. GI losses, post-diuretic use, and post-hypercapnea are all chloride-responsive alkaloses. Chloride-unresponsive alkalosis results in a urine Cl^- concentration >20 mmol/L and is caused by mineralocorticoid excess or active diuretic use.[32]

As with metabolic acidosis, the final step in characterizing a metabolic alkalosis is to determine if a respiratory disorder is also present. The expected arterial pCO_2 in response to a metabolic alkalosis can be determined either using the bicarbonate concentration or the SBE. Measured pCO_2 >2 mmHg more than expected indicates a concomitant respiratory acidosis, whereas measured pCO_2 <2 mmHg less than expected indicates a respiratory alkalosis.[13]

$$pCO_2 = (0.7 \times HCO_3^-) + 21$$
$$pCO_2 = 40 + (0.6 \times SBE)$$

Beware of interpreting the AG in a patient with alkalemia. Alkalemia may increase the AG by as much as 3–5 mEq/L by altering the charges on plasma proteins.[18] Alkalemia may also induce mild hyperlactatemia by stimulating phosphofructokinase activity.[18]

Etiology of metabolic alkalosis

Metabolic alkalosis results from an increase in the SID. There are four mechanisms for this to occur:[37]

1. Severe depletion in free water, which includes a parallel increase in Na^+ and Cl^-. Since the relative concentration of Na^+ >Cl^-, the difference between them increases, increasing the SID.
2. Cl^- is lost from the GI tract or urine in excess of Na^+.
3. Na^+ is administered in excess of Cl^-.
4. Severe deficiency of intracellular cations such as magnesium or potassium. This decreases intracellular Cl^- and, secondarily, total body Cl^- is reduced.

Diuretic use (or abuse) is perhaps the most common reason for metabolic alkalosis. GI losses of Cl^- include vomiting, gastric drainage, and rarely, chloride wasting diarrhea (villous adenoma). For several hours (or longer) following an episode of respiratory failure with elevated pCO_2, a metabolic alkalosis (chloride-responsive) will persist so long as the respiratory failure was chronic enough to induce renal compensation (Cl^- excretion). All forms of mineralocorticoid excess can produce renal Cl^- wasting and metabolic alkalosis. These conditions include primary hyperaldosteronism (Conn's syndrome), secondary hyperaldosteronism, Cushing's syndrome, Liddle's syndrome, Bartter's syndrome, exogenous corticoids, and excessive licorice intake.[38] Administration of nonchloride sodium salts can occur with massive blood transfusions (sodium citrate), parenteral nutrition (sodium acetate), plasma volume expanders (acetate or citrate), Ringer's solution (sodium lactate) or overzealous use of sodium bicarbonate.

Clinical management of metabolic alkalosis

As with other acid–base disorders, the first rule of clinical management is to treat the underlying disorder. This is especially true for the large number of chronic conditions associated with metabolic alkalosis. The chloride-responsive alkaloses are so-named because Cl^- administration can treat them. For patients with diuretic-induced metabolic alkalosis, 0.45% saline is effective for reversing free water deficit and provides a source of Cl^-.

For patients with renal failure and at risk for volume overload, dilute (0.1 N) HCl can be administered through a central venous line.[39] Each liter of this solution contains 100 mmol of Cl^-, and it is advisable to recheck the acid–base status after each liter. For patients with diuretic-responsive volume overload and metabolic alkalosis, KCl can be administered along with loop diuretics. Alternatively, K^+ sparing diuretics (which will also spare Cl^-) can be used. Acetazolamide (250–500 mg twice daily or as a single dose) inhibits carbonic anhydrase and can induce excretion of Na^+ in excess of Cl^- and thus reduce the SID.[40] K^+ excretion is also seen as permitting additional KCl administration. In patients with ongoing gastric losses, H_2-blockers or proton pump inhibitors may prove an important adjunct to therapy.

Chloride unresponsive alkaloses are often more difficult to treat. For neoplastic diseases such as hyperaldosteronism, or Cushing's syndrome, spironolactone may be helpful, but surgery is usually required. Angiotensin-converting enzyme (ACE) inhibitors such as captopril are often effective for secondary hyperaldosteronism. Triamterene may be tried in cases of Bartter's or Liddle's syndrome, though with varying success.[41] Metabolic alkaloses secondary to administration of nonchloride-containing sodium salts are usually self-limited. When additional intravenous (IV) fluids are needed, saline should be used. Parenteral nutrition formulas should be adjusted to maximize chloride (remove citrate and acetate).

Metabolic alkalosis is usually mild and not life-threatening. However, when it is severe (pH >7.6) or when it develops quickly, the condition can produce seizures, decrease cardiac output, depress central ventilation, shift the oxyhemoglobin saturation curve to the left, worsen hypokalemia and hypophosphatemia, and negatively affect the ability to wean patients from mechanical ventilation.[42–44] Table 20.2 lists the known effects of metabolic alkalosis. Just as with severe metabolic acidosis, immediate treatment is with moderation with an appropriate reduction of plasma bicarbonate to 40 mmol/L which should lower the pH to 7.55 or less.[32] Similar to metabolic acidosis, metabolic alkalosis has been found to be associated with increased morbidity and mortality.[45,46]

RESPIRATORY ACIDOSIS

In open systems (when ventilation is present) and in the presence of carbonic anhydrase, pCO_2 is an independent determinant of plasma pH. In plasma, dissolved CO_2 is rapidly converted to carbonic acid and then to HCO_3^- and H^+. In this way, CO_2 is an important biologic acid.[37]

Diagnosis of respiratory acidosis

Pure respiratory acidosis is easily diagnosed, as the pCO_2 will be elevated and arterial pH decreased. Respiratory acidosis may also complicate metabolic acid–base disorders. In metabolic acidosis, the arterial pCO_2 should decrease (respiratory compensation). When the pCO_2 fails to decrease (>2 mmHg more than the estimated pCO_2), respiratory acidosis is also present. For *metabolic acidosis*, the expected pCO_2 can be calculated from either of the following formulas:[13]

$$pCO_2 = 1.5 \times HCO_3^- + 8$$
$$pCO_2 = 40 + SBE$$

In cases of metabolic alkalosis, CO_2 retention occurs and the expected pCO_2 is increased. However, when it is increased >2 mmHg *above* the estimated level, respiratory acidosis is also present. For *metabolic alkalosis*, the expected pCO_2 can be determined by either of the following formulas:[12]

$$pCO_2 = (0.7 \times HCO_3^-) + 21$$
$$pCO_2 = 40 + (0.6 \times SBE)$$

Unlike, respiratory compensation, metabolic compensation takes time (up to 5 days).[47] Therefore, acute and chronic respiratory acid–base disorders will have different patterns of SBE and bicarbonate. In acute respiratory acidosis, SBE is 0 and bicarbonate is determined by the pCO_2, using the following relationship:

$$HCO_3^- = [(pCO_2 - 40)/10] + 24$$

When there is an acute respiratory acidosis, a metabolic acid–base disorder is also present if the SBE is < -3 mEq/L (acidosis) or >3 (alkalosis) or if the measured bicarbonate is different (±2) from expected. When respiratory acidosis is chronic, the SBE and bicarbonate can be estimated from the following formulas:[13]

$$SBE = 0.4 \times (pCO_2 - 40)$$
$$HCO_3^- = [(pCO_2 - 40)/3] + 24$$

Without knowing the history, a patient with a pCO_2 of 60 mmHg and an SBE of +5 mEq/L might have either a pure chronic respiratory acidosis or an acute respiratory acidosis with a superimposed metabolic alkalosis.

Etiology of respiratory acidosis

Respiratory acidosis occurs when CO_2 production exceeds CO_2 elimination. Decreased CO_2 elimination results from either alveolar hypoventilation or increased ventilation/perfusion (V/Q) mismatch. Alveolar hypoventilation results from respiratory depression (e.g. central nervous system (CNS) disease, narcotics), neuromuscular disease, or airway obstruction.[48–51] V/Q mismatch can occur acutely as a result of pulmonary embolism or dynamic hyperinflation (especially when combined with dehydration). Chronic V/Q mismatch can be seen with emphysema and pulmonary fibrosis/vasculitis. When ventilation is fixed (e.g. during general anesthesia), increases in CO_2 production can result in respiratory acidosis.[52] This can be seen with shivering and fever, as oxygen consumption increases to as much as three times normal.[53,54] Large amounts of exogenous CO_2 administration (typically as sodium bicarbonate) can result in hypercarbia when ventilation is fixed.[55]

Chronic respiratory acid–base disorders are those that have been presenting long enough to permit metabolic (primarily renal) compensation. This process generally takes 2–5 days.[47] In general, the decrease in pH with chronic respiratory acidosis is approximately half that seen with acute respiratory acidosis.[47] A patient may present at a time point between acute and chronic that makes classification difficult. Chronic respiratory acidosis is most often caused by chronic lung disease (e.g. chronic obstructive pulmonary disease or COPD) or chest wall disease (e.g. kyphoscoliosis). Rarely, its cause is central hypoventilation or chronic neuromuscular disease.[56,57]

Clinical management of respiratory acidosis

Life-threatening acidosis does not occur from respiratory failure, except when uncontrolled supplemental oxygen is given.[58] This is because fatal hypoxemia will occur prior to pCO_2 reaching critical levels due to decreased ventilatory drive.[59,60] This statement has historical merit; however, a paucity of data and current clinical trials challenge this thinking.[61,62]

However, caution should always be exercised when oxygen therapy is instituted for patients with respiratory insufficiency. pCO_2 and continuous O_2 saturation (goal in low 90% range) should be measured in such cases. Hypercarbia may cause somnolence (CO_2 narcosis) and worsen respiratory depression, precipitating acute respiratory arrest. Intubation and mechanical ventilation should be instituted early in the case of worsening respiratory acidosis, prior to respiratory arrest. Supplemental oxygen should never be withheld from the hypoxemic patient in the fear of precipitating respiratory failure.

When the underlying cause of respiratory acidosis can be addressed quickly (e.g. reversal of narcotics with naloxone), it may be possible to avoid endotracheal intubation. However, more often this is not the case and mechanical ventilation must be initiated. Mechanical support is indicated when the patient is unstable or at risk for instability or when CNS function deteriorates. Furthermore, in patients who are exhibiting signs of respiratory muscle fatigue, mechanical ventilation should be instituted before respiratory failure occurs. Thus, it is not the absolute pCO_2 value that is important, but rather the clinical condition of the patient. Chronic hypercapnia requires treatment when there is an acute deterioration. In this setting, it is important not to try to restore the pCO_2 to 35–45 mmHg, but rather to tailor treatment for the patient's baseline pCO_2 if known. If this is not known, a target pCO_2 of 60 mmHg is perhaps reasonable.

Other options for treatment of hypercarbia include noninvasive positive pressure ventilation (BiPAP). This technique can be useful in the management of some patients, particularly when their sensorium is not impaired.[63] Occasionally, it is useful to reduce CO_2 production. This can be accomplished by reducing carbohydrate in nutritional support, control of temperature in the febrile patient, and sedation of the anxious or combative patient. Treatment of shivering in the postoperative period can reduce CO_2 production. However, it is unusual to control hypercarbia with these techniques alone.

Outcome of respiratory acidosis

Unlike metabolic acidosis, respiratory acidosis does not appear to have the same association with increased mortality. Indeed, controlled respiratory acidosis (permissive hypercapnia) is routinely used in some centers to control airway pressures in patients with acute lung injury.[64] Outcome appears to be related to the underlying disease process. The added risks (or benefits) of respiratory acidosis, per se, have not been adequately evaluated.

In recent years there has been considerable interest in reducing ventilator-associated lung injury. One strategy to reduce lung stretch is to reduce tidal volume and to tolerate a reduced minute ventilation and hence an elevated pCO_2. This practice is often referred to as permissive hypercapnia or controlled hypoventilation.[64] Controversial uncontrolled and controlled studies suggest that this method may reduce mortality in patients with severe acute respiratory distress syndrome (ARDS).[64–67] However, permissive hypercapnia is not without risks. Sedation is mandatory and even neuromuscular blocking agents are frequently required. Intracranial pressure increases, as does transpulmonary pressure, making this technique unusable in patients with brain injury and right ventricular dysfunction.[68,69] Controversy exists as to how low to allow the pH to go. Although some clinicians have reported good results with a pH even lower than 7.0, most authors have advocated more modest pH reductions (above 7.25).[37]

RESPIRATORY ALKALOSIS

In open systems (when ventilation is present) and in the presence of carbonic anhydrase, pCO_2 is an independent determinant of plasma pH. When ventilation is increased, pCO_2 falls and, for a constant rate of CO_2 production, mass action forces the equilibrium in the direction of CO_2 and both HCO_3^- and H^+ are reduced.

Diagnosis of respiratory alkalosis

Pure respiratory alkalosis is easily diagnosed, as the pCO_2 will be reduced and arterial pH increased. Respiratory alkalosis may also complicate metabolic acid–base disorders. In metabolic acidosis, the arterial pCO_2 should decrease (respiratory compensation). However, when the measured pCO_2 is decreased >2 mmHg *below* the estimated pCO_2, respiratory alkalosis is also present. For *metabolic acidosis*, the expected pCO_2 can be calculated from either of the following formulas:[13]

$$pCO_2 = 1.5 \times HCO_3^- + 8$$
$$pCO_2 = 40 + SBE$$

In cases of metabolic alkalosis, CO_2 retention occurs and the expected pCO_2 is increased. When

the pCO_2 fails to increase as expected (>2 mmHg less than the estimated level), respiratory alkalosis is also present. For *metabolic alkalosis*, the expected pCO_2 can be determined by either of the following formulas:[13]

$$pCO_2 = (0.7 \times HCO_3^-) + 21$$
$$pCO_2 = 40 + (0.6 \times SBE)$$

Unlike respiratory compensation, metabolic compensation takes time (up to 5 days).[47] Therefore, acute and chronic respiratory acid–base disorders will have different patterns of SBE and bicarbonate. In acute respiratory alkalosis, SBE is 0 and bicarbonate is determined by the pCO_2, using the following relationship:

$$HCO_3^- = [(40 - pCO_2)/5] + 24$$

When there is an acute respiratory alkalosis, a metabolic acid–base disorder is also present if the SBE is <−3 mEq/L (acidosis) or >3 mEq/L (alkalosis) or if the measured bicarbonate is different (±2) from expected. When respiratory alkalosis is chronic, the SBE and bicarbonate can be estimated from the following formulas:[13]

$$SBE = 0.4 \times (pCO_2 - 40)$$
$$HCO_3^- = [(40—pCO_2)/2] + 24$$

Etiology of respiratory alkalosis

The etiology of respiratory alkalosis is multifactorial, but can be generalized in the following classifications:[31,37]

1. CNS stimulation – pain, anxiety, fever, pregnancy, CNS disease (meningitis, tumor, stroke), hypoxia.
2. Drugs – salicylates, progesterone, nikethamide.
3. Stimulation of chest receptors – cardiac failure, pulmonary embolism.
4. Increased CO_2 production – seizures, recovery from anesthesia.
5. Miscellaneous – sepsis, hepatic failure.

Management of respiratory alkalosis

Respiratory alkalosis may be the presenting manifestation of many serious disorders, including sepsis and pulmonary embolism.[70] Any accompanying hypotension should be aggressively corrected.

Also, severe alkalosis is associated with electrolyte disturbances such as hypokalemia, hypophosphatemia, and hypomagnesemia. One should look for these disturbances and correct them to avoid/treat any accompanying arrhythmias.

The treatment should be directed towards the underlying cause. Most often, simple reassuring, anxiolytics, rebreathing from a bag, or treating the underlying psychological stress is enough to alleviate respiratory alkalosis. Controlling fever, seizure activity, and sepsis will minimize hypocapnia. Sedatives or neurodepressants can decrease ventilatory drive and should not be used prior to evaluation of the underlying cause. Associated electrolyte abnormalities should be corrected in acute settings.[32,37]

Outcome of respiratory alkalosis

Outcome depends on the nature and severity of the underlying cause. However, hypocapnia appears to be a particularly bad prognostic indicator in critically ill patients, especially those with sepsis. Chronic hypocapnia appears to have minimal risk on the health of patients.

CONCLUSION

Acid–base regulation is an important component in the management of the critically ill patient. A strong comprehension of the elements of acid–base disorders is essential in their proper management. By understanding how independent variables, SID, pCO_2, and A_{TOT} interact and contribute to the acid–base disorder, complex derangements can be easily and consistently understood, identified, and treated. Some key points need to be kept in mind while managing acid–base disorders. First of all, when dealing with acid–base problems, a systematic, stepwise approach is key. Secondly, one needs to have a clear understanding that there are three basic methods of solving acid–base interactions, and that all three are similar in their conclusions. However, all three methods have their own limitations and these limitations should be taken into account prior to interpreting and managing acid–base disturbances. Thirdly, calculating the anion gap should be done routinely, even in alkalemic patients, since it often points to the presence of underlying acidemia. However, the anion gap should be always corrected for the patient's serum albumin and phosphorus to avoid misinterpreta-

tion of a falsely normal gap. Finally, extremes of acid–base status are associated with poor clinical outcomes in many clinical subsets. Hence, it may be important to correct these disturbances when clinically appropriate. However, there is insufficient evidence to support the routine use of sodium bicarbonate to correct metabolic acidosis and any therapy should always be titrated so as not to overcorrect the initial disorder.

REFERENCES

1. Stewart PA. How to understand acid–base. In: Stewart PA, ed. A quantitative acid–base primer for biology and medicine. New York: Elsevier; 1981:1–286.
2. Stewart PA. Modern quantitative acid–base chemistry. Can J Physiol Pharmacol 1983;61:1444–61.
3. Kellum JA. Determinants of blood pH in health and disease. Crit Care (London) 2000;4:6–14.
4. Kokko JP. Disturbances in acid–base balance. In: Goldman L, Bennett JC, eds. Cecil Textbook of Medicine. Philidelphia: W.B. Saunders Compan; 2000:558–67.
5. Siggaard-Andersen O. The pH-log pCO_2 blood acid–base nomogram revised. Scand J Clin Lab Invest 1962;14:598–604.
6. Brackett NC, Cohen JJ, Schwartz WB. Carbon dioxide titration curve of normal man. N Engl J Med 1965;272:6–12.
7. Prys-Roberts C, Kelman GR, Nunn JF. Determinants of the in vivo carbon dioxide titration curve in anesthetized man. Br J Anesth 1966;38:500–9.
8. Schlichtig R. Acid–base balance (quantitation). In: Grenvik A, Shoemaker PK, Ayers S, Holbrook P, eds. Textbook of critical care. Philadelphia: WB Saunders; 1999:828–39.
9. Hickling KG, Walsh J, Henderson S, Jackson R. Low mortality rate in adult respiratory distress syndrome using low-volume, pressure-limited ventilation with permissive hypercapnia: a prospective study. Crit Care Med 1994;22:1568–78.
10. Stacpoole PW, Lorenz AC, Thomas RG, Harman EM. Dichloroacetate in the treatment of lactic acidosis. Ann Intern Med 1988;108:58–63.
11. Stacpoole PW, Wright EC, Baumgartner TG, et al. A controlled clinical trial of dichloroacetate for treatment of lactic acidosis in adults. The Dichloroacetate-Lactic Acidosis Study Group. N Engl J Med 1992;327:1564–9.
12. Forsythe SM, Schmidt GA. Sodium bicarbonate for the treatment of lactic acidosis. Chest 2000;117:260–7.
13. Schlichtig R, Grogono AW, Severinghaus JW. Human $PaCO_2$ and standard base excess compensation for acid–base imbalance. Crit Care Med 1998;26:1173–9.
14. Kellum JA, Kramer DJ, Pinsky MR. Closing the gap: a simple method of improving the accuracy of the anion gap. Chest 1996; 110.
15. Gabow PA. Disorders associated with an altered anion gap. Kidney Int 1985;27:472–83.
16. Batlle DC, Hizon M, Cohen E, Gutterman C, Gupta R. The use of the urinary anion gap in the diagnosis of hyperchloremic metabolic acidosis. N Engl J Med 1988;318:594–9.
17. Burkhart KK, Kulig KW. The other alcohols. Methanol, ethylene glycol, and isopropanol. Emerg Med Clin North Am 1990;8: 913–28.
18. Narins RG, Jones ER, Townsend R. Metabolic acid–base disorders: pathophysiology, classification and treatment. In: Arieff AI, DeFronzo RA, eds. Fluid, electrolyte and acid–base disorders. New York: Churchill Livingstone; 1985:269–385.

19. Arieff AI, Carroll HJ. Nonketotic hyperosmolar coma with hyperglycemia: clinical features, pathophysiology, renal function, acid–base balance, plasma–cerebrospinal fluid equilibria and the effects of therapy in 37 cases. Medicine 1972;51:73–94.

20. Gore DC, Jahoor F, Hibbert JM, DeMaria EJ. Lactic acidosis during sepsis is related to increased pyruvate production, not deficits in tissue oxygen availability. Ann Surg 1996;224:97–102.

21. Levraut J, Ciebiera JP, Chave S, et al. Mild hyperlactatemia in stable septic patients is due to impaired lactate clearance rather than overproduction. Am J Respir Crit Care Med 1998;157:1021–6.

22. Stacpoole PW. Lactic acidosis and other mitochondrial disorders. Metabolism 1997;46:306–21.

23. Kellum JA, Kramer DJ, Lee K, et al. Release of lactate by the lung in acute lung injury. Chest 1997;111:1301–5.

24. Kellum JA, Kramer DJ, Pinsky MR. Strong ion gap: a methodology for exploring unexplained anions. J Crit Care 1995;10:51–5.

25. Kirschbaum B. Increased anion gap after liver transplantation. Am J Med Sci 1997;313:107–10.

26. Proudfoot AT. Toxicity of salicylates. Am J Med 1983;75:99–103.

27. Kellum JA, Bellomo R, Kramer DJ, Pinsky MR. Etiology of metabolic acidosis during saline resuscitation in endotoxemia. Shock 1998;9:364–8.

28. Scheingraber S, Rehm M, Sehmisch C, Finsterer U. Rapid saline infusion produces hyperchloremic acidosis in patients undergoing gynecologic surgery. Anesthesiology 1999;90:1265–70.

29. Waters JH, Miller LR, Clack S, Kim JV. Cause of metabolic acidosis in prolonged surgery. Crit Care Med 1999;27:2142–6.

30. Huseby JS, Gumprecht DG. Hemodynamic effects of rapid bolus hypertonic sodium bicarbonate. Chest 1981;79:552–4.

31. Adrogue HJ, Madias NE. Management of life-threatening acid–base disorders. First of two parts [erratum appears in N Engl J Med 1999;340(3):247]. N Engl J Med 1998;338:26–34.

32. Adrogue HJ, Madias NE. Management of life-threatening acid–base disorders. Second of two parts. N Engl J Med 1998; 338:107–11.

33. Bleich HL, Swartz WB. Tris buffer (THAM): an appraisal of its physiologic effects and clinical usefulness. N Engl J Med 1966; 274:782–7.

34. Weil MH, Afifi AA. Experimental and clinical studies on lactate and pyruvate as indicators of the severity of acute circulatory failure (shock). Circulation 1970;41:989–1001.

35. Kellum JA. Fluid resuscitation and hyperchloremic acidosis in experimental sepsis: improved short-term survival and acid–base balance with Hextend compared with saline. Crit Care Med 2002;30:300–5.

36. Madias NE, Bossert WH, Adrogue HJ. Ventilatory response to chronic metabolic acidosis and alkalosis in the dog. J Appl Physiol 1984;56:1640–6.

37. Kellum JA. Diagnosis and treatment of acid–base disorders. In: Shoemaker PK, Ayers S, Grenvik A, Holbrook P, eds. Textbook of critical care. Philiadelphia: WB Saunders; 1999:839–53.

38. Khanna A, Kurtzman NA. Metabolic alkalosis. Respir Care 2001; 46:354–65.

39. Brimioulle S, Berre J, Dufaye P, et al. Hydrochloric acid infusion for treatment of metabolic alkalosis associated with respiratory acidosis. Crit Care Med 1989;17:232–6.

40. Mazur JE, Devlin JW, Peters MJ, et al. Single versus multiple doses of acetazolamide for metabolic alkalosis in critically ill medical patients: a randomized, double-blind trial. Crit Care Med 1999;27:1257–61.

41. Wang C, Chan TK, Yeung RT, et al. The effect of triamterene and sodium intake on renin, aldosterone, and erythrocyte sodium transport in Liddle's syndrome. J Clin Endocrinol Metab 1981; 52:1027–32.

42. Krintel JJ, Haxholdt OS, Berthelsen P, et al. Carbon dioxide elimination after acetazolamide in patients with COPD and metabolic alkalosis. Acta Anaesthiol Scand 1983;27:252–4.

43. Gallagher TJ. Metabolic alkalosis complicating weaning from mechanical ventilation. South Med J 1979;72:784–5.

44. Berthelsen P. Cardiovascular performance and oxyhemoglobin dissociation after acetazolamide in metabolic alkalosis. Intensive Care Med 1982;8:269–74.

45. Anderson LE, Henrich WL. Alkalemia-associated morbidity and mortality in medical and surgical patients. South Med J 1987; 80:729–33.

46. Wilson RF, Gibson D, Pereinal MA, et al. Severe alkalosis in critically ill surgical patients. Arch Surg 1972;105:197.

47. Narins RG, Emmett M. Simple and mixed acid–base disorders: a practical approach. Medicine 1980;59:161–87.

48. Epstein SK, Singh N. Respiratory acidosis. Respir Care 2001;46: 366–83.

49. Langevin B, Petitjean T, Philit F, Robert D. Nocturnal hypoventilation in chronic respiratory failure (CRF) due to neuromuscular disease. Sleep 2000;23(Suppl 4):S204–8.

50. Krachman S, Criner GJ. Hypoventilation syndromes. Clin Chest Med 1998;19:139–55.

51. Martin TJ, Sanders MH. Chronic alveolar hypoventilation: a review for the clinician. Sleep 1995;18:617–34.

52. Scott JC. Investigation of the changes in acid–base equilibrium which occur in neonates and small infants as a result of intermittent positive pressure ventilation performed during general anesthesia. Anaesthesia 1971;26:511.

53. Ciofolo MJ, Clergue F, Devilliers C, Ben-Ammar M, Viars P. Changes in ventilation, oxygen uptake, and carbon dioxide output during recovery from isoflurane anesthesia. Anesthesiology 1989;70:737–41.

54. Just B, Delva E, Camus Y, Lienhart A. Oxygen uptake during recovery following naloxone. Anesthesiology 1992;76:60–4.

55. Steichen JJ, Kleinman LI. Studies in acid–base balance, I: effect of alkali therapy in newborn dogs with mechanically fixed ventilation. J Pediatr 1977;91:287–91.

56. Madias NE, Adrogue HJ. Acid–base disturbances in pulmonary medicine. In: Arieff AI, DeFronzo RA, eds. Fluid, electrolyte, and acid–base disorders. New York: Churchill Livingstone; 1995: 223–53.

57. Adrogue HJ, Tobin MJ. Respiratory pump failure: primary hypercapnia (respiratory acidosis). In: Adrogué HJ, Tobin MJ, eds. Respiratory failure. Cambridge, Mass: Blackwell Science; 1997: 125–34.

58. Chien JW, Ciufo R, Novak R, et al. Uncontrolled oxygen administration and respiratory failure in acute asthma. Chest 2000; 117:728–33.

59. Campbell EJM. The management of acute respiratory failure in chronic bronchitis and emphysema. Am Rev Respir Dis 1967;96:626–39.

60. Campbell EJM. A method of controlling oxygen administration which reduces the risk of carbon dioxide retention. Lancet 1960;1:12–14.

61. Crossley DJ, McGuire GP, Barrow PM, Houston PL. Influence of inspired oxygen concentration on deadspace, respiratory drive, and $PaCO_2$ in intubated patients with chronic obstructive pulmonary disease. Crit Care Med 1997;25:1522–6.

62. Gomersall CD, Joynt GM, Freebairn RC, Lai CK, Oh TE. Oxygen therapy for hypercapnic patients with chronic obstructive pulmonary disease and acute respiratory failure: a randomized, controlled pilot study. Crit Care Med 2002;30:113–16.

63. Evans TW. International Consensus Conferences in Intensive Care Medicine: non-invasive positive pressure ventilation in acute respiratory failure. Organized jointly by the American Thoracic Society, the European Respiratory Society, the European Society of Intensive Care Medicine, and the Societe de Reanimation de Langue Francaise, and approved by the ATS Board of Directors, December 2000. Intensive Care Med 2001;27:166–78.

64. Hickling KG. Low volume ventilation with permissive hypercapnia in the adult respiratory distress syndrome. Clin Intensive Care 1992;3:67–78.

65. Brower RG, Shanholtz CB, Fessler HE, et al. Prospective, randomized, controlled clinical trial comparing traditional versus reduced tidal volume ventilation in acute respiratory distress syndrome patients. Crit Care Med 1999;27:1492–8.

66. Brower RG. Acute Respiratory Distress Syndrome Network: ventilation with lower tidal volumes as compared with traditional tidal volumes for acute lung injury and the acute respiratory distress syndrome. N Engl J Med 2000;342:1301–8.

67. Amato MB, Barbas CS, Medeiros DM, et al. Effect of a protective-ventilation strategy on mortality in the acute respiratory distress syndrome. N Engl J Med 1998;338:347–54.

68. Ropper AH, Rockoff MA. Physiology and clinical aspects of raised intracranial pressure. In: Ropper AH, ed. Neurological and neurosurgical intensive care. New York: Raven; 1993:11–27.

69. Carvalho C, Barbas C, Medeiros D, et al. Temporal hemodynamic effects of permissive hypercapnia associated with ideal PEEP in ARDS. Am J Respir Crit Care Med 1997;156:1458–66.

70. Stein PD, Goldhaber SZ, Henry JW, Miller AC. Arterial blood gas analysis in the assessment of suspected acute pulmonary embolism. Chest 1996;109:78–81.

21

Diuretic use and fluid management

Jerrold S Levine and Jose Iglesias

INTRODUCTION

Decreased perfusion of vital tissues, resulting in inadequate delivery of oxygen and other essential bloodborne nutrients, is a commonly encountered and serious problem for the patient in an intensive care unit (ICU). Hypoperfusion can occur in the setting of either volume depletion, as from gastrointestinal blood loss, or volume overload, as in congestive heart failure (CHF) or cirrhosis. In both cases, the kidney attempts to restore effective tissue perfusion by reabsorbing sodium and increasing extracellular volume (ECV).

The combination of hypoperfusion and volume overload is an especially difficult one to manage, as the physician must balance the need for volume resuscitation and preservation of vital organ function against the risks of volume overload and edema. These risks are magnified in the ICU setting and include pulmonary edema, myocardial edema, hypoxemia, and other organ dysfunction.[1,2] Management is further complicated by the fact that the distribution of fluids between the vascular and extravascular compartments is often abnormal in critically ill patients. Alterations in both capillary permeability and Starling forces lead to transudation of fluid out of the vascular space and further compromises in tissue perfusion.

Given the extent and prevalence of these abnormalities in volume regulation among critically ill patients, it is not surprising that diuretics are one of the most frequently prescribed classes of drugs in the ICU setting.[1,2] Despite their frequent usage, errors in the prescription of diuretics are quite common. Indeed, the administration of diuretics in the ICU setting is beset with particular challenges and problems. For example, the severity and multi-organ nature of the underlying illness fre-

quently alter the pharmacology of these drugs, requiring careful titration of dosage.[3] Moreover, patients may manifest profound resistance to the effects of diuretics, leading to the administration of potentially toxic doses, or they may develop serious electrolyte disturbances or profound prerenal azotemia.[3] All in all, diuretic therapy within the ICU setting should be seen as a double-edged sword – on the one hand, ameliorating volume overload and offering potential benefits, such as earlier weaning from mechanical ventilation, while, on the other hand, reducing intravascular volume and possibly exacerbating hypoperfusion of vital organs.[1,2]

In this chapter, we will first review the pathophysiology and management of alterations in volume, with particular emphasis on those conditions and scenarios commonly encountered in the ICU. We will then review the pharmacology of the various diuretics, as given to critically ill patients, and offer recommendations for their correct usage based on an understanding of their pharmacology and of renal physiology.

DISTURBANCES OF VOLUME

Basic physiology

On average, total body water (TBW) comprises ~60% of lean body weight in men and ~50% in women. TBW is distributed between the intracellular and extracellular compartments, with 60% of TBW residing inside cells and 40% outside cells. ECV is itself divided between two compartments, the extravascular space (predominantly interstitium) and the intravascular space. The intravascular space is the smaller of the two spaces and comprises ~20% of ECV.[4] Thus, in a 70-kg male, TBW is 42 L, with ~40%, or 17 L, making up the ECV. Of these 17 L, only 20%, or ~3 L, circulate as plasma within the vascular space. Red blood cells make up an additional ~2 L of volume.[4] Thus, in summary, for a 70-kg male, the average circulating blood volume is ~5 L, 3 L of plasma and 2 L of red blood cells.[4]

The main part of these 5 L of intravascular blood volume resides in the capacitance vessels of the venous system and therefore does not contribute to tissue perfusion.[4,5] The term effective arterial blood volume (EABV) refers to the ~700 ml of blood volume that lies within the arterial system and is directly responsible for delivery of oxygen and vital nutrients. In effect, it is the EABV that the body seeks to regulate. However, since the body cannot measure EABV directly, it assesses EABV indirectly instead, through such indices as arterial blood pressure (via arterial baroreceptors located in the carotid sinus, cardiac atria, and afferent arterioles of the glomerulus) and delivery of oxygen and other vital nutrients. The body's response to inadequate EABV involves both hemodynamic alterations (such as venoconstriction, increased cardiac contractility, and preferential redistribution of blood flow to more vital organs) and renal retention of sodium (Na) in an effort to increase ECV.[4,6,7]

As discussed in Chapter 22, Na is the predominant extracellular osmole, whereas potassium is the predominant intracellular osmole. Retention of Na will therefore increase ECV; intravascular volume, being a fixed part of ECV, will increase more or less in parallel. Correspondingly, retention of potassium will tend to increase intracellular volume. Thus, although the reasons for inadequate tissue perfusion in disease states such as gastrointestinal blood loss and CHF are widely divergent, the kidney attempts in both cases to restore effective tissue perfusion by reabsorbing Na and increasing EVC and, along with it, EABV.

Hypovolemic states

An acute decrease in intravascular volume with associated hemodynamic instability is a common occurrence in critical illness and a major risk factor for organ failure. The etiologies of intravascular volume depletion are legion, ranging from true loss of blood volume from the body, such as hemorrhagic shock, to states of increased capillary permeability with transudation into the interstitium, such as sepsis or the systemic inflammatory response syndrome (SIRS) (Box 21.1).[5,8]

As EABV decreases, arterial baroreceptors are activated, resulting in increased sympathetic outflow and activation of the renin–angiotensin system.[6,7] The ensuing venoconstriction shifts blood from the venous to the arterial system and helps to restore EABV. Increases in heart rate, cardiac contractility, and cardiac output further help to maintain mean arterial pressure.[6,7] However, with losses that exceed 15% of the total intravascular volume, the compensatory hemodynamic and neurohumoral changes are unable to preserve EABV. At this point, clinical signs of hypovolemia, such as tachycardia and decreased urinary output, appear.[5]

It should be stressed that, in the majority of cases, the kidney is a remarkably sensitive barometer of EABV, and a decrease in urinary output almost always implies a decrease in EABV. There are several exceptions to this rule, including adrenal insufficiency or salt-wasting nephropathies, but by far the most important exception in the ICU setting is osmotic diuresis, as seen in patients with severe hyperglycemia, or malnourished patients receiving large solute loads.[7] Importantly, hypotension is a late finding in hypovolemic states, and is generally not observed until a patient has lost >30% of intravascular volume.[5]

To prevent organ dysfunction and failure, it is essential that hypovolemia, and decreased EABV, be promptly recognized and treated.[5,8] Depending on the clinical setting, patients will have varying degrees of volume loss from each of the different compartments of the body (intracellular, interstitial, and intravascular) (Fig. 21.1). The composition and quantity of fluid used for volume resuscitation will therefore depend on the clinical setting, the volume status of each compartment, and the electrolyte composition of the fluid that has been lost from the body – for example, hemorrhage, diarrheal fluid, nasogastric suctioning, insensible losses.[5]

The effect of fluid composition on the volume status of the various bodily compartments can be understood through a few simple physiologic principles (see Chapter 22). While these principles are the same, irrespective of whether the fluid is lost or administered, our discussion will take place from the perspective of fluid administration. Colloids, such as whole blood, fresh frozen plasma, or human serum albumin, will largely remain within the vascular space, unless there is an abnormality of vascular permeability, in which case oncotically

---

Box 21.1 Etiology of true intravascular volume depletion

True loss of extracellular fluid volume from the body

Gastrointestinal losses:

- Vomiting
- Diarrhea
- Gastrointestinal hemorrhage
- Tube drainage
- Fistulas
- Ostomies

Renal losses:

- Diuretics
- Osmotic diuresis (e.g. hyperglycemia)
- Adrenal insufficiency
- Salt-wasting nephropathies

Skin:

- Burns
- Fever
- Insensible losses

Other

- Hemorrhage

Sequestration of fluid into a 'third space'

Gastrointestinal losses:

- Intestinal obstruction or ileus
- Pancreatitis

- Peritonitis
- Ascites

Pulmonary losses:

- Pleural effusion

Musculoskeletal losses:

- Severe trauma or crush injury
- Skeletal fractures

Edema:[a]

- Nephrotic syndrome
- Malnutrition
- Liver disease
- Severe hypoalbuminemia (<2.0 g/dl)

Increased microvascular permeability and/or states of peripheral vasodilatation

Anaphylaxis

Sepsis

Systemic inflammatory response syndrome (SIRS)

Burns

Adult respiratory distress syndrome

Drugs (e.g. interleukin-2)

[a] As discussed in the text, the presence of edema does not necessarily imply true intravascular volume depletion or even a decrease in effective arterial blood volume (EABV). For example, as many as a third of children with nephrotic syndrome attributable to minimal change disease have increased blood volume, and edema is the result of a primary abnormality in sodium retention by the kidney. We recommend careful clinical assessment, including, if indicated, the placement of a pulmonary artery catheter.

---

active proteins can exit into the interstitium.[5,8] Crystalloids, such as isotonic saline or Ringer's lactate, will distribute uniformly throughout the ECV, with 80% going to the interstitium and only 20% to the intravascular space.[5] The distribution of intravenous crytalloid into the interstitial space occurs with a half-life of 30 minutes.[5,8] Oral water, or its intravenous equivalent D5W, will distribute uniformly throughout TBW, so that 60% will go inside cells and 40% will remain in the ECV, of which just 8% of the total volume will remain in the vascular space. Thus, for example, if one wanted to increase intravascular volume by 1 L, then one could administer 1 L of colloid, 5 L of crystalloid, or 12 L of D5W.[5] The distribution of fluids such as half-isotonic saline may be determined by treating them as a mixture of water and crystalloid, and then

considering separately the distribution of each portion. Although we have included an analysis of the effect of water on the volumes of the various bodily compartments, water should never be used to correct symptomatic hypovolemia.

The debate over the relative benefits of crystalloids vs colloids is ongoing and beyond the scope of this chapter. Suffice it to say that, to date, there has been no convincing evidence that one is superior to the other.[9,10] As long as the volumes of each fluid that remain within the vascular space are comparable – i.e. as long as one administers ~4–5 times as much crystalloid as colloid – then, under most conditions, the two fluids are probably equally effective. Although incompletely studied, several pathophysiologic factors may influence the decision in favor of one or the other. For example,

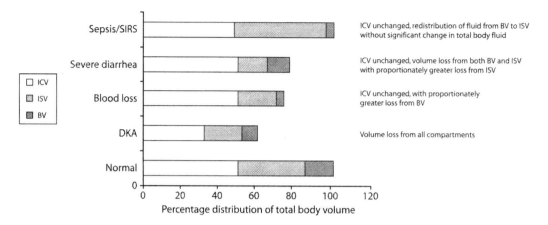

Figure 21.1 Changes in the volume of fluid compartments during various pathologic conditions commonly encountered in the ICU. For each pathophysiologic state, the volume status of each of the three compartments in the body – intracellular (ICV), interstitial (ISV), and intravascular (BV) – are depicted as a percentage of that seen under normal physiologic conditions. Thus, in patients with diabetic ketoacidosis (DKA), blood loss, or severe diarrhea, total body volume is typically reduced, whereas in patients with sepsis/systemic inflammatory response syndrome (SIRS), total body volume is typically normal. In patients with DKA, blood loss, and severe diarrhea, the loss of total body volume differentially affects the various fluid compartments of the body. In patients with sepsis/SIRS, the predominant derangement is a shift of fluid out of the vascular space into the interstitium.

in patients with sepsis, severe burns, or other states associated with systemic inflammation, the presence of profound microcirculatory disturbances, including increased capillary permeability and decreased colloid oncotic pressure, may lead to increased transudation of fluid and marked interstitial edema, if crystalloid solutions are the sole agents used in volume replacement. In contrast, if colloids are the sole agent used in these same patients, then increased colloid oncotic pressure throughout the ECV may lead to intracellular volume depletion. At present, however, these considerations remain largely theoretical. Finally, caution should be exercised in resuscitating trauma patients, as aggressive administration of colloids and/or crystalloids may be harmful, potentially leading to or exacerbating coagulopathy, thereby increasing the risk of continued hemorrhage.[11] Dilutional coagulopathy during large-volume resuscitation may be minimized by monitoring of factor levels and/or empiric administration of plasma.

The benefits and safety of human serum albumin (HSA) have also been debated without resolution. Two meta-analyses have demonstrated an increased mortality among patients given HSA, whereas one meta-analysis and one systematic review found no effect of HSA on mortality.[10,12]

Hydroxyethyl starches (hetastarches) are a synthetic colloid used in volume resuscitation. Although many inexpensive and effective formulations of hetastarch are commercially available, a recent multicenter randomized trial comparing 6% hetastarch (200 kDa, 0.6–0.66 substitution ratio) to 3% gelatin in patients with severe sepsis found a higher incidence of acute renal failure in the hetastarch-treated group.[13] These results need to be confirmed, as acute renal failure was defined by a threshold serum creatinine, and the group receiving hetastarch had a higher serum creatinine at baseline.

Treatment recommendations

If patients present with clinically evident hypovolemia (Box 21.2), but without evidence of respiratory failure, we recommend initial volume expansion with crystalloid, approximately 2 L of isotonic saline or Ringer's lactate, given in boluses of 500 ml. In patients with sepsis, burns, or SIRS, with evident capillary leak, the judicious use of an equivalent volume of colloid (400–500 ml in 100 ml boluses) seems appropriate. If there is no response to initial volume replacement, further therapy should be guided by a pulmonary artery catheter. If patients present with hypotension in the setting of respiratory distress or failure, then initial therapy should consist of respiratory support and vasoactive drugs to optimize perfusion. Fluid management, if indicated, should be guided by hemodynamic monitoring. Patients with

---

Box 21.2   Clinical and laboratory findings suggestive of intravascular volume depletion[a]

Physical findings

Tachycardia

Hypotension

Orthostatic changes:

- Increase in pulse rate $\geq$10–15 beats/min
- Decrease in systolic arterial blood pressure $\geq$10 mmHg

Cold extremities and/or temperature gradient between thighs and knees

Peripheral cyanosis or livedo reticularis

Absence of axillary sweat

Dry mucosa

Decreased skin turgor

Decreased mentation and/or altered sensorium

Decreased central venous pressure (flat neck veins in supine position)

Systolic arterial blood pressure changes during positive pressure ventilation (inspiratory decrease)

Decreased urine output

Laboratory findings

Increased urine osmolality ($\geq$450 mOsm/kg)

Decreased urine sodium concentration ($\leq$10 mEq/L)

Increased ratio of BUN (blood urea nitrogen) to serum creatinine in presence of normal urinalysis ($\geq$20:1)

Hemoconcentration:

- Increased hematocrit
- Increased serum albumin concentration

[a] It is important to note that most of these clinical and laboratory findings are relatively insensitive and nonspecific for the diagnosis of intravascular volume depletion.

---

hemorrhagic shock should be resuscitated by a combination of crystalloid and packed red blood cells. Finally, it is relatively common for critically ill patients with hypovolemia and hypotension to present with concomitant disturbances of osmolality, either hyponatremia or hypernatremia. The primary therapeutic goal for these patients should always be restoration of intravascular volume prior to correction of abnormal osmolality.

Hypervolemia

From a clinical standpoint, edema may be defined as a clinically detectable increase in the volume of interstitial fluid. In the peripheral circulation, edema manifests as palpable swelling, whereas, in the pulmonary circulation, interstitial edema leads to an increase of extravascular lung fluid, eventually flooding the alveolar air spaces.[14] In general,

peripheral edema is not clinically apparent until interstitial volume has increased by approximately 3 L.[14] Thus, the presence of even trace peripheral edema usually indicates an increase of at least 3 L of interstitial fluid, and 3 kg in total body mass. The pathophysiology and mechanisms of edema formation in the major disease states encountered in the ICU setting are reviewed in Box 21.3.

Within the peripheral capillary bed, the exchange of fluid between the intravascular space and the interstitium is determined by the hydrostatic and oncotic pressures in each compartment, as described by the familiar Starling equation:

$$\text{Net filtration} = L_p S \left[(P_{cap} - P_{if}) - \sigma(\pi_{cap} - \pi_{if}) \right]$$

where L_p is the unit permeability of the capillary wall; S is the surface area available for filtration; P_{cap} and P_{if} are the capillary and interstitial hydrostatic pressures, respectively; π_{cap} and π_{if} are the

---

Box 21.3   Etiology of edema

Increased capillary hydrostatic pressure

Increased plasma volume:

- Congestive heart failure
- Cor pulmonale
- Acute renal failure
- Chronic renal failure
- Hepatic cirrhosis (early)
- Nephrotic syndrome (some cases)[a]
- Pregnancy
- Drugs (e.g. nonsteroidal anti-inflammatory drugs, fludrocortisone, minoxidil, diazoxide, estrogens)

Venous obstruction:

- Deep venous thrombosis
- Local venous obstruction
- Hepatic cirrhosis (late)

Impaired cardiac performance:

- Congestive heart failure

Increased capillary permeability

Anaphylaxis and/or angioedema

Sepsis

Systemic inflammatory response syndrome (SIRS)

Burns

Adult respiratory distress syndrome

Drugs (e.g. interleukin-2)

Diabetes mellitus

Trauma

Impaired lymphatic drainage

Malignant lymphadenopathy

Hypothyroidism with myxedema

Lymphatic obstruction

Decreased capillary oncotic pressure

Nephrotic syndrome (some cases)[a]

Malnutrition

Liver disease

Protein-losing enteropathy

Severe hypoalbuminemia ($<$2.0 g/dl)

[a] The development of edema in the nephrotic syndrome is complex and depends upon the clinical situation. In some patients, profound hypoalbuminemia and decreased capillary oncotic pressure lead to the movement of water out of the vascular space into the interstitium, resulting in decreased effective arterial blood volume and avid renal sodium reabsorption. In other patients, poorly understood intrarenal mechanisms within the proteinuric kidney induce avid sodium reabsorption in the face of either a normal or even expanded effective arterial blood volume.

---

capillary and interstitial oncotic pressures, respectively; and σ is the reflection coefficient for proteins across the capillary wall (ranging from 1 for impermeable proteins to 0 for proteins which move freely back and forth across the capillary wall).[14] In the normal state, net filtration is a positive number, and net fluid movement within the capillary beds occurs from the intravascular space into the interstitium. This net movement of fluid into the interstitium from the vascular space is exactly balanced by lymphatic drainage from the interstitium, so that the volume of interstitial fluid remains constant and edema does not develop. An increase in interstitial volume, and edema, will develop only if the volume of fluid entering the interstitium exceeds the capacity of lymphatic drainage. Given this theoretical framework, we may identify four major abnormalities that favor the formation of edema.

Increased capillary hydrostatic pressure

P_{cap} is largely unaffected by changes in arterial pressure. Precapillary sphincters regulate the fraction of arteriolar pressure that is transmitted to the capillaries, so that P_{cap} remains fairly constant even in the face of severe hypertension or hypotension. Therefore, increased P_{cap} virtually always reflects backup from increased venous pressures, occurring as a result of either impaired cardiac performance (CHF), increased intravascular volume (chronic renal failure), or venous obstruction (deep venous thrombosis).[14]

Increased capillary permeability

An increase in L_p promotes the development of edema in two ways, both combining to overwhelm the capacity of lymphatic drainage. First, as a consequence of vascular injury, the capillary wall becomes more porous, permitting a greater flux of fluid out of the vascular space into the interstitium without any change in hydrostatic or oncotic pressures. Secondly, leakage of albumin into the interstitium dissipates the gradient in albumin concentration across the capillary wall and thereby decreases the oncotic pressure, retaining fluid within the vasculature. A large number of disease states lead to vascular injury and increased capillary permeability (see Box 21.3).[14]

Impaired lymphatic drainage

Even in the face of very large interstitial influxes of fluid, edema will not develop until the capacity for lymphatic drainage is exceeded. Thus, any abnormalities leading to impaired lymphatic drainage will predispose patients to edema formation. Such abnormalities may include true lymphatic obstruction (malignant lymphadenopathy) or alterations in the lymph fluid itself (hypothyroidism with myxedema). Recognition of impaired lymphatic drainage as a cause of peripheral edema is critical, since diuretic treatment will lead to loss of fluid from the vascular compartment, with minimal or no effect on interstitial fluid and edema.[14]

Decreased capillary oncotic pressure

Hypoalbuminemia, either as a result of decreased hepatic synthesis or increased urinary losses in the nephrotic syndrome, will lead to a decrease in π_{cap} and impaired retention of fluid in the intravascular space. Although widely touted as a major cause of edema, hypoalbuminemia alone, in the absence of any other concomitant disturbance, is a far less common cause of edema than previously thought. This is because the body has evolved a number of protective mechanisms to protect itself against peripheral edema. Additional factors, such as increased P_{cap} (from overly avid renal Na retention and volume overload) or increased capillary permeability or decreased lymphatic drainage, are generally also present and constitute the major contributing factors to the development of edema in hypoproteinemic states.[14] In general, peripheral edema should not be attributed solely to hypoalbuminemia unless the serum albumin concentration is severely depressed, at least below 2.0 g/dl. At albumin concentrations above this value, lymphatic drainage can usually compensate fully for the increased influx of fluid.[14]

Differences between the peripheral and pulmonary capillary beds

There are several important differences between the peripheral and pulmonary capillary beds that affect the accumulation of fluid within the pulmonary interstitium. First, in the presence of normal cardiac function, the pulmonary capillary hydrostatic pressure pushing fluid into the interstitium is much lower than that in the periphery. Second, and more importantly from a clinical viewpoint, the pulmonary capillary wall is significantly more permeable to proteins, leading to near equalization of protein concentrations between the vascular and interstitial spaces. Hence, there is essentially no oncotic pressure difference in the pulmonary circulation, leading to retention of fluid in the pulmonary vascular space. In terms of pulmonary interstitial fluid volumes, this has both a potentially harmful and an ultimately protective effect. On the negative side, lymphatic drainage must assume an even greater role in protecting the pulmonary interstitium from edema (although lower pulmonary P_{cap} helps to reduce fluid entry). On the positive side, however, the absence of a gradient in protein concentrations between the vascular and interstitial spaces means that the pulmonary interstitium is protected against the effects of hypoalbuminemia. Thus, in the absence of cardiac dysfunction and increased pulmonary P_{cap}, pulmonary edema is rarely, if ever, seen with hypoalbuminemia alone, even at levels associated with profound peripheral edema.[14]

DIURETIC AGENTS

Classification

The proper use of diuretics requires an understanding of the renal reabsorption of Na. Diuretics can be most easily classified according to the portion of the nephron at which they act (Table 21.1). Beginning at the glomerulus, there are four major sites targeted by diuretics:

- proximal tubule (acetazolamide)
- loop of Henle (furosemide, bumetanide, torsemide, ethacrynic acid)
- distal tubule and connecting segment (thiazides, chlorthalidone, metolazone, indipamide)
- cortical collecting duct (spironolactone, amiloride, triamterene).[3,15,16]

Table 21.1 Classification of diuretics according to site of action.

Diuretic class	Major nephron sites of action	Specific diuretics	Mechanism of action	Percentage of normal tubular Na$^+$ absorption at diuretic site of action	Fractional excretion of Na$^+$ at maximal diuretic efficacy
Carbonic anhydrase inhibitors	Proximal tubule	Acetazolamide	Inhibition of carbonic anhydrase leading to decreased cellular H$^+$ available for exchange with tubular Na$^+$ via Na$^+$/H$^+$ exchanger	55–65%	5%
Loop diuretics	Loop of Henle	Furosemide Bumetanide Torsemide Ethacrynic acid	Inhibition of Na$^+$–K$^+$–2Cl$^-$ cotransporter	25–35%	20–25%
Thiazide type	Distal tubule and connecting segment	Chlorothiazide Hydrochlorothiazide Metolazone Indipamide	Inhibition of Na$^+$–Cl$^-$ cotransporter	5–8%	3–5%
Potassium-sparing	Cortical collecting duct	Spironolactone Amiloride Triamterene	Competitive inhibition with aldosterone for aldosterone receptor (spironolactone); inhibition of Na$^+$ channels (amiloride and triamterene)	<5%	2%
Osmotic	Loop of Henle	Mannitol Urea	Increased medullary blood flow, leading to reduced medullary tonicity and reduced passive Na reabsorption in ascending limb of loop of Henle	25–35%	20–25%
B-type natriuretic peptide	Medullary collecting duct	Nesiritide	Multiple interrelated effects, including decreased Na reabsorption, increased glomerular filtration rate, and decreased activity of renin–angiotensin–aldosterone axis	≤5%[a]	~2–5%[b]

[a] This value refers only to that fraction of filtered Na that is normally reabsorbed by the collecting duct, the predominant tubular site of action for nesiritide. Nesiritide has additional hemodynamic and neurohumoral effects (e.g. increased glomerular filtration rate and decreased activity of the renin–angiotensin–aldosterone axis), which can significantly augment Na excretion above this value, especially in patients with congestive heart failure.

[b] These values are an approximation based on limited clinical data. The natriuretic effects of nesiritide seem to differ between healthy controls and patients with congestive heart failure, and individual patients may demonstrate a pronounced natriuresis in response to nesiritide, either alone or in combination with another diuretic.

Basic renal physiology

The crucial role of renal Na reabsorption in maintaining ECV may be appreciated through the following considerations. A normal adult male has a glomerular filtration rate (GFR) of approximately 160 L/day (111 ml/min). Given a serum Na concentration of 150 mEq/L, this means that he will filter 24 000 mEq of Na per day. Assuming a daily Na intake of 120 mEq (~2.75 g of Na), then he must excrete 120 mEq of Na per day in order to maintain an even Na balance. This represents just 0.5% of his daily filtered load. In other words, the kidney must reabsorb >99% of the Na that crosses the glomerulus and enters the lumen of the nephron. Hence, the normal fractional excretion of Na is ≤1%.

Proximal tubule
The bulk of filtered Na (60–65%) is reabsorbed in the proximal tubule through the action of an Na^+/H^+ exchanger located in the luminal brush border.[15] A number of factors, nearly all induced by a decrease in EABV, increase the fraction of filtered Na that is reabsorbed by the proximal tubule. These include angiotensin II and norepinephrine, which act directly through stimulation of the activity of the Na^+/H^+ exchanger as well as indirectly through alterations in peritubular capillary hemodynamics.[15]

Loop of Henle
An additional 25–30% of filtered Na is reabsorbed by the loop of Henle through the action of $Na^+–K^+–2Cl^-$ cotransporter.[15,17] Reabsorption by the loop of Henle is largely dependent on tubular flow, with reabsorption essentially paralleling delivery.[15] An additional factor modulating reabsorption in this segment is so-called 'pressure natriuresis', by which a small increase in arterial pressure leads to a relatively large increase in the excretion of Na and water.[18–20]

Distal tubule and connecting segment
Reabsorption in the distal tubule, like that in the loop of Henle, is mainly flow-dependent.[15,17] These two segments reabsorb about 5% of filtered Na through an $Na^+–Cl^-$ cotransporter.[15]

Cortical collecting duct
The remainder of the filtered Na (~4%) is reabsorbed in the cortical collecting duct through Na^+ channels.[15] Aldosterone and atrial natriuretic peptide increase Na reabsorption in this segment.[3,15]

Clinical pharmacology

The net diuretic, or natriuretic, effect of a diuretic correlates best with the diuretic's site of action along the nephron (see Table 21.1). Loop diuretics acting on the loop of Henle are by far the most potent, increasing the fractional excretion of Na by the kidney from ≤1% up to 25%.[17,21] The maximal natriuretic effect of the other three classes of diuretics is much smaller, in general <5%. Proximal and distal tubular diuretics can increase the fractional excretion of Na up to 5%, whereas cortical collecting duct diuretics can increase fractional Na excretion up to only 2%. Because of their superior potency, as well as their rapid onset of action, loop diuretics are the most commonly administered diuretics in the ICU setting. For this reason, they will be the focus of our discussion.

The potency of a diuretic depends on a large assortment of factors, including:

- the dose, route of administration, frequency of administration, and rate and mechanism of excretion of the diuretic
- the diuretic's site of action along the nephron
- compensatory Na reabsorption at nephron sites not affected by the diuretic
- neurohumoral and other regulatory factors affecting the overall reabsorption of Na, such as norepinephrine, aldosterone, atrial natriuretic factor, and the renin–angiotensin system
- the level of renal function
- co-existent disease states, such as congestive heart failure, cirrhosis, or nephrotic syndrome.

We will discuss several of these factors in greater depth.

Pharmacokinetic considerations

Dependence of the diuretic effect on secretion into the tubular lumen

General pharmacokinetic parameters for all of the commonly used diuretics are given in Table 21.2. It is critical to realize that virtually all diuretics must enter the tubular lumen in order to be effective.[15,21] This is because the transporters and channels inhibited by diuretics are located on the luminal membrane of the nephron, in contact with the tubular fluid and apart from the bloodstream. The sole exception is spironolactone, which competitively inhibits the binding of aldosterone to its receptor located on the blood side of the cortical

Table 21.2 Pharmacologic properties of diuretics.

Diuretic class	Agent	Dosage range	Relative potency[a]	Oral absorption	Half-life	Protein binding	Route of elimination	Side effects and toxicity	Clinical utility	Notes
Carbonic anhydrase inhibitors	Acetazolamide	500 mg iv every 12 h; 250 mg po every 6 h	1	~100%	6–9 h	70–90%	Renal (100%)	Metabolic acidosis; hypokalemia; hepatic encephalopathy in cirrhotic pts	Edematous states with metabolic alkalosis; sequential nephron blockade in diuretic resistance	Efficacy limited by metabolic acidosis and distal reabsorption of Na by loop of Henle and distal nephron; decreases GFR via activation of TGF
Loop diuretics	Furosemide	20–1200 mg/day	1	10–90%	0.3–3.4 h	>90%	Renal (60%) Metabolism (40%)	Metabolic alkalosis; hypokalemia; tinnitus, vertigo, or other ototoxicity; interstitial nephritis; hepatic encephalopathy in cirrhotic pts; hypocalcemia; hypomagnesemia	Diuretic of choice in the ICU setting; because of enhanced ototoxicity, ethacrynic acid should be reserved for pts allergic to furosemide	Ototoxicity most frequently seen with rapid rates of iv infusion; inhibition of TGF, so that, unlike carbonic anhydrase inhibitors, no decrease of GFR seen; venodilation independent of diuresis
	Bumetanide	1–10 mg/day	40	60–90%	0.3–1.5 h	>90%	Renal (65%) Metabolism (35%)			
	Torsemide	10–100 mg/day	3	80–90%	0.8–6.0 h	>90%	Renal (30%) Metabolism (70%)			
	Ethacrynic acid	50–200 mg/day	0.7	~100%	0.5–1.0 h	>90%	Renal (65%) Metabolism (35%)			
Thiazide type	Hydrochlorothiazide	25–100 mg po/day	1	65–75%	2.5 h	40%	Renal (100%)	Metabolic alkalosis; hypokalemia; hyponatremia; hypercalcemia; hypomagnesemia; hyperuricemia	Sequential nephron blockade in diuretic resistance	With exception of metolazone and indipamide, efficacy as solitary agent severely limited in patients whose GFR <30 ml/min; decreases GFR via activation of TGF
	Chlorothiazide	500–1000 mg iv every 12 h	0.1	10–20%	1.5 h	–	Renal (100%)			
	Metolazone	5–20 mg po/day	10	65%	4–5 h	90%	Renal (80%) Metabolism (10%) Biliary (10%)			
	Indipamide	1.25–5.0 mg po/day	20	~100%	10–22 h	70–80%	Metabolism (100%)			

Class	Drug	Dose	Relative potency[a]	Bioavailability	Half-life	Protein binding	Elimination	Adverse effects	Comments
Potassium sparing	Amiloride	5–20 mg/day	1	15–25%	21 h	<10%	Renal (100%)	Hyperkalemia; renal stones (triamterene); glucose intolerance (triamterene); photosensitization (triamterene)	Sequential nephron blockade in diuretic resistance; amelioration of hypokalemia in pts receiving loop or thiazide-type diuretics
	Triamterene	50–200 mg/day	0.1	30–70%	4 h	60–90%	Metabolism (100%)		
Aldosterone antagonist	Spironolactone	25–400 mg po/day	1	60–70%	1.6 h	~100%	Metabolism (100%)	Hyperkalemia; gynecomastia; hirsutism	Sequential nephron blockade in diuretic resistance; amelioration of hypokalemia in pts receiving loop or thiazide-type diuretics; Drug of choice in treatment of ascites; may decrease mortality in pts with congestive heart failure
Osmotic diuretics	Mannitol	50–200 g in 20% solution iv over 24 h 12.5–25 g iv push	1	~0%	0.25–1.7 h; increased to 6–36 h in renal failure	~0%	Renal (100%)	Congestive heart failure and/or pulmonary edema in pts with renal failure; increased plasma osmolality; hypo/hypernatremia; nephrotoxicity with very high doses	Cerebral edema; potential efficacy in treatment of rhabdomyolysis and myoglobinuric renal failure; Higher doses should be used with extreme caution; concomitant volume expansion should be avoided except in pts with rhabdomyolysis at risk for acute renal failure
B-type natriuretic peptide	Nesiritide	2 µg/kg bolus, followed by 0.01 µg/kg/min infusion up to 48–72 h	1	~0%	~0.3 h	~0%	Renal (5–10%) Metabolism (90–95%)	Hypotension; headache	Decompensated congestive heart failure; Should be used with caution in pts with significant aortic stenosis; may increase mortality and the risk of acute renal failure in pts with congestive heart failure

a Relative potencies are applicable only for comparison of agents within a diuretic class.

iv = intravenous; po = orally; pts = patients; ICU = intensive care unit; GFR = glomerular filtration rate; TGF = tubuloglomerular feedback.

collecting duct, and therefore acts while in the blood circulation.

Drugs can enter the tubular lumen through one of two routes: glomerular filtration or tubular secretion. Nearly all commonly used diuretics (the major exceptions being amiloride and osmotic diuretics, such as mannitol) are highly protein-bound, and therefore they are not filtered by the glomerulus. Thus, diuretics are dependent upon secretion for entry into the tubular lumen. Secretion of diuretics occurs in the proximal tubule through specific transporters for organic acids (acetazolamide, loop diuretics, distal diuretics) or ogranic bases (triamterene, amiloride) that directly transport the diuretic from the peritubular capillaries into the tubular lumen.[3,15,21] Thus, the efficacy of diuretics depends critically on the activity of these transporters, which enable diuretics to reach their ultimate site of action. Impaired entry into the lumen, as seen with renal insufficiency, is therefore a major cause of diuretic resistance.[3,21]

Duration of action

With the exception of torsemide, there is no truly long-acting loop diuretic. For example, the duration of action of furosemide is usually 4–6 hours. Because of their relatively short duration of action, loop diuretics must be administered frequently in order to maintain adequate natriuresis. Recognition of this fact is especially pertinent, since the wearing off of diuretic effect is invariably followed by a period of avid Na reabsorption.[3,15,21,22]

Route of administration

Diuretic agents in the ICU setting should be administered intravenously, thereby circumventing absorptive abnormalities frequently encountered in critical illness.[3,21] The sole exceptions are metolazone, indipamide, and spironolactone, which exist only in oral forms, and possibly torsemide and bumetanide, which have excellent oral bioavailability.[3,17,21]

Conversion from intravenous to oral therapy

When converting patients from intravenous to oral therapy, it is important to take into account the oral bioavailability of the diuretic, or that fraction of an oral dose that is absorbed into the blood from the intestine. In normal subjects, the oral bioavailability of furosemide is about 50%.[15] As critically ill patients often have additional abnormalities impairing absorption from the gastrointestinal tract, the oral dose of furosemide should be at least double that of an effective intravenous dose.[15,21]

Oral torsemide and bumetanide have excellent oral bioavailability and usually need no dosage adjustments when converting to oral therapy.[17,21]

Pharmacodynamic considerations

Once a diuretic agent has been secreted into the tubular lumen, its effectiveness is dose-dependent and determined by the degree to which the diuretic binds to and inhibits its target transporter or channel.[3,21] Resistance may arise either because of pharmacokinetic factors, such as decreased renal blood flow or diminished secretion from the blood into the tubular lumen, or because of pharmacodynamic factors, implying a decreased natriuretic effect for a given degree of binding of the diuretic.[3,17] These possibilities may be depicted by a classic pharmacodynamic dose–response curve, in which Na excretion is plotted as a function of diuretic delivery, or, equivalently, urinary excretion of the diuretic (Fig. 21.2).[3,21]

By graphing Na excretion as a function of diuretic excretion, rather than the administered intravenous or oral dose, we can eliminate all pharmacokinetic factors affecting delivery of the diuretic into the tubular lumen, and can therefore consider independently the consequences of the interaction of diuretic with its target. The minimal effective dose of a diuretic is the lowest rate of diuretic excretion that leads to a clinically detectable augmentation of Na excretion. As higher doses of the diuretic are administered, and hence the diuretic excretion rate increases, a greater natriuresis will occur, until finally all binding sites for the diuretic are saturated. Past this point, increasing the dose of diuretic will not produce a further increase in natriuresis. This relationship usually follows a sigmoidal shape.[3,21]

Analysis of such a curve allows one to distinguish the mechanism for diuretic resistance, and impaired natriuretic response.[3] If the problem is solely one of impaired delivery into the tubular lumen, then this curve will be largely unchanged. However, if the problem is one of true renal resistance, as may occur in disease states such as CHF, cirrhosis, or nephrotic syndrome, then the curve will be shifted to the right, so that, even at comparable rates of delivery of the diuretic to its site of action (and presumably comparable degrees of binding of the diuretic to its target transporter or channel), Na excretion will still be diminished.[3,21] The mechanisms for such resistance will be discussed below in reference to specific disease states.

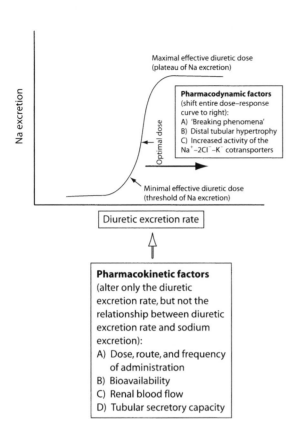

Na excretion

Maximal effective diuretic dose
(plateau of Na excretion)

Pharmacodynamic factors
(shift entire dose–response
curve to right):
A) 'Breaking phenomena'
B) Distal tubular hypertrophy
C) Increased activity of the
Na⁺–2Cl⁻–K⁻ cotransporters

Optimal dose

Minimal effective diuretic dose
(threshold of Na excretion)

Diuretic excretion rate

Pharmacokinetic factors
(alter only the diuretic
excretion rate, but not the
relationship between diuretic
excretion rate and sodium
excretion):
A) Dose, route, and frequency
   of administration
B) Bioavailability
C) Renal blood flow
D) Tubular secretory capacity

Figure 21.2 Pharmacodynamic and pharmacokinetic determinants of diuretic responsiveness. Diuretic efficacy is best represented by a dose–response curve, in which sodium (Na) excretion is plotted as a function of diuretic delivery to its tubular site of action, or, equivalently, urinary excretion of the diuretic. Such a curve has a classic sigmoidal shape. The minimal effective diuretic dose corresponds to the lowest rate of diuretic excretion that yields a clinically detectable increase of Na excretion. The maximal effective diuretic dose corresponds to that rate of diuretic excretion above which no further increase of Na excretion occurs. The optimal dose of a diuretic lies between these two extremes and yields a rate of Na excretion in the mid-range, or steepest, portion of the dose–response curve. Pharmacokinetic factors (white arrow) interfere solely with the ability of the diuretic to get to its site of action, whereas pharmacodynamic factors (black arrows) reflect true resistance of the target cell or transporter to the diuretic effect. In terms of the dose–response curve, pharmacokinetic factors alter only the rate of diuretic excretion, but do not in any way change the shape or location of the sigmoidal curve. Equivalent rates of diuretic delivery yield equivalent rates of Na excretion. In contrast, pharmacodynamic factors usually shift the curve to the right and downward, resulting in a diminished rate of Na excretion despite an equivalent rate of diuretic delivery.

Important non-natriuretic effects of loop diuretics

Within minutes of an intravenous dose, loop diuretics induce venodilation, thereby reducing left ventricular preload, central venous pressure, pulmonary artery pressure, and pulmonary artery wedge pressure.[23,24] The mechanism for these hemodynamic effects is not completely understood, but may be related to the release of vasodilatory mediators, such as prostaglandins and nitric oxide.[25,26] Intrarenal release of these vasodilatory mediators may explain the increased renal blood flow seen following administration of loop diuretics.[25,26]

An additional important effect of loop diuretics is inhibition of tubuloglomerular feedback. Normally, an increase of tubular flow past the macula densa (located just before the distal nephron) stimulates a reflexive decrease in GFR. A major function of tubuloglomerular feedback is to prevent excessive losses of Na and water. However, since the cells of the macula densa sense tubular flow via the same Na⁺–K⁺–2Cl⁻ cotransporter that is inhibited by loop diuretics, tubuloglomerular feedback

cannot occur, and loop diuretic-induced diuresis is not associated with a decrease in GFR.[22] As a result, loop diuretics may continue to induce a significant diuresis, even in the face of severe reductions in EABV.

DIURETIC RESISTANCE

A common scenario in the critically ill patient receiving diuretic therapy is a blunted natriuretic response despite escalating doses of the diuretic. Diuretic resistance within the ICU setting may be defined as a failure to elicit a fractional Na excretion of at least 20–25% following an intravenous dose of 200 mg of furosemide (or the equivalent dose of another loop diuretic). Alternatively, diuretic resistance may be defined as a failure to resolve peripheral edema, ascites, or pulmonary edema despite diuretic therapy and restriction of fluids and Na to less than 1.5 L and 100 mEq/day, respectively.[3,17,21]

In evaluating patients with diuretic resistance, it is crucial to understand the normal hemodynamic and intrarenal compensatory responses that act to restore Na balance following diuretic administration. On the one hand, many of these compensatory factors contribute to the development of diuretic resistance, and knowledge of their mechanism of action allows one to develop strategies for circumvention;[3,27] on the other hand, and perhaps more importantly, a lack of appreciation may lead to improper usage of diuretics and seeming resistance in a normally responsive patient.[3]

Normal compensatory sodium reabsorption in the post-diuretic period

A period of avid Na reabsorption supervenes as soon as tubular diuretic concentrations decline to the point that the natriuretic effects of the diuretic begin to diminish.[15,17] Therefore, unless fluid and Na intake are adequately restricted in the post-diuretic period, net natriuresis may not occur.[3,15,17,21] Indeed, in the absence of proper restriction of Na and fluid intake, diuretic therapy may even worsen volume overload, leading to an erroneous diagnosis of diuretic resistance.[3] Although this problem can be overcome by giving higher and more frequent doses of diuretics, a mainstay of diuretic therapy should be concomitant restriction of Na and volume.

We recommend limiting Na intake to about 100 mEq/day (2.3 g of Na) and fluid intake to about 1.0–1.5 L. Post-diuretic Na reabsorption is of particular importance to the ICU patient, as loop diuretics such as furosemide typically have a short half-life. If effective natriuresis is to be maintained, short-acting diuretics such as furosemide and bumetanide should probably be administered at a minimum of every 8–12 hours.

The mechanisms responsible for post-diuretic avid Na reabsorption are multifactorial (Table 21.3). They may be conveniently divided into short-term factors, which act immediately after urinary elimination of the diuretic, and long-term factors, which require several days before they come into play. In general, short-term factors reflect hemodynamic changes and neurohumoral responses to changes in EABV, whereas long-term factors are the result of intrarenal changes in the number and activity of the Na transporters and channels along the nephron.

Short-term factors
Short-term tolerance to the effect of diuretics is commonly known as the 'braking phenomenon'

and manifests as a gradual decrease in the natriuretic response upon repeated administration of equal doses of the same diuretic.[3,15,17,21] This short-term tolerance occurs in response to decreases in EABV, and is mediated by a wide assortment of interrelated factors, including baroreceptor- and volume-dependent increases in the activity of the renin–angiotensin–aldosterone axis, increased sympathetic outflow, enhanced release of antidiuretic hormone, decreased release of atrial natriuretic peptide, and changes in peritubular hemodynamics leading to enhanced proximal tubular Na reabsorption.[3,17,21,27] These changes in the hemodynamic and neurohumoral milieu can lead to avid Na and water reabsorption at all nephron segments.[3,15] Depending on the degree of decreased EABV, the natriuretic response may fall by as much as 40%.[3,15,17,27]

Long-term factors
Upon chronic administration of loop diuretics, the ongoing intense natriuresis will induce hypertrophy of cells in the distal tubule and connecting segment (sites of action of thiazide diuretics), with concomitant increases in Na reabsorptive capacities.[3,15,27] In addition, the target of the loop diuretics, the $Na^+–K^+–2Cl^-$ cotransporter, may increase in activity and further oppose the effects of loop diuretics.[15] These compensatory tubular effects are a harbinger of diuretic resistance. As discussed below, the development of distal tubular hypertrophy supports the logic of sequential blockade of nephron segments, using a combination of loop and distal tubule diuretics.[3]

Disease-related factors that may blunt the response to diuretics

From a simplistic viewpoint, many of the compensatory factors leading to compensatory Na reabsorption in the post-diuretic period, including both short-term and long-term factors, are also responsible for the development of diuretic resistance. However, disease-related factors may also play an important role in diminishing the natriuretic response to a given dose of a diuretic. Such factors may contribute to diuretic resistance through an independent pharmacokinetic or pharmacodynamic mechanism, or they may augment and exacerbate the normal physiologic adaptations of the post-diuretic period (see Table 21.3).

Table 21.3 Factors contributing to diuretic resistance and potential therapeutic interventions.

Factor	Contributory factors	Therapeutic interventions
Pharmacokinetic factors	1. Inadequate restriction of Na intake 2. Inadequate restriction of fluid intake 3. Dosing interval exceeds metabolic half-life	1. Na restriction to 100 mEq (2.3 g)/day 2. Fluid restriction to 1.0–1.5 L/day 3. More frequent dosing of diuretic
Short-term physiologic factors leading to enhanced post-diuretic renal Na avidity	1. Decreased effective arterial blood volume 2. Increased activity of renin–angiotensin–aldosterone axis 3. Decreased release of atrial natriuretic peptide 4. Enhanced release of antidiuretic hormone 5. Increased sympathetic activity 6. Alterations in peritubular hemodynamics	1. Increased magnitude of diuretic dose 2. Increased frequency of diuretic dosing 3. Continuous intravenous infusion of loop diuretic; consider nesiritide in patients with CHF 4. Sequential nephron blockade
Long-term adaptations leading to enhanced post-diuretic renal Na avidity	1. Hypertrophy of distal tubular and connecting segment cells (target of thiazide diuretics) 2. Increased activity of the Na^+–K^+–$2Cl^-$ cotransporter in loop of Henle	1. Increased magnitude of diuretic dose 2. Increased frequency of diuretic dosing 3. Continuous intravenous infusion of loop diuretic 4. Sequential nephron blockade
Disease-related factors	1. Delayed or decreased intestinal absorption 2. Hypoalbuminemia 3. Proteinuria 4. Decreased delivery of Na to loop of Henle 5. Decreased renal blood flow 6. Accumulation of organic anions in renal failure	1. Increased magnitude of diuretic dose 2. Increased frequency of diuretic dosing 3. Continuous intravenous infusion of loop diuretic 4. Sequential nephron blockade 5. Administration of albumin 6. Administration of albumin–furosemide admixture

CHF = congestive heart failure.

Decreased or delayed intestinal absorption

In many volume-overloaded patients, decreased or delayed intestinal absorption leads to a decreased rate of delivery of the diuretic to proximal tubular secretory sites. This in turn leads to lower intratubular concentrations of the diuretic and, consequently, decreased binding to target transporters and channels. It is important to emphasize that delayed absorption, even in the absence of any change in total absorption, will still lower intratubular concentrations of diuretic (albeit spread out over a longer time), and thereby diminish diuretic efficacy. Decreased intestinal perfusion, alterations in intestinal motility, and bowel wall edema may all play a role in this phenomenon. Such patients will demonstrate typical pharmacokinetic alterations in response to an oral diuretic, including reduced peak concentration and prolonged time to peak concentration of diuretic.[17] As an example of the potential magnitude of this effect, the oral equivalent of a single intravenous dose of 40 mg of furosemide would be about 80 mg in a normal subject and as high as 240 mg in a patient with severe peripheral or pulmonary edema.

Hypoalbuminemia

As previously discussed, nearly all of the commonly used diuretics (with the exception of amiloride and osmotic diuretics) are highly protein-bound. This high degree of protein binding ensures that nearly all the diuretic remains within the vascular space, and therefore that renal delivery of the diuretic is maximized. In patients whose serum albumin is below 2.0 g/dl, however, the fraction of unbound diuretic is increased. Unbound diuretic can diffuse out of the vascular space into the interstitium, thereby decreasing the amount of diuretic that reaches tubular secretory sites.[21,28]

Proteinuria

Under normal circumstances, tubular fluid contains essentially no protein, so that virtually all of the diuretic secreted into the tubular lumen exists in an unbound state and is therefore able to bind to its site of action. Large amounts of intratubular protein, as seen in the nephrotic syndrome, may bind diuretic and prevent the binding of diuretic to its target.[29,30] For example, up to 65% of a loop diuretic may be bound to intratubular protein, resulting in a blunted natriuretic response.[3,15,29]

Decreased delivery of Na to loop of Henle

In some patients with profoundly decreased EABV, as from severe CHF or cirrhosis, the delivery of Na to the loop of Henle is markedly reduced, thereby limiting the natriuretic response to loop diuretics. Decreased delivery is a combined result of decreased renal perfusion, decreased GFR, and enhanced proximal tubular reabsorption of Na. The inhibitory effects of decreased EABV on diuretic efficacy are not restricted to loop diuretics. A decrease in EABV leads to the release of multiple vasoactive mediators (such as norepinephrine, angiotensin II, and aldosterone), the combined effect of which is to enhance Na reabsorption at all nephron segments and reduce the effectiveness of all classes of diuretics.[3,15,27] In patients with profoundly decreased EABV, the addition of a proximal diuretic, such as acetazolamide, may enhance diuresis by increasing delivery of Na to the loop of Henle.[3]

Renal failure

Higher doses of loop diuretics are necessary in patients with acute and chronic renal failure.[17,22]

There are several reasons for the blunted natriuretic response to loop diuretics in patients with a depressed GFR. These include decreased renal blood flow, leading to decreased delivery of diuretics to the secretory pumps in the proximal tubule, plus the accumulation of organic anions such as hippurate that compete with diuretics for entry into the tubular lumen via the secretory pumps.[14,17,21,31]

APPROACH TO DIURETIC RESISTANCE

General strategies

Overcoming diuretic resistance requires a thorough understanding of not only the normal compensatory responses that act to restore Na balance following diuretic administration but also the specific pathophysiologic factors that tend to blunt the renal response to diuretics. We outline here several general strategies that may be adopted to combat diuretic resistance (see Table 21.3).

Sodium and fluid restriction

Failure to restrict the intake of sodium and water can prevent the net loss of fluid, even in the face of an adequate response to diuretics. This simple modality is a frequently neglected aspect in management. We recommend limiting Na intake to about 100 mEq/day (2.3 g of Na) and fluid intake to about 1.0–1.5 L.

Intravenous administration of diuretics

Given the high prevalence of absorptive abnormalities among ICU patients, diuretics should be administered intravenously. The sole exceptions are metolazone, indipamide, and spironolactone, which exist only in oral forms, and possibly torsemide and bumetanide, which have excellent oral bioavailability.

Increased magnitude of dosing

To be effective, diuretics must reach their site of action within the tubular lumen of the kidney. As previously discussed, a number of pharmacokinetic factors may limit delivery of the diuretic to the kidney or reduce proximal secretion of the diuretic into the lumen. Even if the diuretic reaches its target, pharmacodynamic factors (e.g. enhanced distal reabsorption) may reduce the degree of natriuresis for a given level of urinary excretion of the diuretic. As a result, the magnitude of single intravenous boluses of the diuretic may be increased. The benefit of increasing the dose of a single bolus injection above 200 mg for furosemide, or the equivalent dose for other loop diuretics, is marginal, whereas boluses above this amount carry an increased risk for toxicity.

Increased frequency of dosing

A period of avid Na reabsorption ensues once tubular diuretic concentrations decline below a minimal effective concentration. Unless diuretics are administered at an appropriate frequency, post-diuretic Na reabsorption can pose a major obstacle to effective diuresis. This is an especial problem in the case of loop diuretics, such as furosemide, which typically have a short half-life. As a general rule, the interval between successive boluses of an effective diuretic dose should be equal to 1 or 2 half-lives. Alternatively, one may change to a continuous intravenous infusion of the diuretic. In this case, the maximal daily dose should be 2400 mg for furosemide, or the equivalent dose for other loop diuretics.[3,17,21] Beyond this dose, the risk of toxicity outweighs any potential small additional benefit.

Sequential nephron blockade

With chronic administration of loop diuretics, cells in the distal tubule and connecting segment (sites of action of thiazide diuretics) undergo hypertrophy and increase their capacity to reabsorb Na. Enhanced reabsorption of Na distal to the site of action of loop diuretics can offset their efficacy and lead to diuretic resistance. The combined use of a loop and a distal diuretic is an effective means to overcome this problem. Although metolazone has been touted as superior to thiazides, there is little evidence to suggest differences among the distal tubular diuretics, as long as equivalent doses are used. Although the addition of a third diuretic acting at the cortical collecting duct (such as spironolactone, amiloride, or triamterene) leads to only a minor increment in Na excretion, it may help to limit urinary losses of potassium and prevent hypokalemia.

Sequential nephron blockade may also include the proximal tubule. Under normal circumstances the proximal tubule reabsorbs 60–65% of filtered Na. With decreases in EABV, the percentage of filtered Na that is reabsorbed by the proximal tubule can increase to as high as 75–80%. Such enhanced proximal reabsorption of Na, as may occur in patients with severe cirrhosis or CHF, may markedly reduce delivery of Na to the loop of Henle. The addition of a proximal diuretic, such as acetazolamide, may enhance the diuretic response by increasing Na delivery to the loop of Henle.[3]

Administration of albumin or an admixture of albumin plus furosemide

The rationale and efficacy of these strategies in patients with hypoalbuminemia are discussed below in the sections on nephrotic syndrome and cirrhosis.

Specific disease states

We review here several disease states that are commonly associated with diuretic resistance (Table 21.4). We discuss the pathophysiologic reasons underlying resistance as well as any special considerations that pertain to the proper use of diuretics in these conditions.

Congestive heart failure

Decreased EABV among patients with CHF activates all the short-term and long-term compensatory changes discussed above. The net result is enhanced Na reabsorption along all segments of the nephron. Unreliable intestinal absorption necessitates intravenous administration. Short-term diuretic resistance may be overcome by increasing the diuretic dose or switching to a continuous intravenous infusion. Long-term diuretic resistance, as a result of enhanced distal reabsorption of Na, may require sequential nephron blockade, through combined use of loop and distal diuretics.[3]

The acute venodilation seen with loop diuretics would seem to make them ideal agents for patients with CHF. However, in some patients with CHF and severely decreased EABV, the administration of a loop diuretic may induce arteriolar vasoconstriction, with an increase in systemic blood pressure and a decrease in cardiac output.[32] This effect, which can last up to 1 hour after administration, can actually lead to an increase of pulmonary capillary wedge pressure.[32]

Acute and chronic renal failure

Patients with renal failure typically require high doses of diuretics. Decreased renal blood flow limits delivery of diuretics to proximal secretory sites, and the accumulation of organic anions such as hippurate further limits secretion of diuretics into the tubular lumen via competition for the secretory pumps. As a result, single intravenous doses of furosemide as high as 200 mg may be

Table 21.4   Approach to diuretic resistance in particular disease states.

Disease state	Mechanisms of diuretic resistance	Therapeutic interventions
Renal failure	1. Decreased renal blood flow, leading to decreased delivery of diuretics to secretory pumps in proximal tubule 2. Accumulation of organic anions that compete with diuretics for secretory pumps in proximal tubule	1. Increase magnitude of diuretic dose until effective dose achieved 2. Increase frequency of diuretic administration or continuous intravenous infusion of diuretic 3. Sequential nephron blockade
Congestive heart failure	1. Decreased effective arterial blood volume 2. Increased activity of renin–angiotensin–aldosterone axis 3. Decreased release of atrial natriuretic peptide 4. Enhanced release of antidiuretic hormone 5. Increased sympathetic activity 6. Alterations in peritubular hemodynamics 7. Distal tubular hypertrophy 8. Concomitant renal insufficiency 9. Rebound Na reabsorption between diuretic doses	1. Increase magnitude of diuretic dose until effective dose achieved 2. Increase frequency of diuretic administration or continuous intravenous infusion of diuretic 3. Sequential nephron blockade 4. Trial of nesiritide (B-type natriuretic peptide) 5. Maximize cardiac function with inotropic agents 6. Maximize cardiac function with afterload reduction (e.g. angiotensin-converting enzyme inhibitors or angiotensin receptor blockers) 7. Loop diuretic holiday, with initiation of acetazolamide/spironolactone
Nephrotic syndrome	1. Hypoalbuminemia, leading to diffusion of diuretic outside vascular space and decreased delivery to secretory pumps in proximal tubule 2. Proteinuria, leading to binding of diuretic to filtered albumin, thereby limiting the availability of free drug to interact with its receptor on the luminal brush border	1. Increase magnitude of diuretic dose (usually 2–3 times normal starting dose) 2. Increase frequency of diuretic administration or continuous intravenous infusion of diuretic 3. Sequential nephron blockade 4. Administration of albumin 5. Administration of albumin–furosemide admixture
Ascites	1. Decreased effective arterial blood volume 2. Increased activity of renin–angiotensin–aldosterone axis 3. Decreased release of atrial natriuretic peptide 4. Enhanced release of antidiuretic hormone 5. Increased sympathetic activity 6. Alterations in peritubular hemodynamics 7. Hypoalbuminemia 8. Distal tubular hypertrophy 9. Concomitant renal insufficiency 10. Renal vasoconstriction	1. Add spironolactone at doses up to 400 mg/day as tolerated 2. Increase magnitude of dose of loop diuretic until effective dose achieved 3. Increase frequency of administration of loop diuretic or continuous intravenous infusion of loop diuretic 4. Sequential nephron blockade 5. Administration of albumin 6. Administration of albumin–furosemide admixture 7. Consider large volume paracentesis 8. Consider transjugular intrahepatic portosystemic shunt 9. Consider trial of splanchnic vasoconstrictors

required.[15,17,21,31] However, there is very little benefit to increasing the dose of a single bolus injection above 200 mg for furosemide, or the equivalent dose for other loop diuretics.[15] If boluses of loop diuretics are ineffective, one may attempt a continuous infusion of a loop diuretic or add another diuretic that acts at a different portion of the nephron.[3,21] Although some studies have advocated daily doses of furosemide as high as 2400 mg, it should be stressed that such high doses are associated with an enhanced risk of electrolyte disturbances, myalgias, and ototoxicity, with possible permanent deafness.[15,22,33] To minimize the risk of serious toxicity, large boluses of loop diuretics should be infused slowly over 30 minutes.[21]

Among the loop diuretics, ethacrynic acid has the highest risk for ototoxicity. Use of ethacrynic acid should be limited to patients with an allergy to one of the other diuretics, since it is the only loop or distal diuretic that is not derived from a sulfonamide. The extrarenal clearance of bumetamide increases with renal failure, so that, in comparison to furosemide, an equivalent dose of bumetamide must be increased from one-40th that of furosemide in patients with normal renal function to one-20th that of furosemide in patients with advanced renal insufficiency. Finally, with the exception of metolazone and indipamide, thiazide diuretics are generally not effective in patients whose GFR is less than 30 ml/min, unless they are administered with a loop diuretic.[3,15,21]

Nephrotic syndrome

The development of edema in the nephrotic syndrome is complex and depends upon the clinical situation. In some patients, profound hypoalbuminemia and decreased oncotic pressure lead to the movement of water out of the vascular space into the interstitium, resulting in decreased EABV and avid renal sodium reabsorption.[21,28] In other patients, poorly understood intrarenal mechanisms within the proteinuric kidney induce avid sodium reabsorption in the face of either a normal or even expanded EABV.[34] Thus, in this latter group of patients, primary renal sodium retention contributes to edema formation.

Nephrotic patients with severe edema and hypoalbuminemia demonstrate a blunted response to loop diuretics, often requiring two to three times the effective dose for normal individuals.[3] The basis of diuretic resistance is probably multifactorial. First, as in other edematous states, oral bioavailability may be reduced because of bowel wall edema and impaired absorption, necessitating intravenous infusion. Second, in the presence of hypoalbuminemia, furosemide will be incompletely bound to albumin, and therefore diffuse out of the vascular space, resulting in decreased delivery of furosemide to the kidney.[28] Third, even that fraction of furosemide which makes it into the urinary space may be limited in efficacy, as tubular furosemide may bind to filtered albumin, thereby limiting the availability of free drug to interact with its receptor on the luminal brush border.[35] Finally, short- and long-term compensatory changes discussed above, including distal hypertrophy and intrinsic changes to the target of loop diuretics, the $Na^+–K^+–2Cl^-$ cotransporter, may further diminish the diuretic response to furosemide. Although the preceding discussion focused on the loop diuretic furosemide, similar principles apply to all other loop diuretics as well as to the distal tubular and cortical collecting duct diuretics.

A recent study casts doubt on the contribution of urinary protein binding of loop diuretics to diuretic resistance in nephrotic syndrome.[36] In this study, coadministration of sulfisoxazole with furosemide to displace furosemide from binding to urinary albumin failed to enhance the diuretic effect of furosemide. Moreover, despite an observed increase in the volume of distribution of furosemide, there was no reduction in the rate of diuretic excretion, thereby questioning the role of hypoalbuminemia in decreasing delivery of furosemide to the kidney. These results suggest that a primary increase in sodium avidity attributable to the nephrotic syndrome per se and/or normal renal compensatory mechanisms to diuretic use may be more important mechanisms of diuretic resistance in nephrotic patients.

Dosing recommendations for diuretics in nephrotic syndrome are empirically derived and will vary according to the degree of diuretic resistance. As for CHF, short-term diuretic resistance may be overcome by increasing the diuretic dose or switching to a continuous intravenous infusion. Long-term diuretic resistance may require sequential nephron blockade, through combined use of loop and distal diuretics.[3]

Some authors advocate intravenous coadministration of furosemide and albumin for patients with severe refractory edema. The use of such a regimen presumes that pharmacokinetic factors contribute importantly to diuretic resistance. In the most successful study, an equimolar infusion of salt-poor albumin (40 mg of furosemide premixed with 6 g of salt-poor albumin) improved renal delivery of furosemide, as assessed by urinary recovery of the drug, and led to an enhanced diuretic response.[28] More recent studies have yielded less encouraging results. Fliser et al infused 60 mg of furosemide plus 200 ml of 20% human albumin to a group of nephrotic patients.[37] The rate of urinary furosemide excretion was unchanged, suggesting that the observed modest increase in sodium excretion and urine volume was secondary to alterations in renal hemodynamics. Other workers failed to find any potentiation of furosemide by intravenous albumin.[38–40] Some of this lack of effect may be due to the fact that the albumin and furosemide were not admixed prior to infusion or that furosemide was administered at submaximal doses. In addition, in some studies, the diuretic response to furosemide alone was substantial, suggesting that the patients studied may not truly have been diuretic-resistant. Based on current evidence, we recommend that the combination of furosemide and albumin should be reserved for patients with refractory edema. When used in combination, the drugs should be admixed before intravenous administration.

Cirrhosis and ascites

In patients with cirrhosis, arterial vasodilation, particularly of the splanchnic circulation, contributes to a decrease in EABV and leads to avid Na reabsorption along all segments of the nephron.[41] In combination with portal hypertension, enhanced Na reabsorption eventually leads to the formation of both edema and ascites.[41–42] Patients with cirrhosis may demonstrate severe resistance to loop diuretic agents, especially those patients whose spot urinary Na concentration is less than 10 mEq/L.[15,21,43] Indeed, among cirrhotic patients, the maximum natriuresis observed in response to equivalent rates of urinary excretion of the diuretic (implying equivalent rates of delivery to the target transporter) was decreased by as much as 90% in comparison to normal subjects.[15,21,44]

Diuretic resistance in patients with cirrhosis is multifactorial and remains a matter of debate.[15,21,44] Possible mechanisms include the following: systemic hypotension, and hypoperfusion of the kidney; intense renal vasoconstriction; severe hypoalbuminemia; and the accumulation of bile salts or other unknown substances that compete with diuretics for entry into the tubular lumen via the secretory pumps.[15,44,45] Interestingly, spironolactone, the sole diuretic which acts while still in the blood circulation, and therefore does not depend on proximal secretion to reach its site of action, is very effective in the initial management of ascites, and is considered by many to be the drug of choice in this setting.[21,44]

Effective management of ascites includes optimization of central hemodynamics, perhaps guided by insertion of a pulmonary artery catheter, taking care to avoid excessive volume expansion which might precipitate variceal bleeding. Loop diuretics should be administered at higher doses and with increased frequency, or by continuous intravenous infusion.[21,44] Sequential nephron blockade may improve the diuretic response. Proximal diuretics may augment Na delivery to the loop of Henle, whereas distal diuretics may offset enhanced Na reabsorption at sites after the loop of Henle. The combination of furosemide and metolazone has produced adequate results, although high doses of metolazone (100 mg) had to be used.[3] For patients with hypoalbuminemia, especially those whose serum albumin is less than 2.0 g/dl, administration of salt-poor albumin may improve the diuretic response.[45] Although the effectiveness of an admixture of albumin and furosemide has been best studied in nephrotic patients, it seems likely that these results may be extended to hypoalbuminemic patients with ascites.[37–40] An alternative treatment for patients with refractory ascites and diuretic resistance is transjugular intrahepatic portosystemic shunting.[46,47]

Cardiogenic pulmonary edema

The goal in managing patients with cardiac causes of pulmonary edema is to reduce pulmonary capillary hydrostatic pressure. Pulmonary edema is the result of elevations in pulmonary vascular hydrostatic pressure, reflective of increased left ventricular end-diastolic pressure. From a clinical standpoint, the pulmonary artery wedge pressure (PAWP) may be used as an estimate of pulmonary capillary hydrostatic pressures. Cardiogenic pulmonary edema usually develops when the PAWP exceeds 18 mmHg, but may develop at lower values in patients with accompanying pulmonary hypertension or, perhaps, severe hypoalbuminemia.[48,49] It is important to emphasize that, because of the previously discussed differences between the pulmonary and systemic vasculature, pulmonary edema is rarely, if ever, seen with hypoalbuminemia alone, in the absence of cardiac dysfunction, even at levels of hypoalbuminemia associated with profound peripheral edema.

Treatment of cardiogenic pulmonary edema entails the use of effective doses of loop diuretics and methods to decrease left ventricular diastolic pressure, such as morphine sulfate, nitrates, nesiritide, and/or inotropes. Diuretics may improve cardiac performance if diuresis leads to a decrease in left ventricular end-diastolic pressure that is of sufficient magnitude to decrease afterload.[50] The previously discussed non-natriuretic effects of the loop diuretics, including venodilation and occasional transient arteriolar vasoconstriction, are important to bear in mind. A particularly challenging scenario is the development of pulmonary edema in association with diastolic dysfunction, as aggressive diuretic therapy in these patients usually leads to progressive and sometimes severe azotemia.

Noncardiogenic pulmonary edema

In patients with acute respiratory distress syndrome (ARDS), increased permeability of the alveolar capillary membrane leads to the development of pulmonary edema, even in the face of a normal pulmonary capillary hydrostatic pressure.[51] This phenomenon, referred to as noncardiogenic pulmonary edema, may be exacerbated by decreases in serum protein.[52] Studies suggest that positive fluid balance in the setting of ARDS may have an adverse effect on outcome.[51] For example, maintaining the PAWP below 18 mmHg, via fluid restriction and diuretic therapy, as guided by a pulmonary artery catheter,[53] or maintaining extravascular lung water below 7 ml/kg of ideal body weight, as assessed through bedside indicator-dilution measurements,[54] each resulted in fewer days of mechanical ventilation and a shorter stay in the ICU. Similarly, in patients whose serum total protein was less than 5 g/dl, the combination of furosemide-induced diuresis and intravenous administration of serum albumin led to improved oxygenation, improved hemodynamics, and a shorter stay in the ICU.[51] We recommend that management of patients be guided by a pulmonary artery catheter in order to maintain the PAWP as low as possible without causing significant decreases in stroke volume or cardiac output. Diuresis may be effected through the prudent administration of diuretics and possibly albumin.

DIURETICS IN THE PROPHYLAXIS AND MANAGEMENT OF ACUTE RENAL FAILURE

Acute tubular necrosis (ATN) and prerenal azotemia are the most common causes of acute renal failure (ARF) in the ICU setting. In the majority of cases, prerenal azotemia is the result of a decrease in EABV, which, if not rapidly corrected, can lead to ATN.[7] ATN has a multitude of potential causes, but in cases of decreased EABV ultimately reflects an imbalance between oxygen supply and demand. The most common etiologic factors in the ICU setting are renal hypoperfusion from systemic hypotension, nephrotoxic exposure, or the effects of cytokines and other paracrine factors released as a result of sepsis or SIRS on renal autoregulation and blood flow.[55,56]

From a theoretical standpoint, loop diuretics such as furosemide may attenuate or prevent the development of ARF by inducing a decrease in medullary oxygen consumption (via inhibition of energy-requiring transporters) and/or increasing tubular flow (see Table 21.4).[1,2,22,57] Loop diuretics may also be useful in converting oliguric ATN to its nonoliguric states, thereby facilitating fluid management.[2] Nevertheless, despite this strong theoretical basis, and even experimental evidence in animals that loop diuretics may attenuate or prevent ARF, clinical evidence for the efficacy of loop diuretics in humans is thoroughly lacking. The use of loop diuretics had no effect on the incidence of ATN, need for dialysis, or mortality;[33,58-60] e.g. administration of furosemide prior to intravenous contrast failed to prevent the development of contrast nephropathy.[61]

Despite extensive use of the osmotic diuretic mannitol in the prophylactic treatment of myoglobinuric ARF, there has been a paucity of adequately powered clinical trials and supportive data.[62] In lieu of more definitive studies, the judicious use of mannitol in the treatment of rhabdomyolysis would seem to be warranted.[62] A more comprehensive discussion of prophylactic treatment in rhabdomyolysis can be found in Chapter 4.

It is worth noting that diuretics may actually be detrimental in the setting of oliguric ARF.[63] Vasodilation induced by loop diuretics may result in shunting of blood away from the renal medulla, thereby precipitating medullary ischemia. As discussed previously, loop diuretics inhibit tubuloglomerular feedback, which may be a protective mechanism against medullary ischemia. Loop diuretic administration can also increase sympathetic outflow and activate the renin–angiotensin–aldosterone axis, leading to increased systemic vascular resistance and concomitant decreases in cardiac output.[32] Recent evidence from a large observational study revealed that the use of diuretics in critically ill patients with ARF was associated with an increased risk of death and nonrecovery of renal function, although a causal relationship was not established in this study.[63] In light of the underpowered design of previous trials on the effects of diuretics in critically ill patients with ARF, prospective trials are needed to assess the optimal use of diuretics in the ICU.

REFERENCES

1. Kellum JA. The use of diuretics and dopamine in acute renal failure: a systematic review of the evidence. Crit Care 1997;1:53–9.
2. Venkataram R, Kellum JA. The role of diuretic agents in the management of acute renal failure. Contrib Nephrol 2001;132:158–70.
3. Sica DA, Gehr TW. Diuretic combinations in refractory oedema states: pharmacokinetic–pharmacodynamic relationships. Clin Pharmacokin 1996;30:229–49.
4. Guyton AC, Hall JE. Textbook of medical physiology, 9th edn. Philadelphia: WB Saunders; 1996:297–313.
5. Marik PE. Handbook of evidence-based critical care, 1st edn. New York: Springer-Verlag; 2001:109–21.
6. Badr KF, Ichikawa I. Prerenal failure: a deleterious shift from renal compensation to decompensation. N Engl J Med 1988;319:623–9.
7. Blantz RC. Pathophysiology of pre-renal azotemia. Kidney Int 1998;53:512–23.
8. Ragaller MJ, Theilen H, Koch T. Volume replacement in critically ill patients with acute renal failure. J Am Soc Nephrol 2001;17(Suppl 12):S33–9.
9. Schierhout G, Roberts I. Fluid resuscitation with colloid or crystalloid solutions in critically ill patients: a systematic review of randomised trials. Br Med J 1998;316:961–4.
10. Alderson P, Schierhout G, Roberts I, Bunn F. Colloids versus crystalloids for fluid resuscitation in critically ill patients. Cochrane Database Syst Rev 2000;2:CD000567.
11. Bickell WH, Wall MJJ, Pepe PE, et al. Immediate versus delayed fluid resuscitation for hypotensive patients with penetrating torso injuries. N Engl J Med 1994;331:1105–9.
12. Choi PT, Yip G, Quinonez LG, Cook DJ. Crystalloids vs. colloids in fluid resuscitation: a systematic review. Crit Care Med 1999;27:200–10.
13. Schortgen F, Lacherade JC, Bruneel F, et al. Effects of hydroxyethylstarch and gelatin on renal function in severe sepsis: a multicentre randomised study. Lancet 2001;357:911–16.
14. Rose BD, Post TW. Clinical physiology of acid–base and electrolyte disorders, 5th edn. New York: McGraw-Hill; 2001:478–534.
15. Rose BD. Diuretics. Kidney Int 1991;39:336–52.
16. Ellison DH. Diuretic drugs and the treatment of edema: from clinic to bench and back again. Am J Kidney Dis 1994;23:623–43.
17. Brater DC. Clinical pharmacology of loop diuretics in health and disease. Eur Heart J 1992;13(Suppl G):10–14.
18. Liu FY, Cogan MG. Angiotensin II stimulates early proximal bicarbonate absorption in the rat by decreasing cyclic adenosine monophosphate. J Clin Invest 1989;84:83–91.
19. Wright FS. Flow-dependent transport processes: filtration, absorption, secretion. Am J Physiol 1982;243:F1–11.
20. Greger R, Velazquez H. The cortical thick ascending limb and early distal convoluted tubule in the urinary concentrating mechanism. Kidney Int 1987;31:590–6.
21. Brater DC. Diuretic therapy. N Eng J Med 1998;339:387–95.
22. Russo D, Memoli B, Andreucci VE. The place of loop diuretics in the treatment of acute and chronic renal failure. Clin Nephrol 1992;38(Suppl 1):S69–73.
23. Dikshit K, Vyden JK, Forrester JS, et al. Renal and extrarenal hemodynamic effects of furosemide in congestive heart failure after acute myocardial infarction. N Eng J Med 1973;288:1087–90.
24. Johnston GD, Hiatt WR, Nies AS, et al. Factors modifying the early nondiuretic vascular effects of furosemide in man. The possible role of renal prostaglandins. Circ Res 1983;53:630–5.
25. Wilson TW, Loadholt CB, Privitera PJ, Halushka PV. Furosemide increases urine 6-keto-prostaglandin F1 alpha. Relation to natriuresis, vasodilation, and renin release. Hypertension 1982;4:634–41.
26. Gerber JG. Role of prostaglandins in the hemodynamic and tubular effects of furosemide. Fed Proc 1983;42:1707–10.
27. Bock HA, Stein JH. Diuretics and the control of extracellular fluid volume: role of counterregulation. Semin Nephrol 1988;8:264–72.
28. Inoue M, Okajima K, Itoh K, et al. Mechanism of furosemide resistance in analbuminemic rats and hypoalbuminemic patients. Kidney Int 1987;32:198–203.
29. Kirchner KA, Voelker JR, Brater DC. Intratubular albumin blunts the response to furosemide. A mechanism for diuretic resistance in the nephrotic syndrome. J Pharmacol Exp Ther 1990;252:1097–101.
30. Kirchner KA, Voelker JR, Brater DC. Tubular resistance to furosemide contributes to the attenuated diuretic response in nephrotic rats. J Am Soc Nephrol 1992;2:1201–7.
31. Risler T, Kramer B, Muller GA. The efficacy of diuretics in acute and chronic renal failure. Focus on torasemide. Drugs 1991;41(Suppl 3):69–79.
32. Francis GS, Siegel RM, Goldsmith SR, et al. Acute vasoconstrictor response to intravenous furosemide in patients with chronic congestive heart failure. Activation of the neurohumoral axis. Ann Intern Med 1985;103:1–6.
33. Brown CB, Ogg CS, Cameron JS. High dose frusemide in acute renal failure: a controlled trial. Clin Nephrol 1981;15:90–6.
34. Perico N, Remuzzi G. Edema of the nephrotic syndrome: the role of the atrial peptide system. Am J Kidney Dis 1993;22:355–66.
35. Kirchner KA, Voelker JR, Brater DC. Binding inhibitors restore furosemide potency in tubule fluid containing albumin. Kidney Int 1991;40:418–24.
36. Agarwal R, Gorski JC, Sundblad K, Brater DC. Urinary protein binding does not affect response to furosemide in patients with nephrotic syndrome. J Am Soc Nephrol 2000;11:1100–5.
37. Fliser D, Zurbruggen I, Mutschler E, et al. Coadministration of albumin and furosemide in patients with the nephrotic syndrome. Kidney Int 1999;55:629–34.
38. Akcicek F, Yalniz T, Basci A, Ok E, Mees EJ. Diuretic effect of frusemide in patients with nephrotic syndrome: Is it potentiated by intravenous albumin? Br Med J 1995;310:162–3.
39. Sjostrom PA, Odlind BG. Effect of albumin on diuretic treatment in the nephrotic syndrome. Br Med J 1995;310:1537.
40. Chalasani N, Gorski JC, Horlander JC, et al. Effects of albumin/furosemide mixtures on responses to furosemide in hypoalbuminemic patients. J Am Soc Nephrol 2001;12:1010–16.
41. Cardenas A, Gines P. Pathogenesis and treatment of fluid and electrolyte imbalance in cirrhosis. Sem Nephrol 2001;21:308–16.
42. Gines P, Berl T, Bernardi M, et al. Hyponatremia in cirrhosis: from pathogenesis to treatment. Hepatology 1998;28:851–64.
43. Perez-Ayuso RM, Arroyo V, Planas R, et al. Randomized comparative study of efficacy of furosemide versus spironolactone in nonazotemic cirrhosis with ascites. Relationship between the diuretic response and the activity of the renin–aldosterone system. Gastroenterology 1983;84:961–8.
44. Brater DC. Use of diuretics in cirrhosis and nephrotic syndrome. Sem Nephrol 1999;19:575–80.
45. Gentilini P, Casini-Raggi V, Di FG, et al. Albumin improves the response to diuretics in patients with cirrhosis and ascites: results of a randomized, controlled trial. J Hepatol 1999;30:639–45.

46. Gines PU. Transjugular intrahepatic portosystemic shunting versus paracentesis plus albumin for refractory ascites in cirrhosis. Gastroenterology 2000;123:1839–47.

47. Gerbes AL, Gulberg V, Waggershauser T, Holl J, Reiser M. Renal effects of transjugular intrahepatic portosystemic shunt in cirrnosis: comparison of patients with ascites, with refractory ascites, or without ascites. Hepatology 1998;28:683–8.

48. Forrester JS, Diamond G, Chatterjee K, Swan HJ. Medical therapy of acute myocardial infarction by application of hemodynamic subsets. N Eng J Med 1997;295:1356–62.

49. Sibbald WJ, Cunningham DR, Chin DN. Non-cardiac or cardiac pulmonary edema? A practical approach to clinical differentiation in critically ill patients. Chest 1983;84:452–61.

50. Wilson JR, Reichek N, Dunkman WB, Goldberg S. Effect of diuresis on the performance of the failing left ventricle in man. Am J Med 1981;70:234–9.

51. Martin GS, Mangialardi RJ, Wheeler AP, et al. Albumin and furosemide therapy in hypoproteinemic patients with acute lung injury. Crit Care Med 2002;30:2175–82.

52. Mangialardi RJ, Martin GS, Bernard GR, et al. Hypoproteinemia predicts acute respiratory distress syndrome development, weight gain, and death in patients with sepsis. Ibuprofen in Sepsis Study Group. Crit Care Med 2000;28:3137–45.

53. Schuller D, Mitchell JP, Calandrino FS, Schuster DP. Fluid balance during pulmonary edema. Is fluid gain a marker or a cause of poor outcome? Chest 1991;100:1068–75.

54. Mitchell JP, Schuller D, Calandrino FS, Schuster DP. Improved outcome based on fluid management in critically ill patients requiring pulmonary artery catheterization. Am Rev Respir Dis 1992;145:990–8.

55. Breen D, Bihari D. Acute renal failure as a part of multiple organ failure: the slippery slope of critical illness. Kidney Int Suppl 1998;66:S25–33.

56. Lieberthal W. Biology of ischemic and toxic renal tubular cell injury: role of nitric oxide and the inflammatory response. Curr Opin Nephrol Hypertension 1998;7:289–95.

57. Memoli B, Libetta C, Conte G, Andreucci VE. Loop diuretics and renal vasodilators in acute renal failure. Nephrol Dial Transplant 1994;9 (Suppl 4):168–71.

58. Kleinknecht D, Ganeval D, Gonzalez-Duque LA, Fermanian J. Furosemide in acute oliguric renal failure. A controlled trial. Nephron 1976;17:51–8.

59. Lassnigg A, Donner E, Grubhofer G, et al. Lack of renoprotective effects of dopamine and furosemide during cardiac surgery. J Am Soc Nephrol 2000;11:97–104.

60. Shilliday IR, Quinn KJ, Allison ME. Loop diuretics in the management of acute renal failure: a prospective, double-blind, placebo-controlled, randomized study. Nephrol Dial Transplant 1997;12:2592–6.

61. Solomon R, Werner C, Mann D, D'Elia J, Silva P. Effects of saline, mannitol, and furosemide to prevent acute decreases in renal function induced by radiocontrast agents. N Eng J Med 1994;331:1416–20.

62. Better OS, Rubinstein I, Winaver JM, Knochel JP. Mannitol therapy revisited (1940–1997). Kidney Int 1997;52:886–94.

63. Mehta RL, Pascual MT, Soroko S, Chertow GM; PICARD Study Group. Diuretics, mortality, and nonrecovery of renal function in acute renal failure. JAMA 2002;288:2547–53.

22

Water homeostasis

Jerrold S Levine and Rajiv Poduval

INTRODUCTION

The plasma concentration of sodium, or $[Na^+]_p$, and the plasma osmolality are very closely related measures. The correlation between them is so tight that $[Na^+]_p$ is commonly used as a surrogate for plasma osmolality. Indeed, as we shall discuss below, after introducing the concept of effective osmoles, $[Na^+]_p$ may be the physiologically more relevant variable. Disturbances in which $[Na^+]_p$ is reduced, collectively referred to as hyponatremia, are virtually always accompanied by a reduction of plasma osmolality. Similarly, disturbances in which $[Na^+]_p$ is increased, collectively referred to as hypernatremia, are indicative of an elevation of plasma osmolality. Properly understood, both hyponatremia and hypernatremia are not single diseases, but instead syndromes, and each has multiple potential causes. Correct diagnosis and management of these two syndromes depend critically on an understanding of the underlying physiology.

In this chapter, using simple physiologic principles, we construct diagnostic algorithms that enable the clinician to identify the responsible disease state(s) and pathophysiologic mechanism(s). We then use these same physiologic principles to devise a treatment strategy that is based solely on quantitative analysis of the daily balance of sodium, potassium, and water.

BASIC PHYSIOLOGY

Osmoregulation versus volume regulation

One of the more confusing concepts in nephrology is the distinction between regulation of osmolality and regulation of extracellular volume (Table 22.1). Several factors contribute to this confusion.

Concentration versus total quantity of sodium
The first factor is the critical, though distinct, role that sodium plays in the regulation of osmolality vs the regulation of extracellular volume. In the case of osmolality, the regulated variable is the plasma concentration of sodium, while, in the case of extracellular volume, the regulated variable is the total quantity of sodium in the body. Regulation of osmolality and extracellular volume are both essential to the healthy function of tissues and organs. Maintenance of plasma osmolality within a narrow range protects cells from deleterious changes in their intracellular volume or ionic milieu. Regulation of extracellular volume performs a complementary function by insuring an adequate circulating volume so that tissues are effectively perfused with oxygen and vital nutrients.

Osmolality refers to the number of particles of solute dissolved in a given mass of solvent. The mass or charge of the particle, or indeed any other distinguishing feature, is irrelevant. With respect to osmolality, one ion of sodium is equivalent to one molecule of albumin. Therefore, to determine the plasma osmolality, one simply counts the total number of particles, irrespective of identity, dissolved in a given volume of plasma. Since sodium is the predominant extracellular particle, and water is the predominant plasma solvent, osmolality depends largely on the concentration of sodium in water. This intimate relationship between $[Na^+]_p$ and osmolality means that an increase in $[Na^+]_p$ is almost always paralleled by an increase in plasma osmolality, and vice versa.

With respect to regulation of extracellular volume, sodium appears in a different, but no less

Table 22.1	Comparison between the regulation of osmolality and extracellular volume.		
Parameter	Osmolality		Extracellular volume
Homeostatic system	Osmolality of body fluids		Adequacy of tissue perfusion
Primary regulated quantity	Total body H_2O		Total body Na
Relationship to sodium (Na)	Plasma concentration of sodium, $[Na^+]_p$ (ratio of total amount of Na to total amount of H_2O)		Total body content of Na
Sensors	Osmoreceptors (hypothalamus)		Baroreceptors (carotid sinus, cardiac atria)
Hormonal regulators	ADH		Renin–angiotensin Aldosterone Atrial natriuretic peptide Aldosterone Epinephrine–norepinephrine ADH (severe derangements only)
Effector mechanisms	Thirst Renal excretion/retention of H_2O		Renal excretion/retention of Na
Diagnosis			
• Physical examination	Ancillary		Essential
• Laboratory evaluation	Essential		Ancillary

ADH = antidiuretic hormone.

vital, role. In this case, it is the total quantity of sodium in the body that is the critical determinant. Nearly all bodily sodium exists in the form of sodium ions dissolved in extracellular water. Hence, it is the total amount of sodium-containing fluid that determines the volume of extracellular fluid in the body. The exact concentration of sodium in plasma is not important to the perfusion of tissues. Adequate tissue perfusion depends on an adequate extracellular volume, and therefore can take place in the face of normal, reduced, or increased plasma osmolality.

Although a full discussion of the regulation of extracellular fluid volume is beyond the scope of this chapter, it should be emphasized that the major regulated variables are blood pressure and the adequacy of tissue perfusion in terms of delivery of oxygen and other essential blood-borne nutrients. Thus, in disease states as divergent as gastrointestinal blood loss or congestive failure, the kidney attempts to restore effective tissue perfusion by reabsorbing sodium and increasing extracellular volume. In the case of gastrointestinal blood loss, the kidney's response is appropriate and corrective, whereas, in the case of congestive heart failure, the kidney's response leads to further increases of an already expanded extracellular volume. Nonetheless, from a fundamental point of view, the sensors and effectors in these two divergent disease states are responding more or less analogously. For this reason, throughout the rest of this chapter, we will use the phrase 'inadequate tissue perfusion' as a shorthand to denote those pathophysiologic states in which increased absorption of sodium by the kidney occurs in response to a decrease in perceived circulating volume, either appropriately, as in blood loss, or counterproductively, as in congestive heart failure.

This fundamental distinction between the role of sodium in regulation of osmolality vs its role in regulation of extracellular fluid volume leads to a very important point:

Essential Concept #1. Disturbances in osmolality, because they represent changes in the concentration of sodium, can be detected only by a laboratory measurement. In contrast, disturbances in extracellular volume can be detected only by physical examination.

To highlight this point, imagine a glass partially filled with salt water. It should be obvious that measuring the concentration of sodium in the salt water can in no way tell you how full the glass is. Similarly, in evaluating a patient, no simple laboratory test can tell you whether the patient is euvolemic, volume-depleted, or volume-expanded. In assessing the extent of fullness, only direct examination can yield the correct volume. Correspondingly, if you wish to know the concentration of sodium, then only a laboratory measurement can yield that information. Visual examination of the glass (or patient) can in no way tell you the concentration of sodium. As deceptively simple as this concept is, failure to apprehend it often underlies the mismanagement of disorders in $[Na^+]_p$, especially in the setting of an intensive care unit (ICU).

Conflicts between regulation of osmolality and extracellular volume

This brings us to the second, and more subtle, reason for confusion between regulation of osmolality and volume. As would be expected, the body has evolved distinct sensors and effectors by which it regulates osmolality and volume (see Table 22.1). Changes in osmolality are effected almost entirely by changes in water balance, whereas changes in extracellular volume (or its physiologic correlate, tissue perfusion) are effected almost entirely by changes in sodium balance. Under normal circumstances, these two regulatory systems are rarely in conflict, and the body is able to adjust both osmolality and volume with exquisite control and through virtually independent systems.

However, certain pathophysiologic conditions (which we will discuss below) preclude having both a normal osmolality and a normal extracellular volume. This raises the following important question: *'what happens when a conflict exists between these two regulatory systems?'* In other words, if correction of an abnormality in extracellular volume tends to exacerbate, or even engender, a concurrent abnormality in osmolality (or vice versa), which of the two regulatory systems has priority? The answer, while straightforward, is critical to an understanding of disturbances of osmolality:

Essential Concept #2. In all conflicts between regulation of osmolality and regulation of extracellular volume, maintenance of extracellular volume or, more properly put, maintenance of adequate tissue perfusion, always takes precedence.

Intuitively, this concept should make sense, as the body's homeostatic mechanisms always give priority to essential functions required to sustain life, such as adequate perfusion of tissues. In the following section, we explore the mechanism for this hierarchical arrangement.

Antidiuretic hormone – an effector for regulation of both osmolality and extracellular volume

As indicated in Table 22.1, the regulatory systems for osmolality and extracellular volume are almost entirely separate. The sole major overlap occurs for the effector, antidiuretic hormone (ADH), a polypeptide hormone produced in the hypothalamus and transported within axons to the pituitary gland, from which ADH is ultimately released into the blood.[1] The primary effect of ADH is upon water balance and osmolality. As its name suggests, ADH reduces urine volume and promotes the reabsorption of maximal amounts of water from the urine, leading to small volumes of highly concentrated urine.

Secretion of ADH by the pituitary is determined by the summated input from several sources. The two most important are osmoreceptors located in the hypothalamus and baroreceptors located in the blood vessels and heart.[2-4] The osmoreceptors are exquisitely sensitive to changes in osmolality; as little as a 1% increase in osmolality (<2 mEq/L change in $[Na^+]_p$) leads to abundant release of ADH.[2,3] In contrast, the baroreceptors are far less sensitive to changes in effective circulating volume (or tissue perfusion); for example, blood volume depletions on the order of 5–10% are required before ADH is released.[2,5,6] This degree of volume depletion is well in excess of that leading to either activation of the renin–angiotensin system or the release of hormones such as norepinephrine and aldosterone. Thus, while ADH is primarily involved in the regulation of osmolality, ADH functions as an emergency backup for regulation of volume, being marshaled only in situations in which adequate tissue perfusion cannot be maintained by the front-line protectors of extracellular volume.

In patients with both volume depletion and hypo-osmolality, there are conflicting stimuli for ADH release. On the basis of volume depletion, ADH levels should be elevated, whereas, on the basis of hypo-osmolality, ADH levels should be suppressed. As noted in Essential Concept #2, maintenance of adequate tissue perfusion takes priority, and ADH is released.[2,7,8] From a teleological vantage, this dual regulation of ADH is understandable. Improved tissue perfusion, even at the expense of a reduction in plasma osmolality and $[Na^+]_p$, is preferable to continued poor perfusion with a normal osmolality.

The consequences of this dual role for ADH for determining the etiology of disturbances in osmolality are quite profound. Thus, whenever one is faced with a patient with an abnormal plasma osmolality (especially, hypo-osmolality, or hyponatremia), one must first evaluate the patient's volume status. If there is an abnormality of extracellular volume, reflective of inadequate tissue perfusion, then one cannot exclude the possibility that the abnormal osmolality is a direct consequence of the body's homeostatic efforts to restore adequate tissue perfusion at any cost. Stated differently, if one is able to improve tissue perfusion to nearly normal levels, then this alone may lead to complete restoration of a normal osmolality, without the need for any interventions aimed specifically at the osmoregulatory system. Only if a patient's volume status is completely normal, can one state with absolute certainty that an abnormal plasma osmolality is the result of a primary disturbance within the body's osmoregulatory system.

THE KIDNEY'S RESPONSE TO DISTURBANCES IN OSMOLALITY

The kidney represents a final common effector in the regulation of osmolality. By promoting the reabsorption or the excretion of free water, the kidney tightly regulates both $[Na^+]_p$ and plasma osmolality. It is useful to consider separately the responses to either hypernatremia (increased $[Na^+]_p$, and osmolality) or hyponatremia (decreased $[Na^+]_p$, and osmolality).

In the case of hypernatremia, the most straightforward solution is to add water and thereby lower both $[Na^+]_p$ and osmolality. The body brings this about through stimulation of thirst. During thirst-induced ingestion of water, the kidney simultaneously regulates volume by reabsorption or excretion of sodium. Assuming there is no disturbance in effective circulating volume, the kidney will excrete as little water as possible, and may even generate a small amount of free water (see discussion of electrolyte-free water excretion). However, except in very rare situations, the kidney cannot by itself correct hypernatremia, and correction is almost entirely dependent upon the intake or administration of an appropriate volume of free water. Thus, the kidney's role in the correction of hypernatremia is largely ancillary, with stimulation of thirst being the body's major homeostatic response.

In contrast, when it comes to hyponatremia, the kidney takes center stage. To correct hyponatremia, the kidney must remove free water from the body. Without an appropriate renal response, the sole mechanism for elimination of free water would be insensible or other nonrenal losses (e.g. diarrhea or other drainages). Except in extraordinary circumstances, these routes eliminate very little free water, so that $[Na^+]_p$ and osmolality cannot be raised unless oral and intravenous administration of free water is severely restricted to levels below that lost through these nonrenal routes.

Renal requirements for excretion of free water

Given the primary role of the kidney in correction of hyponatremia, it is useful to examine the requirements for effective excretion of free water by the kidney. For every condition or disease associated with hyponatremia, a derangement in the regulation of one or more of these requirements can be found (Table 22.2).[9,10] The three criteria that must be fulfilled in order for the kidney to excrete free water appropriately will now be considered.

Suppression of antidiuretic hormone secretion

In the absence of ADH, the urine is maximally dilute. The normal response to hyponatremia and decreased plasma osmolality is suppression of ADH secretion. However, as previously discussed, in situations of reduced effective circulating volume, maintaining adequate tissue perfusion takes priority over correction of hyponatremia, and ADH is released into the circulation. Other nonosmotic stimuli to ADH release include severe pain or nausea. ADH may also be released from tissues other than the brain as part of a paraneoplastic process or other chronic disease state.

Table 22.2 Common etiologies of hyponatremia grouped according to volume status and urinary osmolar composition.[a]

Condition[b]	Abnormalities impairing free H_2O excretion	Urine osmolality	Urine composition	Diagnostic 'pearls'
Hypovolemia				
$[Na]_u + [K]_u \sim$ or $>[Na]_p$				
Mineralocorticoid deficiency	↓ GFR, ↑ ADH	≥ serum osmolality	Na, urea $[Na]_u >20$ mEq/L	Associated hyperkalemia
Salt-wasting nephropathy	↓ GFR, ↑ ADH	≥ serum osmolality	Na, K, urea $[Na]_u >20$ mEq/L	Associated hypokalemia
Cerebral salt-wasting	↓ GFR, ↑ ADH	≥ serum osmolality	Na, K, urea $[Na]_u >20$ mEq/L	Associated hypokalemia
$[Na]_u + [K]_u << [Na]_p$				
GI losses	↓ GFR, ↑ ADH	≥ serum osmolality	Mostly urea, $[Na]_u <10$ mEq/L	Diarrhea, vomiting, GI bleed, GI drainage
Skin losses	↓ GFR, ↑ ADH	≥ serum osmolality	Mostly urea, $[Na]_u <10$ mEq/L	Burns, marathon runners, cystic fibrosis
Third-spacing	↓ GFR, ↑ ADH	≥ serum osmolality	Mostly urea, $[Na]_u <10$ mEq/L	Intestinal obstruction, pancreatitis, crush injuries, internal bleeding
Loop diuretics[c]	↓ GFR, ↑ ADH, impaired loop	≤ serum osmolality	Na, K, urea $[Na]_u >20$ mEq/L	Associated hypokalemia
Osmotic diuresis (urea, glucose, mannitol)	↓ GFR, ↑ ADH, impaired loop	>300 (~ serum osmolality)	Na, K, urea $[Na]_u >20$ mEq/L	High-protein feeds, saline loading, hyperglycemia
Hypervolemia				
$[Na]_u + [K]_u \sim [Na]_p$				
ARF, CRF	↓ GFR, impaired loop	~ serum osmolality	Variable	
$[Na]_u + [K]_u \leq< [Na]_p$				
CHF	↓ GFR, ↑ ADH	≥ serum osmolality	Mostly urea, $[Na]_u <10$ mEq/L	Depree of hyponatremia correlates with severity of CHF
Cirrhosis	↓ GFR, ↑ ADH	≥ serum osmolality	Mostly urea, $[Na]_u <10$ mEq/L	Stigmata of liver failure
Nephrotic syndrome	↓GFR, ↑ ADH	≥ serum osmolality	Mostly urea, $[Na]_u <10$ mEq/L	Hypoalbuminemia
Euvolemia				
$[Na]_u + [K]_u \sim$ or $\geq [Na]_p$				
SIADH	↑ ADH	≥ serum osmolality	Mostly Na + K	
Glucocorticoid deficiency	↑ ADH	≥ serum osmolality	Mostly Na + K	Cortisol inhibits ADH release

Table 22.2 *Continued.*

Condition[b]	Abnormalities impairing free H$_2$O excretion	Urine osmolality	Urine composition	Diagnostic 'pearls'
'Reset' osmostat[d]	↑ ADH	Variable	Variable	[Na]$_p$ usually 125–130 mEq/L, normal suppression of ADH below altered setpoint
Pregnancy	Reset osmostat	Variable	Variable	Drop in [Na]$_p$ of ~5
Thiazide diuretics[c]	↑ ADH, enhanced Na and K excretion	≥ serum osmolality	Mainly Na + K	Mild hypovolemia, hypokalemia
[Na]$_u$ + [K]$_u$ << [Na]$_p$				
Primary polydipsia	Impaired loop, excess H$_2$O intake	<< serum osmolality	Mainly free H$_2$O	Requires >10 L H$_2$O intake daily
Hypothyroidism	↓ GFR, ↑ ADH	≥ serum osmolality	Mostly urea, [Na]$_u$ <10 mEq/L	Rare in absence of near myxedema, ↓ [Na]$_p$ dependent on cardiac dysfunction and rarely <125 mEq/L
Beer-drinker's potomania, tea-and-toast diet	Inadequate solute in diet	<< serum osmolality	Mainly free H$_2$O	Associated malnutrition
Sick cell syndrome	Redistribution of intracellular H$_2$O into extracellular space	Variable	Variable	Associated with sepsis, increased osmolal gap
Hyperglycemia	Redistribution of intracellular H$_2$O into extracellular space	>300 (~ serum osmolality)	Na, K, urea [Na]$_u$ >20 mEq/L	[Na]$_p$ increases by 2.4 mEq/L for every 100 mg/dl rise in glucose above 200 mg/dl
Severe K depletion ([K]$_p$ <2.0 mEq/L)	Redistribution of intracellular H$_2$O into extracellular space	Variable	Variable	

[a] ADH = antidiuretic hormone; ARF = acute renal failure; CHF = congestive heart failure; CRF = chronic renal failure; GFR = glomerular filtration rate; GI = gastrointestinal; SIADH = syndrome of inappropriate diuretic hormone.

[b] Conditions are grouped according to volume status, as assessed by physical examination. Within each category of volume status, conditions are subdivided according to the ability of the kidney to generate electrolyte-free H$_2$O. For those conditions denoted by [Na]$_u$ + [K]$_u$ << [Na]$_p$, the kidney is able to generate urine which is essentially devoid of electrolytes, but is limited in the volume of urine it can produce. For the remaining conditions, the kidney is impaired in its ability to maximally extract all electrolytes from the urine, and the urine will therefore contain elevated concentrations of Na and/or K. For these latter conditions, under certain circumstances, the sum of [Na]$_u$ and [K]$_u$ may even exceed [Na]$_p$, so that the kidney is actually exacerbating the hyponatremia. To highlight this distinction, we denote these latter conditions by [Na]$_u$ + [K]$_u$ ≥ [Na]$_p$, although in general the sum of [Na]$_u$ and [K]$_u$ will attain a value that, while a significant fraction of [Na]$_p$, does not actually exceed it.

[c] The data given in the table for loop and thiazide diuretics refer to situations in which these diuretics are still exerting their effect upon the kidney. Once the diuretics have been cleared and cease to exert an effect on the kidney, the clinical and laboratory picture will resemble that seen in situations of classic volume depletion, such as that seen with GI losses, skin losses, or third-spacing.

[d] In patients with a reset osmostat, the body's osmoregulatory system functions normally about an abnormally low [Na]$_p$, usually in the range of 125–130 mEq/L. Thus, when [Na]$_p$ is greater than this set point, ADH will be released, urine osmolality will exceed plasma osmolality, and [Na]$_u$ + [K]$_u$ ≥ [Na]$_p$. In contrast, when [Na]$_p$ is less than the set point, ADH will be suppressed, urine osmolality will approach maximal dilution, and [Na]$_u$ + [K]$_u$ << [Na]$_p$.

Functioning loop of Henle

Production of both a maximally concentrated and a maximally dilute urine is dependent on a functioning loop of Henle, through the kidney's countercurrent multiplier system. In the absence of a functioning loop of Henle, the final urine will be essentially isotonic, and the kidney will be unable to effect changes in $[Na^+]_p$ or plasma osmolality. Damage to this portion of the nephron, as in chronic renal failure of any cause, or inhibition of its function, through the use of loop diuretics such as furosemide, will prevent dilution of the urine and excretion of free water.

Adequate glomerular filtration rate

Even if the kidney dilutes the urine appropriately, the free water content of the urine must still exceed the oral and intravenous administration of free water. As an extreme example, imagine that a patient's kidney generates pure water for urine, but that the daily urine volume is only 200 ml per day. Then, this patient can drink no more than 200 ml of water per day, or else the $[Na^+]_p$ will continue to decrease. A major determinant of urine volume is the glomerular filtration rate (GFR). Reductions in GFR, with a consequent decrease in urine volume, are seen in most conditions associated with a decreased effective circulating volume. As we will discuss, for most of these conditions, the extreme example we gave, while quantitatively exaggerated, is an otherwise accurate reflection of the underlying pathophysiology.

DIAGNOSTIC APPROACH TO HYPONATREMIA

Diagnostic algorithm

Hyponatremia is a syndrome with multiple potential causes. A useful approach is to stratify patients according to their volume status (see Table 22.2 and Fig. 22.1). All patients with decreased extracellular fluid volumes on physical examination, as well as most with increased extracellular fluid volumes, have ineffective circulating volumes and inadequate tissue perfusion. As a result, ADH levels are elevated for nonosmotic reasons, with maintenance of tissue perfusion superseding in importance that of osmolality. As a general rule, for hyponatremia to develop, the disturbance in volume status should be clinically apparent by examination and will not at all be subtle. Only for patients who have clinically mild or undetectable changes in extracellular fluid volume can one unequivocally ascribe hyponatremia to a primary disturbance in osmoregulation. For example, patients with true syndrome of inappropriate antidiuretic hormone (SIADH) often accumulate as much as 5 kg of excess weight in water. Because this water is distributed throughout total body water, both intracellularly and extracellularly, its accumulation usually manifests as no more than trace edema. Once patients have been stratified by volume status, then a careful examination of urine osmolality and serum and urine electrolytes will enable establishment of an etiologic diagnosis.

Special considerations for patients in the intensive care unit

Patients in the ICU are at increased risk for developing hyponatremia. Several causes of hyponatremia occur not only with increased severity in ICU patients but also with increased frequency, if not exclusively, in these patients (Table 22.3). We discuss several of these ICU-related causes below.

'Sick cell syndrome'

Critically ill patients, with, for example, sepsis or multi-organ system failure, apparently have an increased permeability of their cell membranes. As a result, intracellular solutes leak out of their cells, generating an osmotic gradient between the extracellular and intracellular compartments. This gradient induces movement of water out of cells in order to restore osmotic equilibrium, thereby diluting extracellular sodium and leading to hyponatremia. A clue to the existence of so-called 'sick cell syndrome' is the presence of an increased osmolal gap, attributable to the intracellular solutes that have leaked from the cells.[11]

Nonosmotic release of antidiuretic hormone

In addition to reduced effective circulating volume, a common occurrence among ICU patients, there are several other important nonosmotic stimuli for ADH release. These include the following:

- severe postoperative or other pain
- severe nausea
- central nervous system pathology, such as infection, hemorrhage, or neoplasm
- pulmonary disease, such as pneumonia or tuberculosis
- ectopic release as part of a paraneoplastic process.[12–20]

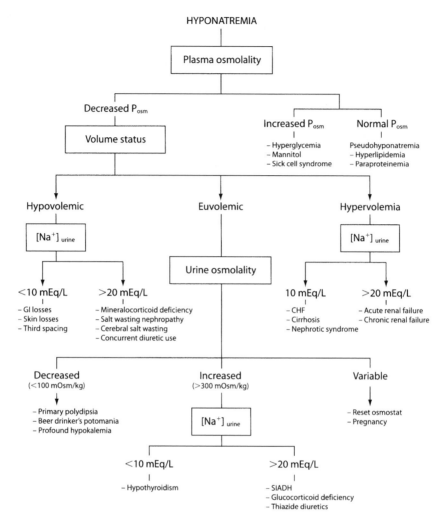

Figure 22.1 Algorithmic approach to hyponatremia. CHF = congestive heart failure; GI = gastrointestinal; SIADH = syndrome of inappropriate diuretic hormone.

Medications

A large number of medications either induce nonosmotic release of ADH or potentiate the effect of released ADH. Given the large number of medications that nearly all ICU patients receive, a careful review of all medications is mandatory. Common culprits include the following:

- neuropyschiatric drugs (haloperidol, thioridazine, monoamine oxidase inhibitors, tricyclic antidepressants, carbamazepine, serotonin uptake antagonists)
- chemotherapeutic agents (cyclophosphamide, vincristine, vinblastine).[21–23]

Diuretics

As discussed above, loop diuretics interfere with free water excretion by preventing maximal dilution of the urine. Although thiazide-type diuretics do not impair renal concentrating or diluting ability, they can produce severe hyponatremia if they are used as the sole diuretic therapy in the presence of increased ADH levels. By inhibiting distal sodium reabsorption, they produce a urine that is not only very concentrated but may also have an electrolyte content exceeding that of plasma (see discussion of electrolyte-free water excretion below).[24,25]

Table 22.3 Causes of hyponatremia in the intensive care unit.

Cause	Volume status (if present as isolated condition)	Mechanism	Diagnostic clues
Nonosmotic release of ADH			
Severe pain	Euvolemia	$\uparrow$ ADH (SIADH)	Inappropriately high urine osmolality
Severe nausea			$[Na^+]_u + [K^+]_u \geq [Na^+]_p$
Pulmonary disease:			
Pneumonia			
Tuberculosis			
Other			
CNS pathology:			
Infection			
Hemorrhage			
Neoplasm			
Other			
Paraneoplastic syndrome:			
Lung cancer			
Mediastinal cancer			
Other			
Medications			
Neuropsychiatric	Euvolemia	$\uparrow$ ADH (SIADH)	Inappropriately high urine osmolality
Haloperidol			$[Na^+]_u + [K^+]_u \geq [Na^+]_p$
Thioridazine			
Monoamine oxidase inhibitors			
Tricyclics			
Carbamazepine			
Serotonin uptake antagonists			
Chemotherapeutic			
Cyclophosphamide			
Vincristine			
Vinblastine			
Diuretics			
Loop diuretics	Hypovolemia	$\downarrow$ GFR, $\uparrow$ ADH, nonfunctioning loop of Henle	
Thiazides	Mild hypovolemia	Impaired urinary dilution	$[Na^+]_u + [K^+]_u \geq [Na^+]_p$
Sepsis	Variable	'Sick cell syndrome'	Increased osmolal gap
Excessive use of hypotonic solutions			
Intravenous drips	Euvolemia	Excessive H_2O intake	Urine osmolality is appropriately low
Irrigations			
Bladder			
Laparoscopy			
Other			
Tap water enemas			

ADH = antidiuretic hormone; CNS = central nervous system; GFR = glomerular filtration rate; SIADH = syndrome of inappropriate antidiuretic hormone.

Excessive use of hypotonic solutions for hydration or irrigation

ICU patients commonly receive large volumes of fluid, often disguised in the form of drips. Over the course of a day, even concentrated drips that have been constituted in hypotonic solutions can accumulate to several liters of administered free water. In addition, irrigation fluids can be absorbed, so that large-volume frequent irrigation with hypotonic solutions can lead to absorption of a substantial volume of free water.[26,27]

A CLINICAL PUZZLE

Traditionally, determination of water balance has focused on urine osmolality. A urine osmolality greater than that of serum indicates the presence of ADH, whereas a urine osmolality less than that of serum indicates suppression of ADH. While correct, this analysis is incomplete and fails to explain several important aspects of water balance, as shown by the following clinical example (Fig. 22.2).

Imagine two patients: one (patient A) with congestive heart failure (CHF) and the other (patient B) with SIADH. Both patients take in 2000 ml of water and 2.75 g of Na/day. Both have a daily urine volume of 1000 ml. Their urine osmolalities are both 600 mOsm/L, approximately twice that of plasma, and apparently indicative of an impairment in the renal excretion of free water. Yet patient B has profound hyponatremia with a $[Na^+]_p$ of 110 mEq/L, whereas patient A has only modest hyponatremia with a $[Na^+]_p$ of 130 mEq/L. How can this be? By traditional analysis, the two patients seem to be identical. And yet the two patients are clearly different. In fact, the greater degree of hyponatremia, with otherwise similar salt and fluid intakes, is well recognized in comparisons of patients with SIADH vs those with CHF.

A: Looks the same at first glance . . .		
	Patient A **(CHF)**	**Patient B** **(SIADH)**
Sodium intake	120 mEq/24 hours	120 mEq/24 hours
Water intake	2 L/24 hours	2L/24 hours
Plasma osmolality	270 mOsm/L	230 mOsm/L
Plasma sodium	130 mEq/L	110 mEql/L
Plasma potassium	4 mEq/L	4 mEq/L
Urine osmolality	600 mOsm/L	600 mOsm/L
Urine volume	1 L/24 hours	1 L/24 hours

B: But look again!		
	Patient A **(CHF)**	**Patient B** **(SIADH)**
Urine osmolality	600 mOsm/L	600 mOsm/L
Urine Na	7 mEq/L	120 MEq/L
Urine K	6 mEq/L	45 mEq/L
Urine urea	500 mOsm/L	200 mOsm/L
Urine [Na + K]	20 mEq/L	165 mEq/L
Plasma [Na + K]	134 mEq/L	114 mEq/L

Figure 22.2 Differences in urinary composition: congestive heart failure (CHF) vs syndrome at inappropriate diuretic hormone (SIADH).

The key to this puzzle is in the composition of the urine. In the case of a patient with SIADH, a large fraction of the osmoles dissolved in the urine are sodium, potassium, and their accompanying anions. In sharp contrast, virtually all of the osmoles in the urine of a patient with CHF derive from urea, and the fraction of electrolytes is very low. This difference in urine composition is critical to explaining the different tendencies towards hyponatremia of these two patients. To understand this, we need to return to some basic physiology.

EFFECTIVE VERSUS INEFFECTIVE OSMOLES

The concept of effective osmoles

From the perspective of renal physiology, not all osmoles are created equally. Some osmoles, such as sodium and potassium, are 'effective', whereas others, such as urea, are 'ineffective'. To understand this distinction, it is best to consider the major homeostatic process for which regulation of osmolality is essential, namely, the maintenance of cell volume. While regulation of cell volume is vital to the function of all cells, brain cells, in particular, are adversely affected by changes in cell volume, with acute increases or decreases of cell volume leading to neurologic abnormalities that range in severity from lethargy or malaise to seizures, coma, or death.

By far the most important determinant of cell volume is the relative movement of water across the cell membrane into and out of cells. Several equilibrium principles guide this movement. First, as long as the cell membrane is permeable to a given solute, the particles of solute will distribute themselves across the membrane so that their concentrations inside and outside the cell are equal. Second, since nearly all cell membranes are freely permeable to water, water will also move in order to equalize its concentration across the cell membrane. Equalization of the concentration of water inside and outside the cell means that the total number of dissolved particles in the water within these two compartments is the same. In other words, water will distribute itself across cell membranes until the intracellular and extracellular osmolalities are equalized.

With these principles in mind, we are now ready to discuss ineffective vs effective osmoles. Ineffective osmoles move freely across cell membranes; as such, they do not affect the distribution of water between the inside and outside of cells, and there-

fore cause no change in cell volume. On the other hand, effective osmoles are unable to cross cell membranes; as a result, the drive to equalize the osmolalities of the intracellular and extracellular compartments causes water to move across the cell membrane, and so cell volume will change.

Let us illustrate these ideas by two simple examples. We consider first the addition of urea, an ineffective osmole, to the extracellular space (Fig. 22.3A). Initially, the concentration of urea outside cells will exceed that inside cells. Since urea is able to move freely across cell membranes, urea

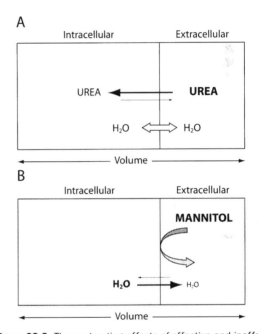

Figure 22.3 The contrasting effects of effective and ineffective osmoles on plasma sodium concentration. (A) Addition of urea, a molecule that can move freely across cell membranes, to the extracellular compartment results in the movement of urea from the extracellular compartment into the intracellular compartment down its concentration gradient. Urea therefore does not generate an osmotic gradient, and, hence, net transfer of water between the extracellular and intracellular compartments does not occur. Urea is therefore an ineffective osmole. Addition of an ineffective osmole to the extracellular compartment has no effect on $[Na^+]_p$. (B) Addition of mannitol, unlike urea, to the extracellular space generates an osmotic gradient, since mannitol cannot move across the cell membrane. Mannitol therefore remains confined to the extracellular compartment, thereby generating an osmotic gradient. This osmotic gradient causes water to move from the intracellular to the extracellular compartment and results in a 'dilutional' hyponatremia. Mannitol is therefore an effective osmole. Addition of an effective osmole to the extracellular space will lower $[Na^+]_p$.

molecules will enter cells until the concentration of urea is the same inside and outside. The intracellular and extracellular osmolalities will both increase, but they will increase by the same amount, and so no net transfer of water will take place across the cell membrane. For this reason, the addition of urea to the extracellular space will have no effect on cell volume. Moreover, it should be clear that, in the absence of any net movement of water, $[Na^+]_p$ will also not change. Thus, the addition of urea to the extracellular fluid has no net effect on $[Na^+]_p$. This is an important point, and we will return to it later, when we consider the effect of urea's leaving the body in the urine.

Next we consider the addition of mannitol, an effective osmole, to the extracellular space (Fig. 22.3B). Since cell membranes are impermeable to mannitol, the intracellular and extracellular concentrations of mannitol cannot be equalized. As a result, the extracellular osmolality will exceed the intracellular osmolality, and water will exit cells until the two osmolalities are once again equal. The net effect will be an increase in extracellular water and a decrease in intracellular water. Thus, the addition of mannitol to the extracellular space leads to a decrease of cell volume. In addition, because sodium ions cannot move across cell membranes, the addition of mannitol will also lower $[Na^+]_p$, as an equivalent number of Na^+ ions will now be dissolved in an increased quantity of water.

We may summarize and generalize these points as follows:

Essential Concept #3. Ineffective osmoles, such as urea, are able to diffuse freely back and forth across cell membranes. Their addition or removal from bodily fluids leads to changes in neither cell volume nor $[Na^+]_p$. In contrast, effective osmoles cannot diffuse across cell membranes. Their addition or removal from the bodily fluids changes both cell volume and $[Na^+]_p$.

Sodium and potassium ions as effective osmoles

Sodium ions, or Na^+, are the main osmoles found in extracellular fluid, while potassium ions, or K^+, are the main osmoles found in intracellular fluid. Cell membranes are essentially impermeable to Na^+ and K^+, so that Na^+ and K^+ both act as effective osmoles, with Na^+ restricted to the outside of cells and K^+ restricted to the inside. The few Na^+

and K^+ that manage to diffuse across the cell membrane down their concentration gradients are restored to their proper locations by the continuous activity of an Na–K ATPase pump, located in cell membranes, that propels the exit of one Na^+ from the cell in exchange for the entry of one K^+.

As previously discussed, $[Na^+]_p$ may be used as a surrogate for plasma osmolality. Correspondingly, $[K^+]_i$ may be used as a surrogate for intracellular osmolality. The free movement of water between the inside and outside of cells guarantees that the osmolality of intracellular fluid equals that of extracellular fluid, and therefore that, under most circumstances, $[Na^+]_p$ is equal to $[K^+]_i$. This simple idea has several implications of major clinical importance.

First, whenever a patient has plasma hypernatremia, the patient virtually always has intracellular hyperkalemia, with $[Na^+]_p$ approximating $[K^+]_i$. The analogous statement is true for hyponatremia, though with one important exception. When hyponatremia is due to the addition to the extracellular fluid of an effective osmole such as glucose or mannitol, then the net transfer of water out of cells will lead to plasma hyponatremia and intracellular hyperkalemia. In all other cases, a close correspondence will exist between $[Na^+]_p$ and $[K^+]_i$. The reader is reminded that we are speaking here of concentrations, and therefore no information can be inferred about the adequacy of extracellular or intracellular fluid volumes.

Second, with respect to $[Na^+]_p$, the loss from the body of one ion of Na^+ is functionally equivalent to the loss of one ion of K^+. This means that, if we were to remove 500 mEq of Na^+ from one patient and 500 mEq of K^+ from a second identical patient, then the final $[Na^+]_p$ of both patients would be exactly the same. This is a very remarkable fact and means that, in all analyses of hyponatremia, we must pay equal attention to losses (or gains) from the body of Na^+ and K^+. As we will discuss shortly, the most important (and easily analyzable) route of loss for both ions is through the urine.

Indeed, appreciation of this concept is so critical to the proper management of hyponatremia that we will demonstrate its validity in two ways. It should be clear that the removal of 500 mEq of Na^+ from the extracellular space will lead to a lowering of plasma osmolality and $[Na^+]_p$. Since extracellular osmolality will now be less than intracellular osmolality, water will enter cells from the extracellular space so as to restore osmotic equilibrium. The net effect will be a lowering of osmolality throughout the body, both inside and outside cells. Correspondingly, if we remove 500 mEq of K^+ from the intracellular space, intracellular osmolality and $[K^+]_i$ will both be decreased. Since intracellular osmolality is now less than extracellular osmolality, water will therefore exit cells to restore equilibrium, the net effect once again being a lowering of osmolality both inside and outside cells. This heuristic argument is lent mathematical precision in Figure 22.4, in which we prove that the final $[Na^+]_p$ is in fact the same for the two cases.

We may summarize as follows:

Essential Concept #4. Na^+ and K^+ are the major effective osmoles in the body. Na^+ is largely restricted to and protects the extracellular volume; similarly, K^+ is restricted to and protects the intracellular volume. Although Na^+ and K^+ are segregated into distinct compartments, the free diffusion of water across cell membranes guarantees that, in the absence of any other effective osmoles (e.g. glucose), $[Na^+]_p$ and $[K^+]_i$ will be coordinately regulated and more or less equal. Furthermore, and even more remarkably, free diffusion of water also entails that the loss or gain from the body of a given number of milliequivalents of K^+ has a quantitatively identical effect on $[Na^+]_p$ as the loss or gain of the same number of milliequivalents of Na^+.

THE CLINICAL PUZZLE SOLVED

We are now in a position to explain the differential susceptibility to hyponatremia in patients with CHF vs SIADH. We consider first the patient with CHF. Of the 600 mOsm (milliosmoles) of solute in this patient's daily liter of urine, nearly all is urea (500 mOsm). As discussed previously, the ability of urea to move freely back and forth across cell membranes means that its removal from the body has no effect on $[Na^+]_p$. On the other hand, excretion of the water within which the urea is dissolved will tend to raise the concentration of $[Na^+]_p$. Once water has moved out of cells to restore equality of $[Na^+]_p$ and $[K^+]_i$, the net effect of urinary excretion in this patient will be to raise the $[Na^+]_p$ and protect against hyponatremia. Thus, in terms of its effect on $[Na^+]_p$, a concentrated urine whose osmolality is predominantly attributable to urea may be regarded as functionally equivalent to pure water. No matter how high the osmolality of the urine, as long as urea is the predominant osmole, excretion of urine will

increase $[Na^+]_p$. From this example, we can see that the problem in patients with CHF is not the quality of the urine produced by the kidney. The kidney is doing a more than adequate job with the urine it is able to produce. Rather, the problem is the quantity of urine. With a urine volume of only 1000 ml/day, excluding insensible losses, this patient can drink no more than 1000 ml of water/day, without further lowering of $[Na^+]_p$. The pathophysiology in this patient with CHF is representative of that in most patients with inadequate tissue perfusion and decreased effective circulating volume.

The situation is quite different for our patient with SIADH. In this case, a large fraction of the 600 Osm is taken up by Na^+, K^+, and their accompanying anions. Recall that, from the point of view of $[Na^+]_p$, the loss of each milliequivalent of K^+ has a quantitatively identical effect as the loss of each milliequivalent of Na^+. Therefore, we may simply add the concentrations of Na^+ and K^+ in the urine to get an idea of the net effect of their loss upon $[Na^+]_p$. Doing so, we find that urinary Na^+ plus urinary K^+, or $[Na^+]_u + [K^+]_u$ equals 165 mEq/L. If we compare this concentration to that of $[Na^+]_p$, or 110 mEq/L, we note that $[Na^+]_u + [K^+]_u$ is significantly greater. Thus, the urine of this patient with SIADH is more concentrated with respect to electrolytes than is plasma, and so the net effect of urinary excretion in this patient with SIADH will be to lower further the $[Na^+]_p$, and so exacerbate the pre-existing hyponatremia. The situation in this patient with SIADH is therefore remarkably different from that of the patient with CHF. In patients with SIADH, the quality of the urine is bad with respect to maintenance and/or restoration of a normal $[Na^+]_p$. These patients are in a no-win situation – in effect, doubly cursed. With every drop of water they drink, they lower their $[Na^+]_p$, and, far too often, with every drop of urine they generate, they tend to lower their $[Na^+]_p$ yet further.

QUANTITATIVE DETERMINATION OF ELECTROLYTE-FREE WATER EXCRETION

In this section, we will lend computational specificity to the ideas generated in our discussion of water balance for patients with CHF or SIADH. For most ICU patients, fluid inputs and outputs are carefully recorded, so that quantitative determination of water balance is a fairly straightforward procedure. To emphasize the importance of

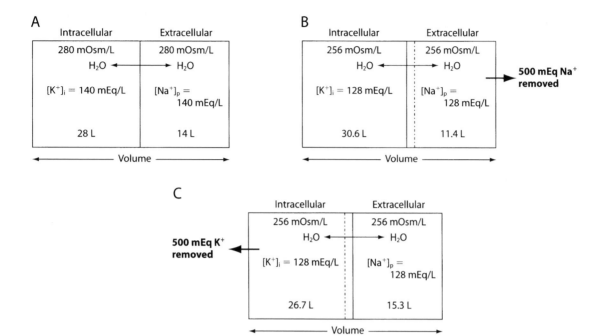

Figure 22.4 Loss of a given number of milliequivalents of K^+ has a quantitatively identical effect on $[Na^+]_p$ as the loss of the same number of milliequivalents of Na^+. We show here that removal from the body of 500 mEq of Na^+ from the extracellular compartment has the same effect on $[Na^+]_p$ as the loss of 500 mEq of K^+ from the intracellular compartment. Surprised? Read on.

(A) Consider a male patient of 70 kg in weight. His total body water (TBW) is 42 L, or 60% of his body weight. Of TBW, two-thirds, or 28 L, is intracellular (ICV), and one-third, or 14 L is extracellular (ECV). Therefore:

> Baseline total body solute = osmolality × TBW = 280 × 42 = 11 760 mOsm
> Baseline extracellular solute = osmolality × EVC = 280 × 14 = 3920 mOsm
> Baseline intracellular solute = osmolality × ICV = 280 × 28 = 7840 mOsm

(B) If we remove 500 mEq of Na^+ (with 500 mEq of accompanying anion) from the extracellular compartment, then:

> New total body solute = 11 760 − 1000 = 10 760 mOsm
> Osmolality = total body solute/TBW = 10760/42 = 256 mOsm/L
> New extracellular solute = 3920 − 1000 = 2920 mOsm
> New ECV = extracellular osmoles/osmolality = 2920/256 = 11.4 L
> New ICV = TBW − ECV = 42 − 11.4 = 30.6 L
> New intracellular osmolality = intracellular osmoles/ICV = 7840/30.6 = 256 mOsm/L (same as ECV)
> New $[Na^+]_p$ = osmolality/2 = 256/2 = 128 mEq/L

(C) Let us repeat the experiment, this time removing 500 mEq of K^+ (with 500 mEq of accompanying anion) from the intracellular compartment:

> New total body solute = 11 760 − 1000 = 10 760 mOsm
> Osmolality = total body solute/TBW = 10 760/42 = 256 mOsm/L
> New extracellular solute = 7840 − 1000 = 6840 mOsm
> New ICV = intracellular osmoles/osmolality = 6840/256 = 26.7 L
> New ECV = TBW − ICV = 42 − 26.7 = 15.3 L
> New extracellular osmolality = extracellular osmoles/ECV = 3920/15.3 = 256 mOsm/L (same as ICV)
> New $[Na^+]_p$ = osmolality/2 = 256/2 = 128 mEq/L

effective osmoles (electrolytes) over ineffective osmoles (urea) in determining $[Na^+]_p$, we will refer to the net urinary excretion of water, as put forth in this chapter, as electrolyte-free water excretion. We recommend the following algorithmic approach:

- STEP #1 = *Compare the sum of the concentration of sodium and potassium in the urine, $[Na^+]_u + [K^+]_u$, to the concentration of plasma sodium, $[Na^+]_p$*

A random urine at any time during the day is usually adequate. If the composition of the urine changes significantly throughout the day, then an aliquot from pooled urine collected over the course of the day should be used. If $[Na^+]_u + [K^+]_u < [Na^+]_p$, then the urine contains electrolyte-free water and the kidney is doing its job towards restoring $[Na^+]_p$ to normal. If $[Na^+]_u + [K^+]_u > [Na^+]_p$, then the kidney is contributing to the hyponatremia, and, with every drop of urine, the kidney is adding free water to the body and further lowering $[Na^+]_p$.

- STEP #2 = *Calculate the net effect of urinary excretion on water balance*

Consider the patient with CHF, whose $[Na^+]_u + [K^+]_u = 13$ mEq/L. Since the patient's $[Na^+]_p$ is 130 mEq/L, the urine contains one-tenth the electrolyte content of plasma, and nine-tenth's of the urine volume is free water. This patient's daily urinary excretion of free water is therefore 0.9×1000 ml, or 900 ml. Next, consider the patient with SIADH, whose $[Na^+]_u + [K^+]_u = 165$ mEq/L. Since this patient's $[Na^+]_p$ is 110 mEq/L, the urine contains $1.5 \times$ the electrolyte content of plasma. To reduce the $[Na^+]_u + [K^+]_u$ in a liter of urine from 165 mEq/L down to 110 mEq/L, we would need to add 500 ml of water. This is exactly how much free water the kidney has generated and added to the body. In the form of an equation, we have the following:

Electrolyte-free water excretion
$$= [\text{24-hour urine volume}] \times \left[1 - \frac{Na_u - K_u}{Na_p} \right] \quad (1)$$

Whenever the value is *positive*, as for the patient with CHF, then the kidney is *removing* water from the body. Whenever the value is *negative*, as for the patient with SIADH, then the kidney is *adding* water to the body.

- STEP #3 = *Repeat this calculation for any other fluids contributing significantly to net daily fluid output*

Eq (1) can also be used to calculate the electrolyte-free water excretion associated with diarrhea, pleural drainage, nasogastric suction, or any other fluid. One need only measure the concentration of Na^+ and K^+ in the relevant fluid, and substitute the values into Eq (1).

- STEP #4 = *Perform an analogous calculation for all daily fluid inputs*

One may similarly use Eq (1) to calculate the free water content of all administered fluids. Alternatively, one may note that, for example, 100% of the volume of D5W (isotonic dextrose) will be free water, or that 50% of the volume of 0.5NS (normal saline) will be free water.

- STEP #5 = *Combine these results to obtain a net daily balance of free water*

Combination of the volumes obtained in *STEPS #2, #3*, and *#4* provides the daily balance for water. The net contribution from insensible water losses plus metabolic generation of water may be estimated as the removal of ~500 ml of water.

We provide a step-by-step example of the application of this algorithm in Figure 22.5.

CLINICAL CONSEQUENCES OF HYPONATREMIA

In the following discussion, we limit ourselves to those clinical settings for which hyponatremia reflects true hypo-osmolality of the extracellular and intracellular compartments. We are therefore excluding those situations in which hyponatremia is due to the addition to the extracellular fluid of an effective osmole such as glucose or mannitol.

The clinical manifestations of hyponatremia are primarily due to neurologic dysfunction. As $[Na^+]_p$ decreases, water will move from the extracellular into the intracellular space in order to maintain equality of osmolality in these two compartments. This movement of water into cells leads to the swelling of brain cells, and consequent cerebral edema. Signs and symptoms of hyponatremia do not usually occur until $[Na^+]_p$ is less than 125 mEq/L. Initial manifestations may include malaise, nausea, and vomiting. With increasing

---

Case

You are asked to consult on a 65-year-old male with small cell cancer of the lung, who was transferred to the ICU for evaluation of altered mental status of 3 days' duration. Initial evaluation reveals an obtunded male who appears to be euvolemic. Neuroimaging studies are negative. His mass is 60 kg. Relevant laboratory data are as follows:

$$[Na^+]_p = 110 \text{ mEq/L}$$
Plasma osmolality = 230 mOsm/L
Urine osmolality = 600 mOsm/L
$$[Na^+]_u = 100 \text{ mEq/L}$$
$$[K^+]_u = 60 \text{ mEq/L}$$
24-hour urine volume = 1L

Evaluation

The patient is currently receiving half-normal saline at 83 ml/min, or 2.0 L/day.

- *STEP #1 = Compare the sum of the concentration of sodium and potassium in the urine, $[Na^+]_u + [K^+]_u$, to the concentration of plasma sodium, $[Na^+]_p$.*

The sum of $[Na^+]_u$ plus $[K^+]_u$ equals 160 mEq/L and exceeds $[Na^+]_p$, which is 110 mEq/L. The kidney is therefore contributing to hyponatremia. With each drop of urine, the kidney is adding free water to the body and further lowering $[Na^+]_p$.

- *STEP #2 = Calculate the net effect of urinary excretion on water balance.*

We apply Eq (1) to calculate the volume of free water generated each day by the kidney.

$$\text{Electrolyte-free water excretion} = [\text{24-hour urine volume}] \times \left[1 - \frac{Na_u + K_u}{Na_p} \right]$$

$$= [1 \text{ L}] \times \left[1 - \frac{160}{110} \right] = -0.45 \text{ L}$$

The negative value means that the kidney has generated and added to the body 450 ml of free water in the process of producing urine.

- *STEP #3 = Repeat this calculation for any other fluids contributing significantly to net daily fluid output.*

The patient does not have any other significant fluid outputs.

- *STEP #4 = Perform an analogous calculation for all daily fluid inputs.*

The sole fluid input is 2.0 L of half-normal saline, 50% of which will be free water. He is therefore receiving 1.0 L of free water per day.

- *STEP #5 = Combine these results to obtain a net daily balance of free water.*

The patient's net daily balance of free water includes the addition of 1000 ml intravenously plus the renal generation of 450 ml. He loses approximately 450 ml of free water daily by insensible means. His net daily balance is therefore the addition of 1000 ml of free water. Assuming no alteration in his management, his $[Na^+]_p$ will decline by approximately 2–3 mEq/L per day.

This patient most likely has SIADH related to his small cell cancer. The presence of neurologic symptoms mandates emergent treatment with hypertonic saline. Moreover, as discussed in the text, the use of any intravenous fluid, including normal saline, is not only ineffective but commonly leads to further lowering of $[Na^+]_p$ in patients with SIADH.

Figure 22.5 A clinical example of the stepwise approach to hyponatremia.

severity of hyponatremia, headaches, lethargy, and obtundation may supervene. Seizures and coma are uncommon unless $[Na^+]_p$ falls below 110 mEq/L.[28,29]

In general, the severity of manifestations depends critically on two factors:

- the degree of hyponatremia

- the rate, or the rapidity, of the decline in $[Na^+]_p$.

Whereas it is easy to understand why the degree of hyponatremia should correlate with the severity of neurologic symptoms and signs, the relationship between the rate of decline in $[Na^+]_p$ and clinical severity is best understood within the context of osmotic adaptation.

Osmotic adaptation to hyponatremia

Brain cells protect themselves against edema from hyponatremia through two major adaptive responses. The first of these occurs immediately and is a direct consequence of the cerebral edema. The increase in intracranial pressure resulting from cerebral edema leads to the transudation of fluid from the interstitium into the cerebrospinal fluid, thereby easing the effects of cerebral edema.

The second adaptive response requires time and represents a specific attempt by each of the brain cells individually to mitigate the increase in its cell volume. By actively transporting solutes from the intracellular to the extracellular space, brain cells reduce their intracellular osmolality, thereby promoting the exit of water and minimizing the degree of cell swelling. A small fraction of these solutes are intracellular electrolytes, such as K^+, but by far the quantitatively most important solutes are organic solutes like inositol and several amino acids.[30] Extrusion of these organic solutes requires the synthesis of new transporters, and therefore takes place over hours to days. For this reason, acute hyponatremia will generally result in greater clinical severity, since brain cells do not have sufficient time to adapt. In contrast, chronic hyponatremia may be clinically silent, even at alarmingly low values of $[Na^+]_p$, as osmotic adaptation is virtually complete within 72 hours.

TREATMENT OF HYPONATREMIA

Optimal management of patients with hyponatremia requires evaluation of the following two areas:

- the degree of hyponatremia, the rapidity of onset, and the presence and severity of clinical signs and symptoms
- the clinical setting, in particular, the patient's volume status, as determined by physical examination.

In general, the first determines whom to treat, whereas the second determines how best to treat (Fig 22.6).

A useful rule of thumb is that restoration to a normal $[Na^+]_p$ should take place over roughly the same period of time as it took for the hyponatremia to develop. If one is uncertain about the time of development, then one should assume that the hyponatremia is chronic ($\geq$72 hours) and full osmotic adaptation has already occurred. Before providing specific recommendations, we need to discuss the considerable risks of therapy in hyponatremic patients.

Risks of treatment

The rate of correction is crucial in patients with chronic hyponatremia for whom osmotic adaptation has been completed. By extruding intracellular solutes, brain cells have returned their cell volume to a pretty much normal level. As treatment commences, and $[Na^+]_p$ and extracellular osmolality increase, water will be drawn out of brain cells. These cells are now confronted with the opposite problem: namely, cell shrinkage and reduced cellular volume. If the rate of correction of hyponatremia is too rapid, then the brain cells lack sufficient time to readapt and reaccumulate the previously extruded solutes. Irreversible neurologic complications may ensue, the most dreaded of which is central pontine myelinolysis (CPM) or osmotic demyelination.[31,32]

CPM is characterized by paraparesis or quadraparesis, dysarthria, dysphagia, coma, and, less commonly, seizures. CPM most probably occurs as a result of abrupt axonal shrinkage, severing the connection of the axons with the surrounding myelin sheaths. The onset of CPM is usually one to several days after treatment. Diagnosis, suggested by clinical findings, can be confirmed by computed tomography or magnetic resonance imaging. Importantly, characteristic radiologic findings may require as long as 4 weeks to appear.[33]

Several risk factors for the development of CPM have been identified. These include:

- correction of the $[Na^+]_p$ by more than 12 mEq/L in the first 24 hours
- overcorrection of the $[Na^+]_p$ to a level greater than 140 mEq/L in the first 48 hours
- hypoxic episodes prior to the initiation of therapy
- malnutrition or hypercatabolism, especially in patients with chronic alcoholism, burns, or severe malignancy.[34]

An unresolved issue is whether water should be given to lower the $[Na^+]_p$ in patients whose hyponatremia has been corrected too rapidly. There are no clinical data addressing this question, but animal studies suggest that, while CPM cannot be reversed by re-lowering the $[Na^+]_p$, the incidence and severity of CPM may be reduced if the $[Na^+]_p$ is re-lowered *before* the onset of neurologic signs or symptoms.

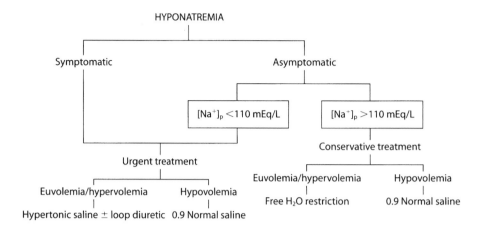

Figure 22.6 Treatment of hyponatremia.

Whom to treat

All patients with hyponatremia require evaluation and appropriate intervention. Treatment may be conservative (e.g. water restriction and correction of hypokalemia) or more aggressive (e.g. administration of hypertonic saline). In this section, we identify those patients requiring nonconservative treatment.

The presence of any neurologic symptoms whatsoever in patients whose $[Na^+]_p$ is less than 125 mEq/L warrants immediate aggressive treatment. The risks of hyponatremia outweigh the risks of treatment, and $[Na^+]_p$ should be raised at a rate of 1.5–2.0 mEq/L/h for 3 or 4 hours, or until neurologic abnormalities resolve.[35,36]

In patients with chronic hyponatremia and no neurologic abnormalities, an $[Na^+]_p$ below 110 mEq/L would seem to warrant intervention, because of the increased risk of seizures and coma. However, correction should be undertaken with extreme caution, and the rate of correction should be kept below 0.5 mEq/L/h, and the target $[Na^+]_p$ should be no higher than 120 mEq/L.

How to treat

Acute volume depletion
Appropriate treatment for patients with hyponatremia is determined by the patient's volume status. In patients with true volume depletion, initial management involves administration of isotonic fluids or colloids to restore adequate tissue perfusion. This will eliminate the nonosmotic stimulus

to ADH secretion, with the result that the concentration of circulating ADH will typically plummet to minimal levels. Urinary flow will then increase, and urinary electrolyte-free water content will approach 100%. The ensuing correction of hyponatremia will be spontaneous and rapid. Fortunately, hyponatremia in patients with true volume depletion is virtually always acute, since sustained tissue underperfusion rarely persists for very long because of its life-threatening implications. As there is insufficient time for osmotic adaptation to occur, the risk of overly rapid correction does not exist.

Nonemergent hyponatremia in patients with normal or increased extracellular fluid volume
The mainstay of treatment for hyponatremic patients whose volume status is normal or increased is the restriction of water intake. The degree of water restriction should be maintained at a level equal to or below that of electrolyte-free water excretion, as calculated by the algorithmic approach described above. Hypokalemia should also be corrected, since deficits in total body potassium can also contribute significantly to lowering of $[Na^+]_p$ (see Fig. 22.4).

Urgent or emergent hyponatremia in patients with normal or increased extracellular fluid volume
Hyponatremic patients with neurologic abnormalities and/or an $[Na^+]_p$ less than 110 mEq/L require more aggressive raising of their $[Na^+]_p$. This may be accomplished through administration of hypertonic saline. Since the rate of increase of $[Na^+]_p$

must be carefully monitored, it is vital to calculate beforehand the exact rate of administration of hypertonic saline that will raise $[Na^+]_p$ at the desired rate.

This is fairly easily accomplished, as long as one bears in mind the physiologic principles discussed in this chapter. Two of these principles merit re-emphasis. First, because of the free movement of water across cell membranes, reduced extracellular osmolality is matched by reduced intracellular osmolality, and $[Na^+]_p$ approximately equals $[K^+]_i$. Therefore, we need to administer enough hypertonic saline not only to increase $[Na^+]_p$ to the desired level but also to increase $[K^+]_i$ to the same level. As long as we use total body water as the relevant volume into which we will be adding the hypertonic saline, we can rely on the free movement of water across cell membranes to take care of both $[Na^+]_p$ and $[K^+]_i$ in parallel. Secondly, from the point of view of $[Na^+]_p$, the effect of every ion of Na^+ is equal to that of every ion of K^+. Although we wish to correct both extracellular hyponatremia and intracellular hypokalemia, administration of hypertonic saline, which contains only Na^+, will achieve both objectives.

We illustrate the calculation through the following clinical example. Imagine a 60 kg patient with symptomatic hyponatremia of 105 mEq/L. We set a target $[Na^+]_p$ of 120 mEq/L. We therefore wish to increase $[Na^+]_p$ by 15 mEq/L. We estimate total body water in liters as 60% of the mass in kilograms, or 36 L. To raise the $[Na^+]_p$ in 36 L by 15 mEq/L, we must add 36 × 15, or 540 mEq of Na^+. Since hypertonic saline (3% sodium chloride) contains 513 mEq of Na^+ per liter, we need to administer just over 1 L of hypertonic saline. At a rate of 1.5–2.0 mEq/L/h, increasing $[Na^+]_p$ by 15 mEq will take 7.5–10 hours. We therefore infuse 1 L of hypertonic saline over 7.5–10 hours. At the end of this infusion, both $[Na^+]_p$ and $[K^+]_i$ will have risen from 105 mEq/L to 120 mEq/L, although the mechanism in each case will differ: $[Na^+]_p$ will have risen because of the addition of Na^+ to the extracellular fluid, whereas $[K^+]_i$ will have risen because of the exit of water from within cells, in response to the rise in extracellular osmolality.

To summarize, the volume of hypertonic saline that needs to be administered can be calculated through the following two equations:

$$\text{Osmolar deficit} = 0.6 \times [\text{weight in kilograms}] \times \{\text{target } [Na^+]_p - \text{patient } [Na^+]_p\} \qquad (2a)$$

$$\text{Volume of hypertonic saline (3\% saline)} = (\tfrac{1}{513}) \times [\text{Osmolar deficit}] \qquad (2b)$$

The role of loop diuretics

A loop diuretic is often given concurrently with hypertonic saline. In the case of patients with CHF, or other types of volume overload, this is necessary in order to prevent complications such as pulmonary edema. Although an essential part of treatment, the effect of a loop diuretic on overall water balance in such patients can be difficult to predict. Examination of Eq (1) helps to explain this element of unpredictability. On the one hand, a loop diuretic will increase the electrolyte content of the urine in patients with CHF or similar conditions, thereby reducing the free water content of the urine. On the other hand, a loop diuretic will increase the overall volume of urine, thereby improving free water excretion. Only careful monitoring, and application of Eq (1), will determine which of these two opposing factors predominates.

Using a loop diuretic in patients with SIADH has a different basis. Recall that the electrolyte content of the urine for patients with SIADH is often greater than $[Na^+]_p$, so that the mere act of urination adds free water to the body. By inhibiting the countercurrent exchange mechanism in the renal medulla, loop diuretics prevent urinary dilution and concentration. ADH is no longer able to concentrate the urine, and therefore the urine of patients with SIADH may be converted from water-generating to water-excreting. In conjunction with hypertonic saline, this is a considerable advantage for patients requiring emergent elevation of their $[Na^+]_p$. However, in the absence of an emergent reason for raising $[Na^+]_p$, we recommend that a loop diuretic not be used in patients with SIADH because of the risk of superimposing the additional problem of hypovolemia onto pre-existing hyponatremia.

The dangers of saline

Except in patients with true volume depletion, infusion of normal saline is ineffective, and even potentially dangerous, in patients with hyponatremia. For patients with CHF or other sodium-retentive states, administration of saline will only compound the degree of volume overload. In patients with SIADH, the problem is subtler. Patients with SIADH are essentially euvolemic and in perfect sodium balance. This means that every milliequivalent of administered Na^+ will be excreted in the urine. The electrolyte content of normal saline is 154 mEq/L. If the electrolyte content of the patient's urine is greater than 154 mEq/L, i.e. if $[Na^+]_u + [K^+]_u > 154$ mEq/L, then all the Na^+ contained within the infused normal saline will be excreted in a volume of urine less than that of the saline. The remaining volume will be added to the body as free water. The end result, therefore, of administering normal saline to a patient with SIADH is to lower the $[Na^+]_p$ further. Hypertonic saline does not have the same effect in patients with SIADH, because the electrolyte content of the urine virtually never exceeds 513 mEq/L (3% saline) or 855 mEq/L (5% saline). Even in the absence of a loop diuretic, excretion of the total quantity of Na^+ will therefore require a volume of urine larger than that of the infused hypertonic saline. The difference between these two volumes equals the net volume of free water removed from the body.

HYPERNATREMIA

Hypernatremia virtually always indicates increased plasma osmolality. Like hyponatremia, hypernatremia is an abnormality in the *concentration* of $[Na^+]_p$ and can be detected only by a laboratory measurement. Patients with hypernatremia may have normal, increased, or decreased extracellular volume, as assessed by physical examination. The free movement of water across cell membranes implies that intracellular osmolality will be increased to a similar extent as extracellular osmolality. In other words, extracellular hypernatremia implies intracellular hyperkalemia, and $[Na^+]_p$ will approximately equal $[K^+]_i$. The physiologic principles underlying the diagnosis and management of hypernatremia are the same as those for hyponatremia, and therefore our discussion of hypernatremia will be abbreviated.

Normal defenses against hypernatremia

The kidney's role in hypernatremia is the converse of that in hyponatremia. Whereas the kidney literally can correct hyponatremia on its own by excreting electrolyte-free water, its job in hypernatremia is more ancillary, in that the kidney cannot itself return the increased $[Na^+]_p$ to normal. Restoration of a normal $[Na^+]_p$ requires an intact thirst mechanism or, in the case of ICU patients, a vigilant team providing an adequate intake of free water. The kidney's sole mandate in hypernatremia is to hold the fort and not exacerbate the problem. This entails the excretion of a minimal volume of electrolyte-free water.

Even in cases where the kidney fails in its mandate, as in diabetes insipidus, thirst is so powerful a drive that $[Na^+]_p$ rarely increases more than a few mEq/L above normal. The problem for ICU patients is either that their thirst mechanism is blunted (e.g. decreased level of consciousness) or that they have essentially no access to water. Thus, hypernatremia in the ICU setting is almost always iatrogenic, and reflects inadequate 'thirst' on the part of the physicians caring for the patient.

Renal requirements for conservation of free water

Excretion by the kidney of a minimal volume of free water has three requirements, which will now be considered.

Increased antidiuretic hormone secretion
In the presence of ADH, the urine is maximally concentrated. The normal response to hypernatremia and increased plasma osmolality is stimulation of ADH secretion. Therefore, as opposed to hyponatremia, there is rarely a conflict between the regulation of osmolality and the regulation of volume for patients with hypernatremia. Whatever the non-osmotic reason for ADH release, whether decreased effective circulating volume or pain or nausea, the increase in circulating ADH will appropriately promote excretion of a maximally concentrated urine. Patients with a failure either to release or to respond to ADH, denoted as central or nephrogenic diabetes insipidus, respectively, will present with polyuria and hypernatremia.

Functioning loop of Henle
In the absence of a functioning loop of Henle, the kidney can neither concentrate nor dilute the urine, irrespective of the presence or absence of ADH. Damage to this portion of the nephron, as in chronic renal failure of any cause, or inhibition of its function, through the use of loop diuretics such as furosemide, will prevent concentration of the urine and retention of free water.

Absence of an increased daily osmotic load
An important, but far too often overlooked, cause of polyuria and hypernatremia is an increased

daily osmotic load. Urinary concentration and dilution are both impaired through multiple inter-related effects on individual nephron segments. Obvious sources of excess osmoles include hyper-glycemia or agents such as mannitol. However, the source of increased osmoles can often be occult. For example, increased urea production, as a result of increased catabolism or overfeeding, both common occurrences in ICU patients, can also produce an osmotic diuresis. Recognition of this problem requires measurement of the daily osmolar excre-tion (urine volume × urine osmolality). Normal osmolar excretion is ~10 mOsm/kg/day.

Diagnostic approach to hypernatremia

Like hyponatremia, hypernatremia is a syndrome with multiple potential causes. Once again, a use-ful approach is to stratify patients according to their volume status (Fig. 22.7). For each of the causes of hypernatremia, we indicate the mecha-nism (Table 22.4). In the case of excessive renal water losses, we indicate which of the require-ments for renal conservation of free water is deranged.

Osmotic adaptation to hypernatremia

The clinical manifestations of hypernatremia are primarily due to neurologic dysfunction. As $[Na^+]_p$ increases, water will move from the intra-cellular into the extracellular space in order to maintain equality of osmolality in these two com-partments. This movement of water out of cells leads to cerebral dehydration and the shrinkage of brain cells. As with hyponatremia, the signs and symptoms of hypernatremia can range from lethargy to seizures, coma, or death.[37] Permanent neurologic dysfunction is uncommon unless $[Na^+]_p$ increases above 158 mEq/L.[38]

In general, the severity of manifestations depends critically on two factors:

- the degree of hypernatremia
- the rate, or the rapidity, of the increase in $[Na^+]_p$.

As for hyponatremia, the relationship between the rate of increase in $[Na^+]_p$ and clinical severity is best understood within the context of osmotic adaptation.

Brain cells protect themselves against shrinkage from hypernatremia by increasing intracellular

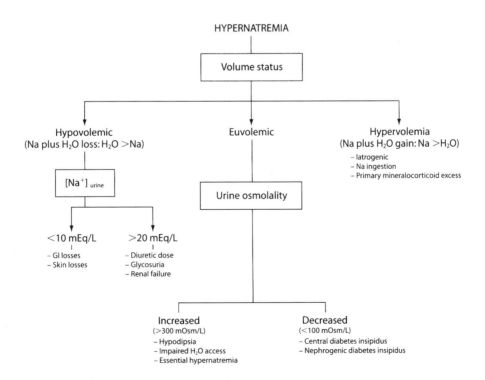

Figure 22.7 Algorithmic approach to hypernatremia. GI = gastrointestinal.

Table 22.4   Causes of hypernatremia.

Etiology	Source	Clinical condition	Mechanism
Water loss	Skin	Burns High fever Post-exercise	Insensible loss
	GI losses	Osmotic diarrhea Vomiting Nasogastric suction Enterocutaneous fistula	Hypotonic losses

	Central diabetes insipidus	Trauma
		Neurosurgery:
		    transsphenoidal
		Malignancy:
		    primary
		    metastatic
		Infection
		Infiltrating disease:
		    sarcoidosis
		    histiocytosis X
		Strokes
		Encephalopathy
			ADH deficiency

	Renal losses	Nephrogenic diabetes insipidus Osmotic diuresis Loop diuretics	ADH resistance Increased osmotic load Nonfunctioning loop
	Central causes	Hypodipsia Essential hypernatremia Stroke/dementia	Thirst center defect Osmoreceptor defect Impaired access to water

Sodium retention	Iatrogenic	Administration of hypertonic fluids:
		    parenteral
		    enteral
			Increased Na load

	Increased NaCl ingestion	? Psychiatric	Increased Na load
	Central causes	Primary mineralocorticoid excess	Reset osmostat
Redistribution of water	Movement of water into cells	Seizures Extreme exercise Rhabdomyolysis	Transient increase in intracellular osmolality

ADH = antidiuretic hormone; GI = gastrointestinal.

osmolality. By actively accumulating intracellular solutes, brain cells promote the retention and entry of water, thereby minimizing the degree of cell shrinkage. A small fraction of the accumulated osmoles are extracellular electrolytes, such as Na$^+$ or K$^+$, that are actively transported from the extra-cellular space into cells. However, by far the quantitatively most important solutes are synthesized by the cells. Such so-called 'idiogenic' osmoles include organic molecules like inositol, glutamine, and glutamate.[39,40] Synthesis of these organic solutes begins within hours, and is usually complete by 24–48 hours. For this reason, acute hypernatremia will generally result in greater clinical severity, since brain cells do not have sufficient time to adapt. In contrast, chronic hypernatremia may be clinically silent, even at alarmingly high values of $[Na^+]_p$.

Risks of treatment of hypernatremia

The rate of correction is just as crucial in patients with chronic hypernatremia, for whom osmotic adaptation has been completed, as it is in patients with chronic hyponatremia. By accumulating intracellular solutes, brain cells have returned their cell volume to a pretty much normal level. As treatment commences, and $[Na^+]_p$ and extracellular osmolality decrease, water will enter brain cells. These cells are now confronted with the opposite problem: namely, cell swelling and increased cellular volume. If the rate of correction of hypernatremia is too rapid, then brain cells lack sufficient time to readapt and rid themselves of the previously accumulated solutes. Irreversible neurologic complications may ensue as a result of the consequent cerebral edema.[41,42]

Treatment of hypernatremia

Treatment of hypernatremia is aimed first at correction of the underlying cause (see Fig. 22.7 and Table 22.4), followed by administration of sufficient water to lower the $[Na^+]_p$ back to the normal range. As for hyponatremia, the rate of correction should not exceed 0.5 mEq/L/h, or 12 mEq/L/day.[43]

Determination of the free water deficit is fairly straightforward. Because of the free movement of water across cell membranes, increased extracellular osmolality is matched by increased intracellular osmolality, and $[Na^+]_p$ approximately equals $[K^+]_i$. Therefore, we need to administer enough free water not only to lower $[Na^+]_p$ to the desired level but also to decrease $[K^+]_i$ to the same level. As long as we use total body water as the relevant volume into which we will be adding the free water, we can rely on the free movement of water across cell membranes to take care of both $[Na^+]_p$ and $[K^+]_i$ in parallel.

We illustrate the calculation through the following clinical example. Imagine a 60 kg patient with hypernatremia to 170 mEq/L. We wish to decrease $[Na^+]_p$ by 12 mEq/L in the first day, so our target

$[Na^+]_p$ is 158 mEq/L. We estimate total body water in liters as 60% of the mass in kilograms, or 36 L. We wish to lower $[Na^+]_p$ and $[K^+]_i$ by 12/158, or ~7%. We therefore need to administer sufficient free water to increase total body water by 7%, or 2.5 L (0.07×36). Taking into account insensible losses, we should therefore administer 3.0 L of free water over the first day. If there are ongoing electrolyte-free water losses through the kidney or other routes (Eq (1)), then these losses need to be added onto the baseline value of 3.0 L. Once we have infused the final calculated volume of free water, both $[Na^+]_p$ and $[K^+]_i$ will have decreased from 170 mEq/L to 158 mEq/L.

To summarize, the volume of free water that needs to be administered can be calculated through the following equation:

$$\text{Free water deficit} = 0.6 \times [\text{weight in kilograms}] \times \left\{ 1 - \frac{[Na]_{target}}{[Na]_{patient}} \right\} \tag{3}$$

The free water can be administered in several different forms, depending upon the patient's volume status. For euvolemic patients, administration of intravenous D5W or enteral water is easiest. In patients with hypernatremia and true volume depletion, first and foremost, adequate tissue perfusion should be restored through administration of isotonic fluids such as normal saline. Only after the circulating volume has been restored to clinically safe levels should correction of hypernatremia be undertaken through administration of free water. The calculated free water deficit can then be given as entirely D5W, as twice the volume of 0.5 NS, or some combination thereof.

Patients with CHF, or another cause of volume overload, warrant special comment. Such patients typically receive inadequate free water, leading to persistence or even worsening of their hypernatremia. Inadequate treatment stems from inappropriate concern over the seemingly large daily volume of free water that needs to be given. It is crucial to remember that the administered free water will distribute evenly over total body water. In the example we gave above, this means that, of the required 3 L of water, 2/3 (2 L) will go to the intracellular space and 1/3 (1 L) will go to the extracellular space. Of the 1 L in the extracellular space, only 1/4 (250 ml) will end up in the vascular space, and 3/4 (750 ml) will end up in the interstitium. Even in a patient with fairly severe CHF, the addition of 250 ml to the vascular space over 24 hours is a relatively safe procedure.

REFERENCES

1. Zimmerman EA, Nilaver G, Hou-Yu A, et al. Vasopressinergic and oxytocinergic pathways in central nervous system. Fed Proc 1984;43:91–6.
2. Baylis PH. Osmoregulation and control of vasopressin secretion in healthy humans. Am J Physiol 1987;253:R671–8.
3. Robertson GL. Physiology of ADH secretion. Kidney Int Suppl 1987;21:S20–6.
4. Zimmerman EA, Ma L-Y, Nilaver G. Anatomical basis of thirst and vasopressin secretion. Kidney Int Suppl 1987;21:S14–19.
5. Bie P, Secher NH, Astrup A, Warberg J. Cardiovascular and endocrine responses to head-up tilt and vasopressin infusions in humans. Am J Physiol 1986;251:R735–8.
6. Goldsmith SR, Francis GS, Cowley AW, et al. Response of vasopressin and norepinephrine to lower body negative pressure in humans. Am J Physiol 1982;243:H970.
7. Mettauer B, Rouleau JL, Bichet D, et al. Sodium and water excretion abnormalities in congestive heart failure. Ann Intern Med 1986;105:161–7.
8. Dunn FL, Brennan TJ, Nelson AE, Robertson GL. The role of blood osmolality and volume in regulating vasopressin secretion in the rat. J Clin Invest 1973;52:3212–19.
9. Derubertis FR Jr, Michelis FM, Bloom ME, et al. Impaired water excretion in myxedema. Am J Med 1971;51:41–53.
10. Raff H. Glucocorticoid inhibition of neurohypophyseal vasopressin secretion. Am J Physiol 1987;252:R635–64.
11. Guglielminotti J, Pernet P, Maury E, et al. Osmolar gap hyponatremia in critically ill patients: evidence for the sick cell syndrome? Crit Care Med 2002;30:1051–5.
12. Ukai M, Moran W Jr, Zimmerman B. The role of visceral afferent pathways on vasopressin secretion and urinary excretory patterns during surgical stress. Ann Surg 1968;168:16–28.
13. Editorial. Nausea and vasopressin. Lancet 1991;337:1133–4.
14. Wijdicks EF, Vermeulen M, Hijdra A, et al. Hyponatremia and cerebral infarction in patients with ruptured intracranial aneurysms: is fluid restriction harmful? Ann Neurol 1985;17:137–40.
15. Glassock RJ, Cohen AH, Danovitch G, et al. Human immunodeficiency virus (HIV) and the kidney. Ann Intern Med 1990;112:35–49.
16. Anderson RJ. Hospital-associated hyponatremia. Kidney Int 1986;29:1237–47.
17. Hill AR, Uribarri J, Mann J, et al. Altered water metabolism in tuberculosis: role of vasopressin. Am J Med 1990;88:357–64.
18. Szatalowicz VL, Goldberg JP, Anderson RJ. Plasma antidiuretic hormone in acute respiratory failure. Am J Med 1982;72:583–7.
19. George JM, Capen CC, Phillips AS. Biosynthesis of vasopressin in vitro and ultrastructure of a bronchogenic carcinoma. J Clin Invest 1972;51:141–8.
20. Osterman J, Calhoun A, Dunham M, et al. Chronic syndrome of inappropriate antidiuretic hormone secretion and hypertension in a patient with olfactory neuroblastoma. Evidence of ectopic production of arginine vasopressin by the tumor. Arch Intern Med 1986;146:1731–5.
21. Peck V, Shenkman L. Haloperidol-induced syndrome of inappropriate secretion of antidiuretic hormone. Clin Pharmacol Therap 1979;26:442–4.
22. Smith NJ, Espir ML, Baylis PH. Raised plasma arginine vasopressin concentration in carbamazepine-induced water intoxication. Br Med J 1977;2:804.
23. Robertson GL, Bhoopalam N, Zelkowitz LJ. Vincristine neurotoxicity and abnormal secretion of antidiuretic hormone. Arch Intern Med 1973;132:717–20.
24. Ashraf N, Locksley R, Arieff AI. Thiazide-induced hyponatremia associated with death or neurologic damage in outpatients. Am J Med 1981;70:1163–8.
25. Szatalowicz VL, Miller PD, Lacher JW, et al. Comparative effects of diuretics on renal water excretion in hyponatremic oedematous disorders. Clin Sci 1982;62:235–8.
26. Sunderrajan S, Bauer JH, Vopat RL, et al. Posttransurethral prostatic resection hyponatremic syndrome: case report and review of the literature. Am J Kidney Dis 1984;4:80–4.
27. Rhymer JC, Bell TJ, Perry KC, et al. Hyponatremia following transurethral resection of the prostate. Br J Urol 1985;57:450–2.
28. Arieff AI, Llach F, Massry SG. Neurological manifestations and morbidity of hyponatremia: correlation with brain water and electrolytes. Medicine 1976;55:121–9.
29. Arieff AI. Hyponatremia, convulsions, respiratory arrest and permanent brain damage after elective surgery in healthy women. N Engl J Med 1986;314:1529–35.
30. Verbalis JG, Gullans SR. Hyponatremia causes large sustained reductions in brain content of multiple organic osmolytes in rats. Brain Res 1991;567:274–82.
31. Sterns RH, Thomas DJ, Herndon RM. Brain dehydration and neurologic dehydration after correction of hyponatremia. Kidney Int 1989;35:69–75.
32. Kleinschmidt-DeMasters BK, Norenberg MD. Rapid correction of hyponatremia causes demyelination: relation to central pontine myelinolysis. Science 1981;211:1068–70.
33. Brunner JE, Redmond JM, Haggar AM, et al. Central pontine myelinolysis and pontine lesions after rapid correction of hyponatremia: a prospective magnetic resonance imaging study. Ann Neurol 1990;27:61–6.
34. Mckee AC, Winkelman MD, Banker BQ. Central pontine myelinolysis in severely burnt patients: relationship to serum hyperosmolality. Neurology 1988;38:1211–17.
35. Berl T. Treating hyponatremia: damned if we do and damned if we don't. Kidney Int 1990;37:1006–18.
36. Cluitmans FH, Meinders AE. Management of hyponatremia: rapid or slow correction. Am J Med 1990;88:161–6.
37. Arieff AI, Guisado R. Effects on the central nervous system of hypernatremic and hyponatremic states. Kidney Int 1976;10:104–16.
38. Morris-Jones PH, Houston IB, Evans RC. Prognosis of the neurological complications of acute hypernatremia. Lancet 1967;2:1385–9.
39. Heilig CW, Stromski ME, Blumenfeld JB, Lee JP, Gullans SR. Characterization of the major brain osmolytes that accumulate in salt-loaded rats. Am J Physiol 1989;257:F1108–16.
40. Lien YH, Shapiro JI, Chan L. Effect of hypernatremia on organic brain osmoles. J Clin Invest 1990;85:1427–35.
41. Pollock AS, Arieff AI. Abnormalities of cell volume regulation and their functional consequences. Am J Physiol 1980;239:F195–205.
42. Hogan G, Dodge PR, Gill S, et al. Pathogenesis of seizures occurring during restoration of plasma tonicity to normal in animals previously chronically hypernatremic. Pediatrics 1969;43:54–64.
43. Blum D, Brasseur D, Kahn A, et al. Safe oral rehydration of hypertonic dehydration. J Pediatr Gastroenterol Nutr 1986;5:232–5.

23

Disorders of potassium homeostasis

Joel Michels Topf and John R Asplin

INTRODUCTION

Potassium is the most common cation in the body. Adults typically have between 3 and 4 moles of potassium, 98% of which is located intracellularly. Potassium's clinical importance comes chiefly from the fact that the ratio of intracellular to extracellular potassium is the primary determinant of the resting membrane potential (E_m). Increased extracellular potassium decreases the $I:E$ ratio and reduces the resting membrane potential; decreased extracellular potassium increases the ratio and hyperpolarizes the membrane (makes E_m more negative). Alterations in the E_m disrupt depolarizing tissues, e.g. neural, cardiac, and muscular.

The fine homeostatic control that the body has over extracellular potassium can be demonstrated by two observations:

1. Since 98% of total body potassium is located intracellularly, the movement of 1–2% of intracellular potassium to the extracellular compartment would increase the serum potassium concentration to a life-threatening 8 mmol/L.
2. The daily dietary potassium intake is roughly equal to the total amount of extracellular potassium. A failure to either shift this dietary potassium to the intracellular compartment or excrete it would double the serum potassium.

Normal serum potassium concentration runs from 3.5 to 5.2 mmol/L. The molecular weight of potassium is 39.1, so a daily potassium intake of 80 mmol is roughly equivalent to 3.1 g of potassium.

NORMAL POTASSIUM METABOLISM

The normal physiologic handling of potassium can be viewed as a three-step process: ingestion, cellular distribution, and excretion. Irregularities at any of these steps can result in pathologic serum potassium concentrations.

Intestinal absorption

Potassium is ubiquitous in the diet, and is found in fruits, vegetables, and meats. Grain products tend to be low in potassium. Normal daily intake is roughly 40–80 mmol. In the United States, people of lower socioeconomic class, African-Americans, and the elderly all have low potassium intake.[1]

Potassium is absorbed rapidly from the small intestine. Data on the relative importance of ileum vs jejunum in normal potassium absorption are inconclusive but patients with short bowel syndrome maintain potassium absorption down to a jejunal length of 50 cm. The studies on the colonic handling of potassium are likewise conflicting, with some studies suggesting a small amount (4 mEq/day) of potassium secretion, whereas others suggest a small amount (4 mEq/day) of potassium absorption.[2,3] Potassium absorption in the gut occurs down an electrochemical gradient and is thought to be paracellular. Net gastrointestinal (GI) absorption (intake − GI losses) is approximately 90%. Typical stool potassium content is 10 mEq/day. Absorption remains near 90% with potassium-rich diets (i.e. there is no adaptive response to reduce potassium absorption in the face of increased dietary potassium). There is a small decrease in fecal potassium loss in response to a potassium-poor diet; stool potassium content falls from an average of 10 mEq/day to 3.5 mEq/day.[4] This reflects decreased dietary potassium rather than an adaptive increase in the fraction of potassium absorbed by the gut.

Lower GI secretions have high concentrations of potassium, 80–90 mmol/L, but due to the limited amount of stool (80–120 g/day), daily GI excretion of potassium is only 10 mEq[5–7] (see Table 23.1). The colonic epithelium is capable of actively excreting potassium, but this does not appear to be clinically significant. Hayes et al reported a large increase in GI potassium excretion, up to 70 mEq/day, in patients with chronic renal failure.[8] Subsequent studies have not been able to replicate this finding and have found only modest increases in potassium excretion (up to 12 mEq/day).[4]

Cell uptake

Following absorption, potassium distributes between the intracellular and extracellular compartment. The intracellular compartment acts as the primary buffer to changes in serum potassium concentration. Disruption of the mechanisms or signals responsible for the transcellular distribution of potassium can cause abrupt changes in serum potassium.

The Na-K-ATPase, a ubiquitous cell surface enzyme, moves potassium into cells while pumping sodium out of cells. The Na-K-ATPase is stimulated by beta-2 adrenergic activity, while alpha-adrenergic activity results in potassium efflux.[9] Insulin stimulates the activity of this pump in adipose, muscle, and hepatic tissue.[10] Insulin's effect on Na-K-ATPase is independent of its hypoglycemic activity.[11] Serum potassium can regulate the secretion of insulin. Hyperkalemia stimulates insulin release and hypokalemia inhibits it.[12,13]

Extracellular pH can affect the cellular distribution of potassium. Various explanations have been proposed, including a direct effect of pH on the Na-K-ATPase, or a H^+–K^+ exchange to maintain electroneutrality. The effect of pH on potassium distribution varies depending on the nature of the acid–base disturbance. Respiratory acidosis and alkalosis have little effect on potassium distribution, as does organic acidosis. Inorganic acidosis can increase serum potassium and metabolic alkalosis can lower potassium. Alkalosis has less effect than acidosis.

Renal excretion of potassium

Though the cellular distribution of potassium provides a temporary respite from alterations in serum potassium, ultimately, ingested potassium must be excreted. Some potassium is lost in GI secretions, but, normally, 90% of potassium excretion is via the kidneys. The kidneys have remarkable flexibility in the excretion of potassium. In potassium-depleted states, urinary losses can be reduced to 5 mEq/day.[14] If ingestion is slowly increased, the kidneys can adapt to excrete over 500 mEq of potassium/day.[15]

Regardless of the serum potassium level, essentially all of the filtered potassium is reabsorbed in the proximal tubule and loop of Henle. Essentially, all of the potassium that is excreted in the urine is secreted by the distal tubule.[16] Because of this phenomenon, the study of renal potassium handling can focus on the distal tubule.

The secretion of potassium in the distal tubule is governed by two phenomena: tubule flow and aldosterone activity.

The secretion of potassium by the principal cells of the collecting duct is passive and depends on a

Table 23.1 Potassium concentration in gastrointestinal secretions and sweat.	
Fluid	**Potassium content[4,136,137]**
Sweat	4.5 mmol/L
Stool water	83–95 mmol/L. Potassium concentration falls with increasing stool volume, diarrhea. In severe cholera, stool potassium concentration is <10 mmol/L
Stomach	10 (10–32) mmol/L
Biliary drainage	5 (3–12) mmol/L
Duodenum secretions	5 mmol/L
Ileum secretions	5 (2–8) mmol/L

favorable electrochemical gradient. Rapid tubular flow provides this favorable electrochemical gradient in two ways. First, tubular flow provides a continuous supply of potassium-depleted fluid, which maintains the chemical gradient favoring potassium secretion. Secondly, rapid tubular flow is synonymous with high tubular sodium delivery. Sodium enters the tubular cell without either an associated anion or secretion of a cation, so reabsorption of sodium generates a negative charge in the tubule. Some of this negative charge is lost by concurrent reabsorption of chloride, but since sodium reabsorption is faster than chloride reabsorption, a net negative charge remains. The luminal electronegativity increases the electrical gradient in favor of potassium secretion. Any factor that enhances sodium reabsorption (e.g. aldosterone, loop diuretics) or decreases chloride delivery (e.g. metabolic alkalosis: bicarbonate replaces much of the chloride normally delivered to the collecting tubule so that less chloride is available to be reabsorbed) will enhance potassium secretion. Factors that decrease sodium reabsorption (potassium sparing diuretics) or increase chloride reabsorption will decrease potassium secretion[17] (Fig. 23.1).

Aldosterone is a steroid hormone produced in the zona glomerulosa of the adrenal gland. Its principal site of action is the connecting segment and collecting tubules of the distal nephron. In the principal cells of the cortical collecting duct (CCD), aldosterone increases the reabsorption of sodium and the secretion of potassium. Aldosterone stimulates the production and activity of Na-K-ATPases, sodium channels, and potassium channels.[18] Aldosterone also has a small but measurable effect on increasing GI potassium excretion.[4]

The fact that potassium secretion is dependent on both tubular flow and aldosterone means that renal potassium handling is independent of volume status despite the fact that both tubular flow and aldosterone are intimately tied to volume status. With volume depletion, increased angiotensin II stimulates the release of aldosterone, which increases potassium secretion; however, in volume depletion, decreases in glomerular filtration rate (GFR) and increases in proximal tubule reabsorption result in decreased tubular flow, which decreases the potassium secretion. These two influences neatly oppose each other. In the case of volume overload, the decrease in aldosterone results in decreased secretion of potassium that is compensated by an increase in tubular flow.

The two primary stimuli for the release of aldosterone are angiotensin II and serum potassium. Angiotensin II is released in response to volume depletion.[19] Aldosterone release is sensitive to potassium levels, such that even modest increases in potassium (0.1–0.2 mmol/L) can cause significant increases in aldosterone release.[20]

HYPOKALEMIA

Hypokalemia is defined as a serum potassium concentration below 3.5 mmol/L. Hypokalemia has been reported to occur in 20% of hospitalized patients. However, this high number probably does not reflect total body potassium depletion. In a review of 70 hospitalized patients with potassium concentrations below 2.8 mmol/L, the potassium concentration rose toward normal regardless of whether the patients were given potassium or not, although the use of intravenous (IV) potassium was associated with a faster rate of recovery. The authors suggested that hospitalization for acute illness was associated with increased adrenergic stimulation, resulting in intracellular movement of potassium and transient hypokalemia.[21] Hypokalemia is also common in outpatients treated with diuretics. Hypokalemia was found in 11% of patients on 50 mg of hydrochlorothiazide.[22]

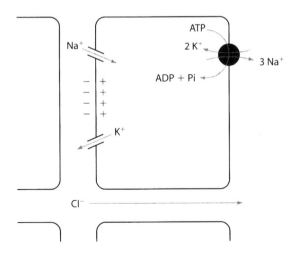

Figure 23.1 Potassium handling in the cortical collecting duct. The reabsorption of sodium creates a negatively charged tubule lumen. This charge helps drive the secretion of potassium. Chloride reabsorption decreases the negative charge, so increased chloride reabsorption decreases potassium secretion.

Etiology

For the causes of hypokalemia see Table 23.2.

Decreased dietary intake

Normal potassium intake is 40–80 mEq/day. The kidney is able to reduce the excretion of potassium to as little at 5–15 mEq/day. So, in order for decreased intake alone to cause significant potassium depletion, the diet must contain less than 5–10 mEq of potassium and be continued for a prolonged period of time. Poor diet can contribute to hypokalemia in cases of increased potassium loss, e.g. with diarrhea, vomiting or diuretics. A study of 945 outpatients with eating disorders (the cohort included a mixture of patients with anorexia nervosa and/or bulimia) found serum potassium below 3.5 in only 4.6% and a potassium below 3.0 in less than 2%. All of the patients with hypokalemia were abusing cathartics or inducing vomiting. None of the cases of hypokalemia were due to restricted caloric intake alone, despite the fact that the restricted calorie subgroup was the most nutritionally deprived of all the subgroups.[23]

Dietary insufficiency often contributes to hypokalemia in alcoholics. Beer and liquor contain little potassium. People who get much of their calories from alcoholic beverages are at risk for hypokalemia. Alcoholics often have additional processes that predispose them to potassium depletion, including vomiting, malabsorption, hypomagnesemia and increased adrenergic activity in cases of alcohol withdrawal.[24]

Cellular shifts

Increased movement of potassium into cells can result in a transient hypokalemia. The central actor here is the Na-K-ATPase. Increased activity of this

Table 23.2 Causes of hypokalemia.

Decreased potassium intake	Cellular shift	Increased potassium loss
Anorexia	Beta-adrenergic activity:	Extra-renal losses:
Malnutrition/malabsorption	Endogenous	Chronic diarrhea
Alcoholism	Albuterol	Fistulas and ostomies
Ingestion of gray clay	Dobutamine	Renal losses:
	Terbutaline	Loop diuretics
	Fenoterol	Thiazide diuretics
	Insulin	Osmotic diuretics
	Alkalemia	Acetazolamide
	Periodic paralysis:	Type I and II RTA
	Thyrotoxicosis	Metabolic alkalosis
	Familial	Bicarbonaturia (vomiting)
	Xanthines:	Ketonuria
	Theophylline toxicity	Hypomagnesemia
	Caffeine	Carbenicillin
	Barium toxicity	Bartter's and Gitelman's syndrome
	Treatment of anemia	Hyperaldosteronism:
	(rapid cell proliferation)	Exogenous steroids
		Adrenal adenoma
		Adrenal hyperplasia (Conn's syndrome)
		Syndrome of apparent mineralocorticoid excess
		Liddle syndrome
		Congenital adrenal hyperplasia
		Renal artery stenosis
		Renin-secreting tumor

RTA = renal tubular acidosis.

enzyme can result in increased movement of potassium into cells. Though the hypokalemia is transient and may not be associated with total body potassium depletion, it can still cause clinically significant symptoms.

Activation of beta-adrenergic receptors increases Na-K-ATPase activity. Any physiologic stress that releases epinephrine or norepinephrine can result in a transient decrease in serum potassium. Patients undergoing withdrawal from alcohol classically are hyperadrenergic and can become hypokalemic. Use of primarily beta-adrenergic catecholamines, such as dobutamine, in the treatment of heart failure or the diagnosis of coronary disease can cause transient hypokalemia.[25] The beta-agonist fenoterol, a tocolytic agent, lowered potassium from 4.10 to 2.88 mmol/L within 2 hours of treatment.[26]

Hypokalemia is common during acute myocardial infarctions (MIs), and has been explained by the high prevalence of diuretic use among these patients. An alternative hypothesis is the hyperadrenergic response to the infarction stimulates the Na-K-ATPase, causing an intracellular shift of potassium. This hypokalemia predisposes to post-infarction arrhythmias and sudden cardiac death. The use of beta-blockers blunts this intracellular shift and may be part of the reason that beta-blockers reduce fatalities following MIs.

Insulin reliably stimulates Na-K-ATPase and lowers serum potassium.[11] Eating presents the body with a simultaneous carbohydrate and potassium load. The release of insulin in response to a carbohydrate load triggers the movement of both glucose and potassium into cells. Clinically, drops in potassium with insulin can be seen in the treatment of diabetic ketoacidosis (DKA) and nonketotic hyperosmolar coma. Intravenous infusion of dextrose solutions has been associated with a fall in serum potassium.[27] Refeeding syndrome is a classic cause of hypokalemia due to the release of insulin. It is seen in patients who are given a carbohydrate-rich diet or parenteral nutrition following prolonged starvation.[28]

Increases in extracellular pH are buffered by the movement of hydrogen ions from the intracellular to the extracellular compartment. Potassium moves into cells to maintain electroneutrality. Simultaneously, increases in filtered load of bicarbonate lead to increased renal potassium excretion. Some early studies on metabolic alkalosis failed to account for the increased renal losses and, hence, overestimated the transcellular effect of alkalemia.[29] Studies in nephrectomized dogs show a modest but measurable decrease in serum potassium of less than 0.3 mmol/L for an increase in pH of 0.1 (although these data did not account for a significant increase in serum osmolality).[30] The common association of alkalosis and hypokalemia is primarily due to enhanced renal excretion of potassium rather than a transcellular shift of potassium.

Hypokalemic periodic paralysis is an unusual clinical entity where transcellular shifts in potassium result in paralysis. These patients develop sudden, severe drops in serum potassium associated with skeletal muscle paralysis. Triggers include carbohydrates, exercise, and changes in body temperature. Many of the cases show autosomal dominant inheritance with a defect mapped to the dihydropyridine-sensitive calcium channel gene on chromosome 1q.[31] Acetazolamide can decrease the frequency and severity of symptoms in some families, but worsens them in others.[32,33] Oral potassium can be used to treat acute paralysis, but patients often develop rebound hyperkalemia.[34] A sporadic form of periodic paralysis exists, which is associated with thyrotoxicosis, and most commonly affects Asian men. Often, the hypokalemia and muscle weakness precedes any symptoms of hyperthyroidism.[34] Nonselective beta-blockers have been shown to reverse the paralysis and increase serum potassium.[35]

Xanthines can stimulate the movement of potassium into cells. Theophylline toxicity is associated with hypokalemia.[36] Explanations include increased beta-adrenergic activity, increased insulin, and increased renal losses from protracted vomiting.

Increased potassium loss

The cortical collecting duct is the critical site of renal potassium handling. The important factors in the secretion of potassium are delivery of sodium to the collecting duct, the potential difference across the tubule epithelium, and aldosterone activity in the principal cells. Normally, aldosterone activity and sodium delivery to the CCD are balanced so that when one is elevated the other is decreased (i.e. increases in aldosterone due to volume deficiency are associated with decreased delivery of sodium to the CCD due to volume deficiency). Renal potassium excretion leads to hypokalemia when there are simultaneous increases in both aldosterone and sodium delivery to the CCD.

Most diuretics increase the distal delivery of sodium. Thiazide and loop diuretics directly block sodium absorption in the distal convoluted tubule and the thick ascending limb of the loop of Henle (TALH), respectively. Osmotic diuretics such as mannitol or conditions such as hyperglycemia block sodium reabsorption throughout the entire nephron. Enhanced sodium loss results in volume deficiency and the body responds by increasing aldosterone (i.e. secondary hyperaldosteronism). Thus, diuretics cause simultaneous increases in aldosterone activity and sodium delivery, leading to hypokalemia.[37]

Thiazide diuretics, despite being less potent diuretics than loop diuretics, cause greater renal potassium losses. Average fall in potassium for thiazide-type diuretics was 0.6 mmol/L compared with 0.3 mmol/L for furosemide.[38] This may be due to the shorter duration of action of loop diuretics that allows renal retention of potassium between doses.

In a comprehensive study of diuretics and hypokalemia, Licht et al found that 11.0% of patients on 50 mg of hydrochlorothiazide were hypokalemic vs 3.8% on 40 mg of furosemide. The addition of potassium supplements (average dose 37 mEq/day) to patients on 50 mg of hydrochlorothiazide increased the average serum potassium (from 3.92 to 4.08 mmol/L) but did not change the prevalence of hypokalemia (11.6%). Pairing hydrochlorothiazide with potassium-sparing diuretics was effective at decreasing the prevalence of hypokalemia (triamterene with hydrochlorothiazide, 5.3%; spironolactone with hydrochlorothiazide, 0.0%).[22]

Unregulated increases in aldosterone cause hypertension and hypokalemia. The hypokalemia is due to the simultaneous increase in aldosterone activity and sodium delivery to the distal nephron. The increased sodium delivery is due to a phenomenon known as *aldosterone escape*. Aldosterone increases the distal reabsorption of sodium, resulting in volume expansion and hypertension. Aldosterone escape is a spontaneous diuresis, which occurs despite continued sodium retention in the distal tubule. Evidence suggests that the diuresis is triggered by hypertension, which suppresses sodium reabsorption proximal to the distal tubule. A full discussion of the causes of increased aldosterone activity is beyond the scope of this text; however, a list is included in Table 23.2.

Normally, the primary anion in the tubular fluid is chloride. Various conditions can result in chloride being replaced by an unreabsorbable anion. Anions that are not reabsorbed prevent sodium from being reabsorbed and increase sodium and tubular fluid delivery to the distal nephron. Additionally, unreabsorbable anions increase tubule electronegativity, which increases potassium secretion by the principal cells. This is essentially the same as increasing aldosterone activity. Thus, unreabsorbable anions cause simultaneous increases in aldosterone activity and sodium delivery, which causes hypokalemia.

The most common example of an unreabsorbable anion resulting in hypokalemia is bicarbonate. Normally, all of the filtered bicarbonate is reabsorbed by the proximal tubule. Increases in serum bicarbonate can overwhelm the reabsorptive capacity of the proximal tubule (Tm), so that residual, unreabsorbed bicarbonate is delivered to the distal tubule. This occurs when serum bicarbonate rises above 26 mmol/L, the Tm for bicarbonate. Unreabsorbed bicarbonate increases sodium delivery and luminal electronegativity in the CCD. An important cause of this is vomiting or gastric drainage.[29] Proximal renal tubular acidosis (RTA) also increases the distal delivery of bicarbonate. In this disorder, congenital or acquired defects in the proximal tubule prevent it from efficiently reabsorbing bicarbonate, so that the Tm for bicarbonate is decreased from 26 to 16–18 mmol/L. If the serum bicarbonate is raised above the Tm for bicarbonate, incomplete proximal reabsorption will result in increased bicarbonate in the cortical collecting tubule.[39]

DKA increases delivery of the unreabsorbable anion β-hydroxybutyrate to the distal tubule. Hippurate is an unreabsorbable anion produced following toluene exposure from glue or solvent inhalation. High-dose oxacillin or carbenicillin therapy increases renal potassium loss by acting as unreabsorbable anions.[40]

Hypomagnesemia is associated with hypokalemia that is resistant to therapy. Decreased magnesium increases renal potassium losses by two mechanisms. Since magnesium is a critical cofactor for the Na-K-ATPase, hypomagnesemia decreases Na-K-ATPase activity, resulting in intracellular potassium leaking into the extracellular space. This increase in potassium stimulates renal potassium excretion and leads to decreased total body potassium. The second effect is to decrease the activity of the ATP-dependent ROMK channel in the TALH. Loss of this channel slows the activity of the Na–K–2Cl channel, increasing distal delivery of sodium.[41]

Distal RTAs (type 1 RTA) are also associated with hypokalemia, but the etiology is probably multifactorial. Normally, some hydrogen secretion in the intercalated cells of the collecting tubule is due to an H–K exchanger in the apical membrane. Decreased activity of this enzyme in distal RTA would decrease potassium reabsorption, increasing renal losses.[42] Another mechanism is due to the general decrease in hydrogen secretion in the intercalated cells. This decreased outward movement of a cation results in a relative increase in the electronegativity of the tubule, enhancing potassium secretion by the principal cells.

Nephrotoxic drugs generally affect GFR, but some toxins affect tubular function, which results in electrolyte abnormalities. Cisplatin, amphotericin B, and aminoglycosides can all increase renal potassium losses, independent of any effect on GFR. Amphotericin B damages the integrity of the tubular cell epithelium, so that potassium is able to flow down its concentration gradient from the cell into the collecting duct lumen.[43] Aminoglycosides may cause hypokalemia secondary to tubular damage, resulting in magnesium wasting; the hypomagnesemia then causes abnormal renal potassium wasting.[44]

Despite an elevated concentration of potassium in lower GI secretions, 85–95 mmol/L, GI potassium losses are typically modest, 10 mEq/day.[6] Chronic diarrhea can cause hypokalemia, but the mechanism appears to be more complex than simple GI loss of potassium. In cases of experimental diarrhea, daily GI potassium loss was never higher than 24 mEq/day, a level well below average daily potassium intake.[45] In addition, studies on diarrhea show that as stool volume increases, stool potassium concentration falls, ultimately reaching a level similar to plasma in cases of severe cholera.[4] Explanations for the commonly seen association of diarrhea and hypokalemia include secondary hyperaldosteronism, diminished intake of potassium, or transcellular shifts of extracellular potassium.

Hypokalemia from chronic diarrhea is most frequent in neuroendocrine tumors.[4] In a group of 311 patients with moderately severe chronic diarrhea (average stool weight 707 g/day, normal is 125 g/day), only 10% had a potassium concentration below 3.5 mmol/L. Of note, the correlation of daily GI potassium loss to serum potassium was relatively weak.

Gastric secretions have potassium concentration similar to plasma, at 5–8 mmol/L. Gastric losses result in severe metabolic alkalosis and secondary hyperaldosteronism, both of which enhance renal losses of potassium. So, although upper GI losses do cause hypokalemia, it is a result of enhanced renal excretion of potassium rather than GI loss of potassium.

Clinical consequences

Potassium depletion has numerous effects throughout the body. The most life-threatening symptoms are found in the cardiovascular and nervous systems. Metabolic and gastrointestinal effects may predominate in some individuals.

Cardiovascular effects
The effect of hypokalemia on hypertension is underrecognized. Controlled human trials in both hypertensive and normotensive patients have shown that low potassium diets (10 mEq/day) were associated with a significant increase in systolic, diastolic, and mean arterial pressure. Low potassium diets also increased salt sensitivity.[46,47] The addition of KCl to patients who became hypokalemic on thiazide diuretics resulted in an increase in serum potassium and a decrease in blood pressure.[48] The hypotensive effect of potassium supplementation is more pronounced in African-Americans.[49]

Decreased potassium is a well-known risk factor for cardiac arrhythmia. In various clinical scenarios, hypokalemia has been associated with ventricular and atrial arrhythmias.

In a study of men with hypertension, hydrochlorothiazide-induced hypokalemia was associated with increased ventricular ectopy in one-third of patients, 90% of whom were asymptomatic. The mean serum potassium concentration in affected patients was 2.9 mmol/L.[50] Whereas some workers have been able to replicate these findings, others have failed to find an increased risk of arrhythmia.[51–53] In a study of patients undergoing elective coronary artery bypass grafting (CABG), preoperative hypokalemia increased the intraoperative and postoperative risk of ventricular and atrial arrhythmias.[54] In a prospective study of initial potassium concentration and acute MI, patients with hypokalemia had almost twice the rate of ventricular fibrillation (24.4% vs 13.0% $p = 0.04$).[55] In a retrospective analysis of over 1000 acute MIs, hypokalemia at admission was associated with a higher prevalence of atrial fibrillation, ventricular tachycardia, ventricular flutter, or ventricular fibrillation (34% for K $\leq$3.5 mmol/L, 24% for K $>$3.5 mmol/L). Ventricular fibrillation was increased the most by hypokalemia (16% for K $\leq$3.5 mmol/L, 7% for K $>$3.5 mmol/L).[56]

Hypokalemia has long been implicated as a risk factor for arrhythmia in patients on digitalis. In a study of 79 consecutive admissions for arrhythmias consistent with cardiac glycoside toxicity, the average digoxin level for patients with normal serum potassium (mean K = 4.7 mmol/L) was 3.7 ng/ml, whereas the average level for patients who were hypokalemic (mean K = 3.0 mmol/L) was 1.1 ng/ml, a level traditionally thought to be nontoxic.[57]

Muscular complications

A drop in extracellular potassium increases the potential difference across the plasma membrane. It hyperpolarizes the muscle cells, which can prevent myocytes from depolarizing. Clinically, this can lead to weakness, fatigue, cramping, and myalgia. Severe cases can result in paralysis. Numerous case reports of respiratory muscle weakness and respiratory failure have been reported with hypokalemia due to DKA. Severe hypokalemia can cause rhabdomyolysis. Alcoholics may be particularly prone to proximal muscle weakness due to rhabdomyolysis.[58,59]

Other complications

Hypokalemia can cause polyuria due to two effects: low potassium stimulates thirst and it prevents the concentration of urine by causing a mild nephrogenic diabetes insipidus.[60,61] The etiology of the concentrating defect is multifactorial, but primarily represents decreased renal response to antidiuretic hormone (ADH).

Gastrointestinal complications are primarily related to decreased gut motility associated with hypokalemia. Serum potassium concentration of less than 3.0 mmol/L is associated with constipation. Paralytic ileus can occur as potassium concentration falls below 2.5 mmol/L.

Patients with liver disease are at risk for a unique complication of hypokalemia. Decreases in serum potassium stimulates ammoniagenesis in the proximal tubule. Patients predisposed to hepatic encephalopathy can develop encephalopathy from the increased ammonia load.[62]

Diagnosis

Hypokalemia is defined as a serum potassium concentration less than 3.5 mmol/L. Once hypokalemia has been established, the primary diagnostic goal is differentiating whether it is due to inappropriate renal potassium wasting or extrarenal potassium loss/decreased intake. In the latter situation, the kidneys are potassium avid, whereas in the former, urine studies show increased potassium loss.

Three studies may be used to differentiate these states:

- spot urine potassium concentration
- 24-hour urine potassium
- transtubular potassium gradient (TTKG).

The spot urine is the simplest test to use. The urine potassium should be less than 20 mmol/L in the face of hypokalemia. If the spot potassium is greater than 40 mmol/L, renal potassium wasting should be suspected. Urine potassium of 20–40 mmol/L is considered nondiagnostic.[63] There are two primary problems with this test: the first problem is that it fails to control for changes in the water content of urine. Increased ADH activity will increase the concentration of all solutes, including potassium, while not materially affecting the renal excretion of potassium. The second problem is that spot samples provide information for only a single moment in time. Patients with diuretic-induced hypokalemia become potassium avid after the diuretic has cleared and spot urine potassium concentrations will show intact renal potassium handling. One study found spot urine potassium to have a sensitivity of only 40%.[64]

The 24-hour urine potassium test avoids both of the above problems at the expense of increased complexity and a 24-hour delay. Patients with hypokalemia should reduce urinary potassium losses to less than 15 mEq/day. Potassium losses greater than that indicate inappropriate renal losses. The 24-hour urine provides no information on the renal potassium handling prior to the urine collection. Surreptitious diuretic use which is stopped before the 24-hour collection will show a potassium-avid kidney.

The TTKG calculates the ratio of tubular potassium to venous potassium at the end of the CCD. The CCD is responsible for potassium excretion, so increases in the TTKG indicate renal wasting of potassium, whereas decreases indicate renal sparing of potassium. Since it is impossible to measure the tubular potassium content at the cortex, urine potassium is used. Changes in the tubular potassium concentration after the CCD are assumed to be solely due to the reabsorption of water in the medullary collecting duct. TTKG compensates for the reabsorption of water by dividing the urinary potassium by the ratio of urine osmolality to serum osmolality (Figs 23.2 and 23.3).

When serum potassium and renal potassium handling are normal, the TTKG runs from 5 to 8.[63,65] In the face of hypokalemia, the CCD should minimize the excretion of potassium. This is

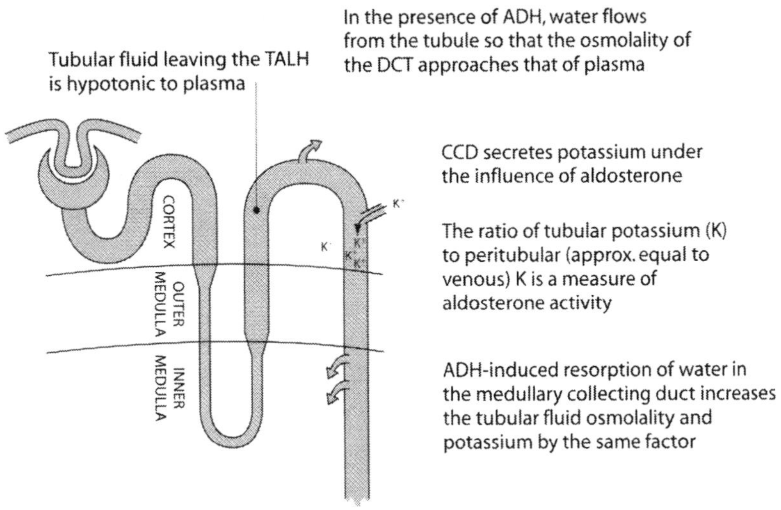

Figure 23.2 Physiology of the transtubular potassium gradient (TTKG). The TTKG measures the ratio of tubular potassium to interstitial potassium and quantifies the renal excretion of potassium. ADH = antidiuretic hormone; CCD = cortical collecting duct; DCT = distal convoluted tubule; TALH = thick ascending limb of the loop of Henle.

$$TTKG = \frac{Urine\ K \div \dfrac{Urine\ Osm}{Plasma\ Osm}}{Plasma\ K}$$

Figure 23.3 The transtubular potassium gradient (TTKG) equation.

reflected in a reduced TTKG. After only 2 days on a potassium-depleted diet, the TTKG fell from 5 to <2 in nine of nine patients.[65] In 73 patients with hypokalemia due to periodic paralysis, the mean TTKG was 2.3 mmol/L.[64] Patients with mineralocorticoid excess often have a TTKG greater than 10, even in the presence of hypokalemia.[66] Diuretic-induced hypokalemia has shown conflicting results, with some studies reporting increases and others decreases in the TTKG.[66,67] Vomiting resulted in hypokalemia without a change in the TTKG. An unchanged or normal TTKG in the face of hypokalemia is consistent with increased renal potassium losses, which is exactly what occurs with vomiting.[66]

The TTKG has two assumptions that must be met prior to using this formula:[68]

- There must be ADH activity to ensure that the osmolality of the tubular fluid approximates the osmolality of blood by the end of the CCD. ADH activity is assured by only using the formula when urine osmolality exceeds serum osmolality.

- There must be adequate tubular sodium to allow the CCD to secrete potassium. The test should only be done if the urine sodium concentration is greater than 25 mmol/L.

Treatment

The treatment of hypokalemia can be broken down into three questions: when to treat, what type of potassium to give, and how much potassium to give. The National Council on Potassium in Clinical Practice has published clinical practice guidelines on potassium replacement. The guidelines recommend correcting potassium in any patient with potassium concentration below 3.0 mmol/L and in select patients with serum potassium below 3.5 mmol/L. They specified the more aggressive treatment regimen for patients with hypertension, congestive heart failure, and increased risk for, or history of, cardiac arrhythmias or stroke.[69]

Determining the dose of potassium to correct hypokalemia is difficult because there is not a firm relationship between serum potassium and total body potassium depletion. Most balance studies have concluded that potassium is disproportionately lost from the extracellular compartment rather than total body potassium. For example, a decrease in serum potassium of 25% (a drop from 4.0 to 3.0 mmol/L) reflects less than a 25% decrease in total body potassium. Sterns et al analyzed the results of 7 balance studies and found a linear relationship for potassium deficit and serum potassium ($r = 0.893$). The loss of 100 mmol of potassium lowered the serum potassium by 0.27 mmol/L, so that a fall from 4 to 3 mmol/L represented 370 mmol deficit of potassium.[70] In Scribner and Burnell's review, they estimated that a drop in potassium from 4 to 3 mmol/L represented a loss of 100–200 mmol of potassium and a drop in serum potassium from 3 to 2 mmol/L represented an additional 200–400 mmol loss.[71] These estimates do not account for altered cellular distribution of potassium. In DKA, for example, the lack of insulin and solute drag cause the serum potassium to overestimate total body potassium, while the use of albuterol in status asthmaticus causes an intracellular shift of potassium so that serum potassium underestimates total body potassium. In most cases of hypokalemia due to cellular redistribution, experts advise not to treat, as the hypokalemia is typically transient and treatment predisposes the patient to hyperkalemia. One exception to this is symptomatic periodic paralysis. Patients can develop life-threatening respiratory failure due to hypokalemia and emergent IV potassium is indicated. Caution should still be used, as rebound hyperkalemia is common, particularly in thyrotoxicosis-associated periodic paralysis.

The form of potassium used in repletion is most often potassium chloride. The chloride anion has some advantages over alternatives such as phosphate, bicarbonate, or citrate. The chloride anion is primarily an extracellular anion, which minimizes the movement of potassium into the cell, maximizing the change in serum potassium. Chloride also does not increase the secretion of potassium at the collecting duct. The use of alternate potassium salts should be reserved for specific clinical scenarios where there is an indication for the anion (metabolic acidosis or hypophosphatemia).

Oral

In patients who are asymptomatic, oral replacement is generally recommended and doses from 40 to 100 mEq of KCl are typically sufficient to correct the hypokalemia over multiple days.[69] Increasing intake of potassium-rich foods is less effective than potassium chloride supplements because the anions associated with dietary potassium are primarily phosphate and citrate.

Potassium chloride can be given as a liquid, powder (often marketed as a salt substitute), or pill

with multiple formulations and coatings. The bioavailability of all these formulations is identical, with greater than 70% absorption.[72] The liquid formulation has the fastest absorption, although in one study of patient compliance it had the lowest adherence of all the potassium formulations (thought to be related to the bad taste).[73] Wax-matrix extended-release tablets have been associated with GI tract ulcers and stenotic lesions. The microencapsulated, extended-release formulations have the best compliance and low rates of GI side effects.[69,73]

Parenteral repletion

Parenteral potassium is commonly used to correct hypokalemia in patients with symptoms or when patients are unable to take oral medications: 20–40 mmol KCl/L isotonic saline or 5% dextrose is a typical solution. Both saline and dextrose solutions can cause problems. Dextrose solutions stimulate insulin release, which can result in acute worsening of the hypokalemia.[27,74] The use of saline with dilute concentrations of potassium means that patients must get multiple liters of saline to correct even modest potassium deficits.

The use of concentrated potassium solutions has generated fears about the possibility of precipitating arrhythmias from local, transient hyperkalemia near the infusion site or causing peripheral vein irritation from caustic potassium solutions. Despite these concerns, the use of concentrated potassium infusions, 200 mmol/L, at a rate of 20 mEq/h in the intensive care unit (ICU) was shown to be safe and efficacious in both a retrospective study of 495 infusions and a prospective study of 40 patients:[75,76] 20 mEq of KCl increased the serum potassium by 0.25 mmol/L 1 hour after the infusion finished. The peak rise in serum potassium, 0.48 mmol/L, was at the end of the infusion. Electrocardiogram (ECG) monitoring showed no change, except for decreased ventricular ectopy. Potassium was infused safely through both peripheral and central sites. Burning was documented in 2.6% of peripheral infusions.

Other issues in the treatment of hypokalemia

Hypomagnesemia is a common cause of treatment failure. Patients who are resistant to potassium supplementation should have serum magnesium measured and, if low, repleted. Patients with diuretic-induced hypokalemia often benefit from the initiation of a potassium-sparing diuretic. Amiloride has also been shown to mitigate magnesium losses associated with loop and thiazide diuretics.

Patients on amphotericin B often become hypokalemic. Both spironolactone (100 mg twice a day) and amiloride (5 mg twice a day) have been shown to increase serum potassium and decrease the use of potassium supplements in randomized prospective trials.[77,78]

In patients with recalcitrant vomiting (i.e. bulimia) and associated hypokalemia, one treatment strategy is to decrease the loss of hydrogen ions with a proton pump inhibitor or H_2-blocker. In one case a bulemic patient was started on lansoprazole and the patient's alkalosis and hypokalemia improved. In addition, the patient remained normokalemic for the following year despite continued vomiting.[79] Proton pump inhibitors may have a similar role in ameliorating hypokalemia associated with gastric suction.

Preoperative hypokalemia due to anxiety-induced beta-adrenergic activity can be eliminated with clonidine. In a double-blind, placebo-controlled, randomized trial 0.3 mg of clonidine, 2 hours prior to surgery, reduced the incidence of hypokalemia from 50% to 0%.[80]

HYPERKALEMIA

Etiology

The ability of the kidney to excrete potassium is flexible and adaptable. If dietary ingestion of potassium is increased over a number of days, the kidney increases daily potassium excretion to match. Because of this, dietary loads of potassium do not result in hyperkalemia unless they are sudden, or paired with a defect in renal potassium handling. Likewise, conditions associated with the movement of intracellular potassium to the extracellular space are associated with only transient hyperkalemia because either the kidneys excrete or the cells reuptake the excess potassium. Decreases in the ability of the kidney to excrete potassium increase susceptibility to hyperkalemia from increased potassium intake or transcellular shifts. Table 23.3 lists the causes of hyperkalemia.

Increased potassium intake

Dietary potassium is typically in the range of 40–80 mEq/day. Large amounts of potassium are found in dried fruits, citrus fruits, and legumes. Hyperkalemia has been reported to follow the use of potassium chloride salt substitutes, even in the presence of normal renal function.[81] One teaspoon of potassium chloride contains 50–65 mEq of potassium. Enteral nutrition supplements may be rich sources of potassium. Ensure Plus at 100 ml/h, provides 130 mEq potassium/day. Other sources of enteral potassium include potassium supplements, which are often given routinely to patients on diuretics.[82] Citrate, which is used to treat metabolic acidosis, is available as a potassium or sodium salt. Use of the potassium salt in patients with renal insufficiency can result in hyperkalemia.

Parenteral potassium sources include penicillin, which may be prepared as a potassium salt and contains 1.7 mEq of potassium per 1 000 000 units. Red blood cell (RBC) transfusions can have extracellular potassium concentration as high as 70 mmol/L.[83] The risk of hyperkalemia from transfusions rises as the age of the transfusions increases (Table 23.4). Use of 'washed' packed red blood cells (PRBCs) reduces the risk of transfusion-associated hyperkalemia. In one case, the use of an autotransfusion device to 'wash' the RBC (2 ml of saline for 1 ml of blood) lowered the average potassium from 39.6 mmol/L to 2.3 mmol/L.[84] Errors in the preparation of parenteral nutrition, hemofiltration replacement fluid, or peritoneal dialysate can all provide occult potassium loads.

Intracellular redistribution of potassium

The intracellular compartment contains 98% of total body potassium. The movement of a small proportion of this potassium can cause life-threatening hyperkalemia. Release of intracellular potassium can be secondary to changes in plasma osmolality, decreased activity of the Na-K-ATPase, and cell death.

Increases in plasma osmolality are most often due to hyperglycemia. In the absence of insulin, glucose acts as an effective osmole and draws water from the intracellular compartment. Along with water, potassium moves out of the cell as part of a phenomenon known as solute drag. Mannitol increases extracellular osmolality and results in hyperkalemia by the same mechanism. In healthy volunteers, using mannitol to increase serum osmolality 5% (from 283 to 300 mmol/kg) resulted in a 18% increase in serum potassium (4.4 to 5.2 mmol/L).[85]

A lack of insulin also increases serum potassium by slowing the Na-K-ATPase. The classic example of this is the hyperkalemia found with DKA

Table 23.3 Causes of hypokalemia.

Increased potassium intake	Cellular shift	Decreased potassium excretion
Oral:	Beta-blockers	Decreased tubular flow:
Dietary	Lack of insulin	Renal insufficiency
K supplements	Acidemia (inorganic)	Prerenal azotemia
Salt substitutes	Digitalis toxicity	• Volume depletion
Ingestion of red clay	Succinylcholine	• CHF
Enteral feeding supplements	Periodic paralysis:	• Cirrhosis
Parenteral:	Hyperkalemic	NSAID
Medical error	Hypertonicity:	Decreased stimulation of aldosterone:
• TPN	Hyperglycemia	Type IV RTA (hyporeninism)
• CVVH replacement fluid	Mannitol	ACE inhibitor
• Peritoneal dialysis fluid	Cell destruction:	Angiotensin receptor blocker
Old blood transfusions	Ischemia	Decreased synthesis of aldosterone:
Treatment of hypokalemia	Necrosis	Adrenal insufficiency, primary
Penicillin (K formulations)	Hemolysis	Ketoconazole
	Rhabdomyolysis	Heparin
	Tumor lysis syndrome:	Congenital adrenal hyperplasia
	• Chemotherapy	Decreased aldosterone activity:
	• Radiation therapy	Spironolactone
	• Spontaneous	Trimethoprim
		Amiloride
		Triamterene
		Cyclosporin A
		Tacrolimus
		Type I RTA, hyperkalemic variety SLE,
		obstruction, sickle cell
		Decreased GI excretion:
		Constipation in ESRD patients

ACE = angiotensin-converting enzyme; CHF = congestive heart failure; CVVH = continuous venovenous hemofiltration; ESRD = end-stage renal disease; GI = gastrointestinal; NSAID = nonsteroidal anti-inflammatory drug; RTA = renal tubular acidosis; SLE = systemic lupus erythematosus; TPN = total parenteral nutrition.

despite total body potassium depletion. This also plays a role in fasting hyperkalemia that can occur in patients with end-stage renal disease (ESRD). Allon et al demonstrated that when ESRD patients fasted for 18 hours they had an increase in serum potassium of over 0.5 mmol/L. Providing basal levels of insulin and glucose abolished the effect.[86]

The Na-K-ATPase is critical in preventing intracellular potassium from causing hyperkalemia. Any factor that decreases the activity of this enzyme will cause potassium to leak from cells. Beta-blockers predictably inhibit the Na-K-ATPase activity and are associated with a mild increase in serum potassium. They also prevent adrenergic-induced intracellular shifts in potassium. Exercise causes a transient, physiologic, hyperkalemia due to the release of potassium from muscle. Following exercise, muscle cells rapidly absorb potassium, restoring eukalemia. During vigorous exercise, potassium can rise by 1.2 mmol/L. Pretreatment with the beta-blocker propranolol increases exercise-induced hyperkalemia by 50%.[9] Uremia reduces Na-K-ATPase activity. Decreased Na-K-ATPase activity puts uremic patients at risk of hyperkalemia by reducing their ability to use the intracellular compartment to buffer potassium loads. Digitalis is a Na-K-ATPase antagonist and its use is associated with mild increases in serum

Table 23.4 Potassium concentration in red blood cell transfusions.		
Age (days)	Plasma potassium (mmol/L)[132]	Extracellular potassium (mmol) per 250 ml of PRBCs (hematocrit 60%)
0	1.6	0.2
7	17	1.7
14	27	2.7
35	44	4.4
42	46	4.6

PRBCs = packed red blood cells.

potassium. Digitalis toxicity can cause severe hyperkalemia. Removing digitalis with binding antibodies restores Na-K-ATPase activity and allows rapid correction of the hyperkalemia.[87]

Inorganic acids increase serum potassium. The increase in serum potassium is due to a transcellular exchange of hydrogen for potassium. Attempts to predict the change in potassium from changes of pH have shown tremendous variability (0.3–1.1 mmol/L for a decrease in pH of 0.1) and are considered unreliable.[85] Decreases in pH due to respiratory or organic acidosis have minimal effect on serum potassium.

Cell death releases intracellular potassium. Wide-scale cell death can cause fatal hyperkalemia. Tissue necrosis and hyperkalemia can be seen with rhabdomyolysis of any etiology. Tissue ischemia, likewise, can cause cell death and release large amounts of potassium. Bowel and limb ischemia may be occult causes of hyperkalemia. Hemolysis causes hyperkalemia by releasing the intracellular potassium of RBCs. Tumor destruction with chemotherapy results in release of intracellular contents. Tumor lysis syndrome is hyperphosphatemia, hyperuricemia, hyperkalemia and hypocalcemia associated with acute renal failure. The prophylactic use of allopurinol has nearly eliminated acute renal failure, which is due to uric acid nephropathy. The syndrome most often occurs with poorly differentiated neoplasms such as Burkitt's lymphoma and acute leukemias, but it has been reported with medulloblastoma, breast, ovarian and lung cancer. In some rapidly growing tumors, spontaneous lysis occurs prior to therapy. Hyperkalemia in tumor lysis syndrome is more common in patients with premorbid renal insufficiency.[88]

Succinylcholine is a depolarizing paralytic. It can cause hyperkalemia by two unique mechanisms. The first occurs after muscle damage from burns, trauma, or disuse (often from denervation, prolonged ICU stay, or central nervous system lesion, i.e. stroke, Gullain–Barré syndrome). The muscle damage causes up-regulation of the nicotinic acetylcholine receptors so that subsequent exposure to succinylcholine causes massive potassium efflux and hyperkalemia. The second mechanism is a drug-induced rhabdomyolysis. Nearly all of the reported cases of rhabdomyolysis occurred in patients with a pre-existing myopathy, often a form of muscular dystrophy (Duchenne's or Becker's).[89]

Renal dysfunction

Increased intake and cellular redistribution cause transient increases in potassium because the kidneys are so efficient at excreting potassium. Persistent hyperkalemia is almost always associated with a defect in renal potassium clearance. Renal potassium excretion is dependent on adequate tubular flow and adequate aldosterone activity. Besides dramatic decreases in renal function, defects in renal potassium clearance can always be traced back to one of these two problems.

Decreases in GFR from chronic renal insufficiency or prerenal azotemia reduce the flow through the distal tubule and can cause hyperkalemia. Decreases in renal function not associated with oliguria do not typically cause hyperkalemia. Examples of this include aminoglycoside toxicity (usually associated with hypokalemia) and chronic interstitial nephritis.

Inadequate aldosterone activity can be due to pathology at any point in the aldosterone axis. Inadequate renin production causes hypoaldosteronism and, subsequently, type IV RTA. Angiotensin-converting enzyme (ACE) inhibitors and angiotensin receptor blockers prevent angiotensin II from stimulating the release of aldosterone. Since serum potassium itself can directly stimulate aldosterone release, most patients can maintain potassium homeostasis despite the loss of angiotensin II. However, patients with other defects in potassium handling (e.g. renal insufficiency, decreased insulin) can become hyperkalemic.[90]

Drugs can antagonize aldosterone activity by multiple mechanisms. Drugs such as ketoconazole and heparin decrease aldosterone synthesis. Spironolactone is a competitive inhibitor of aldosterone. Cyclosporin A causes hyperkalemia in a subset of transplant patients, possibly by inducing tubular insensitivity to aldosterone.[91] Similar findings have been found with tacrolimus.[92]

Defects in the absorption of sodium at the CCD antagonize aldosterone activity by preventing the generation of the electronegative tubule. This is most commonly seen with potassium-sparing diuretics such as amiloride and triamterene. The antibiotic trimethoprim can also block sodium channels. Hyperkalemia is most often seen with high-dose IV therapy, although standard doses in the elderly have been implicated.[93] Distal RTAs usually cause hypokalemia; however, one subtype causes hyperkalemia due to a defect in sodium reabsorption at the CCD. This condition is unique from type IV RTA and does not respond to supplemental mineralocorticoid. This defect has been reported in chronic urinary tract obstruction, lupus, and sickle cell anemia.[94,95]

Clinical consequences

The potassium concentration inside and outside of the cell is the primary determinant of the cellular resting membrane potential (E_m). Changes in the extracellular concentration can have dramatic effects on the resting membrane potential and the cell's ability to depolarize. As extracellular potassium rises, the normally negative E_m increases toward zero; this allows easier depolarization, i.e. increased excitability. However, this excitability is short-lived, as chronic hyperkalemia ultimately inactivates the sodium channels critical to producing an action potential. Hyperkalemia shortens the refractory period following depolarization by facilitating faster potassium uptake.

In the myocardium, inactivated sodium channels slow conduction velocity, and high serum potassium speeds repolarization. Clinically, this is evidenced by widened QRS complexes (slowed conduction velocity) and shortened ST intervals with tented T waves (rapid repolarization). The slowed conduction associated with rapid repolarization predisposes the myocardium to ventricular fibrillation.

Whereas animal models and experimental protocols document a stepwise progression of ECG changes, from peaked T waves to widened QRS to disappearance of P waves, and ultimately a sinusoidal ECG, clinically, patients may develop symptomatic arrhythmias without prior ECG changes.[96] Rapid increases in potassium, hyponatremia, hypocalcemia, and metabolic acidosis all increase the likelihood of arrhythmia.[97–100]

Neuromuscular toxicity from hyperkalemia is another concern. Ascending paralysis, mimicking Guillain–Barré syndrome, has been documented with a serum potassium of 7 mmol/L. In a review of all published cases of hyperkalemic paralysis (excluding hereditary periodic paralysis), the average potassium was 9 mmol/L. The use of potassium-sparing diuretics was the etiology of the hyperkalemia in over half of the cases. Electromyograms showed the paralysis to be due to abnormal nerve depolarization rather than muscle pathology.[101]

Diagnosis

Because of the large amount of potassium inside cells, artifacts are a common cause of hyperkalemia. The most common is hemolysis after the blood is drawn, and this should be reported by the laboratory, as it is easy to detect. Increased platelets or white cells can also release potassium, especially if the specimen is allowed to clot. Thrombocytosis greater than 1 000 000 platelets or leukocytosis over 100 000 increase the likelihood of pseudohyperkalemia. Rarely, counts as low as 600 000 platelets or 70 000 leukocytes have been reported to cause the same phenomena.[102] The other major cause of pseudohyperkalemia is fist pumping prior to phlebotomy. Forearm exercise in the presence of a tourniquet can falsely elevate potassium by 1.4 mmol/L.[103]

In the diagnosis of hyperkalemia, urine chemistries have a limited role. Spot urine potassium measurements in isolation provide little information. In addition, 24-hour urine potassium in a patient with persistent hyperkalemia will merely inform the physician that the patient has inadequate renal potassium excretion. The only time the 24-hour urine is helpful is in the unusual case where it is greater than 80 mEq. This is consistent with increased intake or rapid cell death as the etiology of hyperkalemia. It must be stressed, however, that these are unusual causes of persistent hyperkalemia in the absence of a defect in the renal excretion of potassium.

An important diagnostic test is the TTKG. High levels (>10) indicate increased aldosterone activity, which is expected with hyperkalemia. An inappropriately low TTKG (<7) is consistent with inadequate aldosterone activity in the setting of hyperkalemia (i.e. type IV RTA, primary adrenal insufficiency, ACE inhibitors/angiotensin receptor blockers, spironolactone, sodium channel antagonists). Patients with low tubular flow or increased potassium intake should have an appropriately elevated TTKG.

Treatment

The decision of when and how to treat hyperkalemia should be based on physical signs, clinical situation, and serum potassium. Individual tolerances of hyperkalemia can vary dramatically and are influenced by pH, calcium concentration, rate of potassium rise, and underlying heart disease. Patients with rapid increases in serum potassium or hypocalcemia may have arrhythmias at serum potassium levels as low as 7 mmol/L, while new-borns regularly tolerate potassium concentrations of that level. Patients with muscle weakness or ECG changes consistent with hyperkalemia should be urgently treated. Modestly elevated potassium in the absence of ECG or muscle weakness can be treated more conservatively (Table 23.5).

The initial therapy for hyperkalemia should be stopping any and all potassium sources. Total parenteral nutrition (TPN), potassium supplements, transfusions, and medications containing potassium should be stopped. Patients already on peritoneal dialysis with potassium added to the peritoneal fluid should be switched to potassium-free fluid. Patients on continuous renal replacement therapies need to have the replacement fluid potassium verified.

Table 23.5 Time course, expected decrement of potassium, and side effects of each therapy.

Treatment	Dose	Onset	Duration	Magnitude	Side effects
Calcium[133]	1 g (10 ml) of 10% calcium gluconate or calcium chloride. May repeat	Immediate (doumented normalization of ECG as early as 15 s)	30–60 min		Caution/contraindicated in hypercalcemia and digoxin toxicity
Insulin and glucose[108]	10 units of regular insulin and 50 g of glucose. Can omit the glucose if the patient is hyperglycemic	Significant reduction at 15 min,[114] peak action at 60 min[134]	Greater than 6 h (potassium still decreased by 0.76 mmol/L at 6 h)[118]	1 mmol/L	Hypoglycemia and hyperglycemia. Hyperglycemia may increase serum potassium through solute drag
Albuterol IV[111]	0.5 mg in 100 ml of 5% dextrose solution infused over 15 min	Onset and peak action at 30 min	6 h	1–1.5 mmol/L	Tachycardia, variable changes in BP, tremor. Rise in blood glucose and insulin. Rise in serum potassium in the first minute after Albuterol MDI use. Rise averaged only 0.15 mmol/L but 59% had a rise of at least 0.1 mmol/L and 2 had a rise of >0.4 mmol/L
Albuterol nebulized[110]	10–20 mg in 5 ml of normal saline inhaled over 10–15 min	5–10 min with peak action at 30–120 min	3–6 h		
Albuterol MDI with spacer[109]	1200 µg MDI	3–5 min with potassium falling at end of study	Only one study and test ended at 60 min, potassium was still trending down	1–1.5 mmol/L	
Sodium bicarbonate	4 mEq/min drip for a total of 400 mEq (Note: lower doses, 50–100 mEq have been shown to be ineffective)	240 min[135] (Note: the prolonged time for onset of hypokalemic effect)	Potassium was still falling at end of 6 h study	0.6 at 4 h 0.74 mmol/L at 6 h	May precipitate tetany by decreasing ionized calcium. May antagonize cardioprotective effect of calcium

BP = blood pressure; ECG = electrocardiogram; IV = intravenous; MDI = metered-dose inhaler; MDI-S = MDI with spacer.

Calcium

Calcium reverses the ECG changes seen in hyperkalemia and decreases the risk of arrhythmia. Both calcium chloride and calcium gluconate can be used, but the chloride formulation has three times as much elemental calcium (0.225 mmol/ml vs 0.68 mmol/ml of a 10% solution). Since the cardioprotective effect of calcium has been shown to be dose-dependent, it is presumed that the chloride salt is more effective than the gluconate.[104] The downside of calcium chloride is that it is more irritating to veins. Both compounds can cause tissue necrosis if extravasated, so a functioning IV access must be assured prior to infusion. The onset of action is immediate, and duration is approximately 1 hour. Doses can be repeated. In animal studies the cardioprotective effect of calcium is ablated by verapamil.[104,105]

Calcium may be contraindicated in hypercalcemia and cardiac glycoside toxicity.[106] Digitalis toxicity is associated with intracellular hypercalcemia. Theoretically, additional calcium can worsen the toxicity and precipitate arrhythmias. Clinical data to support this are scant. Bower and Mengle reported two cases of cardiovascular collapse and death following the administration of calcium in digitalized patients, but no information on digitalis levels, serum calcium, or potassium concentrations was provided.[107] Digoxin toxicity with hyperkalemia should be treated with digoxin Fab to rapidly remove the drug (improvement within 2 hours).

Transcellular redistribution

The fastest method to reduce serum potassium is to induce a transcellular shift. Insulin is a reliable way to do this. It is typically given with glucose to prevent hypoglycemia. Insulin should be given IV to maximize the speed of potassium shift. Onset of action is within 15 minutes and the hypokalemic effect has persisted for 6 hours in some trials.[108] This can be repeated. The primary side effect is hypoglycemia.

Albuterol has been used to stimulate beta-2 receptors and produce a transcellular shift of potassium. Albuterol has been shown to be effective when given IV, by nebulizer, or by metered-dose inhaler (MDI) with spacer.[109–111] One concern is the beta-selectivity of albuterol. Alpha-agonists increase serum potassium. Two studies that looked at potassium immediately after administration of albuterol showed a brief increase in serum potassium.[109,112] A short-lived predominance of alpha activity immediately following administration of albuterol may account for the increase in serum potassium.

Combining therapies is additive but not synergistic. Combining albuterol and insulin/glucose is particularly appealing, as albuterol decreases the incidence of hypoglycemia. In one trial of combined modalities, the addition of albuterol to insulin regimens eliminated hypoglycemia as a complication. (This treatment protocol used only 5 g of glucose for 10 units of insulin.[113]) In a well-controlled trial the use of insulin and glucose with albuterol was twice as efficacious as either drug alone (1.2 mmol/L at 1 hour vs 0.6 mmol/L).[114]

Bicarbonate has long been listed as a way to induce an intracellular potassium shift based primarily on case reports and small trials.[115,116] Recent data have shown bicarbonate to be an ineffective agent for the treatment of hyperkalemia. Blumberg et al found an increase in potassium of 0.2 mmol/L following bicarbonate infusions regardless of whether isotonic or hypertonic bicarbonate was used.[117] Bicarbonate also failed to demonstrate synergy with insulin/glucose or nebulized albuterol. Sodium bicarbonate also did not help in patients with low serum bicarbonate. Additionally, increases in pH lower ionized calcium, which increases the risk of arrhythmia with hyperkalemia.

Other strategies to induce a transcellular shift include epinephrine infusions and aminophylline; however, both of these therapies are less effective than insulin and glucose.[117,118]

In patients with cardiac arrest requiring external cardiac massage, the ability to induce a transcellular shift is reduced:[119] this may be due to a redistribution of blood flow to the heart and brain and away from skeletal muscle and liver, the tissues primarily involved in cellular redistribution.[120]

Enhanced gastrointestinal clearance of potassium

In addition to inducing a transcellular shift of potassium, patients with increases in total body potassium require specific therapy to remove potassium from the body. Cation exchange resins can enhance intestinal potassium excretion. Sodium polysterene (SPS) resins bind approximately 1 mEq of potassium per gram of resin. SPS maximally absorbs potassium when given orally, but enemas are effective.[121] When given at doses of 20–40 g, SPS resins can be effective at treating acute hyperkalemia after calcium and intracellular shift treatments have been initiated. Two recent studies have questioned the effectiveness of SPS resins, but until larger studies corroborate these findings, SPS resins remain part of the therapy for acute hyperkalemia.[106,122] SPS and sorbitol usage have rarely been associated with intestinal necrosis; whether this is due to sorbitol, the resin, or other factors is unclear.[123–125]

Enhanced renal clearance of potassium

In patients with decreased renal excretion of potassium, but adequate GFR, the kidneys may be used to increase potassium excretion. The best way to increase renal potassium excretion is to increase distal delivery of sodium and increase tubular flow by increasing sodium intake and using loop diuretics. Potassium-sparing diuretics should be stopped.

Dialysis

In cases of severe hyperkalemia, dialysis is the best method of removing potassium from the body. In a study comparing various therapeutic regimens for hyperkalemia, Blumberg et al found hemodialysis to be faster than insulin and glucose. The use of a 1 mmol/L potassium bath for 1 hour lowered the serum potassium by 1.34 mmol/L.[117] Higher serum potassium concentrations enhance dialytic clearance of potassium. A 4-hour dialysis session with a potassium bath of 1 mmol/L can be expected to remove between 60 and 140 mmol of potassium.[126] Following dialysis, the serum concentration rises significantly. Therapies that shift potassium into cells decrease the effectiveness of dialysis and increase the post-rebound serum potassium.[126] There is concern that dialyzing patients prone to cardiac arrhythmias (patients on digoxin, coronary artery disease, left ventricular hypertrophy, etc.) with low potassium dialysate may precipitate arrhythmias. In a randomized controlled trial, potassium modeling (stepwise lowering of the potassium bath during treatment) reduced premature ventricular complexes (PVCs) and PVC couplets during dialysis.[127]

Continuous renal replacement therapies are also effective at reducing potassium and are generally better tolerated than intermittent hemodialysis in unstable patients. Peritoneal dialysis has been used successfully to treat hyperkalemia. Patients with cardiac arrest requiring external cardiac massage may be particularly appropriate candidates for peritoneal dialysis, as this modality does not depend on systemic blood pressure.[119] Continuous hemofiltration has gained acceptance in the ICU and has been used to successfully treat hyperkalemic asystole.[128]

The use of intermittent dialysis techniques in the face of cardiac arrest may be possible. In one case of ventricular fibrillation due to hyperkalemia, cardiopulmonary resuscitation (CPR) provided adequate blood pressure to dialyze the patient. Cardiac function was restored after 25 minutes of dialysis.[129]

Other issues in the treatment of hypokalemia

An important factor to consider when adopting a treatment strategy for hyperkalemia is whether the source of potassium is transient (e.g. potassium overdose) or continuous (e.g. limb or gut ischemia). In the latter situation, the use of intermittent hemodialysis will provide temporary correction followed by recurrent hyperkalemia. Continuous renal replacement therapy offers a unique advantage in this situation as it prevents rebound hyperkalemia. In cases of severe hyperkalemia from a continuous potassium leak, one should consider mixed modalities of dialysis. Using intermittent hemodialysis will allow rapid correction of hyperkalemia, and then initiating continuous venovenous hemofiltration will prevent rebound hyperkalemia.

There are multiple cases in the literature of patients with remarkable neurologic recovery despite prolonged resuscitative efforts. Jackson et al reported an adolescent who developed hyperkalemic asystole and required 3½ hours of external cardiac massage before restoring cardiac function. There were no permanent neurologic deficits.[119] Quick and Bastani reported a case of hyperkalemia that appeared to be fatal: after 26 minutes of Advanced Cardiac Life Support (ACLS), the patient was pronounced dead; 8–10 minutes later spontaneous recovery occurred and the patient was ultimately discharged with intact neurologic function.[130] Lin and Huang reported no neurologic or cardiac sequelae after 80 minutes of CPR as part of the resuscitation from hyperkalemic cardiac arrest.[131] Patients with hyperkalemic cardiac arrest may have better outcomes than generally associated with cardiac arrest and deserve aggressive and prolonged resuscitative efforts.

REFERENCES

1. Council NR. Diet and health: implications for reducing chronic disease risk. Report of the Committee on Diet and Health, Food and Nutrition Board. Washington, DC: National Academy Press; 1989.

2. Kanaghinis T, Lubran M, Coghill NF. The composition of ileostomy fluid. Gut 1963;4:322–38.

3. Phillips SF, Giller J. The contribution of the colon to electrolyte and water conservation in man. J Lab Clin Med 1973;81:733–46.

4. Agarwal R, Afzalpurkar R, Fordtran JS. Pathophysiology of potassium absorption and secretion by the human intestine. Gastroenterology 1994;107:548–71.

5. Cummings JH, Bingham SA, Heaton KW, et al. Fecal weight, colon cancer risk, and dietary intake of nonstarch polysaccharides (dietary fiber). Gastroenterology 1992;103:1783–9.

6. Bjork JT, Soergel KH, Wood CM. The composition of 'free' stool water. Gastroenterology 1976;70:864.

7. Deitrick JE, Whedon GD, Shorr E. Effects of immobilization upon various metabolic and physiologic functions in normal men. Am J Med 1948;4:3–32.

8. Hayes CP, McLeod ME, Robinson RR. An extrarenal mechanism for the maintenance of potassium balance in severe chronic renal failure. Trans Am Soc Artif Int Organs 1965;11:242–6.

9. Williams ME, Gervino EV, Rosa RM, et al. Catecholamine modulation of rapid potassium shifts during exercise. N Engl J Med 1985;312:823–7.

10. DeFronzo RA, Sherwin RS, Dillingham M, et al. Influence of basal insulin and glucagon secretion on potassium and sodium metabolism. Studies with somatostatin in normal dogs and in normal and diabetic human beings. J Clin Invest 1978;61:472–9.

11. Zierler KL, Rabinowitz D. Effect of very small concentrations of insulin on forearm metabolism. Persistence of its action on potassium and free fatty acids without its effects on glucose. J Clin Invest 1964;43:950.

12. Martinez R, Rietberg B, Skyler J, et al. Effect of hyperkalemia on insulin secretion. Experientia 1991;47:270–2.

13. Rowe JW, Tobin JD, Rosa RM, et al. Effects of experimental potassium deficiency on glucose and insulin metabolism. Metabolism 1980;29:498–502.

14. Squires RD, Huth EJ. Experimental potassium depletion in normal human subjects. I. Relation of ionic intakes to the renal conservation of potassium. J Clin Invest 1959;38:1134–48.

15. Rabelink TJ, Koomans HA, Hené RJ, et al. Early and late adjustment to potassium loading in humans. Kidney Int 1990;38:942.

16. Malnic G, Klose RM, Giebisch G. Micropuncture study of distal tubular potassium and sodium transport in rat nephron. Am J Physiol 1966;211:529.

17. Halperin ML, Kamel KS. Potassium.Lancet 1998;352:135–40.

18. Sanson S, Muto S, Giebisch G. Na-dependent effects of DOCA on cellular transport properties of CCDs from ADX rabbits. Am J Physiol 1987;253:F753–9.

19. Ames R, Borkowski A, Sicinski A, et al. Prolonged infusions of angiotensin II and norepinephrine on blood pressure, electrolyte balance, and aldosterone and cortisol secretion in normal man and in cirrhosis with ascites. J Clin Invest 1965;44:1171.

20. Himathongkam T, Dluhy RG, Williams GH. Potassium–aldosterone–renininterrelationships. J Clin Endocrinol Metab 1975;41:153–9.

21. Morgan DB, Young RM. Acute transient hypokalemia: new interpretation of a common event. Lancet 1982;8301:751–2.

22. Licht JM, Haley RJ, Pugh B, et al. Diuretic regimens in essential hypertension. A comparison of hypokalemic effects, BP control, and cost. Arch Intern Med 1983;143:1694–9.

23. Greenfeld D, Mickley D, Quinlan DM, et al. Hypokalemia in outpatients with eating disorders.Am J Psychiatry 1995;152:60–3.

24. Elisaf M, Liberopoulos E, Bairaktari E, et al. Hypokalaemia in alcoholic patients. Drug Alcohol Rev 2002;21:73–6.

25. Coma-Canella I. Changes in plasma potassium during the dobutamine stress test. Int J Cardiol 1991; 33:55–9.

26. Hildebrandt R, Weitzel HK, Gundert-Remy U. Hypokalaemia in pregnant women treated with the beta 2-mimetic drug fenoterol – a concentration and time dependent effect. J Perinat Med 1997; 25:173–9.

27. Kunin AS, Surawicz B, Sims EAH. Decrease in serum potassium concentrations and appearance of cardiac arrhythmias during infusion of potassium with glucose in potassium-depleted patients. N Engl J Med 1962;266:228–33.

28. Crook MA, Hally V, Panteli JV. The importance of the refeeding syndrome. Nutrition 2001;17:632–7.

29. Kassirer JP, Schwartz WB. The response of normal man to selective depletion of hydrochloric acid. Am J Med 1966;40:19–26.

30. Swan RC, Axelrod DR, Seijs M, et al. Distribution of sodium bicarbonate infused into nephrectomized dogs. J Clin Invest 1975; 34:1795–801.

31. Ptacek LJ, Tawil R, Griggs RC, et al. Dihydropyridine receptor mutations cause hypokalemic periodic paralysis. Cell 1994;77:863–8.

32. Johnsen T. Trial of the prophylactic effect of diazoxide in the treatment of familial periodic hypokalemia. Acta Neurol Scand 1977;56:525–32.

33. Vern BA, Danon MJ, Hanlon K. Hypokalemic periodic paralysis with unusual responses to acetazolamide and sympathomimetics. J Neurol Sci 1987;81:159–72.

34. Ko GT, Chow CC, Yeung VT, et al. Thyrotoxic periodic paralysis in a Chinese population. QJM 1996;89:463–8.

35. Lin SH, Lin YF. Propranolol rapidly reverses paralysis, hypokalemia, and hypophosphatemia in thyrotoxic periodic paralysis. Am J Kidney Dis 2001;37:620–3.

36. Shannon M, Lovejoy FH. Hypokalemia after theophylline intoxication. The effects of acute vs chronic poisoning. Arch Intern Med 1989;149:2725–9.

37. Greger R. Why do loop diuretics cause hypokalaemia? Nephrol Dial Transplant 1997;12:1799–801.

38. Morgan DB, Davidson C. Hypokalemia and diuretics: an analysis of publications. BMJ 1980;280:905–8.

39. Sebastian A, McSherry E, Morris RC. Renal potassium wasting in renal tubular acidosis (RTA): its occurrence in types 1 and 2 RTA despite sustained correction of systemic acidosis. J Clin Invest 1971;50:677–8.

40. Lipner HI, Ruzany F, Dasgupta M, et al. The behavior of carbenicillin as a nonreabsorbable anion. J Lab Clin Med 1975;86:183–94.

41. Kelepouris E, Kasama R, Agus ZS. Effects of intracellular magnesium on calcium, potassium and chloride channels. Miner Electrolyte Metab 1993;19:277–81.

42. Wingo CS, Smolka AJ. Function and structure of H-K-ATPase in the kidney. Am J Physiol 1995;269:F1–F16.

43. Douglas JB, Healy JK. Nephrotoxic effects of amphotericin B, including renal tubular acidosis. Am J Med 1969;46:154.

44. Patel R, Savage A. Symptomatic hypomagnesemia associated with gentamicin therapy. Nephron 1979;23:50–2.

45. Hammer HF, Santa Ana CA, Shiller LR, et al. Studies of osmotic diarrhea induced in normal subjects by ingestion of polyethylene glycol and lactulose. J Clin Invest 1989;84:1056–62.

46. Krishna GG, Miller E, Kapoor SC. Potassium depletion elevates blood pressure in normotensives. N Engl J Med 1989;320:1177–82.

47. Krishna GG, Kapoor SC. Potassium depletion exacerbates essential hypertension. Ann Intern Med 1991;115:77–83.

48. Kaplan NM, Carnegie A, Raskin P, et al. Potassium supplementation in hypertensive patients with diuretic-induced hypokalemia. N Engl J Med 1985;312:746–9.

49. Svetkey LP, Yarger WE, Feussner JR, et al. Double-blind, placebo-controlled trial of potassium chloride in the treatment of mild hypertension. Hypertension 1987;9:444–50.

50. Holland OB, Nixon JV, Kuhnert L. Diuretic-induced ventricular ectopic activity. Am J Med 1981;70:762–8.

51. Hollifield JW, Slaton PE. Thiazide diuretics, hypokalemia and cardiac arrhythmias. Acta Med Scand 1981;647:67–75.

52. Counsil MR. Working party on mild to moderate hypertension. Ventricular extrasystoles during thiazide treatment: substudy of MRC mild hypertension trial. BMJ 1983;287:1249–58.
53. Madias JE, Madias NE, Gavras HP. Nonarrhythmogenicity of diuretic-induced hypokalemia. Arch Intern Med 1984;144: 2171–6.
54. Parks R, Boisvert D, Comunale M, et al. Preoperative serum potassium levels and perioperative outcomes in cardiac surgery patients. JAMA 1999;281:2203–10.
55. Madias JE, Shah B, Chintalapally G, et al. Admission serum potassium in patients with acute myocardial infarction: its correlates and value as a determinant of in-hospital outcome. Chest 2000;118:904–13.
56. Nordrehaug JE. Malignant arrhythmias in relation to serum potassium values in patients with an acute myocardial infarction. Acta Med Scand 1981;Suppl 647:101–7.
57. Shapiro W. Correlative studies of serum digitalis levels and the arrhythmias of digitalis intoxication. Am J Cardiol 1978;41:852–9.
58. Sharief MK, Robinson SF, Swash M. Hypokalaemic myopathy in alcoholism. Neuromuscul Disord 1997;7:533–5.
59. Finsterer J, Hess B, Jarius C, et al. Malnutrition-induced hypokalemic myopathy in chronic alcoholism. J Toxicol Clin Toxicol 1998;36:369–73.
60. Berl T, Linas SL, Aisenbrey GA, et al. On the mechanism of polyuria in potassium depletion. The role of polydipsia. J Clin Invest 1977;60:620–5.
61. Rubini M. Water excretion in potassium-deficient man. J Clin Invest 1961;40:2215–24.
62. Gabuzda GJ, Hall PW. Relation of potassium depletion to renal ammonium metabolism and hepatic coma. Medicine 1966;45:481.
63. West ML, Marsden PA, Richardson RM, et al. New clinical approach to evaluate disorders of potassium excretion. Miner Electrolyte Metab 1986;12:234–8.
64. Lin SH, Lin YF, Halperin ML. Hypokalaemia and paralysis. QJM 2001;94:133–9.
65. Ethier JH, Kamel KS, Magner PO, et al. The transtubular potassium concentration in patients with hypokalemia and hyperkalemia. Am J Kidney Dis 1990;15:309–15.
66. Joo KW, Chang SH, Lee JG, et al. Transtubular potassium concentration gradient (TTKG) and urine ammonium in differential diagnosis of hypokalemia. J Nephrol 2000;13:120–5.
67. Haris A, Rado JP. Patterns of potassium wasting in response to stepwise combinations of diuretics in nephrotic syndrome. Int J Clin Pharmacol Ther 1999;37:332–40.
68. West ML, Bendz O, Chen CB, et al. Development of a test to evaluate the transtubular potassium concentration gradient in the cortical collecting duct in vivo. Miner Electrolyte Metab 1986; 12:226–33.
69. Cohn JN, Kowey PR, Whelton PK, et al. New guidelines for potassium replacement in clinical practice: a contemporary review by the National Council on Potassium in Clinical Practice. Archf Intern Med 2000;160:2429–36.
70. Sterns RH, Cox M, Feig PU, et al. Internal potassium balance and the control of the plasma potassium concentration. Medicine 1981;60:339–54.
71. Scribner BH, Burnell JH. Interrpretation of the serum potassium concentration. Metabolism 1956;5:468–79.
72. Skoutakis VA, Acchiardo SR, Wojciechowski NJ, et al. The comparative bioavailability of liquid, wax-matrix, and microencapsulated preparations of potassium chloride. J Clin Pharmacol 1985; 25:619–21.
73. Halpern MT, Irwin DE, Brown RE, et al. Patient adherence to prescribed potassium supplement therapy. Clin Ther 1993;15: 1133–45.
74. Agarwal A, Wingo CS. Treatment of hypokalemia [erratum appears in N Engl J Med 1999;340(8):663]. N Engl J Med 1999; 340:154–5.
75. Kruse JA, Carlson RW. Rapid correction of hypokalemia using concentrated intravenous potassium chloride infusions. Arch Intern Med 1990;150:613–17.
76. Kruse JA, Clark VL, Carlson RW, et al. Concentrated potassium chloride infusions in critically ill patients with hypokalemia. J Clin Pharmacol 1994;34:1077–82.
77. Ugur UA, Avcu F, Cetin T, et al. Spironolactone: is it a novel drug for the prevention of amphotericin B-related hypokalemia in cancer patients? Eur J Clin Pharmacol 2002;57:771–3.
78. Smith SR, Galloway MJ, Reilly JT, et al. Amiloride prevents amphotericin B related hypokalemia in neutropenic patients. J Clin Pathol 1988;41:494–7.
79. Eiro M, Katoh T, Watanabe T. Use of a proton-pump inhibitor for metabolic disturbances associated with anorexia nervosa. N Engl J Med 2002;346:140.
80. Hahm TS, Cho HS, Lee KH, et al. Clonidine premedication prevents preoperative hypokalemia. J Clin Anesth 2002;14:6–9.
81. Schim vdLHJ, Strack vSRJ, Thijs LG. Cardiac arrest due to oral potassium intake. Intensive Care Med 1988;15:58–9.
82. Lawson DH. Adverse reactions to potassium chloride. QJM 1974; 43:433–40.
83. de Silva M, Seghatchian MJ. Is depletion of potassium in blood before transfusion essential? Lancet 1994;344:136.
84. Knichwitz G, Zahl M, Van AH, et al. Intraoperative washing of long-stored packed red blood cells by using an autotransfusion device prevents hyperkalemia. Anesth Analg 2002;95:324–5.
85. Kurtzman NA, Gonzalez J, DeFronzo R, et al. A patient with hyperkalemia and metabolic acidosis. Am J Kidney Dis 1990; 15:333–56.
86. Allon M, Takeshian A, Shanklin N. Effect of insulin-plus-glucose infusion with or without epinephrine on fasting hyperkalemia. Kidney Int 1993;43:212–17.
87. Carlebach M, Hasdan G, Shimoni T, et al. Vomiting, hyperkalaemia and cardiac rhythm disturbances. Nephrol Dial Transplant 2001;16:169–70.
88. Hande KR, Garrow GC. Acute tumor lysis syndrome in patients with high-grade non-Hodgkin's lymphoma. Am J Med 1993; 94:133–9.
89. Gronert GA. Cardiac arrest after succinylcholine: mortality greater with rhabdomyolysis than receptor upregulation. Anesthesiology 2001;94:523–9.
90. Brater DC. Effects of nonsteroidal anti-inflammatory drugs on renal function: focus on cyclooxygenase-2-selective inhibition. Am J Med 1999;107:65S–70S; discussion 70S–1S.
91. Kamel KS, Ethier JH, Quaggin S, et al. Studies to determine the basis for hyperkalemia in recipients of a renal transplant who are treated with cyclosporine. J Am Soc Nephrol 1992;2:1279–84.
92. Oishi M, Yagi T, Urushihara N, et al. A case of hyperkalemic distal renal tubular acidosis secondary to tacrolimus in living donor liver transplantation. Transplant Proc 2000;32:2225–6.
93. Marinella MA. Trimethoprim-induced hyperkalemia: an analysis of reported cases. Gerontology 1999;45:209–12.
94. Batlle DC, Arruda JA, Kurtzman NA. Hyperkalemic distal renal tubular acidosis associated with obstructive uropathy. N Engl J Med 1981;304:373–80.
95. Batlle D, Itsarayoungyuen K, Arruda JA, Kurtzman NA. Hyperkalemic hyperchloremic metabolic acidosis in sickle cell hemoglobinopathies. Am J Med 1982;72:188–92.
96. Sakemi T, Ikeda Y, Rikitake O. Tonic convulsion associated with sinus arrest due to hyperkalemia in a chronic hemodialysis patient. Nephron 1996;73:370–1.
97. Roberts KE, Magida MG. Electrocardiographic alterations produced by an increase in plasma pH, bicarbonate and sodium as compared with those produced by an increase in potassium. Circulation 1953;1:206.

98. Braun HA, Van Horne R, Bettinger JC, et al. The influence of hypocalcemia induced by sodium ethylenediamine tetraacetate on the toxicity of potassium. J Lab Clin Med 1955;46:544–8.

99. Surawicz B, Chlebus H, Mazzoleni A. Hemodynamic and electrocardiographic effects of hyperpotassemia. Differences in response to slow and rapid increases in concentration of plasma K. Am Heart J 1967;73:647–64.

100. Surawicz B, Lepeschkin E. The electrocardiogram in hyperpotassemia. Heart Bull 1961;10:66.

101. Evers S, Engelien A, Karsch V, et al. Secondary hyperkalaemic paralysis. J Neurol Neurosurg Psychiatry 1998;64:249–52.

102. Howard MR, Ashwell S, Bond LR, et al. Artefactual serum hyperkalaemia and hypercalcaemia in essential thrombocythaemia. J Clin Pathol 2000;53:105–9.

103. Don BR, Sebastian A, Cheitlin M, et al. Pseudohyperkalemia caused by fist clenching during phlebotomy. N Engl J Med 1990; 322:1290–2.

104. Bisogno JL, Langley A, Von DMM. Effect of calcium to reverse the electrocardiographic effects of hyperkalemia in the isolated rat heart: a prospective, dose-response study. Crit Care Med 1994;22:697–704.

105. Nugent M, Tinker JH, Moyer TP. Verapamil worsens rate of development and hemodynamic effects of acute hyperkalemia in halothane-anesthetized dogs: effects of calcium therapy. Anesthesiology 1984;60:435–9.

106. Emmett M. Non-dialytic treatment of acute hyperkalemia in the dialysis patient. Semin Dial 2000;13:279–80.

107. Bower JO, Mengle HAK. The additive effect of calcium and digitalis. A warning and a report of two deaths. JAMA 1936;106: 1151–3.

108. Allon M, Shanklin N. Effect of bicarbonate administration on plasma potassium in dialysis patients: interactions with insulin and albuterol. Am J Kidney Dis 1996;28:508–14.

109. Mandelberg A, Krupnik Z, Houri S, et al. Salbutamol metered-dose inhaler with spacer for hyperkalemia: how fast? How safe? Chest 1999;115:617–22.

110. Montoliu J, Almirall J, Ponz E, et al. Treatment of hyperkalaemia in renal failure with salbutamol inhalation. J Intern Med 1990; 228:35–7.

111. Montoliu J, Lens XM, Revert L. Potassium-lowering effect of albuterol for hyperkalemia in renal failure. Arch Intern Med 1987;147:713–17.

112. Du PWJ, Hay L, Kahler CP, et al. The dose-related hyper- and hypokalaemic effects of salbutamol and its arrhythmogenic potential. Br J Pharmacol 1994;111:73–6.

113. Ngugi NN, McLigeyo SO, Kayima JK. Treatment of hyperkalaemia by altering the transcellular gradient in patients with renal failure: effect of various therapeutic approaches. East African Med J 1997;74:503–9.

114. Allon M, Copkney C. Albuterol and insulin for treatment of hyperkalemia in hemodialysis patients. Kidney International 1990;38:869–72.

115. Schwarz KC, Cohen BD, Lubash GD, et al. Severe acidosis and hyperpotassemia treated with sodium bicarbonate infusion. Circulation 1959;19:215–20.

116. Burnell JM, Villamil MF, Uyeno BT, et al. The effect in humans of extracellular pH change on the relationship between serum potassium concentration and intracellular potassium. J Clin Invest 1956;35:935–9.

117. Blumberg A, Weidmann P, Shaw S, et al. Effects of various therapeutic approaches on plasma potassium and major regulating factors in terminal renal failure. Am J Med 1988;85:507–12.

118. Mahajan SK, Mangla M, Kishore K. Comparison of aminophylline and insulin-dextrose infusions in acute therapy of hyperkalemia in end-stage renal disease patients. J Assoc Physicians India 2001;49:1082–5.

119. Jackson MA, Lodwick R, Hutchinson SG. Hyperkalaemic cardiac arrest successfully treated with peritoneal dialysis. BMJ 1996;312:1289–90.

120. Schummer WJ, Schummer C. Hyperkalemic cardiac arrest: the method chosen depends on the local circumstances. Crit Care Med 2002;30:1674–5.

121. Evans BM, Hughes Jones NC, Milne MD, et al. Ion exchange resins in the treatment of anuria. Lancet 1953;791–5.

122. Gruy-Kapral C, Emmett M, Santa ACA, et al. Effect of single dose resin-cathartic therapy on serum potassium concentration in patients with end-stage renal disease. J Am Soc Nephrol 1998; 9:1924–30.

123. Wootton FT, Rhodes DF, Lee WM, et al. Colonic necrosis with Kayexalate enemas after renal transplantation. Ann Intern Med 1989;111:947–9.

124. Rashid A, Hamilton SR. Necrosis of the gastrointestinal tract in uremic patients as a result of sodium polystyrene sulfonate (Kayexalate) in sorbitol: an underrecognized condition. Am J Surg Pathol 1997;21:60–9.

125. Gerstman BB, Kirkman R, Platt R. Intestinal necrosis associated with postoperative orally administered sodium polystyrene sulfonate in sorbitol. Am J Kidney Dis 1992;20:159–61.

126. Ahmed J, Weisberg L. Hyperkalemia in dialysis patients. Semin Dial 2001;14:348–56.

127. Redaelli B, Locatelli F, Limido D, et al. Effect of a new model of hemodialysis potassium removal on the control of ventricular arrhythmias. Kidney Int 1996;50:609–17.

128. Torrecilla C, de la Serna JL. Hyperkalemic cardiac arrest, prolonged heart massage and simultaneous hemodialysis. Intensive Care Med 1989;15:325–6.

129. Lin JL, Huang CC. Successful initiation of hemodialysis during cardiopulmonary resuscitation due to lethal hyperkalemia. Crit Care Med 1990;18:342–3.

130. Quick G, Bastani B. Prolonged asystolic hyperkalemic cardiac arrest with no neurologic sequelae. Ann Emerg Med 1994; 24:305–11.

131. Lin JL, Huang CC. Successful initiation of hemodialysis during cardiopulmonary resuscitation due to lethal hyperkalemia. Crit Care Med 1990;18:342–3.

132. Murthy BV. Hyperkalaemia and rapid blood transfusion. Anaesthesia 2000;55:398.

133. Campieri C, Fatone F, Mignani R, et al. Terminal arrhythmia due to hyperkalemia corrected by intravenous calcium infusion. Nephron 1987;47:312.

134. Lens XM, Montoliu J, Cases A, et al. Treatment of hyperkalaemia in renal failure: salbutamol v. insulin. Nephrol Dial Transplant 1989;4:228–32.

135. Blumberg A, Wiedmann P, Ferrari P. Effect of prolonged bicarbonate administration on plasma potassium in terminal renal failure. Kidney Int 1992;41:369–74.

136. Shires G, Barber A, Shires GT. Fluid and electrolyte management of the surgical patient. In: Schwartz SI, Brunicardi FC, Andersen DK et al, eds. Schwartz's Principles of Surgery, 7th edn. New York: McGraw-Hill; 1999:53–74.

137. Patterson MJ, Galloway SD, Nimmo MA. Effect of induced metabolic alkalosis on sweat composition in men. Acta Physiol Scand 2002;174:41–6.

24

Disorders of calcium, phosphorus, and magnesium

Joel Michels Topf and Elaine Worcester

CALCIUM

Calcium is a divalent cation that regulates cellular movement, hormone release, enzyme activity, and coagulation. Calcium also plays a role in cell injury and death.[1] Ninety-nine percent of total body calcium is located in the bones and teeth. Normally, cytosolic calcium is very low, with a ratio of extracellular to intracellular ionized calcium of 10 000:1.[2]

MEASURING CALCIUM

Normal serum calcium concentration is 8.8–10.3 mg/dl. The molecular weight of calcium is 40; in SI units the normal range is 2.2–2.6 mmol/L (4.4–5.2 mEq/L). Forty percent of serum calcium is protein-bound, primarily to albumin; an additional 10–15% is complexed to serum anions, such as bicarbonate, phosphate, and citrate. The remaining 45% is the physiologically active, *ionized* fraction.[3] Normal ionized calcium is 4.0–5.2 mg/dl (1.0–1.3 mmol/L). Decreases in albumin lower total serum calcium without affecting ionized calcium. Likewise, increases in albumin or dramatic increases in globulins cause meaningless increases in total calcium, while the calcium regulatory mechanism maintains a normal ionized calcium.[4,5] Increases in pH enhance calcium binding to albumin, lowering ionized calcium, whereas decreases in pH have the opposite effect. Free fatty acids, either from lipid infusions or endogenous lipolysis, increase calcium binding by albumin, lowering ionized calcium.[6] Despite widespread use of formulas to adjust total calcium for albumin and pH, these have been shown to be poor predictors of ionized calcium. In patients where total calcium is borderline or there is suspicion of disordered protein–calcium binding, an ionized calcium should be checked.[7,8]

NORMAL REGULATION

A complex web of hormones tightly regulates the concentration of serum calcium. Unlike most electrolytes, the regulation of calcium balance begins with control of dietary absorption. In most situations 300–400 mg of dietary calcium is absorbed but since 200 mg is lost in gastrointestinal (GI) secretions, the net daily absorption is only 100–200 mg (Fig. 24.1). When patients are in calcium balance, all of that calcium is excreted in the urine. Calcium metabolism is under the influence of parathyroid hormone (PTH), calcitriol, calcitonin, estrogen, and testosterone. The effect of estrogen and testosterone are complex, poorly understood, and will not be further discussed (Fig. 24.2).

PTH is a peptide hormone released from the parathyroid glands in response to ionized hypocalcemia. Elevated calcium, magnesium, and calcitriol all suppress PTH release. PTH minimizes urinary calcium excretion by increasing calcium resorption in the thick ascending limb of the loop of Henle (TALH) and the distal convoluted tubule. PTH also stimulates the conversion of 25-hydroxyvitamin D to 1,25-dihydroxyvitamin D (calcitriol) by the kidney. PTH, in conjunction with calcitriol, mobilizes calcium from bone.

Vitamin D is ingested or synthesized in the skin. In order for vitamin D to become metabolically active it must be hydroxylated, first in the liver and then in the kidney, to form calcitriol. Calcitriol increases dietary absorption of calcium and phosphorus, is active in bone metabolism, and can

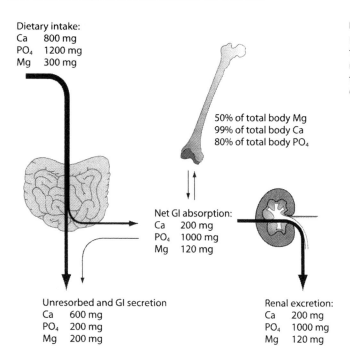

Dietary intake:
Ca   800 mg
PO₄   1200 mg
Mg   300 mg

50% of total body Mg
99% of total body Ca
80% of total body PO₄

Net GI absorption:
Ca   200 mg
PO₄   1000 mg
Mg   120 mg

Unresorbed and GI secretion
Ca   600 mg
PO₄   200 mg
Mg   200 mg

Renal excretion:
Ca   200 mg
PO₄   1000 mg
Mg   120 mg

Figure 24.1 Calcium (Ca), phosphorus (as phosphate PO_4), and magnesium (Mg) have unique patterns of dietary intake, absorption, degree of mineralization, and renal excretion. Values are typical for adult males on an American diet. GI = gastrointestinal.

increase calcium reabsorption by the distal convoluted tubule. Calcitriol feeds back on the parathyroids to decrease PTH synthesis.

Calcitonin is a 32-amino acid peptide that decreases serum calcium.

RENAL HANDLING OF CALCIUM

Both the ionized fraction and the complexed calcium, representing 55–60% of total calcium, are freely filtered at the glomerulus. Nearly all of this filtered calcium (98%) is reabsorbed by the tubules (Fig. 24.3). In the proximal tubule calcium is reab-

sorbed in concert with sodium. Increased proximal sodium reabsorption, as seen with volume depletion, increases calcium reabsorption. Typically two-thirds of filtered calcium is reabsorbed by the proximal tubules. Calcium reabsorption in the TALH is primarily passive down an electrical gradient created by the Na–K–2Cl carrier and the ROMK channel (Fig. 24.4). The distal convoluted tubule (DCT) is the only area where calcium can be reabsorbed independent of sodium. PTH stimulates calcium reabsorption at the TALH by increasing the calcium permeability of the paracellular junctions. PTH and calcitriol both increase calcium reabsorption in the DCT by complex mechanisms.

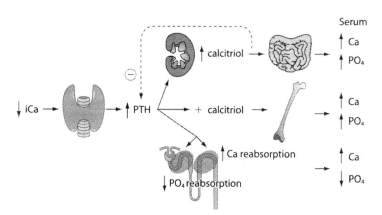

Serum
↑ Ca
↑ PO₄

↑ Ca
↑ PO₄

↑ Ca

↓ PO₄

↓ iCa → ↑ PTH → + calcitriol
↑ calcitriol
↑ Ca reabsorption
↓ PO₄ reabsorption

Figure 24.2 Decreased ionized calcium (Ca) stimulates parathyroid hormone (PTH) release from the parathyroid gland. PTH acts on three targets: it stimulates 1-alpha-hydroxylase to increase calcitriol synthesis, which increases gastrointestinal Ca and phosphate (PO_4) absorption (calcitriol also inhibits PTH secretion); in concert with calcitriol, PTH stimulates bone resorption, releasing Ca and PO_4; PTH increases tubular reabsorption of Ca and decreases tubular reabsorption of PO_4, increasing serum calcium and lowering serum PO_4.

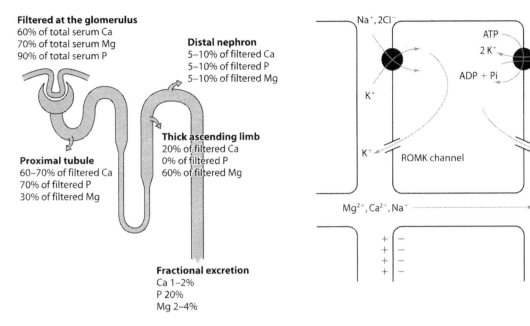

Filtered at the glomerulus
60% of total serum Ca
70% of total serum Mg
90% of total serum P

Distal nephron
5–10% of filtered Ca
5–10% of filtered P
5–10% of filtered Mg

Proximal tubule
60–70% of filtered Ca
70% of filtered P
30% of filtered Mg

Thick ascending limb
20% of filtered Ca
0% of filtered P
60% of filtered Mg

Fractional excretion
Ca 1–2%
P 20%
Mg 2–4%

Figure 24.3 Renal handling of calcium (Ca), phosphorus (P), and magnesium (Mg) varies in each segment of the nephron.

Figure 24.4 The thick ascending limb of the loop of Henle (TALH). Calcium (Ca^{2+}) and magnesium (Mg^{2+}) are both reabsorbed through the paracellular space down an electrical gradient. The Na–K–2Cl carrier paired with the apical potassium channel, ROMK, generates the positive potential difference. The Na–K–2Cl carrier itself is not electrogenic because the two cations are balanced by the 2 chloride anions, but since potassium is recycled through the ROMK channel, the net movement of charge is one anion leaving the tubule, which generates a positive potential difference. Factors which block either the Na–K–2Cl carrier (e.g. furosemide) or the ROMK channel (e.g. hypercalcemia, magnesium depletion) increase renal excretion of calcium and magnesium.

HYPOCALCEMIA

Hypocalcemia is common among intensive care unit (ICU) patients with prevalence variously reported to be 70–90%.[8] Ionized hypocalcemia is only slightly less common, with prevalence ranging from 20 to 88%.[8–10] The frequency of ionized hypocalcemia increases with increasing severity of illness and is associated with increased mortality.[9,10]

Etiologies

Broadly speaking, hypocalcemia occurs when calcium moves out of the vascular space faster than it can be repleted by the mobilization of skeletal calcium. Calcium moves into the vascular space via dietary absorption and bone resorption. Calcium leaves the vascular space via excretion by the kidneys or due to deposition in bones or soft tissue. In addition, increases in pH or chelation by anions can acutely drop the ionized calcium. The etiologies of hypocalcemia are summarized in Table 24.1.

Calcium deposition
Deposition of calcium in tissues can occur with sudden increases in phosphorus.[11] Tumor lysis syndrome releases a large amount of intracellular phosphorus, which binds ionized calcium. Phosphorus overdoses from enemas (especially if mistakenly taken orally) cause hypocalcemia due to the hyperphosphatemia.[11–13] Pancreatitis results in increased serum lipase, resulting in increased free fatty acids that chelate ionized calcium. In addition, pancreatitis is associated with increased calcitonin and decreased PTH, both of which contribute to the hypocalcemia.

The citrate used to preserve blood transfusions can bind calcium and cause ionized hypocalcemia. It is normally rapidly metabolized and well tolerated, despite transient decreases in calcium (10% of patients transiently have ionized calcium levels less than 1 mmol/L).[14] Factors that inhibit citrate metabolism (liver failure, kidney failure, hypothermia) or rapid or large transfusions predispose patients to hypocalcemia. Plasmapheresis also uses large amounts of plasma and citrate and can predispose patients to symptomatic hypocalcemia.

Table 24.1 Etiologies of hypocalcemia.		
Decreased intestinal absorption	**Increased renal excretion**	**Tissue deposition/serum complexes**
25-Hydroxy vitamin D deficiency:	Hypoparathyroidism	Citrate
Low sunlight exposure	Congenital:	EDTA
Liver disease	• Mutations of CaS receptor	Radiocontrast agents (gadolinium
Phenytoin	• DiGeorge syndrome	causes a pseudohypocalcemia)[160]
Phenobarbital	• Pseudohypoparathyroidism	Pancreatitis
Malabsorption	Acquired:	Hyperphosphatemia
Nephrotic syndrome	• Surgical hyparathyroidism	Hungry bone syndrome
Gastrectomy[157]	• Autoimmune polyendocrinopathy	Osteoblastic metastatic lesions:
1,25-Dihydroxy vitamin D deficiency:	candidiasis ectodermal dystrophy	Breast cancer
Renal failure	syndrome	Pancreatic cancer
Ketoconazole	(APECED)	
Hydroxychloroquine	• Hypermagnesemia	**Other:**
5-Fluorouracil and leucovorin	• Hypomagnesemia	Pentamidine
	• Hemochromatosis	Asparaginase
	• Granulomatous diseases	Doxorubicin
	• Neoplastic infiltration	Fluoride
	• Amyloidosis	
	• Wilson's disease	
	• Hyperthyroidism (thyroid crisis)[158]	
	• Cimetidine[159]	

Citrate-induced hypocalcemia that results in cardiac arrest has been reported.[15]

Hypoparathyroidism

Hypoparathyroidism is an important cause of acute hypocalcemia because it removes calcium from the vascular space via increased renal excretion and prevents mobilizing skeletal calcium. The most common cause of acquired hypoparathyroidism is neck surgery. Following thyroidectomy, the parathyroid gland may stop releasing PTH. It often regains function after a few days but may remain permanently dysfunctional. Hypoparathyroidism can follow radiation therapy, autoimmune, infiltrative and granulomatous diseases. Following parathyroidectomy for primary or tertiary hyperparathyroidism, there may be widespread osteoblastic activity, resulting in hypocalcemia, hypomagnesemia, and hypokalemia. This is termed hungry bone syndrome and is due to the rapid mineralization of osteoid. The hypocalcemia can last for months.

Disorders of magnesium can decrease PTH activity. Modest hypomagnesemia decreases end-organ responsiveness to PTH, whereas more severe hypomagnesemia suppresses PTH release.[16] Low magnesium levels were correlated with low ionized calcium levels in one cohort of ICU patients.[10] Magnesium, at high concentrations (>5 mg/dl), can bind the calcium receptor on the parathyroid gland, directly suppressing PTH release.

Vitamin D deficiency

Acute hypocalcemia with vitamin D deficiency occurs because of the inability to mobilize skeletal reserves of calcium. Vitamin D deficiency is very common among nursing home patients, alcoholics, and malnourished patients. Increased hepatic metabolism of vitamin D occurs in patients on phenytoin and phenobarbital. The nephrotic syndrome is commonly associated with hypocalcemia, though most of this is due to hypoalbuminemia. Ionized hypocalcemia also can occur with the nephrotic syndrome and may be due to the loss of 25-hydroxyvitamin D and its binding protein in the urine. Decreased activation of 25-hydroxyvitamin D occurs with renal failure and hypoparathyroidism.

Critical illness

Hypocalcemia is a pervasive disorder in the ICU. Although hypocalcemia was thought to be limited to patients with sepsis, Zivin et al have shown it to be frequent in all patients with severe illness.[10] Despite careful assessment, however, a definitive etiology can be found in less than half of the patients.[9] Some authors believe that ICU-associated hypocalcemia (ICU-H) is an adaptive, beneficial, response to critical illness, as it may prevent intracellular hypercalcemia and associated tissue damage.[17]

While not describing all patients with ICU-H, most patients have elevated levels of PTH and low levels of calcitriol.[18,19] Elevated levels of procalcitonin have also been found in ICU-H, leading some authors to wonder if this supposedly calcium neutral precursor to calcitonin may exert a hypocalcemic effect.[19] Septic patients with renal failure have lower ionized calcium than matched patients without renal failure. Renal failure decreases the production of calcitriol and results in hyperphosphatemia, both of which predispose patients to hypocalcemia.

Zaloga and Chernow found a striking association of hypocalcemia with Gram-negative sepsis: 30% of the patients with Gram-negative septicemia had hypocalcemia as opposed to none of the patients with Gram-positive septicemia.[18] Alberts et al had similar findings: 16 of 17 hypocalcemic patients had Gram-negative infections, whereas none had Gram-positive infections.[20]

Clinical sequelae

The primary manifestation of hypocalemia is neuromuscular irritability, ranging from perioral numbness and acral paresthesias to severe tetany and seizures. Seizures can occur in the absence of any other neuromuscular irritability. Grand mal, petit mal, and focal seizures have all been reported.

Tetany classically affects the upper extremities followed by the lower extremities. Patients typically demonstrate elbow extension, wrist flexion, and metacarpophalangeal flexion.[12] Tetany can cause laryngospasm or bronchospasm, resulting in respiratory failure. The classic signs of latent tetany are Trousseau's sign (carpal spasm after inflation of a blood pressure cuff on the arm for 3 minutes) and Chvostek's sign (facial spasm induced by tapping on the facial nerve at the temple). The sensitivity of both is poor and the specificity of Chvostek's is particularly poor (a partial Chvostek's sign is found in 25% of eucalcemic individuals).[21] Tetany may be masked by anticonvulsant therapy.

Other findings include movement disorders (extrapyramidal signs), dementia, and myopathy. Papilledema and optic neuritis have also been reported. Psychiatric disturbances, including anxiety, depression, and psychosis, have been demonstrated.

Acute hypocalcemia can cause heart failure. Even modest hypocalcemia can precipitate heart failure and hypotension in patients with latent cardiac damage. These serious findings can precede tetany.[22] The classic electrocardiogram (ECG) findings of hypocalcemia are bradycardia, prolonged QT interval, and inversion of the T wave.[15] Heart block and cardiac arrest have also been documented. The ECG is not a sensitive marker of hypocalcemia and may be normal during life-threatening hypocalcemia.

Hypotension can occur following loss of vascular tone. In one ICU study, decreased ionized calcium correlated with decreased mean arterial pressures. Digitalis acts by increasing intracellular calcium. Hypocalcemia is a cause of digitalis resistance. Patients can sometimes tolerate toxic digitalis levels with concurrent hypocalcemia. Correction of this protective hypocalcemia can precipitate arrhythmias due to digitalis toxicity.

Treatment

When to treat
Unique to calcium among all electrolyte disorders is the theory that hypocalcemia may be an adaptive response to critical illness and, because of this, the treatment of ICU-H is controversial.[17] Care must be taken not to extrapolate this controversy to patients in whom the etiology of their hypocalcemia is understood (e.g. acute hypoparathyroidism, tumor lysis syndrome, acute renal failure). Patients with chronic hypocalcemia and myocardial dysfunction should be given a trial of calcium supplementation. Patients with asymptomatic hypocalcemia secondary to surgical hypoparathyroidism had improved cardiac function with calcium infusions.[23] Calcium should be repleted in cases of seizures, tetany, laryngospasm, and hyperkalemia.[24] Among asymptomatic patients, the risk of significant clinical symptoms rises as the ionized calcium falls below 3 mg/dl, and treatment is warranted in these patients.[2]

The controversy regarding the treatment of ICU-H is born of in-vitro data that show intracellular calcium to be a mediator of cell injury in reperfusion and sepsis models. Abbott et al looked at calcium in relation to reperfusion in isolated rat hearts and found that calcium infusion immediately following reperfusion increased mitochondrial damage and decreased cardiac function.[25] In addition, animal studies have repeatedly shown that administering calcium to hypocalcemic, septic rats improves blood pressure but *increases mortality*.[26,27] The increased mortality was not reproduced in septic pigs and more recent research has questioned the appropriateness of the rat as an animal model for human sepsis.[28,29]

In critically ill, hypocalcemic, patients with life-threatening hypotension resistant to other therapies (e.g. pressors, volume resuscitation, and inotropes), trials of intravenous (IV) calcium have been undertaken. In a study of 12 hypocalcemic patients with bacterial sepsis, 7 were hypotensive despite volume resuscitation, dopamine, and norepinephrine infusions. Correcting hypocalcemia restored normal blood pressure in all 7 patients. Cardiac output, systemic vascular resistance, and urine output all improved following the calcium.[18]

We would like to emphasize that all of the negative data on replacing calcium come from studies of sepsis in animals. The applicability to the human population with ICU-H is unclear. In the limited human data on the treatment of ICU-H, the primary hemodynamic outcome improved but the clinically important outcome of mortality was not addressed. The mutifactorial etiology of ICU-H is accepted and it is likely that benefits of treatment vary with the etiology. However, until human studies have been completed to assess the effect of treating ICU-H, treatment should be considered experimental and quite possibly harmful.

How to treat

Patients with asymptomatic, mild hypocalcemia (ionized calcium >3.2 mg/dl), can be treated with increased dietary calcium (Table 24.2). Increases of 1000 mg/day are appropriate. The 25-hydroxy-vitamin D level should be checked and patients placed on vitamin D if low. In patients with renal failure, treating the hyperphosphatemia and decreased calcitriol levels will help correct the hypocalcemia.

Severe or symptomatic hypocalcemia should be treated with an infusion of 100–200 mg of elemental calcium. This should be given over 10–20 minutes to avoid cardiac toxicity. This initial infusion tends to suppress symptoms longer than it maintains a normal calcium level. In order to prevent rebound hypocalcemia, a calcium infusion should be started at 0.5–1.5 mg elemental calcium/kg/h (Table 24.3).

Two forms of parenteral calcium are commonly available: calcium gluconate and calcium chloride. Concerns that calcium gluconate would require hepatic metabolism to release the calcium have not been borne out.[30] In a randomized, double-blind trial of the two calcium salts in critically ill children, the chloride salt resulted in a higher and more consistent rise in ionized calcium levels (100% of patients receiving the chloride salt had an increase in ionized calcium vs 65% of the gluconate group).[31] Calcium chloride is caustic to veins and should be reserved for central access. Calcium gluconate can safely be infused peripherally. Both calcium compounds can cause tissue necrosis if extravasated.

Other treatment issues

Treatment of hypocalcemia can precipitate arrhythmias, especially in patients on digitalis. Other complications reported from treating hypocalcemia include bradycardia, pancreatitis, and vasospasm.[32]

When hypocalcemia is due to hyperphosphatemia, there is concern that providing calcium could accelerate metastatic soft tissue calcification.

Table 24.2 Oral calcium formulations.

Agent	Elemental calcium	How supplied
Calcium glubionate	64 mg/g	1.8 g/5 ml
Calcium gluconate	90 mg/g	500–1000 mg tablets
Calcium lactate	130 mg/g	325–650 mg tablets
Calcium citrate	211 mg/g	950 mg tablets
Calcium acetate	253 mg/g	667 mg tablets
Calcium carbonate	400 mg/g	650–1500 mg tablets

Table 24.3 Parenteral calcium formulations.

Agent	Supplied	Elemental Ca per ml	Elemental Ca per gram	
Calcium gluconate	1 g in 10 ml	9 mg/ml	90 mg	4.5 mEq
Calcium chloride	1 g in 10 ml	27.2 mg/ml	272 mg	13.6 mEq
Calcium gluceptate	1 g in 5 ml	18 mg/ml	90 mg	4.5 mEq

The degree to which this occurs is unclear. In the face of hyperphosphatemia, calcium should be given in order to reverse serious toxicity (laryngospasm, arrhythmias) and full correction of hypocalcemia should be delayed until the phosphorus is normalized.[11]

Hypomagnesemia can contribute to hypocalcemia; therefore, patients should have their magnesium checked and repleted if low.[16] Reports of magnesium-responsive hypocalcemia despite normal serum magnesium levels are thought to be due to total body magnesium depletion despite normal serum levels (see Diagnosis section of Hypomagnesemia for details).

The principal therapy for hypocalcemia due to citrate toxicity is metabolism of the citrate. Citrate metabolism occurs via temperature-dependent enzymes; therefore, correcting hypothermia improves hepatic metabolism. Steps to improve hypotension and hepatic blood flow should be taken. Saline loading in order to increase renal clearance may speed recovery, but be aware that saline loading will also increase renal calcium excretion. About 20% of citrate is excreted unmetabolized in the urine.

HYPERCALCEMIA

Etiologies

Hypercalcemia, a relatively common clinical finding, occurs when calcium enters the vascular compartment faster than it can be excreted. There are two mechanisms by which calcium enters the vascular space: vitamin D mediated absorption from the gut and bone resorption. Likewise, there are two means by which calcium is removed from the vascular space: deposition in tissue and excretion in urine.

The most common cause of hypercalcemia is primary hyperparathyroidism, with malignancy a distant second. Among hospitalized patients, however, this ratio is reversed, with cancer accounting for 65% of cases and hyperparathyroidism 25%. One series found milk-alkali syndrome to account for up to 12% of patients hospitalized for hypercalcemia.[33] A summary of the etiologies of hypercalcemia is listed in Table 24.4.

Increased intake
Increased dietary intake alone rarely causes hypercalcemia because the kidney is able to increase calcium excretion dramatically. Increased intake causes hypercalcemia in patients with renal failure or in patients where the kidney is prevented from excreting calcium.

Milk-alkali syndrome. The milk-alkali syndrome (MAS) is defined by three concurrent findings – hypercalcemia, metabolic alkalosis, and renal insufficiency – and is due to the ingestion of calcium and alkali.[33] In the modern era, patients are typically women being treated for osteoporosis with calcium carbonate, which supplies both the calcium and the alkali. Historically, MAS was characterized by hyperphosphatemia due to the high phosphorus content of milk. In modern MAS, the calcium is a pharmaceutical product without phosphorus and patients tend to be hypophosphatemic, which stimulates calcitriol production, increasing calcium absorption. The hypercalcemia typically responds to stopping the alkali and calcium. Additionally, saline infusions and loop diuretics have been shown to be particularly effective treatments.[33]

Hypervitaminosis D. Vitamin D intoxication causes hypercalcemia. This occurs from iatrogenic vitamin overdoses or inadvertent overfortification of milk.[34] Since vitamin D and 25-hydroxyvitamin D have half-lives of weeks, the hypercalcemia will be long-lasting.

Endogenous calcitriol production. Calcitriol synthesis can be increased by chronic granulomatous disorders, lymphomas, and acromegaly.[35,36] Of the

Table 24.4 Etiologies of hypercalcemia.

Increased intestinal intake	Increased bone resorption	Decreased renal excretion
Increased calcium intake:	Hyperparathyroidism:	Thiazide diuretics
Renal failure (often with vitamin	Primary:	Familial hypocalciuric hypercalcemia
D supplementation)	● Adenoma	Hyperparathyroidism
Milk-alkali syndrome	● Hyperplasia	
Hypervitaminosis D:	Tertiary	
Increased intake of vitamin D or	MEN I	
metabolites	MEN IIA	
● Calcipotriol (topical treatment for	Lithium therapy[166]	
psoriasis is structurally similar	Malignancy:	
to 1,25-dihydroxyvitamin D)[161]	PTH-rP (humoral hypercalcemia)	
Chronic granulomatous disorders:	Metastasis to the bones:	
Sarcoidosis	● breast cancer	
Leprosy	● prostate cancer	
Tuberculosis	● Langerhans cell histiocytosis[167]	**Miscellaneous**
Berylliosis	Hyperthyroidism	Phenochromocytoma
Histoplasmosis	Immobilization	Adrenal insufficiency
Silicon-induced granulomas[162]	Paget's disease	Rhabdomyolysis
Disseminated candidiasis	Estrogen and antiestrogens in	Theophylline toxicity
Wegener's granulomatosis[163]	metastatic breast cancer	Coccidioidomycosis[170]
Brucellosis	Hypervitaminosis A	Pseudohypercalcemia due to
Talc granulomatosis[164]	Retinoic acid	thrombocytosis[171]
Cat-scratch disease[165]	PTH-rP in pregnancy and lactation[168]	Human growth hormone[172]
Hodgkin's/non-Hodgkin's lymphoma[36]	Vitamin A toxicity[169]	Recovery of rhabdomyolysis-induced
Acromegaly		acute renal failure[173]

MEN = multiple endocrine neoplasia; PTH-rP = parathyroid hormone-related protein.

chronic granulomatous disorders, sarcoidosis is the most common. Macrophages, found in the granulomas, convert 25-hydroxyvitamin D to 1,25-dihydroxyvitamin D despite low PTH levels, the normal regulator of alpha 1-hydroxylase. Both Hodgkin's disease and non-Hodgkin's lymphoma can cause hypercalcemia by endogenous production of 1,25-dihydroxyvitamin D.

Increased bone resorption

Malignancy is the most common cause of inpatient hypercalcemia: 10–20% of patients with cancer get hypercalcemia. The most common associated malignancies are breast cancer, lung cancer, and multiple myeloma. There are three primary mechanisms for increased bone resorption in malignancy:

● local osteolysis from bone metastasis

● tumor secretion of PTH-related peptide (PTH-rP), often called humoral hypercalcemia
● tumor-induced hydroxylation of 25-hydroxyvitamin D to calcitriol.

Local osteolytic hypercalcemia follows bone metastasis and, hence, is most often seen in cancers with a predilection for bone: small-cell lung cancer, breast cancer, and myeloma.

The most common cause of hypercalcemia of malignancy is PTH-rP. This physiologic protein is normally secreted by nonmalignant cells and is involved in the synthesis and development of cartilage. PTH-rP binds to PTH receptors because they share 13 amino acids at the amino terminal. PTH-rP stimulates all of the normal PTH actions but, compared with PTH, has less effect on calcitriol production and bone resorption. PTH-rP's primary mechanism of hypercalcemia is increased renal reabsorption of calcium. PTH-rP is not measured by PTH assays and requires a specific blood test. PTH-rP production is most common in nonmetastatic solid tumors but also occurs in non-Hodgkin's lymphoma, chronic myeloid leukemia (blast phase), and adult T-cell lymphoma.

Hyperparathyroidism

Primary hyperparathyroidism is the most frequent cause of hypercalcemia. Mild hypercalcemia, hypophosphatemia, and elevated PTH are the hallmarks of this condition. Generally, patients have three normal parathyroid glands, with one large gland containing a functional adenoma. However, in 15% of cases, there will be four-gland hyperplasia. Parathyroid cancer accounts for less than 1% of primary hyperparathyroidism. Surgery to remove the autonomous gland is the preferred treatment and in cases of diffuse, four-gland enlargement, three and a half glands are removed. For patients who are not surgical candidates, symptomatic treatment is appropriate. Rarely, extreme, symptomatic hypercalcemia can occur with hyparathyroidism. This is called parathyroid crisis and is characterized by mental status changes, severe hypercalcemia, and very high PTH levels. Surgical removal of the parathyroid tissue is indicated.

Secondary hyperparathyroidism is an increase in PTH due to normal stimuli, i.e. hypocalcemia and low calcitriol levels. This commonly occurs in chronic renal failure and results in high PTH levels associated with low or normal ionized calcium. Correcting the hypocalcemia and/or replacing the calcitriol suppresses the release of PTH. Long-standing secondary hyperparathyroidism may progress to tertiary hyperparathyroidism. In tertiary hyperparathyroidism the glands no longer respond to normal stimuli and autonomously secrete PTH. These patients, as in primary hyperparathyroidism, are hypercalcemic. Unlike primary hyperparathyroidism, the patients typically have four-gland hyperplasia. Surgery is the usual therapy.

Clinical sequelae

Mild hypercalcemia is associated with relatively mild, nonspecific symptoms. Patients with primary hyperparathyroidism are generally asymptomatic but may complain of weakness, fatigue, anorexia, depression, vague abdominal pain, and constipation. Gastrointestinal side effects become more severe at higher calcium levels. Hypercalcemia has been associated with increased gastrin secretion and may predispose patients to peptic ulcers. Severe hypercalcemia can cause pancreatitis. The hypothesized mechanism is inappropriate activation of trypsinogen within the pancreatic parenchyma.

Hypercalcemia can cause multiple forms of renal dysfunction. Long-standing hypercalcemia predisposes patients to nephrolithiasis. Hypercalcemia causes a renal concentrating defect by reducing sodium reabsorption in the TALH and decreasing the renal response to antidiuretic hormone (ADH), predisposing patients to volume depletion. Hypercalcemia also causes renal insufficiency. Primarily this is due to volume deficiency but calcium-induced vasoconstriction reduces renal blood flow. If the hypercalcemia is long-standing, calcification and ischemia result in irreversible renal insufficiency.

Mental status changes from mild confusion to psychosis or coma can occur in severe cases of hypercalcemia. Mental status impairment can persist for 1–2 days following correction of hypercalcemia.[37]

Shortened QT interval occurs with hypercalcemia and is generally considered a benign finding.[38] Bradycardia, responsive to atropine, has been reported.[39]

Treatment

The best treatment for hypercalcemia is to correct the underlying etiology. In situations where this is not possible or specific hypocalcemic therapy is needed, the treatment should focus on the three legs of calcium physiology: calcium reabsorption in the kidney, calcium mobilization by the bones, and calcium absorption by the gut. A summary of therapies can be found in Table 24.5.

Renal reabsorption of filtered calcium occurs primarily in the proximal tubule and TALH. Calcium reabsorption is generally tied to sodium reabsorption, so that interventions that reduce sodium reabsorption also reduce calcium reabsorption. The most effective way to do this is to infuse saline. Saline also treats the volume depletion found with hypercalcemia. Following volume repletion, loop diuretics can further reduce calcium reabsorption. The goal of therapy is a brisk diuresis of 250–300 ml/h; however, this may be difficult to achieve and poses significant risk to patients.[40] Care should be given to monitor the patient's volume status and electrolytes. Saline and diuretics are short-term

Table 24.5   Treatment of hypercalcemia.

Drug	Dose	Onset	Effectiveness	Duration	Concerns
Saline and furosemide	Infuse saline at a rate high enough to achieve urine output of 250–300 ml/h	24–48 h	0.5–2.0 mg/dl. Frequent treatment failures	3 days	Volume overload, electrolyte abnormalities
Calcitonin	4–8 IU/kg SC or IV b.i.d.–q.i.d. for 1–2 days	4 h	2–3 mg/dl	1–4 days	Tachyphylaxis, nausea, rash flushing malaise
Hemodialysis	3 h with low calcium dialysate (0–1 mmol/L)	Significant decrease in calcium at 1 h	4–6 mg/dl in 3 h	Variable. May be repeated as needed	Cardiovascular instability from rapid decrease in calcium
Plicamycin (mithramycin)	25 µg/kg IV over 4–6 h, repeat q.d.	12–72 h	1–2 mg/dL per dose	2–14 days	Hepatic, renal, bone marrow toxicity. Thrombocytopenia
Pamidronate[46]	Single infusion over 2, 4, or 24 h. 30 mg for Ca < 12. 60 mg for Ca 12–13.5. 90 mg for Ca >13.5	48 h with normocalcemia at 96 h	30 mg lowered Ca by 2.2 mg/dl 60 mg lowered Ca by 3.3 mg/dl 90 mg lowered Ca by 3.9 mg/dl	10–30 days Dosing every 2 weeks increased maintenance of normocalcemia	Limit to 30 mg in patients with renal failure. Fever in 20%. Hypocalcemia (asymptomatic)
Zoledronate[48]	4 mg given over 5 min. 8 mg for relapse or refractory hypercalcemia	96 h Calcium was not assessed prior to 96 h	50% remission at 4 days 88% at 7 days	32 days for 4 mg 43 days for 8 mg	Fever. Rare (1–2%) renal insufficiency
Chloroquine[45]	250 mg b.i.d.	1–3 days	Able to normalize serum calcium in sarcoidosis	Maintenance chloroquine	Only used in patients with increased 1,25-dihydroxyvitamin D. Ineffective in hypercalcemia of malignancy
Corticosteroids	Hydrocortisone 200–400 mg/ day for 3–5 days	4–7 days	0.5–3 mg/dl	3–4 days	Hyperglycemia, immunosuppression, electrolyte abnormalities

initial therapies, but significant hypercalcemia usually requires additional therapy.

In hypercalcemia due to granulomatous diseases, conservative therapy consists of minimizing sun exposure, avoiding supplemental vitamin D, and discouraging calcium-rich diets.[41] Corticosteroids reduce serum and urinary calcium levels within days by blocking calcium absorption at the gut and reducing extrarenal formation of calcitriol.[42] Failure of prednisone (20–40 mg/day) to correct the hypercalcemia within 2 weeks should prompt exploration for an alternative diagnosis.[41] Chloroquine and hydroxychloroquine can block peripheral production of calcitriol and have been shown to be an effective treatment for sarcoidosis-induced hypercalcemia;[43,44] however, they were ineffective in calcitriol-induced hypercalcemia from lymphoma.[45] Ketoconazole has also been used in the treatment of calcitriol-induced hypercalcemia.

There are multiple pharmacologic strategies designed to block calcium resorption from bone. The most effective are the bisphosphonates, which are pyrophosphate analogues that bind to hydroxyapatite crystals, and following uptake by osteoclasts, prevent further bone resorption. The bisphosphonates are effective at correcting hypercalcemia of malignancy regardless of the etiology.[46] Pamidronate has achieved widespread use and has been shown to be superior in both efficacy and convenience to etidronate and clodronate.[47] Zoledronate, a newer bisphosphonate, has been shown to be superior to the maximum dose of pamidronate in two randomized controlled trials.[48] However, some clinicians have questioned the validity of these data due to the poor performance of pamidronate compared to prior trials. It is unclear if zoledronate will eclipse pamidronate as the standard of care.

Salmon calcitonin can rapidly lower serum calcium by inhibiting osteoclastic bone resorption. It also increases renal excretion of calcium. It can be given IV or subcutaneously (SQ) and reduces serum calcium by 1–2 mg/dl within hours of administration. Unfortunately, it only works in just over half of patients with hypercalcemia of malignancy, and tachyphylaxis is common after 2–3 days.

Mithramycin (now called plicamycin) was a primary therapy for hypercalcemia prior to the development of bisphosphonates. It blocks DNA transcription in osteoclasts. It works reliably, but has largely been dropped due to its significant hepatic and bone marrow toxicity.

Dialysis
Dialysis should be considered in patients with severe symptomatic hypercalcemia that is unresponsive to drug therapy. Low calcium hemodialysis (dialysate calcium of 0–0.5 mmol/L) has repeatedly been shown to rapidly correct hypercalcemia. Calcium clearance for hemodialysis ranges from 270–680 mg/h. Although there is a risk of

rebound hypercalcemia, many patients are able to maintain normocalcemia with drug therapy following a single dialysis session.[49] Peritoneal dialysis has been used for hypercalcemia but calcium clearance was unsatisfactory (average 60 mg/h, compared with 82 mg/h with saline and furosemide). Continuous renal replacement therapy (CRRT) has been used in cases where rebound hypercalcemia has been a problem. CRRT can be paired with citrate regional anticoagulation, which chelates free calcium, allowing rapid and durable control of hypercalcemia.[50]

Overview
Treatment of hypercalcemia may utilize multiple modalities. Initially, calcium and vitamin D preparations should be stopped. The next action should be to administer saline to restore euvolemia. In cases of endogenous calcitriol excess, steroids are an effective acute treatment and chloroquine/hydroxychloroquine or ketoconazole may be used as long-term therapies. In patients with hyperparathyroidism, surgical treatment is the definitive therapy and seldom is additional therapy required. Using bisphosphonates prior to surgery may result in severe hypocalcemia postoperatively (hungry bone syndrome). In hypercalcemia of malignancy, bisphosphonates are the standard of care, but since onset of action can be delayed up to 48 hours, calcitonin may be used as a bridge. In recalcitrant cases, saline and lasix to create a brisk diuresis may be tried with careful monitoring; however, if patients are severely symptomatic, dialysis should be initiated.

PHOSPHORUS

NORMAL PHYSIOLOGY

In medicine, phosphate and phosphorus are often used interchangeably, although, using strict nomenclature, phosphorus refers to the element and phosphate to the PO_4^{2-} anion. Inorganic phosphorus exists as a weak acid with 3 protons which can dissociate: H_3PO_4, $H_2PO_4^-$, HPO_4^{2-}, PO_4^{3-}. At a pH of 7.4 the ratio of HPO_4^{2-} to $H_2PO_4^-$ is 4:1. (H_3PO_4 and PO_4^{3-} are essentially nonexistent at physiologic pH.) Clinical laboratories report the concentration of elemental inorganic phosphorus which exists almost exclusively as phosphate (e.g. organic phospholipids and phosphorylated proteins, which represent two-thirds of serum phosphorus, are not measured in the laboratory assay).

The normal range of phosphorus is 3–4.5 mg/dl. The molecular weight is 31, so the normal concentration in SI units is 1–1.5 mmol/L (1.7–2.6 mEq/L). Normal values of phosphorus vary with age (higher levels in younger people). The upper limit of normal in infants is 6.5 mg/dl and adult ranges are not found until late adolescence.

Phosphate is a multivalent anion that powers a wide range of chemical reactions as part of the high-energy molecule, adenosine triphosphate. Phosphate is also important in regulating enzyme activity and the oxygen avidity of hemoglobin. The majority (80%) of phosphorus is mineralized in bone, with almost all of the remainder in the intracellular compartment. Only 0.1% of total body phosphorus is in the extracellular compartment.

Dietary absorption

The recommended daily allowance for phosphorus is 800 mg. Although the bioavailability of phosphorus varies widely, it is generally well absorbed by the jejunum. Meats contain organic phosphorus that is readily absorbed. Cow's milk contains casein, a phosphopeptide, which decreases bioavailability. Grains also have lower phosphorus bioavailability (see Fig. 24. 1).

Renal handling of phosphorus

The kidney filters 90% of serum phosphorus and then reabsorbs 75–99% of filtered phosphorus, depending on current phosphorus and PTH levels. Most of the filtered phosphorus (70%) is reabsorbed in the proximal tubule by two unique Na–P co-transporters. Additional phosphorus is reabsorbed in the distal convoluted tubule. PTH causes the Na–P transporters to be internalized, decreasing phosphate reabsorption.[51] Metabolic acidosis decreases transporter activity, increasing renal excretion of phosphorus. Since phosphorus reabsorption is concurrent with sodium, any factor that decreases sodium reabsorption will decrease the tubular reabsorption of phosphorus. A drop in dietary phosphorus increases renal reabsorption of phosphorus before measurable decreases in serum phosphorus occur[52] (see Fig. 24.3).

Phosphorus regulation

Normal phosphorus concentrations are maintained by adjusting intestinal absorption and renal excretion. Normally, people absorb 80% of dietary phosphorus.[53] PTH decreases renal reabsorption of phosphorus (increases renal phosphate excretion). Hypophosphatemia stimulates alpha-1 hydroxylase, which converts 25-hydroxyvitamin D to calcitriol. For details on the effects of PTH and calcitriol, see the subsections Normal regulation and Renal handling of calcium in the Calcium section (see Figs 24.2 and 24.5).

HYPOPHOSPHATEMIA

Modest degrees of hypophosphatemia are common and of little consequence. Severe hypophosphatemia, however, is rare. In a retrospective review of 55 000 serum phosphorus measurements, phosphorus levels less than 1.5 mg/dl were found in only 0.4%. Half of these samples were isolated findings, so that the rate of severe, persistent, hypophosphatemia was 0.2%.[54] However, hypophosphatemia was much more prevalent among patients with chronic obstructive pulmonary disease (COPD) exacerbations and patients admitted to the ICU. Twenty percent of patients with COPD exacerbations had a phosphorus <2.5 mg/dl and 10% had a phosphorus <2.0 mg/dl.[55] In a

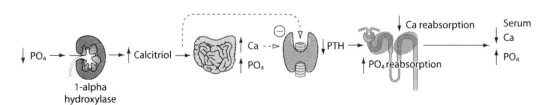

Figure 24.5 Decreased phosphorus directly stimulates the production of calcitriol by the kidney. Calcitriol has two principal actions: it increases gut absorption of calcium (Ca) and phosphate (PO₄) and suppresses parathyroid hormone (PTH) release (the increased calcium from gut absorption also suppresses PTH release). The decreased PTH increases renal reabsorption of phosphorus. Increased serum phosphorus feeds back and inhibits calcitriol production.

prospective study of surgical intensive care unit (SICU) patients, 29% were found to be hypophosphatemic.[56] Because only a tiny proportion of the total body phosphorus is found in the vascular space, the serum phosphorus is not a reliable indicator of total body phosphorus. Isolated hypophosphatemia without intracellular depletion is of little consequence and is usually a transient phenomenon. Severe symptoms from hypophosphatemia are due to total body phosphorus depletion. There are four primary etiologies of hypophosphatemia: pseudohypophosphatemia, transcellular redistribution, decreased GI absorption, and increased renal loss (Table 24.6).

Table 24.6   Etiologies of hypophosphatemia.

Intracellular shift of phosphorus	Decreased phosphorus absorption	Increased renal excretion
Carbohydrate infusions:	Dietary insufficiency	Alcoholism
Fructose	Malabsorption	Volume expansion/natriuretic states:
Glucose	Phosphate binders:	IV bicarbonate
Glycerol	Calcium	Bicarbonaturia
Lactate	Magnesium	Glucosuria
Calcitonin	Aluminum	Diuretics:
Catecholamines:	Sevelamer	• Acetazolamide is the most
Epinephrine	Lanthium	phosphaturic
Dopamine	Steatorrhea	• Thiazides
Terbutaline[60]		• Loop diuretics[55]
Albuterol	Vitamin D deficiency	• Osmotic diuretics
Insulin[75]	Glucocorticoids	High salt diet or saline infusion
Respiratory alkalosis	**Miscellaneous**	Hyperaldosteronism
Rapid cell proliferation:	Hungry bone syndrome	SIADH
Treatment of anemia	Burns	Fanconi syndrome:
CML in blast crisis	Acetaminophen overdose	Multiple myeloma
AML	Bisphosphonates	Aminoglycosides
AMML	Gallium nitrate	Heavy metal toxicity
Refeeding syndrome		Chinese herbs
Rewarming hypothermia		Congenital
		Ifosfamide
		Cisplatin
		Cystinosis
		Wilson's disease
		Hereditary fructose intolerance
		Glucocorticoids
		Hyperparathyroidism
		Hypercalcemia
		Metabolic acidosis
		Paraneoplastic syndrome:
		PTH-rP
		Tumor-induced osteomalacia
		Renal transplantation
		Acute malaria (falciparum)
		X-linked hypophosphatemic rickets
		(vitamin D resistant rickets)
		Xanthines

AML = acute myelogenous leukemia; AMML = acute myelomonocytic leukemia; CML = chronic myelogenous leukemia; IV = intravenous; PTH-rP = parathyroid hormone-related protein; SIADH = syndrome of inappropriate antidiuretic hormone.

Etiologies

Transcellular redistribution

Transcellular redistribution is movement of phosphorus into cells. This is usually transient and, in the face of normal total body phosphorus, is harmless. However, in the face of pre-existing phosphorus depletion, this transcellular movement can provoke serious symptoms, and death.[57] The most severe cases of hypophosphatemia due to transcellular distribution are found with refeeding syndrome. Starvation decreases total body phosphorus due to decreased dietary intake. Despite the phosphorus depletion, however, serum phosphorus typically remains normal as phosphorus leaks out of cells. With refeeding, insulin moves phosphorus into cells and phosphorus is consumed to phosphorylate carbohydrates as part of glycolysis. These processes rapidly unmask the total body phosphorus depletion.

Refeeding syndrome is seen during treatment of anorexia, and during the use of IV dextrose solutions or total parenteral nutrition (TPN) for patients who are not being fed. Refeeding syndrome is probably responsible for the high rate of hypophosphatemia seen among post-surgical patients: 34% of ICU patients experienced refeeding-associated hypophosphatemia after being NPO (nothing by mouth) for as little as 48 hours.[58]

Alcoholics admitted to the hospital may get severe refeeding syndrome. Alcoholics are often poorly nourished and have a renal phosphorus leak, resulting in total body phosphorus depletion. After admission, the use of dextrose fluids causes an intracellular redistribution of phosphorus. Additional factors predisposing this population to hypophosphatemia include respiratory alkalosis from associated liver disease, and increased adrenergic activity from alcohol withdrawal, resulting in intracellular movement of phosphorus.

One of the most common causes of intracellular phosphorus redistribution is respiratory alkalosis.[54] The drop in pCO_2 results in intracellular alkalemia. The increased pH stimulates glycolysis, which consumes phosphorus.[59] Renal excretion of phosphorus drops to nearly zero due to the decreased filtered load of phosphorus and PTH resistance secondary to the alkalemia. Metabolic alkalosis rarely causes the intracellular alkalemia that is essential for the phenomenon.

Inadequate phosphorus intake

Dietary insufficiency of phosphorus is rare, as phosphorus is ubiquitous in the diet and the body is efficient at reducing renal losses to nearly zero. Unfortunately, GI losses of 100–200 mg/day continue despite decreased intake and result in a negative phosphorus balance. However, the decreased body phosphorus is usually occult, because transcellular shifts maintain normal serum phosphorus levels. Malnourished patients with a predominantly carbohydrate diet can have hypophosphatemia due to insulin-induced intracellular shifts.

Steroids reduce phosphorus absorption by the gut and increase renal phosphorus wasting. Hypophosphatemia due to corticosteroids occurs with both therapeutic steroids and Cushing's disease. Antacids that contain magnesium, calcium, or aluminum bind dietary phosphorus and prevent its absorption.

Vitamin D deficiency decreases intestinal absorption of phosphorus and the lack of calcitriol increases PTH release. Vitamin D deficiency most often occurs with steatorrhea or other malabsorptive conditions. Hereditary vitamin D resistance results in hypophosphatemia that is independent of nutritional supplies of vitamin D.

Increased renal excretion of phosphorus

Phosphorus is primarily reabsorbed in the proximal and distal tubules (see Fig. 24.3). The common causes of pathologic renal phosphorus loss are increased PTH (primary and secondary hyperparathyroidism, vitamin D deficiency) or increased PTH-rP as part of a paraneoplastic syndrome.

Since phosphate is reabsorbed in conjunction with sodium, any process that decreases sodium reabsorption in the proximal and distal tubules decreases phosphorus reabsorption. Volume expansion, osmotic diuretics, glucosuria, and diuretics all increase renal phosphorus excretion. Diuretics that act in the proximal tubules, such as osmotic diuretics and carbonic anhydrase inhibitors, have particularly potent phosphaturic effects because they block the primary site of phosphate reabsorption.

Hypophosphatemia also occurs during therapy for acute bronchospasm. Beta-2 agonists, steroids, and IV fluids all increase renal excretion of phosphorus.[60] Since a growing body of evidence indicates that hypophosphatemia weakens the ability to breathe, monitoring and replacing phosphorus in patients with obstructive pulmonary disease is prudent.[61]

Because the kidney must reabsorb 75–99% of filtered phosphate, it is not surprising that tubular disorders result in hypophosphatemia. Fanconi's syndrome is characterized by proximal tubule dysfunction and has marked phosphaturia as one of its components. Alcoholics develop a renal leak of phosphorus, that is reversible following weeks of abstinence.[62]

Clinical sequelae

Severe hypophosphatemia in the presence of intracellular phosphate depletion can result in significant cellular dysfunction. The oxygen affinity of hemoglobin is regulated by 2,3-diphosphoglycerate (2,3-DPG). Severe hypophosphatemia lowers 2,3-DPG, increasing hemoglobin's affinity for oxygen and thereby decreasing oxygen delivery to tissues. Since phosphate is a substrate for glycolysis, intracellular phosphate depletion can prevent the utilization of glucose. Phosphate depletion also results in decreased adenosine triphosphate (ATP) levels. Hypophosphatemia without intracellular phosphate depletion is typically benign.[63]

Modest hypophosphatemia is also devoid of clinical symptoms. Symptomatic hypophosphatemia generally becomes apparent as phosphorus falls below 1.0 mg/dl.

Central nervous system (CNS) symptoms include weakness, tremors, and paresthesias. Progressive hypophosphatemia can cause delirium, seizures, coma, and death. CNS symptoms are particularly prominent with refeeding syndrome.

Myopathy can occur and is attributed to decreased myocyte ATP. This can present as proximal muscle weakness, ileus, and respiratory failure.[64] Patients with decreased total body phosphorus who undergo an intracellular shift of phosphorus and develop severe hypophosphatemia can develop rhabdomyolysis. This classically occurs in alcoholics following hospital admission. The rhabdomyolysis can result in acute renal failure.[65] Since tissue lysis releases phosphorus, patients may have normal phosphorus that obscures the diagnosis.

Cardiomyopathy can occur with hypophosphatemia, possibly due to depletion of myocyte ATP. Phosphate repletion has been shown to restore cardiac contractility.[56,66] Schwartz and colleagues looked at the incidence of arrhythmias in septic patients and found a higher rate among patients with low phosphorus levels.[67]

Hemolysis can rarely occur with severe hypophosphatemia. Lack of red blood cell ATP decreases cellular compliance, predisposing to lysis.[68]

Metabolic effects of hypophosphatemia are primarily due to increased calcitriol production, suppressing PTH release. Hypoparathyroidism can lead to hypocalcemia, hypomagnesemia, and osteomalacia.

Diagnosis

Determining the etiology of hypophosphatemia is usually obvious from the history. Rarely, some clinical scenarios will result in spurious laboratory results. Mannitol, multiple myeloma, and hyperbilirubinemia (>3 mg/dl) can all interfere with some phosphorus assays, resulting in artifactual hypophosphatemia. Patients with very high white blood cell counts can have spurious hypophosphatemia if the specimen is allowed to clot. Heparinized blood samples avoid this error.

Occasionally it is important to separate patients with extrarenal phosphorus losses from renal losses. Patients with extrarenal losses and transcellular distribution of phosphorus should have less that 100 mg (3.3 mmol) of phosphorus in a 24-hour collection. Determining the fractional reabsorption of phosphorus ($FrPO_4$) on a spot urine can give similar information. Whereas $FrPO_4$ normally varies from 75–99%, in the face of hypophosphatemia, a $FrPO_4$ less than 95% indicates renal wasting (see Fig. 24.6).

Treatment

Patients with hypophosphatemia and depletion of phosphorus should be treated. Patients with hypophosphatemia due *solely* to a transcellular shift (e.g. respiratory alkalosis) do not need repletion of phosphorus. One should be particularly aggressive about treating hypophosphatemia in patients with septic shock. Hypophosphatemia is common in sepsis and patients with lower phosphorus have

$$FrPO_4 = 100 \times \left(1 - \frac{sCr \times uPO_4}{sPO_4 \times uCr}\right)$$

Figure 24.6 The fractional reabsorption of phosphorus (Fr PO_4) can be used to determine if hypophosphatemia is due to abnormal renal phosphorus loss or extrarenal phosphorus loss. An $FrPO_4$ less than 95% in the face of hypophosphatemia indicates abnormal renal phosphorus wasting. sCr = serum creatinine, uCr = urine creatinine, sPO_4 = serum phosphorus.

higher rates of arrhythmia.[67] Animal data suggest that hypophosphatemia decreases response to vasopressors.[69] Human data have shown increased left ventricular (LV) function, systolic blood pressure, and pH following normalization of phosphorus.[56,70]

Enteral replacement

Oral replacement of phosphorus is appropriate for patients with low serum phosphorus and no acute symptoms. Dietary phosphorus can be used, but care should be taken not to give phosphorus with an abundance of carbohydrates, which could precipitate an intracellular shift, worsening the hypophosphatemia. In patients with refeeding syndrome and severe hypophosphatemia, in addition to supplementing phosphorus, an important aspect of treatment is to decrease the delivery of carbohydrates (increased lipids or proteins can be used to replace the carbohydrates). Skim milk has a safe ratio of phosphorus to carbohydrates, along with the potassium, calcium, and protein needed in malnourished patients (Table 24.7).

Patients should receive 1000–4000 mg (30–130 mmol) of phosphorus/day divided into three or four doses. This should replace most phosphorus deficits over 7–10 days. Dividing the daily dose reduces diarrhea. Since it is impossible to know the exact degree of phosphorus depletion, patients should have periodic laboratory monitoring.

Parenteral replacement

Patients with signs or symptoms consistent with hypophosphatemia should be given IV phosphorus. Various regimens recommend giving 2.5–5 mg/kg over 6 hours.[71] Larger and faster doses (620 mg in 1 hour or 25 mg/kg in 30 minutes) have been shown

to be safe and effective.[56,70] Continued vigilance is important, as hypophosphatemia returns in most patients. After completing IV therapy, using oral phosphates to replenish body stores is indicated.

While therapy is generally safe, it is not without complications. In a randomized controlled trial of phosphorus replacement in diabetic ketoacidosis (DKA), no benefit from treatment was found in terms of speed of recovery, mental status, oxygen-carrying capacity, or 2,3-DPG levels. The only significant finding was decreased ionized calcium in the phosphorus group.[72] Complications due to therapy for hypophosphatemia include:

* hyperphosphatemia with or without associated hypocalcemia
* hyperkalemia from potassium preparations
* volume overload or hypernatremia from sodium preparations.[73]

HYPERPHOSPHATEMIA

The kidney is responsible for excreting excess phosphorus and is so effective at this that it is able to compensate for huge increases in daily phosphate intake. Essentially, the study of hyperphosphatemia can be limited to acute phosphorus loads, generalized renal failure, and specific failure in the kidney's ability to excrete phosphorus.

Etiologies

Increased intake of phosphorus

The ability to maintain phosphorus balance in the face of massive phosphorus loads (4000 mg/day)

Table 24.7 Phosphorus supplements.			
Phosphate source	Phosphate	Sodium	Potassium
Oral formulations:			
Skim cow's milk	1 mg/ml (0.032 mmol/ml)	28 mEq/L	38 mEq/L
Neutra-Phos	250 mg/pkg (8 mmol)	7.1 mEq/pkg	7.1 mEq/pkg
Phospho-Soda	150 mg/ml (5 mmol/ml)	4800 mEq/L	
Neutra-Phos K	250 mg/cap (8 mmol)		14.25 mEq/cap
K-Phos	150 mg/cap (5 mmol)		3.65 mEq/cap
K-Phos Neutral	250 mg/tablet (8 mmol)	13 mEq/tab	1.1 mEq/tab
Parenteral formulations:			
Potassium phosphate	93 mg/ml (3 mmol/ml)		4.4 mEq/ml
Sodium phosphate	93 mg/ml (3 mmol/ml)	4.4 mEq/ml	

Table 24.8 Etiologies of hyperphosphatemia.		
Exogenous phosphorus intake	**Endogenous phosphorus loads**	**Decreased renal clearance of phosphorus**
Fleets enemas	Cell death:	Renal failure
Oral phosphorus overdose	Tumor lysis syndrome	Hypoparathyroidism:
Parenteral phosphate	Rhabdomyolysis	Acquired:
Vitamin D intoxication	Tissue infarction	• Post-surgical
White phosphorus burns	Malignant hyperthermia	• Hypomagnesemia
	Neuroleptic malignant syndrome	• Radiation treatment
	Heat stroke	• Hemochromatosis
	Transcellular movement:	Congenital:
	Metabolic acidosis	• Pseudohypoparathyroidism
	• Ketoacidosis	• Hypoparathyroidism
	• Lactic acidosis	• DiGeorge syndrome
	Respiratory acidosis	Acromegaly
		Growth hormone therapy
		Tumoral calcinosis
		Bisphosphonates

depends on the phosphorus load being spread over time. Sudden loads can overwhelm renal phosphate clearance, resulting in hyperphosphatemia. Phosphorus loads can be exogenous or endogenous (Table 24.8). Exogenous intake can be from diet, phosphate enemas, or parenteral sources. Fleets enemas contain 130 mg (4.15 mmol) of phosphorus per milliliter. Dietary intake of phosphorus can be enhanced by vitamin D toxicity. Calcitriol enhances gut absorption of phosphorus. In addition, these patients are hypercalcemic, which, along with the increased calcitriol, suppresses PTH. The low PTH decreases renal phosphorus clearance.

Phosphorus can be absorbed through the skin. Cutaneous phosphate absorption follows industrial exposures and white phosphorus burns. White phosphorus is found in munitions and fireworks. Patients often develop severe symptomatic hyperphosphatemia from relatively small burns. Local wound care is considered critical to preventing phosphorus absorption.[74]

Endogenous sources of phosphate are due to release from cells. Phosphorus is the primary anion in cells, and cell death or transcellular distribution of phosphorus can result in hyperphosphatemia. Patients who present with DKA are usually hyperphosphatemic despite total body phosphorus depletion.[75] This is due to the lack of insulin, which decreases the movement of phosphorus into cells, and metabolic acidosis, which slows glycolysis.

Tumor lysis syndrome is due to destruction of large bulky tumors with chemotherapy or radiation therapy. These cells release phosphorus, resulting in acute hyperphosphatemia. In addition to hyperphosphatemia, both potassium and uric acid rise and calcium falls. All of the electrolyte abnormalities can be worsened by associated acute renal failure from uric acid nephropathy. For more information, see discussion of hyperkalemia in Chapter 23.

Decreased renal clearance of phosphorus

Since the kidney is the primary means of excreting phosphorus, renal failure of any etiology is associated with hyperphosphatemia. The kidney maintains phosphorus balance by filtering serum phosphorus and then adjusting the fractional reabsorption of phosphorus via PTH. Both decreased glomerular filtration rate (GFR) and increased serum phosphorus ultimately stimulate PTH release, which decreases the fractional reabsorption of phosphorus.

In some cases, the kidneys fail to excrete phosphorus despite adequate GFR. The primary cause of this is hypoparathyroidism. The most common causes of acquired hypoparathyroidism are surgical removal of the parathyroids or neck surgery. In the former the hypoparathyroidism is permanent, whereas in the latter it is usually a temporary stunning of the gland. Patients develop hypocalcemia in addition to hyperphosphatemia. Other causes of hypoparathyroidism are discussed under etiologies of hypocalcemia (see Table 24.1).

Clinical sequelae

The primary clinical consequence of hyperphosphatemia is hypocalcemia and its metabolic manifestations. Increased serum phosphorus binds ionized calcium, lowering the biologically active fraction of calcium.[76]

Severe hyperphosphatemia can result in metastatic calcification in soft tissues. In rare cases this may contribute to acute renal failure or cardiac arrhythmias.[77] The risk of calcification increases as the calcium–phosphorus product rises above 70 mg/dl². In patients with end-stage renal disease, empiric data have shown that mortality is decreased in patients whose calcium–phosphorus product was less than 52 mg/dl². In the same study, prolonged hyperphosphatemia was an independent predictor of increased mortality.[78]

Diagnosis

Artifactual hyperphosphatemia can occur with a hemolyzed blood specimen or in patients with thrombocytosis. Some patients with multiple myeloma have a serum protein that interferes with the phosphorus assay, resulting in a falsely elevated serum phosphorus.[79]

Treatment

Hyperphosphatemia in patients with intact renal function is usually transient and self-correcting. Infusing saline to induce natriuresis can enhance renal clearance of phosphorus. Acetazolamide can increase renal clearance by blocking phosphate reabsorption in the proximal tubule.[80] However, the use of acetazolamide increases urine pH, which decreases the solubility of calcium phosphate, predisposing to renal calcium deposition.

If there is decreased renal function or symptomatic hypocalcemia, dialysis is essential. A 4-hour dialysis session can remove 625–937 mg (20–30 mmol) of phosphorus. The calcium content of the dialysate does not affect phosphorus clearance.

Continuous renal replacement strategies have been shown to provide better control of hyperphosphatemia and hypocalcemia.[81]

In tumor lysis syndrome the use of sodium bicarbonate to alkalinize the urine can be detrimental. Alkalinization has been used to increase solubility of uric acid in the urine; however, urinary phosphorus solubility decreases with higher urine pH. The use of sodium bicabonate predisposes to renal calcium deposition. In addition, raising the pH exacerbates the ionized hypocalcemia found in tumor lysis syndrome. In the modern era, the use of allopurinol and uricase prevents the hyperuricemia, decreasing the need for aggressive alkalinization.

Phosphate binders are regularly used in patients with chronic renal failure to reduce the absorption of dietary phosphorus. Although they primarily act to decrease absorption of dietary phosphorus, they have a small but measurable ability to bind phosphorus in gut secretions and may have a role in acute hyperphosphatemia.[82] Patients with acute hyperphosphatemia should have a low phosphorus diet and be started on phosphorus binders (i.e. calcium salts, aluminum salts, lanthanum carbonate or sevelamer). In the face of severe hypercalcemia, a noncalcium-containing binder should be used to prevent metastatic calcification.

MAGNESIUM

MAGNESIUM PHYSIOLOGY

Magnesium is the second most prevalent intracellular cation. It is a critical cofactor in any reaction powered by ATP, so deficiency of this ion can have dramatic effects on metabolism. Magnesium also acts as a calcium channel antagonist and plays a key role in the modulation of any activity governed by intracellular calcium (e.g. muscle contraction, insulin release).[83] The atomic weight of magnesium is 24.3. Half of total body magnesium is mineralized in bone. Almost all of the remainder is localized in the intracellular compartment, with only 1% of total body magnesium in the extracellular space.[84] Normal plasma magnesium concentration is 1.8–2.3 mg/dl (0.75–0.95 mmol/L, 1.5–1.9 mEq/L). Magnesium exists in three states: ionized magnesium (60% of total magnesium), protein bound (30%, mostly albumin), and complexed to serum anions (10%).[85,86] Only the ionized magnesium is physiologically active; however, it is not routinely measured. Patients with low serum albumin may have low serum magnesium levels with normal ionized magnesium levels.[87]

Magnesium balance

Dietary sources of magnesium are primarily whole grain cereals, green vegetables, soybeans, nuts, and seafood.[88] Typical magnesium ingestion is 300 mg/day. The entire length of bowel, including the colon, is capable of absorbing magnesium. Net daily magnesium intake is 100 mg (see Fig. 24.1).

The kidneys are responsible for maintaining magnesium balance. The bulk of magnesium reabsorption (60–70%) occurs in the TALH (see Fig. 24.3). The resorption of magnesium in the TALH is inversely related to flow, so that any situation associated with increased tubular flow reduces magnesium resorption. Similarly, any factor that abolishes the positive luminal charge (e.g. loop diuretics, hypercalcemia) opposes the resorption of magnesium.

Renal reabsorption of magnesium varies widely to maintain magnesium homeostasis. Fractional reabsorption of filtered magnesium can decline to nearly zero in the presence of hypermagnesemia or reduced GFR. In response to magnesium depletion or decreased intake, the fractional reabsorption of Mg^{2+} can rise to 99.5% in order to minimize urinary losses. Renal magnesium losses can be reduced to as little as 12 mg/day.[89]

HYPOMAGNESEMIA

Hypomagnesemia is common. Among ICU patients, the prevalence of hypomagnesemia ranges from 11% to 65%.[90–92] When present, hypomagnesemia is usually undetected. In a prospective study, 47% of patients undergoing clinical blood testing for electrolyte concentrations had hypomagnesemia, but physicians ordered magnesium levels in only 10% of these patients.[93]

Etiologies

Decreased intake

Magnesium is found in a wide variety of foods and, consequently, hypomagnesemia due purely to a magnesium-deficient diet is rare. Hospitalized patients receiving enteral or parenteral nutrition often become hypomagnesemic. Although decreased intake plays a role in the pathogenesis of hypomagnesemia, increased losses are more important. A retrospective study of 305 patients on nutritional support found 11.5% to have plasma magnesium below 1.5 mg/dl; increased loss was perceived to be the primary cause of hypomagnesemia[94] (Table 24.9).

Alcoholics are commonly hypomagnesemic (30% in one study).[62] Alcoholics have magnesium-poor diets and suffer from increased urinary magnesium wasting from alcohol intoxication. During alcohol intoxication, urinary magnesium increases 2.7 to 3.6 times the baseline level; this effect is reversible with abstinence.[62] Alcoholics are also predisposed to malabsorption, diarrhea, and acute and chronic pancreatitis, all of which can cause magnesium depletion.[95]

Malabsorption of magnesium

Any condition associated with severe steatorrhea or diarrhea can cause hypomagnesemia.[96] Short bowel syndrome can cause malabsorption;[97] Hessov et al studied patients with bowel resections due to Crohn's disease and found muscle magnesium depletion only in patients with loss of more than 75 cm of bowel.[98] GI magnesium wasting is proportional to the stool fat content. Fat may form insoluble magnesium soaps, blocking its absorption. Inflammation of the small intestine also decreases the absorption of magnesium.

Hypomagnesemia has been reported to occur in 40% of patients with burns.[99] In a careful analysis, Berger et al showed that although these patients had higher than expected renal losses of magnesium, the exudative skin losses accounted for the bulk of the magnesium loss. In fact, skin losses of magnesium were fourfold higher than renal losses and were proportional to the surface area of the burn.[100]

Bone sequestration

Hungry bone syndrome following parathyroidectomy can cause symptomatic hypomagnesemia. The sudden drop in parathyroid hormone level results in acute mineralization of osteoid. This causes an acute drop in serum calcium, magnesium, and potassium. Hungry bone syndrome can result in seizures and tetany.[101]

Renal losses

There are two major causes of congenital magnesium wasting: Bartter's syndrome and Gitelman's syndrome. Both conditions are characterized by hypokalemia, metabolic alkalosis, and normotension. Patients have elevated renin, aldosterone,

Table 24.9 Etiologies of magnesium disturbances.

Hypomagnesemia	Hypermagnesemia

Extrarenal causes
Gastointestinal:
  Diarrhea
  Steatorrhea
  Congenital malabsorption
  Protein calorie malnutrition
  Alcoholism
  Enteral nutrition
  Inflammatory bowel disease[174]
  Gastric suction
  Vomiting
  Short bowel syndrome[98]
  Sprue
  Intestinal bypass for obesity[175]
  Chronic pancreatitis[176]
Skin:
  Burns
  Toxic epidermal necrolysis
Bone:
  Hungry bone syndrome
Other:
  Pancreatitis
 	
Renal losses
Drugs:
  Aminoglycoside toxicity
  Pentamidine toxicity
  Amphotericin B toxicity
  Thiazide diuretics
  Calcineurin inhibitors
  Foscarnet
  Cisplatin
Loop of Henle:
  Loop diuretics
  Hypercalcemia
Increased tubular flow:
  Osmotic diuresis
  Diabetes type I and II
  Hyperaldosteronism[106]
  Volume expansion
  DKA
Tubular dysfunction:
  Recovery from ATN
  Recovery from obstruction
  Recovery from transplantation
  Congenital renal magnesium wasting
  Bartter's syndrome (one-third of cases)
  Gitelman's syndrome (universal)
	Decreased renal excretion of magnesium
	Renal insufficiency
	  Any etiology with a GFR <10 ml/min
	Lithium
	Hypocalciuric, hypercalcemia[110]
	
	Magnesium ingestion
	Parenteral:
	  Dosing error
	  Treatment of pre-eclampsia
	  Treatment of torsades de pointes or myocardial infarction
	Oral:
	  Damage to the intestinal lining may increase magnesium absorption
	  Mg^{2+}-containing antacids:
	  • Gaviscon ($Al(OH)_3$ and $MgCO_3$)
	  • Mylanta ($CaCO_3$ and $MgCO_3$)
	  • Milk of Magnesia ($Mg(OH)_2$)
	  • Maalox ($Al(OH)_3$ and $Mg(OH)_2$)
	  Epsom salts ($MgSO_4$)
	  Mg^{2+}-containing cathartics:
	  • Magnesium citrate
	  • Milk of Magnesia ($Mg(OH)_2$)
	  Magnesium-containing enemas:
	  • Magnesium citrate
	  Aspiration
	  • Dead Sea near drowning
	
	Other
	Theophylline toxicity[151]

ATN = acute tubular necrosis; DKA = diabetic ketoacidosis; GFR = glomerular filtration rate.

and prostaglandin levels.[102] The primary differentiating factor is the urinary calcium, which is elevated in Bartter's syndrome and typically decreased in Gitelman's syndrome.[103] Magnesium wasting is seen in about one-third of Bartter's syndrome cases, but is a universal finding in Gitelman's syndrome, where magnesium typically runs just over 1 mg/dl.[104]

Renal tubular damage can result in inappropriate renal magnesium wasting. The recovery phases of acute tubular necrosis (ATN), urinary tract obstruction, and delayed renal allograft function have all been reported to cause symptomatic hypomagnesemia.[105] In all of the reported cases of hypomagnesemia associated with the recovery from acute renal failure the patients had dramatic polyuria. Polyuria is also the likely mechanism behind the magnesium depletion associated with DKA.

Volume expansion due to saline infusions, hyperaldosteronism, and syndrome of inappropriate antidiuretic hormone (SIADH) all increase tubular flow, resulting in hypomagnesemia.[106] Although loop diuretics have been implicated as a cause of hypomagnesemia, actual clinical data to support this are scant. Multiple small series of patients on loop diuretics have failed to find an association with hypomagnesemia.[107–109] Sutton and Domrongkitchaiporn theorized that the short duration of action of the loop diuretics allowed the kidneys to reduce renal magnesium losses below normal for much of the day to compensate for the increased losses while the drug is active.[110] If this theory is correct, patients on frequent doses, or infusions, of loop diuretics may be at increased risk of hypomagnesemia. Thiazide diuretics have been shown to cause hypomagnesemia.[111] Amiloride and spironolactone have each been shown to decrease renal excretion of magnesium.[107,112]

Cisplatin reliably causes magnesium wasting that is dose-related and can become irreversible. The magnesium wasting is independent of its effect on GFR.[113] Amphotericin B results in increased renal magnesium loss.[114] The frequency and severity of the magnesium loss increase with higher doses but can be seen at a cumulative dose of only 200 mg. Amiloride has been used to decrease renal potassium losses, and it has a similar effect on Mg^{2+} wasting.[115,116] Aminoglycosides can cause tubular damage, resulting in renal magnesium wasting. Typically, symptomatic hypomagnesemia is delayed for a couple of weeks, and presents following the completion of therapy. Hypomagnesemia can persist for months. All of the above-mentioned toxins induce magnesium wasting independent of any effect on GFR.[117]

Clinical sequelae

Hypomagnesemia is usually asymptomatic. In a retrospective review of 1576 consecutive admissions to a geriatric facility in Scotland, 169 patients with hypomagnesemia (≤1.6) showed no difference in duration of stay, survival to discharge, or 6-month survival.[118] However, a prospective study done in an inpatient setting showed a tremendous impact of hypomagnesemia on survival. Although there was no difference in APACHE II scores at admission, patients with a serum magnesium <1.5 mg/dl had a dramatically higher mortality rate than patients with normal magnesium (31% vs 22%).[119]

Determining the clinical consequences of isolated hypomagnesemia is difficult because patients with hypomagnesemia typically also have hypokalemia, hypocalcemia, and hyponatremia. Symptoms due to hypomagnesemia have been reported at modest degrees of depletion but, in general, symptoms become more common as serum magnesium falls below 1.2 mg/dl[120] (Table 24.10).

Neuromuscular effects
Neuromuscular irritability is a common sign of magnesium depletion. Patients can develop Trousseau's and Chvostek's signs despite normal ionized calcium. Severe depletion can cause weakness, fatigue, vertical nystagmus, tetany and seizures.[89] Cortical blindness due to magnesium deficiency has been reported; sight returns following treatment of the hypomagnesemia.[121,122]

Metabolic effects
Hypokalemia is commonly associated with hypomagnesemia. One series reported it to occur in 40% of patients with hypomagnesemia. The converse is also true – 60% of patients with hypokalemia are hypomagnesemic.[93] One explanation for this phenomenon is that many of the etiologies of hypomagnesemia (diuretics, alcoholism, diarrhea, etc.) also result in hypokalemia. In addition, there is renal potassium wasting as a direct consequence of hypomagnesemia. This renal potassium wasting is refractory to potassium supplementation until magnesium is adequately repleted. The mechanism for potassium depletion is multifactorial. Decreased intracellular magnesium slows ATP production, which decreases Na^+-K^+-ATPase

Table 24.10   Clinical sequelae of magnesium disturbances.

mg/dl	Magnesium concentration mEq/L	mmol/L	Manifestation
<1.2	<1	<0.5	Tetany Seizures Arrhythmias
1.2–1.8	1.0–1.5	0.5–0.75	Neuromuscular irritability Hypocalcemia Hypokalemia
1.8–2.5	1.5–2.1	0.75–1.05	Normal magnesium level
2.5–5.0	2.1–4.2	1.05–2.1	Typically asymptomatic
5.0–7.0	4.2–5.8	2.1–2.9	Lethargy Drowsiness Flushing Nausea and vomiting Diminished deep tendon reflex
7.0–12	5.8–10	2.9–5	Somnolence Loss of deep tendon reflexes Hypotension Electrocardiogram changes
>12	>10	>5	Complete heart block Cardiac arrest Apnea Paralysis Coma

activity, resulting in the loss of intracellular potassium. In the TALH and CCD the loss of ATP increases the number of potassium channels on the apical membrane.[123] Intracellular potassium flows downs its concentration gradient into the tubule and is lost in the urine.

Hypocalcemia has been reported in 12–50% of patients with hypomagnesemia.[94,118] Hypomagnesemia suppresses the release of PTH and causes end-organ resistance to PTH. The hypocalcemia is refractory to calcium supplementation until the magnesium deficit is corrected.[16]

Cardiovascular effects

Hypomagnesemia has been associated with a variety of atrial and ventricular arrhythmias.[101] Zuccala et al prospectively studied 52 elderly patients undergoing hip surgery. They noted an association of higher rates of arrhythmias with greater perioperative drops in magnesium. The arrhythmogenic association of magnesium depletion was independent of changes in serum calcium

and potassium.[124] Of special importance are ventricular arrhythmias caused by hypomagnesemia, some of which do not respond to conventional therapy and require magnesium supplementation.[125] This phenomenon led to the 1993 American Heart Association recommendation for empiric magnesium infusions for *torsades de pointes*. ECG findings with hypomagnesemia include flattened T waves, U waves, prolonged QT interval, and widened QRS complexes: all of these effects are also found with hypokalemia, and may be secondary to changes in potassium.

Since both magnesium depletion and digitalis inhibit the Na-K-ATPase, it is not surprising that hypomagnesemia aggravates digitalis toxicity. In fact, hypomagnesemia was the most frequent electrolyte abnormality in a study of digitalis toxicity.[126]

Symptomatic mitral valve prolapse (MVP) has been associated with hypomagnesemia. In the largest study to date, patients with highly symptomatic MVP had an average magnesium concentration of 1.56 mg/dl vs healthy controls who had a magnesium concentration of 1.84 mg/dl. These patients underwent a randomized, double-blind, placebo-controlled trial of oral magnesium. The supplements reduced the frequency of symptoms (faintness, chest pain, palpitations, dyspnea, and anxiety) by half.[127]

Diagnosis

Hypomagnesemia can be divided into extrarenal and renal causes, which can be readily distinguished by determining if the kidney is in a magnesium-avid or magnesium-wasting state (see Table 24.9). There are two ways to determine renal magnesium avidity: 24-hour urine collection and fractional excretion of magnesium (FeMg).

The 24-hour urine collection for total magnesium is a useful indication of renal magnesium avidity. Urinary magnesium loss of under 20 mg is consistent with an intact renal response to hypomagnesemia and implicates decreased intake or extrarenal losses as the cause of hypomagnesemia. In the presence of hypomagnesemia, a 24-hour urinary magnesium above 24 mg indicates abnormal renal wasting.

The FeMg provides a rapid assessment of the renal response to hypomagnesemia. In the best study on the accuracy of the FeMg, using a cutoff of 4% correctly separated the patients with inappropriate renal magnesium wasting (FeMg >4%) from the patients with decreased magnesium absorption (FeMg <4%)[128] (Fig. 24.7).

Measured plasma magnesium levels often do not reflect total body magnesium content. Clinical sequelae of altered magnesium content are more dependent on tissue magnesium levels than blood magnesium concentration. One method to infer the tissue magnesium level in patients with normal serum magnesium is a physiologic test that measures the renal response to a magnesium load.

$$FeMg = 100 \times \frac{sCr \times uMg}{(0.7 \times sMg) \times uCr}$$

Figure 24.7 The fractional excretion of magnesium (FeMg) differentiates between magnesium-avid and magnesium-wasting states. An FeMg greater than 4%, in the presence of hypomagnesemia indicates abnormal renal magnesium wasting. FeMg = fractional excretion of magnesium, sCr = serum creatinine, uCr = urine creatinine, sMg = serum magnesium, uMg = urine magnesium, sPO_4 = serum phosphorus.

Patients who retain over 30% of an 800 mg load of IV magnesium are thought to be magnesium depleted, whereas those who retain less than 20% are said to be magnesium replete:[129] this will only work in patients with normal renal function and normal renal magnesium handling.

Treatment

Patients with symptomatic hypomagnesemia should be treated with intravenous magnesium. The most common formulation is magnesium sulfate ($MgSO_4 \cdot 7H_2O$): 1 g of magnesium sulfate contains 0.1 g of elemental magnesium. Acute symptomatic hypomagnesemia (e.g. seizures, tetany, arrhythmias) should be treated with 2 g IV over 1–5 minutes. In order to restore intracellular magnesium stores, the acute bolus should be followed by 8 g over 24 hours and 4–6 g/day for 3 or 4 days.[101,125,130]

Intravenous magnesium therapy is advocated in some acutely ill patients without documented magnesium depletion. The American College of Cardiology and the American Heart Association (AHA) recommend 1–2 g of magnesium sulfate as an IV bolus over 5 minutes for treatment of *torsades de pointes*. Because early studies demonstrated a benefit of magnesium in acute myocardial infarction (AMI), the AHA currently recommends administration of 2 g of $MgSO_4$ over 15 minutes, followed by 18 g over 24 hours for AMI in the elderly or patients for whom reperfusion therapy is contraindicated. However, the MAGIC trial failed to show any benefit (or harm) from the use of magnesium in AMI; therefore we expect the AHA to rescind any recommendations for using magnesium in AMI.[131]

Magnesium replacement should be done cautiously in patients with renal insufficiency; doses should be reduced by 50–75%. Patients should be monitored during infusions for decreased deep tendon reflexes and magnesium levels should be checked at regular intervals.

Oral supplementation with 360 mg of elemental magnesium per day (divided three times a day) was effective at treating magnesium depletion.[132] Trials at lower doses were not effective.[133] Patients with significant GI magnesium wasting who fail to raise their magnesium on one formulation of Mg^{2+} may respond to another.[134]

Potassium-sparing diuretics may be helpful in patients with chronic renal magnesium wasting. Diuretics that block the sodium channel in the

DCT, such as amiloride and triamterene, reduce magnesium wasting in some patients.[107,135]

HYPERMAGNESEMIA

Normally, the kidney excretes only 2–4% of the filtered magnesium, but is capable of increasing fractional excretion to nearly 100% in the face of decreased GFR or increased serum magnesium levels.[110] Because of this renal reserve, hypermagnesemia is rarely seen. In a study that looked for magnesium levels greater than 6 mg/dl, only 8 were found among nearly 20 000 non-obstetric patients who had magnesium levels checked.[136]

Differential diagnosis

Decreased renal excretion of magnesium
The most common cause of hypermagnesemia is renal insufficiency. Patients with progressive renal insufficiency maintain magnesium balance by increasing the FeMg. Patients with severe renal insufficiency have essentially no resorption of magnesium. This allows preservation of magnesium balance until the GFR is less than 30 ml/min.[137]

Increased intake

Parenteral magnesium. Symptomatic hypermagnesemia (despite normal renal function) has been reported with magnesium infusions. The typical setting is the treatment of preterm labor or pre-eclampsia/eclampsia. Protocols (4–6 g load followed by 1–2 g/h) typically result in serum magnesium levels of 4–8 mg/dl.[138] Patients suffering accidental parenteral magnesium overdoses usually have good outcomes, despite significant short-term morbidity and magnesium levels as high as 24 mg/dl.[139,140]

Oral magnesium. Hypermagnesemia due to oral ingestion of magnesium is unusual in the absence of renal insufficiency. Reported causes include antacids, laxative abuse, magnesium cathartics used to treat overdoses, and accidental ingestion of Epsom salts.[141–143] Chronic oral ingestions of magnesium result in more severe symptoms and death than acute ingestions.

In a retrospective study of hypermagnesemia, excluding obstetric admissions, all cases were due to known or suspected oral ingestion of magnesium. All but one of the patients had GI disturbances (constipation, ulcers, GI bleeding, gastritis, colitis). These GI disturbances may have led the patients to ingest over-the-counter magnesium preparations (i.e. cathartics, antacids) or may have allowed enhanced mucosal absorption of magnesium. Other contributory predisposing factors included advanced age and renal insufficiency (average creatinine was 4.8 mg/dl).[136]

Other causes. Hypermagnesemia has been repeatedly reported following the use of magnesium-containing enemas, including one fatality.[144–146]

Clinical sequelae

Neuromuscular toxicity
Magnesium can block synaptic transmission of nerve impulses. Hypermagnesemia causes loss of deep tendon reflexes, and may lead to flaccid paralysis and apnea.[136,139,147,148] Neuromuscular toxicity also affects smooth muscle, resulting in ileus and urinary retention.[149] In cases of oral intoxication, the development of ileus can slow intestinal transit times, increasing absorption of magnesium.[141] Hypermagnesemia has also been reported to cause parasympathetic blockade, resulting in fixed and dilated pupils, mimicking brainstem herniation.[139] Other neurologic signs include lethargy, confusion, and coma[136,139,148] (see Table 24.10).

Cardiovascular toxicity
Magnesium acts as a calcium channel blocker and, in cardiac tissue, also blocks potassium channels needed for repolarization. Cardiac manifestations of hypermagnesemia initially include bradycardia and hypotension.[136,141,148] Higher magnesium levels cause PR interval prolongation, increased QRS duration, and prolonged QT interval.[136] Extreme cases can result in complete heart block or cardiac arrest. One case of ventricular fibrillation has been reported with an Mg^{2+} level of 9.7 mg/dl.[140]

Metabolic disturbances
Hypocalcemia can occur, although it is typically mild and asymptomatic.[136,138] As with hypomagnesemia, inhibition of PTH release has been proposed as the cause of the hypocalcemia seen in hypermagnesemia, although some studies have found elevations in PTH in this setting.[138,150]

Hyperkalemia has variably been reported in hypermagnesemic case series.[136,142,151,152] This may be due to blockade of potassium channels in the apical membranes of principal cells of the CCD. In addition, multiple studies have found suppression of plasma renin activity in pregnant patients treated with magnesium sulfate.[152–154]

Treatment

The first principle of treatment is prevention. Patients with renal insufficiency should not be given magnesium-containing antacids or cathartics. In cases of hypermagnesemia, stopping the infusion or supply of magnesium will allow patients with intact renal function to recover.

Calcium salts can reverse hypotension and respiratory depression.[155] Patients are typically given 100–200 mg of elemental calcium IV over 5–10 minutes.

To speed the renal clearance of magnesium, loop diuretics and saline diuresis are intuitive options, although we could find no literature to support their use. Clark and Brown suggested adding calcium gluconate (15 mg/kg over 4 hours) to augment renal clearance of magnesium, although we could find no data to support this approach.[136]

In patients with severe renal dysfunction, dialysis offers a way to rapidly clear magnesium. Although both peritoneal and hemodialysis can lower magnesium in an acute situation, hemodialysis is the preferred modality.[136,141,156] CRRT is also effective at lowering serum magnesium, but is slower than hemodialysis.[148]

REFERENCES

1. Marban E, Koretsune Y, Corretti M, et al. Calcium and its role in myocardial cell injury during ischemia and reperfusion. Circulation 1989;80:IV17–22.
2. Zaloga GP. Hypocalcemia in critically ill patients. Crit Care Med 1992;20:251–62.
3. Ladenson JH, Lewis JW, Boyd JC. Failure of total calcium corrected for protein, albumin, and pH to correctly assess free calcium status. J Clin Endocrinol Metab 1978;46:986–93.
4. Lindgarde F, Zettervall O. Hypercalcemia and normal ionized serum calcium in a case of myelomatosis. Ann Intern Med 1973;78:396–9.
5. Side L, Fahie-Wilson MN, Mills MJ. Hypercalcemia due to calcium binding in Waldenstrom's macroglobulinaemia. J Clin Pathol 1995;48:961–2.
6. Zaloga G, Willey S, Tomasic P, et al. Free fatty acids alter calcium binding: a cause for misinterpretation of serum calcium values and hypocalcemia in critical illness. J Clin Endocrinol Metab 1987;64:1010–14.
7. Taylor B, Sibbald WJ, Edmonds MW, et al. Ionized hypocalcemia in critically ill patients with sepsis. Can J Surg 1978;21:429–33.
8. Zaloga G, Chernow B, Cook D, et al. Assessment of calcium homeostasis in the critically ill surgery patient. The diagnostic pitfalls of the McLean–Hastings nomogram. Ann Surg 1985;202:587–94.
9. Desai TK, Carlson RW, Geheb MA. Prevalence and clinical implications of hypocalcemia in acutely ill patients in a medical intensive care setting. Am J Med 1988;84:209–14.
10. Zivin JR, Gooley T, Zager RA, et al. Hypocalcemia: a pervasive metabolic abnormality in the critically ill. Am J Kidney Dis 2001;37:689–98.
11. Sutters M, Gaboury CL, Bennett WM. Severe hyperphosphatemia and hypocalcemia: a dilemma in patient management. J Am Soc Nephrol 1996;7:2056–61.
12. Edmondson S, Almquist TD. Iatrogenic hypocalcemic tetany. Ann Emerg Med 1990;19:938–40.
13. Craig JC, Hodson EM, Martin HC. Phosphate enema poisoning in children. Medi J Australia 1994;160:347–51.
14. Howland WS, Schweizer O, Jascott D, et al. Factors influencing the ionization of calcium during major surgical procedures. Surg Gynecol Obstet 1976;143:895–900.
15. Bashour TT, Ryan C, Kabbani SS, et al. Hypocalcemic acute myocardial failure secondary to rapid transfusion of citrated blood. Am Heart J 1984;108:1040–2.
16. Hermans C, Lefebvre C, Devogelaer JP, et al. Hypocalcaemia and chronic alcohol intoxication: transient hypoparathyroidism secondary to magnesium deficiency. Clin Rheumatol 1996;15:193–6.
17. Zaloga GP. Ionized hypocalcemia during sepsis. Crit Care Med 2000;28:266–8.
18. Zaloga GP, Chernow B. The multifactorial basis for hypocalcemia during sepsis. Studies of the parathyroid hormone–vitamin D axis. Ann Intern Med 1987;107:36–41.
19. Lind L, Carlstedt F, Rastad J, et al. Hypocalcemia and parathyroid hormone secretion in critically ill patients. Crit Care Medi 2000;28:93–9.
20. Alberts DS, Serpick AA, Thompson WL. Hypocalcemia complicating acute leukemia. Med Pediatr Oncol 1975;1:289–95.
21. Hofmann E. The Chvostek sign: a clinical study. Am J Surg 1958;96:33–5.
22. Shinoda T, Aizawa T, Shirota T, et al. Exacerbation of latent heart failure by mild hypocalcemia after parathyroidectomy in a long-term hemodialysis patient. Nephron 1992;60:482–6.
23. Wong CK, Lau CP, Cheng CH, et al. Hypocalcemic myocardial dysfunction: short- and long-term improvement with calcium replacement. Am Heart J 1990;120:381–6.
24. Chernow B. Calcium: does it have a therapeutic role in sepsis? Crit Care Med 1990;18:895–6.
25. Abbott AJ, Hill R, Shears L, et al. Effects of calcium chloride administration on the postischemic isolated rat heart. Ann Thorac Surg 1991;51:705–10.
26. Zaloga G, Sager A, Black KW. Low dose calcium administration increases mortality during septic peritonitis in rats. Circ Shock 1992;37:226–9.
27. Malcolm D, Zaloga G, Holaday J. Calcium administration increases the mortality of endotoxic shock in rats. Crit Care Med 1989;17:900–3.
28. Carlstedt F, Eriksson M, Kiiski R, et al. Hypocalcemia during porcine endotoxemic shock: effects of calcium administration. Crit Care Med 2000;28:2909–14.
29. Steinhorn D, Sweeney M, Layman L. Pharmacodynamic response to ionized calcium during acute sepsis. Crit Care Med 1990;18:851–7.
30. Martin TJ, Kang Y, Robertson KM, et al. Ionization and hemodynamic effects of calcium chloride and calcium gluconate in the absence of hepatic function. Anesthesiology 1990;73:62–5.
31. Broner CW, Stidham GL, Westenkirchner DF, et al. A prospective, randomized, double-blind comparison of calcium chloride and calcium gluconate therapies for hypocalcemia in critically ill children. J Pediatr 1990;117:986–9.

32. Jankowski S, Vincent JL. Calcium administration for cardiovascular support in critically ill patients: when is it indicated? J Intensive Care Med 1995;10:91–100.

33. Beall DP, Scofield RH. Milk-alkali syndrome associated with calcium carbonate consumption: report of 7 patients with parathyroid hormone levels and an estimate of prevalence among patients hospitalized with hypercalcemia. Medicine 1995;74:89–96.

34. Polyxeni K, Chen TC, Holick MF. Vitamin D intoxication associated with an over-the-counter supplement. N Engl J Med 2001;345:66–7.

35. Lemann J, Gray RW. Calcitriol, calcium, and granulomatous disease. N Engl J Med 1984;311:1115–16.

36. Seymour JF, Gagel RF, Hagemeister FB, Dimopoulos MA, Cabanillas F. Calcitriol production in hypercalcemic and normocalcemic patients with non-Hodgkin lymphoma. Ann Intern Med 1994;121:633–40.

37. Cardella CJ, Birkin BL, Rapoport A. Role of dialysis in the treatment of severe hypercalcemia: report of two cases successfully treated with hemodialysis and review of the literature. Clin Nephrol 1979;12:285–90.

38. Bronsky D, Dubin A, Kushner DS, et al. Calcium and the Electrocardiogram. The relationship of the intervals of the electrocardiogram to the levels of serum calcium. Am J Cardiol 1961;7:840–3.

39. Badertscher E, Warnica JW, Ernst DS. Acute hypercalcemia and severe bradycardia in a patient with breast cancer. Can Med Assoc J 1993;148:1506–8.

40. Davidson TG. Conventional treatment of hypercalcemia of malignancy. Am J Health System Pharm 2001;58:S8–15.

41. Sharma OP. Vitamin D, calcium and sarcoidosis. Chest 1996;109:535–9.

42. Seymour JF, Gagel RF. Calcitriol: the major humoral mediator of hypercalcemia in Hodgkin's disease and non-Hodgkin's lymphoma. Blood 1993;82:1383–94.

43. O'Leary TJ, Jones G, Yip A, et al. The effects of chloroquine on serum 1,25 dihydroxyvitamin D and calcium metabolism in sarcoidosis. N Engl J Med 1986;315:727–30.

44. Adams JS, Diz MM, Sharma OP. Effective reduction in the serum 1,25-dihydroxyvitamin D and calcium concentration in sarcoidosis-associated hypercalcemia with short-course chloroquine therapy. Ann Intern Med 1989;111:437–8.

45. Adams JS, Kantorovich V. Inability of short-term, low-dose hydroxychloroquine to resolve vitamin D-mediated hypercalcemia in patients with B-cell lymphoma. J Clin Endocrinol Metab 1999;84:799–801.

46. Nussbaum SR, Younger J, Vandepol CJ, et al. Single-dose intravenous therapy with pamidronate for the treatment of hypercalcemia of malignancy: comparison of 30-, 60-, and 90-mg dosages. Am J Med 1993;95:297–304.

47. Ralston SH, Patel U, Fraser WD, et al. Comparison of three intravenous bisphosphonates in cancer-associated hypercalcemia. Lancet 1989;8673:1180–2.

48. Major P, Lortholary A, Hon J, et al. Zoledronic acid is superior to pamidronate in the treatment of hypercalcemia of malignancy: a pooled analysis of two randomized, controlled clinical trials. J Clin Oncol 2001;19:558–67.

49. Kaiser W, Biesenbach G, Kramar R, et al. Calcium free hemodialysis: an effective therapy in hypercalcemic crisis – report of 4 cases. Intensive Care Med 1989;15:471–4.

50. Sramek V, Novak I, Matejovic M, et al. Continuous venovenous hemodiafiltration (CVVHDF) with citrate anticoagulation in the treatment of a patient with acute renal failure, hypercalcemia, and thrombocytopenia. Intensive Care Med 1998;24:262–4.

51. Kempson SA, Lotscher M, Kaissling B, et al. Parathyroid hormone action on phosphate transporter mRNA and protein in rat renal proximal tubules. Am J Physiol 1995;268:F784–91.

52. Kronenberg HM. NPT2a – the key to phosphate homeostasis. N Engl J Med 2002;347:1022–4.

53. Ramirez JA, Emmett M, White MG, et al. The absorption of dietary phosphorus and calcium in hemodialysis patients. Kidney Int 1986;30:753–9.

54. Halevy J, Bulvik S. Severe hypophosphatemia in hospitalized patients. Arch Intern Med 1988;148:153–5.

55. Fiaccadori E, Coffrini E, Ronda N, et al. Hypophosphatemia in course of chronic obstructive pulmonary disease. Prevalence, mechanisms, and relationships with skeletal muscle phosphorus content. Chest 1990;97:857–68.

56. Zazzo JF, Troche G, Ruel P, et al. High incidence of hypophosphatemia in surgical intensive care patients: efficacy of phosphorus therapy on myocardial function. Intensive Care Med 1995;21:826–31.

57. Weinsier RL, Krumdieck CL. Death resulting from overzealous total parenteral nutrition: the refeeding syndrome revisited. Am J Clin Nutr 1981;34:393–9.

58. Marik PE, Bedigian MK. Refeeding hypophosphatemia in critically ill patients in an intensive care unit. A prospective study. Arch Surg 1996;131:1043–7.

59. Brautbar N, Leibovici H, Massry SG. On the mechanism of hypophosphatemia during acute hyperventilation: evidence for increased muscle glycolysis. Miner Electrolyte Metab 1983;9:45–50.

60. Brady HR, Ryan F, Cunningham J, et al. Hypophosphatemia complicating bronchodilator therapy for acute severe asthma. Arch Intern Med 1989;149:2367–8.

61. Farber M, Carlone S, Palange P, et al. Effect of inorganic phosphate in hypoxemic chronic obstructive lung disease patients during exercise. Chest 1987;92:310–12.

62. De Marchi S, Cecchin E, Basile A, et al. Renal tubular dysfunction in chronic alcohol abuse – effects of abstinence. N Engl J Med 1993;329:1927–34.

63. Subramanian R, Khardori R. Severe hypophosphatemia. Pathophysiologic implications, clinical presentations, and treatment. Medicine (Baltimore) 2000;79:1–8.

64. Newman JH, Neff TA, Ziporen P. Acute respiratory failure associated with hypophosphatemia. N Engl J Med 1977;296:1101–3.

65. Wada S, Nagase T, Koike Y, et al. A case of anorexia nervosa with acute renal failure induced by rhabdomyolysis; possible involvement of hypophosphatemia or phosphate depletion. Intern Med 1992;31:478–82.

66. O'Connor LR, Wheeler WS, Bethune JE. Effect of hypophosphatemia on myocardial performance in man. N Engl J Med 1977;297:901–3.

67. Schwartz A, Gurman G, Cohen G, et al. Association between hypophosphatemia and cardiac arrhythmias in the early stages of sepsis. Eur J Intern Med 2002;13:434.

68. Melvin JD, Watts RG. Severe hypophosphatemia: a rare cause of intravascular hemolysis. Am J Hematol 2002;69:223–4.

69. Saglikes Y, Massry SG, Iseki K, et al. Effect of phosphate depletion on blood pressure and vascular reactivity to norepinephrine and angiotensin II in the rat. Am J Physiol 1985;248:F93–9.

70. Bollaert PE, Levy B, Nace L, et al. Hemodynamic and metabolic effects of rapid correction of hypophosphatemia in patients with septic shock. Chest 1995;107:1698–701.

71. Shiber JR, Mattu A. Serum phosphate abnormalities in the emergency department. J Emerg Med 2002;23:395–400.

72. Fisher JN, Kitabchi AE. A randomized study of phosphate therapy in the treatment of diabetic ketoacidosis. J Clin Endocrinol Metab 1983;57:177–80.

73. Winter RJ, Harris CJ, Phillips LS, et al. Diabetic ketoacidosis. Induction of hypocalcemia and hypomagnesemia by phosphate therapy. Am J Med 1979;67:897–900.

74. Chou TD, Lee TW, Chen SL, et al. The management of white phosphorus burns. Burns 2001;27:492–7.

75. Kebler R, McDonald FD, Cadnapaphornchai P. Dynamic changes in serum phosphorus levels in diabetic ketoacidosis. Am J Med 1985;79:571–6.

76. Eisenberg E. Effect of intravenous phosphate on serum strontium and calcium. N Engl J Med 1970;282:889–92.

77. Isotalo PA, Halil A, Green M, et al. Metastatic calcification of the cardiac conduction system with heart block: an under-reported entity in chronic renal failure patients. J Forensic Sci 2000;45:1335–8.

78. Block GA, Hulbert-Shearon TE, Levin NW, et al. Association of serum phosphorus and calcium × phosphate product with mortality risk in chronic hemodialysis patients: a national study. Am J Kidney Dis 1998;31:607–17.

79. Larner AJ. Pseudohyperphosphatemia. Clin Biochem 1995;28: 391–3.

80. Yamaguchi T, Sugimoto T, Imai Y, et al. Successful treatment of hyperphosphatemic tumoral calcinosis with long-term acetazolamide. Bone 1995;16:247S-50S.

81. Tan HK, Bellomo R, M'Pis DA, et al. Phosphatemic control during acute renal failure: intermittent hemodialysis versus continuous hemodiafiltration. Int J Artif Organs 2001;24:186–91.

82. Schiller LR, Santa Ana CA, Sheikh MS, et al. Effect of the time of administration of calcium acetate on phosphorus binding. N Engl J Med 1989;320:1110–13.

83. Sanders GT, Huijgen HJ, Sanders R. Magnesium in disease: a review with special emphasis on the serum ionized magnesium. Clin Chem Lab Med 1999;37:1011–33.

84. Yu ASL. Disturbances of magnesium metabolism. In: Brenner BM, eds. The kidney. Philadelphia: WB Saunders; 2000:1055–70.

85. Kulpmann WR, Gerlach M. Relationship between ionized and total magnesium in serum. Scand J Clin Lab Invest Suppl 1996;224:251–8.

86. Thienpont LM, Dewitte K, Stockl D. Serum complexed magnesium – a cautionary note on its estimation and its relevance for standardizing serum ionized magnesium. Clin Chem 1999;45:154–5.

87. Saha H, Harmoinen A, Karvonen AL, et al. Serum ionized versus total magnesium in patients with intestinal or liver disease. Clin Chem Lab Med 1998;36:715–18.

88. Marier JR. Magnesium content of the food supply in the modern-day world. Magnesium 1986;5:1–8.

89. Shils ME. Experimental human magnesium depletion. Medicine 1969;48:61–85.

90. Broner CW, Stidham GL, Westenkirchner DF, et al. Hypermagnesemia and hypocalcemia as predictors of high mortality in critically ill pediatric patients. Crit Care Med 1990;18:921–8.

91. Ryzen E, Wagers PW, Singer FR, et al. Magnesium deficiency in a medical ICU population. Crit Care Med 1985;13:19–21.

92. Hebert P, Mehta N, Wang J, et al. Functional magnesium deficiency in critically ill patients identified using a magnesium-loading test. Crit Care Med 1997;25:749–55.

93. Whang R, Ryder KW. Frequency of hypomagnesemia and hypermagnesemia: requested vs routine. JAMA 1990;263:3063–4.

94. Dickerson RN, Brown RO. Hypomagnesemia in hospitalized patients receiving nutritional support. Heart Lung 1985;14:561–9.

95. Rivlin RS. Magnesium deficiency and alcohol intake: mechanisms, clinical significance and possible relation to cancer development (a review). J Am Coll Nutr 1994;13:416–23.

96. Lim P, Jacob E. Tissue magnesium level in chronic diarrhea. J Lab Clin Invest 1972;80(3):313–21.

97. Nielsen JA, Thaysen EH. Acute and chronic magnesium deficiency following extensive small gut resection. Scand J Gastroenterol 1971;6:663–6.

98. Hessov I, Hasselblad C, Fasth S, et al. Magnesium deficiency after ileal resections for Crohn's disease. Scand J Gastroenterol 1983;18:643–9.

99. Cunningham JJ, Anbar RD, Crawford JD. Hypomagnesemia: a multifactorial complication of treatment of patients with severe burn trauma. JPEN J Parenter Enteral Nutr 1987;11:364–7.

100. Berger MM, Rothen C, Cavadini C, et al. Exudative mineral losses after serious burns: a clue to the alterations of magnesium and phosphate metabolism. Am J Clin Nutri 1997;65:1473–81.

101. Al-Ghamdi SM, Cameron EC, Sutton RA. Magnesium deficiency: pathophysiologic and clinical overview. Am J Kidney Dis 1994;24:737–52.

102. Kurtz I. Molecular pathogenesis of Bartter's and Gitelman's syndromes. Kidney Int 1998;54:1396–410.

103. Bettinelli A, Bianchetti MG, Girardin E, et al. Use of calcium excretion values to distinguish two forms of primary renal tubular hypokalemic alkalosis: Bartter and Gitelman syndromes. J Pediatr 1992;120:38–43.

104. Bettinelli A, Bianchetti MG, Borella P, et al. Genetic heterogeneity in tubular hypomagnesemia–hypokalemia with hypocalcuria (Gitelman's syndrome). Kidney Int 1995;47:547–51.

105. Davis BB, Preuss HG, Murdaugh HVJ. Hypomagnesemia following the diuresis of post-renal obstruction and renal transplant. Nephron 1975;14:275–80.

106. Massry SG, Coburn JW, Chapman LW, et al. The effect of long-term deoxycorticosterone acetate administration on the renal excretion of calcium and magnesium. J Lab Clin Invest 1968;71:212–19.

107. Ng LL, Garrido MC, Davies JE, et al. Intracellular free magnesium in lymphocytes from patients with congestive cardiac failure treated with loop diuretics with and without amiloride. Br J Clini Pharmacol 1992;33:329–32.

108. Ralston MA, Murnane MR, Kelley RE, et al. Magnesium content of serum, circulating mononuclear cells, skeletal muscle, and myocardium in congestive heart failure. Circulation 1989;80:573–80.

109. Barton CH, Vaziri ND, Martin DC, et al. Hypomagnesemia and renal magnesium wasting in renal transplant recipients receiving cyclosporine. Am J Med 1987;83:693–9.

110. Sutton RA, Domrongkitchaiporn S. Abnormal renal magnesium handling. Miner Electrolyte Metab 1993;19:232–40.

111. Lim P, Jacob E. Magnesium deficiency in patients on long-term diuretic therapy for heart failure. BMJ 1972;3:620–2.

112. Dyckner T, Wester PO. Renal excretion of electrolytes in patients on long-term diuretic therapy for arterial hypertension and/or congestive heart failure. Acta Med Scand 1985;218:443–8.

113. Lam M, Adelstein DJ. Hypomagnesemia and renal magnesium wasting in patients treated with cisplatin. Am J Kidney Dis 1986;8:164.

114. Barton CH, Pahl M, Vaziri ND, et al. Renal magnesium wasting associated with amphotericin B therapy. Am J Med 1984;77:471–4.

115. Bearden DT, Muncey LA. The effect of amiloride on amphotericin B-induced hypokalaemia. J Antimicrob Chemother 2001;48:109–11.

116. Wazny LD, Brophy DF. Amiloride for the prevention of amphotericin B-induced hypokalemia and hypomagnesemia. Ann Pharmacother 2000;34:94–7.

117. Green CG, Doershuk CF, Stern RC. Symptomatic hypomagnesemia in cystic fibrosis. J Pediatr 1985;107:425–8.

118. Martin BJ, Black J, McLelland AS. Hypomagnesaemia in elderly hospital admissions: a study of clinical significance. Q J Med 1991;78:177–84.

119. Rubeiz GJ, Thill-Baharozian M, Hardie D, et al. Association of hypomagnesemia and mortality in acutely ill medical patients. Crit Care Med 1993;21:203–9.

120. Kingston ME, Al-Siba'i MB, Skooge WC. Clinical manifestations of hypomagnesemia. Criti Care Med 1986;14:950–4.

121. Al-Tweigeri T, Magliocco AM, DeCoteau JF. Cortical blindness as a manifestation of hypomagnesemia secondary to cisplatin therapy: case report and review of literature. Gynecol Oncol 1999;72:120–2.

122. Vlasveld LT, Cornelissen JJ, Dellemijn PL, et al. [Cortical blindness during treatment with cyclosporin]. Nederlands Tijdschrift voor Geneeskunde 1994;138:2057–61 [in Dutch].

123. Kelepouris E, Kasama R, Agus ZS. Effects of intracellular magnesium on calcium, potassium and chloride channels. Miner Electrolyte Metab 1993;19:277–81.

124. Zuccala G, Pahor M, Lattanzio F, et al. Detection of arrhythmogenic cellular magnesium depletion in hip surgery patients. BJA: Br J Anaesth 1997;79:776–81.

125. Ramee SR, White CJ, Svinarich JT, Watson TD, Fox RF. Torsades de pointes and magnesium deficiency. Am Heart J 1985;109:164–7.

126. Young IS, Goh EM, McKillop UH, et al. Magnesium status and digoxin toxicity. Br J Clin Pharmacol 1991;32:717–21.

127. Lichodziejewska B, KloS J, Rezler J, et al. Clinical symptoms of mitral valve prolapse are related to hypomagnesemia and attenuated by magnesium supplementation. Am J Cardiol 1997;79:768–72.

128. Elisaf M, Panteli K, Theodorou J, et al. Fractional excretion of magnesium in normal subjects and in patients with hypomagnesemia. Magnes Res 1997;10:315–20.

129. Gullestad L, Dolva LO, Waage A, et al. Magnesium deficiency diagnosed by an intravenous loading test. Scand J Clin Lab Invest 1992;52:245–53.

130. Brucato A, Bonati M, Gaspari F, et al. Tetany and rhabdomyolysis due to surreptitious furosemide – importance of magnesium supplementation. J Toxicol Clin Toxicol 1993;31:341–4.

131. Magnesium in Coronaires (MAGIC) Trial Investigators. Early administration of intravenous magnesium to high-risk patients with acute myocardial infarction in the Magnesium in Coronaries (MAGIC) trial: a randomised controlled trial. Lancet 2002;360:1189–96.

132. Gullestad L, Oystein DL, Birkeland K, et al. Oral versus intravenous magnesium supplementation in patients with magnesium deficiency. Magnesium & Trace Elements 1991;10:11–16.

133. Costello RB, Moser-Veillon PB, DiBianco R. Magnesium supplementation in patients with congestive heart failure J Am Coll Nutr 1997;16:22–31.

134. Ross JR, Dargan PI, Jones AL, et al. A case of hypomagnesaemia due to malabsorption, unresponsive to oral administration of magnesium glycerophosphate, but responsive to oral magnesium oxide supplementation. Gut 2001;48:857–8.

135. Ryan MF. The role of magnesium in clinical biochemistry: an overview. Ann Clin Biochem 1991;28:19–26.

136. Clark B, Brown R. Unsuspected morbid hypermagnesemia in elderly patients. Am J Nephrol 1992;12:336–43.

137. Wacker WE, Parisi AF. Magnesium metabolism. N Engl J Med 1968;278:772–6.

138. Cruikshank DP, Pitkin RM, Reynolds WA, et al. Effects of magnesium sulfate treatment on perinatal calcium metabolism. I. Maternal and fetal responses. Am J Obstet Gynecol 1979;134:243–9.

139. Rizzo MA, Fisher M, Lock P. Hypermagnesemic pseudocoma. Arch Intern Med 1993;153:1130–2.

140. Morisaki H, Yamamoto S, Morita Y, et al. Hypermagnesemia-induced cardiopulmonary arrest before induction of anesthesia for emergency cesarean section. J Clini Anesth 2000;12:224–6.

141. Weber C, Santiago R. Hypermagnesemia: a potential complication during treatment of theophylline intoxication with oral activated charcoal and magnesium-containing cathartics. Chest 1989;95:56–9.

142. Gren J, Woolf A. Hypermagnesemia associated with catharsis in a salicylate-intoxicated patient with anorexia nervosa. Ann Emerg Med 1989;18:2:200–3.

143. McGuire JK, Kulkarni MS, Baden HP. Fatal hypermagnesemia in a child treated with megavitamin/megamineral therapy. Pediatrics 2000;105:18.

144. Ashton MR, Sutton D, Nielsen M. Severe magnesium toxicity after magnesium sulphate enema in a chronically constipated child. BMJ 1990;300:541.

145. Collinson PO, Burroughs AK. Severe hypermagnesaemia due to magnesium sulphate enemas in patients with hepatic coma [erratum appears in Br Med J (Clin Res Ed) 1986;293(6556):1222]. Br Med J Clin Res Ed. 1986;293:1013–14.

146. Outerbridge EW, Papageorgiou A, Stern L. Magnesium sulfate enema in a newborn. Fatal systemic magnesium absorption. JAMA 1973;224:1392–3.

147. Castelbaum A, Donofrio PD, Walker FO, et al. Laxative abuse causing hypermagnesemia, quadriparesis, and neuromuscular junction defect. Neurology 1989;39:746–7.

148. Schelling JR. Fatal hypermagnesemia. Clin Nephrol 2000;53:61–5.

149. Razavi B, Somers D. Hypermagnesemia-induced multiorgan failure. Am J Med 2000;108:686–7.

150. Cholst IN, Steinberg SF, Tropper PJ, et al. The influence of hypermagnesemia on serum calcium and parathyroid hormone levels in human subjects. N Engl J Med 1984;310:1221–5.

151. Eshleman SSH, Shaw LM. Massive theophylline overdose with atypical metabolic abnormalities. Clin Chem 1990;36:398–9.

152. Spital A, Greenwell R. Severe hyperkalemia during magnesium sulfate therapy in two pregnant drug abusers. South Med J 1991;84:919–21.

153. Sipes SL, Weiner CP, Gellhaus TM. The plasma renin–angiotensin system in preeclampsia: effects of magnesium sulfate. Obstet Gynecol 1989;56:934–7.

154. Outerbridge EW, Papageorgion A, Stem L. Angiotensin-converting enzyme activity in hypertensive subjects after magnesium sulfate therapy. Am J Obstet Gynecol 1987;56:1375–9.

155. Meltzer SJ, Auer J. The antagonistic action of calcium upon the inhibitory effect of magnesium. Am J Physiol 1908;21:400–19.

156. Porath A, Mosseri M, Harmon I, et al. Dead Sea water poisoning. Ann Emerg Me 1989;18:2:187–91.

157. Efstathiadou Z, Bitsis S, Tsatsoulis A. Gastrectomy and osteomalacia: an association not to be forgotten. Horm Res 1999;52:295–7.

158. Yamaji Y, Hayashi M, Suzuki Y, et al. Thyroid crisis associated with severe hypocalcemia. Jpn J Med 1991;30:179–81.

159. Edwards H, Zinberg J, King TC. Effect of cimetidine on serum calcium levels in an elderly patient. Arch Surg 1981;116:1088–9.

160. Lin J, Idee JM, Port M, et al. Interference of magnetic resonance imaging contrast agents with the serum calcium measurement technique using colorimetric reagents. J Pharm Biomed Anal 1999;21:931–43.

161. Hardman KA, Heath DA, Nelson HM. Drug points: hypercalcemia associated with calcipotriol (Dovonex) treatment. BMJ 1993;306:896.

162. Kozeny GA, Barbato AL, Bansal VK, et al. Hypercalcemia associated withh silicone-induced granulomas. N Engl J Med 1984;311:1103–5.

163. Bosch X, Lopez-Soto A, Morello A, et al. Vitamin D metabolite-mediated hypercalcemia in Wegener's granulomatosis. Mayo Clin Proc 1997;72:440–4.

164. Woywodt A, Schneider W, Goebel U, et al. Hypercalcemia due to talc granulomatosis. Chest 2000;117:1195–6.

165. Bosch X. Hypercalcemia due to endogenous overproduction of active vitamin D in identical twins with cat-scratch disease. JAMA 1998;279:532–4.

166. Bendz H, Sjordin L, Toss G, et al. Hyperparathyroidism and long-term lithium therapy: a cross sectional study and the effect of lithium withdrawl. J Intern Med 1996;240:357–65.

167. McLean TW, Pritchard J. Langerhans cell histiocytosis and hypercalcemia: clinical response to indomethacin. J Pediatr Hematol Oncol 1996;18:318–20.

168. Lepre F, Grill V, Ho PWM, et al. Hypercalcemia in pregnancy and lactation associated with parathyroid hormone-related protein. N Engl J Med 1993;328:666–7.

169. Fishbane S, Frei GL, Finger M, et al. Hypervitaminosis A in two hemodialysis patients. Am J Kidney Dis 1995;25:346–9.

170. Westphal SA. Disseminated coccidioidomycosis associated with hypercalcemia. Mayo Clin Proc 1998;73:893–4.

171. Howard RA, Ashwell S, Bond LR, et al. Artefactual serum hyperkalemia and hypercalcemia in essential thrombocythemia. J Clin Pathol 2000;53:105–9.

172. Knox JB, Demling RH, Wilmore DW, et al. Hypercalcemia associated with the use of human growth hormone in an adult surgical intensive care unit. Arch Surg 1995;130:442–5.

173. Meneghini LF, Oster JR, Camacho JR, et al. Hypercalcemia in association with acute renal failure and rhabdomyolysis. Case report and literature review. Miner Electrolyte Metab 1993;19:1–16.

174. Galland L. Magnesium and inflammatory bowel disease. Magnesium 1988;7:78–83.

175. Lipner A. Symptomatic magnesium deficiency after small-intestinal bypass for obesity. BMJ 1977;1:148.

176. Papazachariou IM, Martinez-Isla A, Efthimiou E, Williamson RC, Girgis SI. Magnesium deficiency in patients with chronic pancreatitis identified by an intravenous loading test. Clin Chim Acta 2000;302:145–54.

25

Nutrition in the intensive care unit

John W Drover, Eduard A Iliescu, and Daren K Heyland

In this chapter our goal is to outline the current knowledge and understanding of the literature as it pertains to the management of nutritional support for the critically ill patient. Following a discussion of the metabolic response to critical illness and acute renal failure (ARF), we review general principles applicable to patients in the intensive care unit (ICU) and identify the issues that are specific to the critically ill patient with renal dysfunction. Acute renal failure in the critical care setting usually occurs as part of multiple organ system dysfunction resulting from the underlying disease process. The general principles of nutritional management of critically ill patients with ARF are not significantly different from those of patients without ARF. There are, however, specific metabolic consequences of ARF and renal replacement therapy (RRT) that require special consideration.

In order to bring forward the best-available evidence for making decisions about nutritional support in critically ill patients we have conducted a systematic review of the literature, the details of which can be found elsewhere.[1] In brief, we systematically searched Medline and Cinahl, Embase, and the Cochrane Library for randomized controlled trials and meta-analyses of randomized controlled trials that evaluated any form of nutrition support in critically ill adults. We also searched reference lists and personal files. Data on methodologic quality and outcomes were extracted from the primary papers. When data were missing or unclear, the primary investigators were contacted and requested to provide further information. Where we have combined data to estimate risk ratios (RRs) and their confidence intervals (CIs), these were estimated using the random effects model of DerSimonian and Laird,[2]

as implemented in RevMan4.1.[3] We considered $p < 0.25$ to be supportive of a trend and $p < 0.05$ to be statistically significant.

METABOLIC RESPONSE TO CRITICAL ILLNESS AND ACUTE RENAL FAILURE

The response to injury can be defined by the physiologic derangements that are mediated through neuroendocrine pathways. The degree of response is in proportion to the degree of injury. Energy expenditure rises in response to the injury and there is accelerated breakdown of glycogen and proteins in preference to lipid stores. This first catabolic phase of the physiologic response after injury may be as short as 24–72 hours following an uncomplicated major surgery or it may last indefinitely if the insult continues. As the insult abates, the neuroendocrine response begins to reduce and the patient enters an anabolic or convalescent phase of illness.

In the absence of nutritional intake, the individual will suffer the results of starvation, with protein and calorie deficiency. In the case of the individual who has suffered an injury, the loss of body stores is accelerated. The eventual outcome of starvation is death. Nutritional support is instituted to avoid this outcome. Issues about when, how, and what to feed patients will be addressed in this chapter.

Acute renal failure is associated with increased protein catabolism and negative nitrogen balance that cannot be suppressed effectively by administration of nutritional substrates.[4] Metabolic acidosis is a major cause of protein catabolism and causes protein degradation in muscle through a steroid-dependent ubiquitin–proteasome mediated mechanism.[5,6] Correction of acidosis in dialysis patients has been shown to decrease protein degradation.[7] Another important cause of protein catabolism in ARF is insulin resistance. Insulin has an antiproteolytic effect via the ubiquitin–proteasome pathway and insulin resistance in ARF is associated with increased protein degradation in muscle.[8,9] Other factors that contribute to protein degradation in ARF include hormonal derangements such as hyperparathyroidism, circulating proteases, and inflammatory mediators.[4] The dialysis process itself contributes to the negative nitrogen balance through loss of amino acids and protein that is greater with convection than with diffusion.[10,11] Depending on the serum protein concentration and the nature of solute removal (convection vs diffusion), protein losses with continuous renal replacement therapy (CRRT) can vary from 1.2 to 7.5 g/day.[10]

Other pertinent metabolic consequences of ARF include hyperlipidemia, micronutrient deficiencies, electrolyte abnormalities, and increased extracellular fluid volume (ECFV). Abnormal lipid metabolism, specifically impaired lipolysis, occurs within a few days of the onset of ARF and is not influenced by residual renal function, urine output, or duration of renal failure.[12] Acute renal failure is associated with deficiency of a variety of micronutrients including vitamins A, C, 1,25-dihydroxyvitamin D_3, E, selenium, and zinc.[13,14] Micronutrient deficiencies are consequences of systemic inflammatory response and losses associated with RRT and are not necessarily specific to ARF. Abnormalities of polyvalent ion metabolism occur early in ARF and include hypocalcemia, hyperphosphatemia, hypermagnesemia, and elevation in parathyroid hormone level.[15]

ESTIMATING METABOLIC REQUIREMENTS

The appropriate target for delivery of nutrients has been elusive in the critically ill patient. In the clinical setting there are methods that can be used to measure metabolic activity as well as formulas that can be used to estimate energy requirements. Indirect calorimetry can be done with a bedside monitoring device to measure oxygen consumption and CO_2 production. These currently can be stand-alone devices or incorporated with ventilator software. This device can give feedback to the clinician on the metabolic rate and possible targets for the patient's nutrition support.[16]

There are many empiric formulas that are available for estimating energy expenditure. The most widely known formula is the Harris–Benedict equation, which accounts for the variables of height, weight, and age. The equation was established on the basis of healthy adults, and adjustments for the increased metabolic rate of patients can be performed with correction using activity factors and injury factors.[17] These equations are readily available. Another common method of estimating caloric requirements is to calculate the estimated expenditure based on the weight of the individual: this has the advantage of being easily applied at the bedside.

It is not clear that any one of these methods is superior to another based on differences in significant patient outcomes. One study of nutrition support in burned patients evaluated the effect of measuring metabolic rate on outcome. Patients were randomized to have their target enteral nutrition based on the Currerri formula or indirect calorimetry. There was no difference in mortality or hyperglycemia among the group.[18] Although the method of estimating nutritional requirements may not affect outcome, it is important to use some method of monitoring the provision of calories to avoid complications of overfeeding.[19]

PARENTERAL NUTRITION OR ENTERAL NUTRITION

Patients receiving nutrition support during their stay in the ICU may receive the nutrition parenterally or enterally. Given parenterally, this procedure generally entails central venous access to deliver adequate amounts of calories and protein in a restricted volume. Enteral feeds in this population generally mean feeding through a tube placed in the gastrointestinal tract. In recent reviews of the literature, some authors have taken the stance that enteral nutrition (EN) is superior to parenteral nutrition (PN) in most patients, whereas others have argued that they are perhaps equal apart from the possibility that there is a difference in cost.[20,21] In a systematic review of the literature, we identified 12 studies that evaluated EN compared with PN.[22] These studies evaluated a diverse group of critically ill patients, including patients with head injury (4),[23–25] trauma (3),[26–28] patients in general ICU (3),[29–31] high-risk surgical patients (1),[32] and pancreatitis (1).[33] All of these studies reported on mortality, and meta-analysis showed no difference between the groups receiving enteral nutrition or parenteral nutrition (RR 1.08, 95% CI 0.70–1.65, $p = 0.7$).[1] Of the studies, six reported infectious complications. When these were aggregated, with meta-analysis there was significant reduction in infectious complications with EN compared to PN (RR 0.64, 95% CI 0.47–0.87, $p = 0.004$) (Fig. 25.1).

The largest study addressing this question was published by Moore et al.[32] It was a meta-analysis that combined individual patient data from eight separate studies. The majority of patients were victims of trauma, although a proportion was also high-risk elective surgical patients. The study showed there was no significant difference between mortality rates of the two groups, with the group receiving parenteral nutrition having a mortality rate of 10% and the enteral group having a mortality rate of 7% at 30 days ($p = 0.48$). Infectious complications in the parenteral nutrition group were 35% and in the enterally fed group 16% for an absolute risk reduction of 19% ($p = 0.01$). The authors did not report on caloric or protein intake.

The five studies that report amount of intake found that parenteral nutrition was associated with a higher delivery of calories.[27,31,34–36] Three studies reporting on the incidence of hyperglycemia found significantly fewer instances of hyperglycemia associated with enteral nutrition[25,26,33] and also reduced cost with enteral nutrition compared to parenteral nutrition.

When there is the opportunity to choose between parenteral or enteral nutrition for a patient in the ICU, it would appear that the reduced risk of infection and lower cost would favor the use of enteral nutrition. There does not seem to be an effect on mortality. We recommend the use of enteral nutrition for critically ill patients with an intact functioning gastrointestinal tract.

EARLY VERSUS DELAYED NUTRITIONAL SUPPORT

There is some debate as to the appropriate timing of initiation of enteral feeding. As discussed earlier, ongoing starvation eventually leads to metabolic collapse and death. The goals of early enteral nutrition are to support organ function and modulate the inflammatory response to illness rather than meet the nutritional requirements. Eight randomized trials addressing the issue of early nutritional support have been published.[37–44] They have studied patients with trauma (5), burns (1), secondary peritonitis (1), and pancreatitis (1). There was no standard definition for early enteral nutrition. In the studies quoted above the most common definition fell within 48 hours, although one study used 60 hours[43] and one study used completion of resuscitation[40] as the point of initiating feeding. Similarly, delayed nutritional support is difficult to define exactly. In the studies noted, this ranged from 24 hours after admission to the use of intravenous fluids only waiting for the reintroduction of an oral diet. Overall, a reasonable definition for early nutritional support is that which is introduced within 48 hours of admission to an ICU.

All of these studies reported on mortality. When the results are aggregated, early enteral nutrition was associated with a trend towards reduced mortality (RR 0.52, 95% CI 0.25–1.08, $p = 0.08$)[1] (Fig. 25.2). The aggregated data of the three studies[37,41,43] that reported on the number of patients with infection showed a trend to reduced infection

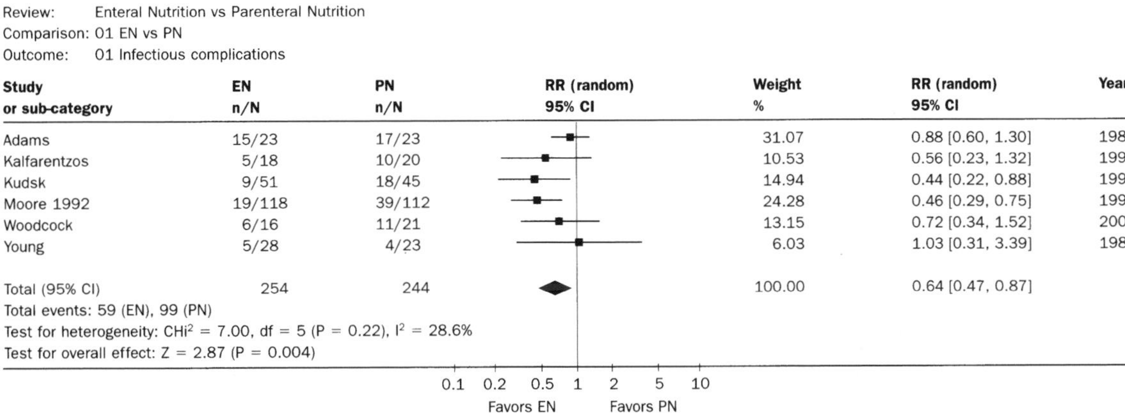

Review: Enteral Nutrition vs Parenteral Nutrition
Comparison: 01 EN vs PN
Outcome: 01 Infectious complications

Study or sub-category	EN n/N	PN n/N	RR (random) 95% CI	Weight %	RR (random) 95% CI	Year
Adams	15/23	17/23		31.07	0.88 [0.60, 1.30]	1986
Kalfarentzos	5/18	10/20		10.53	0.56 [0.23, 1.32]	1997
Kudsk	9/51	18/45		14.94	0.44 [0.22, 0.88]	1992
Moore 1992	19/118	39/112		24.28	0.46 [0.29, 0.75]	1992
Woodcock	6/16	11/21		13.15	0.72 [0.34, 1.52]	2001
Young	5/28	4/23		6.03	1.03 [0.31, 3.39]	1987
Total (95% CI)	254	244		100.00	0.64 [0.47, 0.87]	

Total events: 59 (EN), 99 (PN)
Test for heterogeneity: CHi^2 = 7.00, df = 5 (P = 0.22), I^2 = 28.6%
Test for overall effect: Z = 2.87 (P = 0.004)

0.1 0.2 0.5 1 2 5 10
Favors EN   Favors PN

Figure 25.1 Studies comparing parenteral nutrition (PN) with enteral nutrition (EN): effect on infectious complications.[22]

Review: Early Enteral Nutrition vs delayed nutrient intake
Comparison: 01 Early EN vs delayed nutrient intake
Outcome: 01 Mortality

Study or sub-category	Early EN n/N	Delayed n/N	RR (random) 95% CI	Weight %	RR (random) 95% CI	Year
Chiarelli	0/10	0/10			Not estimable	1990
Chuntrasakul	1/21	3/17		11.15	0.27 [0.03, 2.37]	1996
Eyer	2/19	2/19		15.29	1.00 [0.16, 6.38]	1993
Kompan	0/27	1/25		5.28	0.31 [0.01, 7.26]	1999
Minard	1/12	4/15		12.44	0.31 [0.04, 2.44]	2000
Moore	1/32	2/31		9.52	0.48 [0.05, 5.07]	1986
Pupelis	1/30	7/30		12.71	0.14 [0.02, 1.09]	2001
Singh	4/21	4/22		33.62	1.05 [0.30, 3.66]	1998
Total (95% CI)	172	169		100.00	0.52 [0.25, 1.07]	

Total events: 10 (Early EN), 23 (Delayed)
Test for heterogeneity: CHi^2 = 4.07, df = 6 (P = 0.67), I^2 = 0%
Test for overall effect: Z = 1.77 (P = 0.08)

```
0.01    0.1     1      10    100
   Favors Early EN   Favors delayed
```

Figure 25.2 Studies comparing early vs delayed nutrient intake: effect on mortality.[1] Reprinted from Heyland DK, Dhaliwal R, Drover JW, Gramlich L, Dodek P; Canadian Critical Care Clinical Practice Guidelines Committee. Canadian clinical practice guidelines for nutrition support in mechanically ventilated, critically ill adult patients. JPEN J Parenter Enteral Nutr 2003;27: 359, with permission from the American Society for Parenteral and Enteral Nutrition (A.S.P.E.N.). A.S.P.E.N. does not endorse the use of this material in any form other than its entirety.

associated with early enteral nutrition (RR 0.62, 95% CI 0.41–0.93, p = 0.02).[45] One study reported early enteral feeding was associated with reduced hospital length of stay[38] and one reported early enteral feeding was associated with an increased ICU length of stay.[43] For all of the studies reporting on nutritional endpoints, early enteral feed was associated with a significant improvement in caloric intake,[39–41,43,44] protein intake,[39] percentage of goal achieved,[42] or faster achievement of nitrogen balance.[38,41]

There is the potential for causing iatrogenic complications related to the early delivery of enteral feeding. A prospective cohort study evaluated upper digestive intolerance in patients receiving gastric feeding.[46] They found that high gastric residual volumes occurred early and were associated with infusion of sedative agents or catecholamines. The high gastric residual volumes were associated with an increased ICU length of stay and a higher incidence of nosocomial pneumonia and ICU mortality. A pseudorandomized study evaluating early enteral feeding compared to late enteral feeding in medical ICU patients demonstrated that early EN was associated with higher rates of infectious complications and increased ICU and hospital length of stay.[47] There was no difference in mortality between the groups.

We recommend that critically ill patients receive early enteral feeding, defined as being within 48 hours of admission. For individual patients, it is important to choose management strategies that reduce the potential for complications: this includes, but is not restricted to, starting feeds after the acute phase of resuscitation, using small bowel feeding[48] and nursing in the semirecumbent position.[49]

IMMUNONUTRITION

Immune-modulating enteral formulas have received considerable attention in the past decade. The most common nutrients assessed in human trials are arginine, glutamine, nucleotides, and omega-3 fatty acids, either alone or in combination. These agents have been studied in a variety of patient groups, but a large number of the studies have focused on surgical patients. Although these patients may be managed in an ICU they are systematically different to the general ICU population, which have multiple organ failure that may include renal failure. We will concentrate on the literature that addresses the critically ill patient.

The most common commercially available enteral formulas combine arginine, nucleotides, and omega-3 fatty acids. Data regarding critically ill patients have recently been reported in a meta-analysis.[50] When all studies of critically ill patients were pooled, there was no effect on mortality or infectious complications. Subgroup analysis studies with higher methodologic scores demonstrated a significantly higher mortality (RR 1.46, 95% CI 1.01–2.11) and a reduction of infectious complications (RR 0.8, 95% CI 0.64–1.01) associated with the use of immunonutrition. There is concern that there may be an adverse effect on mortality of the combination of arginine, nucleotides, and omega-3 fatty acids.[51] The largest trial that has studied this type of formula in the general ICU population did not demonstrate beneficial effects on clinical outcomes.[52] We recommend that these combined formulas not be used routinely in critically ill patients.

The amino acid glutamine plays a central role in nutrition transport within the body. Glutamine represents the greatest individual amino acid loss in CRRT;[11,53] it has been studied in critically ill patients without renal failure, and an aggregation of these data was recently reported in a meta-analysis.[54] In critically ill patients, there was no difference in infectious complications or length of hospital stay. There was a trend toward reduced mortality associated with the use of glutamine (RR 0.77, 95% CI 0.57–1.03). In subgroup analyses, the mortality benefit of glutamine supplementation was seen when it was given parenterally in higher doses (>0.2 g/kg/day) to critically ill patients on PN.

The use of glutamine supplementation, particularly for doses higher than 0.2 g/kg/day given by the parenteral route, should be considered for use in critically ill patients on PN. It is important to recognize that the safety of large doses of glutamine in patients with renal failure has not been studied in randomized controlled trials.

POST-PYLORIC FEEDING

Enteral feedings delivered by a tube may be instilled into the stomach or by various means into the small bowel. This topic has recently been reviewed.[48] In this meta-analysis no difference in mortality was reported. Nine randomized trials have compared the effect of small bowel feeding with gastric feeding.[45] When these data are combined (Fig. 25.3), post-pyloric feeding was associated with a reduced incidence of pneumonia (RR 0.77, 95% CI 0.60–1.00, $p = 0.05$).[45] Several studies found that patients fed into the small bowel received more protein and energy,[43,55–57] and time to reach target amount was shorter than with patients fed into the stomach.[58] There may be issues locally that influence the ability to access the small bowel and complications associated with small bowel feeding have been reported.[59]

A large proportion of ICU patients will tolerate and receive adequate nutrition when delivered into the stomach. Providing effective nutritional support into the stomach requires attention to certain aspects of care. Gastric residual volumes, as a marker of feeding intolerance, have not been validated. If they are used, a volume of greater than 200 ml is probably a reasonable cutoff.[60] Delivering feeds following a targeted aggressive algorithm can improve success of reaching energy and protein targets and reduce complications.[55] Using prokinetic agents can also improve success at gastric feeding and may be as good as our current methods of delivering small bowel feeds.[61] Enteral feeding in the supine position increases the risk of nosocomial pneumonia and having the patient in the semirecumbent position with the head elevated to 45° can reduce this risk.[49]

We recommend the use of small bowel feedings in units where gaining access to the small bowel is

Review: Small Bowel vs Gastric
Comparison: 01 Small Bowel vs Gastric
Outcome: 01 Pneumonia

Study or sub-category	Small Bowel n/N	Gastric n/N	RR (random) 95% CI	Weight %	RR (random) 95% CI	Year
Davies	2/31	1/35		1.19	2.26 [0.22, 23.71]	2002
Day	0/14	2/11		0.76	0.16 [0.01, 3.03]	2001
Kearns	4/21	3/23		3.48	1.46 [0.37, 5.78]	2000
Kortbeek	10/37	18/43		16.28	0.65 [0.34, 1.22]	1999
Minard	6/12	7/15		10.74	1.07 [0.49, 2.34]	2000
Montecalvo	4/19	6/19		5.50	0.67 [0.22, 1.99]	1992
Montejo	16/50	20/51		23.51	0.82 [0.48, 1.39]	2002
Neumann	1/30	0/30		0.66	3.00 [0.13, 70.83]	1999
Taylor	18/41	26/41		37.88	0.69 [0.46, 1.05]	1999
Total (95% CI)	255	268		100.00	0.77 [0.60, 1.00]	

Total events: 61 (Small Bowel), 83 (Gastric)
Test for heterogeneity: CHi^2 = 4.79, df = 8 (P = 0.78), I^2 = 0%
Test for overall effect: Z = 1.96 (P = 0.05)

0.01   0.1   1   10   100
Favors Small bowel   Favors Gastric

Figure 25.3 Studies comparing small bowel vs gastric feeding: effect on ventilator-associated pneumonia.[45] Reprinted from Heyland DK, Drover JW, Dhaliwal R, Greenwood J. Optimizing the benefits and minimizing the risks of enteral nutrition in the critically ill: role of small bowel feeding. JPEN J Parenter Enteral Nutr 2002;26(Suppl):S51–S57, with permission from the American Society for Parenteral and Enteral Nutrition (A.S.P.E.N.). A.S.P.E.N. does not endorse the use of this material in any form other than its entirety.

feasible. Obtaining access to the small bowel should not unduly delay the initiation of enteral nutrition.

ROLE OF PARENTERAL NUTRITION

Parenteral nutrition may be effective in meeting nutritional goals. However, a recent meta-analysis[62] suggested that PN, compared with standard care, may be associated with increased complications and mortality. In subgroup analyses, the rate of major complications was significantly lower among malnourished patients receiving PN (RR 0.52, 95% CI 0.30–0.91) compared to PN in adequately nourished patients (RR 1.02, 95% CI 0.75–1.41) ($p = 0.05$). In studies that did not use lipids, there were significantly fewer complications (RR 0.59, 95% CI 0.38–0.90), although this was just short of statistical significance when compared with the complication rate in studies that used lipids (RR 0.96, 95% CI 0.69–1.34) ($p = 0.09$). This is consistent with the findings of a randomized trial of PN with lipids compared to PN without lipids in critical trauma patients that demonstrated a lower complication rate in the group that did not receive lipids.[63]

If patients have a contraindication to EN, we recommend that PN be used in such a way that maximizes the benefits and minimizes the risks in critically ill patients. We recommend that lipids not be used as a source of energy in the short term (<10 days) and that serum blood sugars be monitored closely and controlled with insulin infusion.[64]

SUPPLEMENTAL PARENTERAL NUTRITION

Even when patients can be fed by the enteral route, it is sometimes challenging to achieve targets for protein and calorie delivery. This has led to the practice of supplementing the enteral feedings with parenteral nutrition to achieve these targets until goal rates of enteral feeding are met, either at initiation of EN or after several days of hypocaloric EN. Combining both forms of nutrition support can lead to complications and there is also a greater possibility of overfeeding because of the unrestricted ability to give calories and protein. Five randomized trials have evaluated the combination of parenteral nutrition started with enteral nutrition as compared to enteral nutrition alone.[28,65–68] These studies were done in patients with burns (2), trauma (1), and ICU patients (2).

Of the studies evaluating combined parenteral and enteral nutrition, three reported that the combined group received significantly more calories compared to the enteral nutrition group.[65,66,68] Only two studies reported on infections, blood sugars, and cost.[67,68] Bauer et al reported that blood sugars were higher in the combined group, but this only occurred on day 7. Overall, there was no difference in infections noted but the combined group was associated with higher cost.

When the data are combined to assess mortality, there is no effect associated with supplemental parenteral nutrition (RR 1.27, 95% CI 0.82–1.94, $p = 0.30$).[69] One study reported a significant increase in mortality associated with parenteral nutrition in burn patients.[66] It appears that adding parenteral nutrition to enteral nutrition increases the cost of therapy without improving clinically important outcomes. When initiating nutrition support in critically ill patients, we recommend that parenteral nutrition not be routinely added to enteral nutrition solely for the purpose of reaching target goals of protein and calories. In the patient who is not tolerating adequate enteral nutrition, there are insufficient data to put forward a recommendation about when parenteral nutrition should be initiated. Practitioners will have to weigh the safety and benefits of initiating PN in patients not tolerating EN on an individual case-by-case basis. We recommend that PN not be started in critically ill patients until all strategies to maximize EN delivery (such as small bowel feeding tubes, motility agents) have been attempted.

A recent study demonstrated improved mortality of critically ill surgical patients managed with insulin infusion to achieve tight glycemic control (blood sugar 4.4–6.1 mmol/L) compared to standard glycemic control.[64] The majority were elective cardiac surgery patients and all received a dextrose load of 300 g in the first day of their ICU stay followed by enteral feeding and most (60%) also received supplemental PN. The generalizability of these results is limited because of the narrow patient population studied and the aggressive use of parental dextrose. We recommended that for critically ill surgical patients receiving this type of nutrition support that tight glycemic control be targeted. Given the degree of insulin resistance apparent in critically ill patients, we do not recommend that parenteral glucose or nutrition be used in this manner. There are insufficient data to make recommendations about tight glycemic control for other groups of critically ill patients.

NUTRITIONAL MANAGEMENT OF ACUTE RENAL FAILURE

The nutritional management of ARF has been the subject of recent in-depth reviews.[70,71] Due to the paucity of data, particularly from randomized trials focusing on clinically important outcomes in patients with ARF, it is not possible to make specific evidence-based recommendations on the nutritional management of ARF. In general, the guidelines for nutritional management of critically ill patients without ARF are applied to the management of patients with ARF, with consideration of the physiologic changes associated with ARF and the nutritional losses associated with RRTs. The presence of renal disease in a critically ill patient should not lead to restrictions in nutritional support.[70] Regardless of the modality of RRT employed, the dose of dialysis should be sufficient to control the metabolic and ECFV changes associated with the appropriate nutritional regimen.

PROTEIN DOSING

Protein catabolism is perhaps the most significant metabolic consequence of ARF. Macias et al examined the impact of the nutritional regimen on protein catabolism and nitrogen balance in 40 critically ill patients with ARF on continuous venovenous hemofiltration and estimated that protein administration rates of 1.5–1.7 g/kg/day are necessary to achieve nitrogen balance.[72] A number of studies have shown that, in practice, no amount of protein administration will achieve a neutral or positive nitrogen balance in the majority of catabolic patients with ARF because higher protein doses are associated with increased protein catabolism. For example, Bellomo et al compared protein dosing directed by the attending physician (1.2 g/kg/day) and a fixed high dose of protein (2.5 g/kg/day) in two consecutive cohorts of critically ill patients with ARF on CRRT.[73] The high protein dose had a favorable impact on nitrogen balance that did not reach statistical significance (−1.9 g/kg/day vs −5.5 g/kg/day, N/S). The high protein cohort required a higher dose of dialysis and had higher levels of plasma urea, absolute nitrogen losses, and absolute protein turnover. The potential benefit of high protein doses must be balanced against the risks, including increased urea formation, increased fluid administration, and the need for increased dialysis dose. Accordingly, Druml has suggested that catabolic patients with

ARF should receive 1.2–1.5 g/kg/day of protein or amino acids.[71] These calculations include the losses induced by intermittent hemodilaysis (IHD), CRRT, or peritoneal dialysis. In the most recent review, Bellomo has recommended that critically ill patients with ARF should receive 1.5–2.0 g/kg/day of protein:[70] a dose of 1.5 g/kg/day of protein or amino acids appears to be a reasonable compromise. The use of enteral formulas designed for patients with renal failure can reduce the administration of water and electrolytes, such as potassium and phosphate, but should not restrict the delivery of protein.

ENERGY, LIPIDS, AND MICRONUTRIENTS

Energy requirements in patients with acute renal failure are determined by the concomitant illnesses. Energy expenditure is not increased in isolated acute renal failure, but is increased 1.3-fold in the presence of catabolic illness such as sepsis.[74]

Accordingly, a caloric intake of 25–35 kcal/kg/day has been recommended for critically ill patients with ARF, depending on the estimated energy expenditure of individual patients.[70,71] In regards to lipid abnormalities in ARF, when lipid emulsions are used in the setting of PN, as much as 1 g/kg/day of fat will not significantly increase plasma triglyceride levels.[71] In regards to vitamins, the recommended daily allowance (RDA) for vitamins and trace elements should be administered while limiting the vitamin C intake to below 200 mg/day.[70,71] If CRRT is employed, twice the RDA of folate and vitamin B_6 should be administered and supplementation of zinc and selenium should be considered.[70] Selenium replacement in patients with systemic inflammatory response syndrome may improve clinical outcomes and reduce the incidence of acute renal failure requiring hemodialysis.[75] In the general ICU population, selenium supplementation may be associated with decreased mortality.[76]

SUMMARY

When considering nutrition support in critically ill patients, we strongly recommend that EN be used in preference to PN. We recommend that enteral feeding be initiated within 24–48 hours of admission and that arginine-containing enteral products not be used. Strategies to optimize delivery of EN (use of small bowel feeding) and minimize the risks of EN (elevating the head of the bed) should be considered. When initiating EN, we strongly recommend that PN not be used in combination with EN. When PN is utilized, we recommend it be supplemented with glutamine. There are insufficient data to generate treatment recommendations specifically for patients with ARF. Consideration will need to be given to individual patient characteristics and the associated pathophysiologic changes.

REFERENCES

1. Heyland DK, Dhaliwal R, Drover JW, Gramlich L, Dodek P, Canadian Critical Care Clinical Practice Guidelines Committee. Canadian clinical practice guidelines for nutrition support in mechanically ventilated, critically ill adult patients. JPEN J Parenter Enteral Nutr 2003;27(5):255–73.
2. DerSimonian R, Laird N. Meta-analysis in clinical trials. Control Clin Trials 1986;7(3):177–88.
3. Clarke M, Moustgaard R, Ris J. RevMan 4.1 User's guide. The Cochrane Collaboration. Copenhagen. 2000;71–5.
4. Druml W. Protein metabolism in acute renal failure. Miner Electrolyte Metab 1998;24(1):47–54.
5. May RC, Kelly RA, Mitch WE. Metabolic acidosis stimulates protein degradation in rat muscle by a glucocorticoid-dependent mechanism. J Clin Invest 1986;77(2):614–21.
6. Price SR, England BK, Bailey JL, Van Vreede K, Mitch WE. Acidosis and glucocorticoids concomitantly increase ubiquitin and proteasome subunit mRNAs in rat muscle. Am J Physiol 1994;267(4 Pt 1):C955–60.
7. Graham KA, Reaich D, Channon SM, Downie S, Goodship TH. Correction of acidosis in hemodialysis decreases whole-body protein degradation. J Am Soc Nephrol 1997;8(4):632–7.
8. May RC, Clark AS, Goheer MA, Mitch WE. Specific defects in insulin-mediated muscle metabolism in acute uremia. Kidney Int 1985;28(3):490–7.
9. Price SR, Bailey JL, Wang X, et al. Muscle wasting in insulinopenic rats results from activation of the ATP-dependent, ubiquitin–proteasome proteolytic pathway by a mechanism including gene transcription. J Clin Invest 1996;98(8):1703–8.
10. Mokrzycki MH, Kaplan AA. Protein losses in continuous renal replacement therapies. J Am Soc Nephrol 1996;7(10):2259–63.
11. Maxvold NJ, Smoyer WE, Custer JR, Bunchman TE. Amino acid loss and nitrogen balance in critically ill children with acute renal failure: a prospective comparison between classic hemofiltration and hemofiltration with dialysis. Crit Care Med 2000;28(4):1161–5.
12. Druml W, Laggner A, Widhalm K, Kleinberger G, Lenz K. Lipid metabolism in acute renal failure. Kidney Int Suppl 1983;16:S139–42.
13. Story DA, Ronco C, Bellomo R. Trace element and vitamin concentrations and losses in critically ill patients treated with continuous venovenous hemofiltration. Crit Care Med 1999;27(1):220–3.
14. Druml W, Schwarzenhofer M, Apsner R, Horl WH. Fat-soluble vitamins in patients with acute renal failure. Miner Electrolyte Metab 1998;24(4):220–6.
15. Massry SG, Arieff AI, Coburn JW, Palmieri G, Kleeman CR. Divalent ion metabolism in patients with acute renal failure: studies on the mechanism of hypocalcemia. Kidney Int 1974;5(6):437–45.
16. McClave SA, McClain CJ, Snider HL. Should indirect calorimetry be used as part of nutritional assessment? J Clin Gastroenterol 2001;33(1):14–19.
17. Long CL, Schaffel N, Geiger JW, Schiller WR, Blakemore WS. Metabolic response to injury and illness: estimation of energy and protein needs from indirect calorimetry and nitrogen balance. JPEN. J Parenter Enteral Nutr 1979;3(6):452–6.
18. Saffle JR, Larson CM, Sullivan J. A randomized trial of indirect calorimetry-based feedings in thermal injury. J Trauma 1990;30(7):776–82.
19. McClave SA, Lowen CC, Kleber MJ, et al. Are patients fed appropriately according to their caloric requirements? JPEN. J Parenter Enteral Nutr 1998;22(6):375–81.
20. Braunschweig CL, Levy P, Sheean PM, Wang X. Enteral compared with parenteral nutrition: a meta-analysis. Am J Clin Nutr 2001;74(4):534–42.
21. Lipman TO. Grains or veins: is enteral nutrition really better than parenteral nutrition? A look at the evidence. JPEN J Parenter Enteral Nutr 1998;22(3):167–82.
22. Gramlich L, Kichian K, Pinilla J, et al. Does enteral nutrition compared to parenteral nutrition result in better outcomes in critically ill adult patients? A systematic review of the literature. Nutrition 2004;20(10):843–8.
23. Young B, Ott L, Twyman D, et al. The effect of nutritional support on outcome from severe head injury. J Neurosurg 1987;67(5):668–76.
24. Hadley MN, Grahm TW, Harrington T. Nutritional support and neurotrauma: a critical review of early nutrition in forty-five acute head injury patients. Neurosurgery 1986;19(3):367–73.
25. Borzotta AP, Pennings J, Papasadero B, et al. Enteral versus parenteral nutrition after severe closed head injury. J Trauma 1994;37(3):459–68.
26. Adams S, Dellinger EP, Wertz MJ. Enteral versus parenteral nutritional support following laparotomy for trauma: a randomized prospective trial. J Trauma 1986;26(10):882–91.
27. Kudsk KA, Croce MA, Fabian TC, et al. Enteral versus parenteral feeding: effects on septic morbidity after blunt and penetrating abdominal trauma. Ann Surg 1992;215(5):503–13.
28. Dunham CM, Frankenfield D, Belzberg H, et al. Gut failure–predictor of or contributor to mortality in mechanically ventilated blunt trauma patients? J Trauma 1994;37(1):30–4.
29. Cerra FB, McPherson JP, Konstantinides FN, Konstantinides NN, Teasley KM. Enteral nutrition does not prevent multiple organ failure syndrome (MOFS) after sepsis. Surgery 1988;104(4):727–33.
30. Hadfield RJ, Sinclair DG, Houldsworth PE, Evans TW. Effects of enteral and parenteral nutrition on gut mucosal permeability in the critically ill. Am J Respir Crit Care Med 1995;152(5):1545–8.
31. Woodcock NP, Zeigler D, Palmer MD, et al. Enteral versus parenteral nutrition: a pragmatic study. Nutrition 2001;17(1):1–12.
32. Moore FA, Feliciano DV, Andrassy RJ, et al. Early enteral feeding, compared with parenteral, reduces postoperative septic complications: the results of a meta-analysis. Ann Surg 1992;216(2):172–83.
33. Kalfarentzos F, Kehagias J, Mead N, Kokkinis K, Gogos CA. Enteral nutrition is superior to parenteral nutrition in severe acute pancreatitis: results of a randomized prospective trial. Br J Surg 1997;84(12):1665–9.
34. Rapp RP, Young DB, Twyman D. The favorable effect of early parenteral feeding on survival in head-injured patients. J Neurosurg 1983;58(6):906–12.
35. Young B, Ott L, Haack D. Effect of total parenteral nutrition upon intracranial pressure in severe head injury. J Neurosurg 1987;67(1):76–80.
36. Moore FA, Moore EE, Jones TN, McCroskey BL, Peterson VM. TEN versus TPN following major abdominal trauma – reduced septic morbidity. J Trauma 1989;29(7):916–23.

37. Moore EE, Jones TN. Benefits of immediate jejunostomy feeding after major abdominal trauma – a prospective, randomized study. J Trauma 1986;26(10):874–81.
38. Chiarelli A, Enzi G, Casadei A, et al. Very early nutrition supplementation in burned patients. Am J Clin Nutr 1990;51:1035–9.
39. Eyer SD, Micon LT, Konstantinides FN, et al. Early enteral feeding does not attenuate metabolic response after blunt trauma. J Trauma 1993;34(5):639–44.
40. Chuntrasakul C, Siltharm S, Chinswangwatanakul V, et al. Early nutritional support in severe traumatic patients. J Med Assoc Thai 1996;79(1):21–6.
41. Singh G, Ram RP, Khanna SK. Early postoperative enteral feeding in patients with nontraumatic intestinal perforation and peritonitis. J Am Coll Surg 1998;187(2):142–6.
42. Kompan L, Kremzar B, Gadzijev E, Prosek M. Effects of early enteral nutrition on intestinal permeability and the development of multiple organ failure after multiple injury. Intensive Care Med 1999;25(2):157–61.
43. Minard G, Kudsk KA, Melton S, Patton JH, Tolley EA. Early versus delayed feeding with an immune-enhancing diet in patients with severe head injuries. JPEN J Parenter Enteral Nutr 2000;24(3):145–9.
44. Pupelis G, Selga G, Austrums E, Kaminski A. Jejunal feeding, even when instituted late, improves outcomes in patients with severe pancreatitis and peritonitis. Nutrition 2001;17(2):91–4.
45. Clinical Practice Guidelines Website: http//www.criticalcare-nutrition.com. Date last accessed: July 2005.
46. Mentec H, Dupont H, Bocchetti M, et al. Upper digestive intolerance during enteral nutrition in critically ill patients: frequency, risk factors, and complications. Crit Care Med 2001;29(10):1955–61.
47. Ibrahim EH, Mehringer L, Prentice D, et al. Early versus late enteral feeding of mechanically ventilated patients: results of a clinical trial. JPEN J Parenter Enteral Nutr 2002;26(3):174–81.
48. Heyland DK, Drover JW, Dhaliwal R, Greenwood J. Optimizing the benefits and minimizing the risks of enteral nutrition in the critically ill: role of small bowel feeding. JPEN J Parenter Enteral Nutr 2002;26:51–7.
49. Drakulovic MB, Torres A, Bauer TT, et al. Supine body position as a risk factor for nosocomial pneumonia in mechanically ventilated patients: a randomised trial. Lancet 1999;354(9193):1851–8.
50. Heyland DK, Novak F, Drover JW, et al. Should immunonutrition become routine in critically ill patients? A systematic review of the evidence. JAMA 2001;286(8):944–53.
51. Heyland DK. Immunonutrition in the critically ill patient: putting the cart before the horse? Nutr Clin Pract 2002;17:267–72.
52. Kieft H, Ross A, Van Drunen, et al. Clinical outcome of immunonutrition in a heterogeneous intensive care population. Intensive Care Med 2005;31(4):524–32.
53. Novak I, Sramek V, Pittrova H, et al. Glutamine and other amino acid losses during continuous venovenous hemodiafiltration. Artif Organs 1997;21(5):359–63.
54. Novak F, Heyland DK, Avenell A, Drover JW, Su X. Glutamine supplementation in serious illness: a systematic review of the evidence. Crit Care Med 2002;30(9):2022–9.
55. Taylor SJ, Fettes SB, Jewkes C, Nelson RJ. Prospective, randomized, controlled trial to determine the effect of early enhanced enteral nutrition on clinical outcome in mechanically ventilated patients suffering head injury. Crit Care Med 1999;27(11):2525–31.
56. Montecalvo MA, Steger KA, Farber HW, et al. Nutritional outcome and pneumonia in critical care patients randomized to gastric versus jejunal tube feedings. The Critical Care Research Team. Crit Care Med 1992;20(10):1377–87.
57. Kearns PJ, Chin D, Mueller L, et al. The incidence of ventilator-associated pneumonia and success in nutrient delivery with gastric versus small intestinal feeding: a randomized clinical trial. Crit Care Med 2000;28(6):1742–6.
58. Kortbeek JB, Haigh PI, Doig C. Duodenal versus gastric feeding in ventilated blunt trauma patients: a randomized controlled trial. J Trauma 1999;46(6):992–6.
59. Drover JW, Dhaliwal R, Heyland DK. Post pyloric enteral feeding: not all it is cracked up to be! Int J Intensive Care 2002;9:139–45.
60. McClave SA, Snider HL. Clinical use of gastric residual volumes as a monitor for patients on enteral tube feeding. JPEN J Parenter Enteral Nutr 2002;26:43–50.
61. Boivin MA, Levy H. Gastric feeding with erythromycin is equivalent to transpyloric feeding in the critically ill. Crit Care Med 2001;29(10):1916–19.
62. Heyland DK, MacDonald S, Keefe L, Drover JW. Total parenteral nutrition in the critically ill patient: a meta-analysis. JAMA 1998;280(23):2013–19.
63. Battistella FD, Widergren JT, Anderson JT, et al. A prospective, randomized trial of intravenous fat emulsion administration in trauma victims requiring total parenteral nutrition. J Trauma 1997;43(1):52–60.
64. van den Berghe G, Wouters P, Weekers F, et al. Intensive insulin therapy in the critically ill patients. N Engl J Med 2001;345(19):1359–67.
65. Herndon DN, Stein MD, Rutan TC, Abston S, Linares H. Failure of TPN supplementation to improve liver function, immunity, and mortality in thermally injured patients. J Trauma 1987;27(2):195–204.
66. Herndon DN, Barrow RE, Stein M, et al. Increased mortality with intravenous supplemental feeding in severely burned patients. J Burn Care Rehabil 1989;10(4):309–13.
67. Chiarelli AG, Ferrarello S, Piccioli A, et al. [Total enteral nutrition versus mixed enteral and parenteral nutrition in patients at an intensive care unit.] Minerva Anestesiol 1996;62(1–2):1–7. [in Italian]
68. Bauer P, Charpentier C, Bouchet C, et al. Parenteral with enteral nutrition in the critically ill. Intensive Care Med 2000;26(7):893–900.
69. Dhaliwal R, Jurewitsch B, Harrietha D, Heyland DK. Combination enteral and parenteral nutrition in critically ill patients: harmful or beneficial? A systematic review of the evidence. Intensive Care Med 2004;30(8):1666–71.
70. Bellomo R. How to feed patients with renal dysfunction. Blood Purif 2002;20(3):296–303.
71. Druml W. Nutritional management of acute renal failure. Am J Kidney Dis 2001;37(1 Suppl 2):S89–S94.
72. Macias WL, Alaka KJ, Murphy MH, et al. Impact of the nutritional regimen on protein catabolism and nitrogen balance in patients with acute renal failure. JPEN J Parenter Enteral Nutr 1996;20(1):56–62.
73. Bellomo R, Seacombe J, Daskalakis M, et al. A prospective comparative study of moderate versus high protein intake for critically ill patients with acute renal failure. Ren Fail 1997;19(1):111–20.
74. Schneeweiss B, Graninger W, Stockenhuber F, et al. Energy metabolism in acute and chronic renal failure. Am J Clin Nutr 1990;52(4):596–601.
75. Angstwurm MW, Schottdorf J, Schopohl J, Gaertner R. Selenium replacement in patients with severe systemic inflammatory response syndrome improves clinical outcome. Crit Care Med 1999;27(9):1807–13.
76. Heyland D, Dhaliwal R, Suchner U, Berger M. Antioxidant nutrients: a systematic review of trace elements and vitamins in the critically ill patient. Intensive Care Med 2005;31(3):327–37.

26

Hypertensive disorders in the intensive care unit

Munavvar Izhar and William J Elliott

INTRODUCTION

Blood pressure (BP) sometimes can be elevated to such levels that blood vessels and target organs (brain, heart, kidneys, and other vascular beds) become damaged acutely. In these circumstances, blood pressure must be swiftly and effectively reduced, typically in an intensive care unit (ICU) with parenterally delivered drugs, to prevent further deterioration of organ function. More frequently, patients present with very high blood pressures, but without evidence of acute target organ damage (TOD); this situation is considered a 'hypertensive urgency' and need not be treated either in hospital or with intravenous medication. A primary and critical function of the physician initially evaluating a person with distinctly elevated blood pressures is to distinguish between these two situations, for two major reasons. The route of administration of drug therapy is different (intravenous therapy is typical for emergencies, whereas oral therapy can be given for urgencies), and hospitalization (usually in the ICU) is almost always necessary for hypertensive emergencies, but seldom required for hypertensive urgencies.

HISTORICAL PERSPECTIVE

The term, 'malignant hypertension' has been used since the early 1900s when there was no effective therapy for high blood pressure.[1] This diagnosis was given to patients who presented with severely elevated blood pressures and signs or symptoms of acute TOD. Because the short-term mortality rate in such patients was very high (mean survival was only 6 months after diagnosis), the prognosis

with this form of hypertension rivaled that of many cancers.

The phrase *malignant hypertension* has been largely replaced by *hypertensive crisis*, or more specifically, *hypertensive emergency or urgency*. Most authorities,[2,3] including the authors of the Seventh Report of the Joint National Committee on Prevention, Detection, Evaluation, and Treatment of High Blood Pressure[4] have accepted this revised terminology.

The occurrence of hypertensive crises not only depends on the prevalence of treated hypertension but also on socioeconomic and demographic variables and on the availability of antihypertensive medications. Early National Health and Nutrition Examination Surveys performed in the USA estimated that less than 2% of the population had a diastolic BP in excess of 115 mmHg.[4,5] Medicaid claims data from Georgia, USA, a few years later, suggested that the incidence of malignant hypertension was less than 0.2% of the population.[6]

Hypertensive emergencies were much more common in the 1960s and 1970s, when one in three beds in hospitals were occupied by patients with hypertension or related complications. Many factors have been identified that predispose to hypertensive emergencies. Discontinuation or reduction in dose or frequency of antihypertensive therapy because of side effects without a physician's advice is the most common clinical situation leading to a hypertensive emergency. Although elevated plasma renin levels have been implicated in some cases, higher plasma adrenomedullin and natriuretic peptide concentrations have been found in patients with hypertensive emergencies than in either chronically hypertensive or normotensive controls.[7] Lack of a primary care physician or an inability to obtain prescription refills due to financial reasons was also an important risk factor for presenting to an Emergency Department with severely elevated blood pressure.[8]

Patients with hypertensive crises have a higher prevalence of secondary hypertension than the general hypertensive population. Renovascular hypertension,[9] and especially pheochromocytoma, are the most common types; hyperaldosteronism is rare.[10,11] Most authorities recommend a formal evaluation for secondary hypertension after successful lowering of blood pressure. Although exacerbation of chronic renal impairment frequently occurs during and after treatment of hypertensive emergencies, renal function may recover gradually over days to weeks when blood pressure is adequately controlled.[12,13] A history of pregestational chronic hypertension in a pregnant patient is a risk factor for the development of a hypertensive crisis,[14,15] but this is relatively rare. Although high doses formerly used in oral contraceptives were previously identified as a risk factor for the development of hypertensive emergency,[16] the lower doses in current use appear not to have this problem. Occasionally, withdrawal of antihypertensive medications (especially alpha$_2$-agonists) or ingestion of substances that raise BP[8,17] can be identified as a proximal cause of a hypertensive emergency.

PATHOGENESIS

Abnormalities of autoregulation in vascular beds appear to be the basic pathophysiologic problem that leads to TOD in hypertensive crises. Autoregulation refers to the ability of blood vessels to dilate or constrict in order to maintain normal organ perfusion. Normal arteries in normotensive individuals can maintain flow over a wide range of mean arterial pressures. Many studies in animal models, usually of the cerebral circulation, and a few experiments in humans,[18] have shown that chronic elevations in BP cause compensatory functional and structural changes in the arterial circulation. This alteration in pressure–flow relationships in hypertensive patients allows them to maintain normal perfusion. When BP increases above the autoregulatory range, tissue damage occurs, either due to excessive vasoconstriction and resultant ischemia or due to complete loss of vascular integrity, resulting in hemorrhage. The autoregulatory range and the structural compensatory changes help explain why chronically hypertensive patients can often tolerate very high BPs without problems, and why normotensive

patients, or patients with only a recent onset or rapidly increasing BP, can develop hypertensive crises at relatively low BP levels.

This pathophysiologic paradigm also has important implications for therapy, since the sudden lowering of BP into a range that would otherwise be considered 'normal' may reduce BP below the autoregulatory capacity of the circulation in a chronically hypertensive person. This phenomenon explains the hypoperfusion of vital organs and the development of acute renal failure and/or cerebral ischemia and infarction, too often seen in patients when BP is lowered too far or too fast.

In the later stages of hypertensive crises, and especially in fatal cases, pathologists can often demonstrate cerebral edema and both acute and chronic inflammation of the medium and small arteries and arterioles, often associated with necrosis called 'fibrinoid necrosis'. This was frequently seen in the 1950s; because of therapeutic advances in the last five decades, this pathologic entity is much rarer now. When hypoperfusion occurs in the renal circulation, relative ischemia in the juxtaglomerular apparatus leads to progressively increasing secretion of renin, raising BP further, and causing a pressure diuresis and hypovolemia, both of which provide additional stimuli to renin secretion. Ischemia can also be seen in other vascular beds, including the retina, the heart, and the brain. In a sizeable minority of patients with hypertensive crises, microangiopathic hemolytic anemia occurs.

CLINICAL MANIFESTATIONS

The association of an extremely elevated BP with physical examination and/or laboratory findings indicative of acute TOD most easily defines a hypertensive crisis. The organs that require special attention during the initial evaluation of the patient with very high BPs include the brain, eyes, heart, kidneys, and peripheral vasculature.

In a patient with very elevated BP and neurologic findings or an altered mental status, a thorough inspection of the optic fundi is essential, and may be very helpful in distinguishing among the various types of neurologic crises. Hypertensive encephalopathy is a diagnosis of exclusion in a patient with elevated BP readings, altered mental status, and no other cause of the neurologic disturbance. Hypertensive encephalopathy is essentially always associated with significant hypertensive retinal findings: seldom just arteriovenous (A-V) nicking (grade II), most commonly acute hemorrhages (grade III), or somewhat less often, papilledema (grade IV). Patients with either new hemorrhages/exudates or papilledema also represent a hypertensive crisis, as their prognosis is similar.[19] The fundi can sometimes provide a clue about the etiology of hypertension, since patients with underlying renovascular hypertension presenting with hypertensive emergency frequently have grade III or IV retinopathy.[9] This association is particularly strong in whites.

A careful neurologic examination should be performed early and repeated often during the first few hours after presentation. Mental status should be carefully assessed, since the level of cognition is one of the most important determinants of the success or failure of therapy. A thorough cardiac examination is essential to detect abnormalities such as cardiac ischemia, dysrhythmias, heart failure, and coarctation of the aorta or dissecting aortic aneurysm. The presence of any of these abnormalities helps to guide the choice of parenteral antihypertensive drug therapy.

Examination of the abdomen and peripheral vasculature is also necessary, not only to look for TOD, but also to screen for a secondary cause of hypertension. The presence of an abdominal bruit is still the most reliable and cost-effective physical sign of renovascular hypertension. The radio-radial pulse delay (as in Takayasu's arteritis) and the radio-femoral pulse delay (due to a coarctation of the aorta) should not be missed because they were not sought. Occasionally, palpation of a pheochromocytoma can initiate a typical paroxysm of hypertension and other symptoms that suggest the diagnosis.

It is very important to compare a serum creatinine level drawn from the patient at presentation with the most recent corresponding value, because an acute deterioration in renal function that is temporally correlated with very elevated BP is a hypertensive crisis.[2–4,13] The presence of gross or microscopic hematuria at presentation suggests acute glomerular injury that may be due to very elevated BPs. However, red cell casts and significant proteinuria generally mean that acute glomerulonephritis is the cause of the elevated BP and perhaps also the hypertensive crisis.

Another hypertensive emergency most often encountered by nephrologists is scleroderma renal crisis, which is defined as the onset of accelerated arterial hypertension and/or rapidly progressive renal failure; it is a surprisingly common initial presentation of scleroderma. This situation requires hospitalization and parenteral drug therapy and has a lifetime risk of about 10–25% of patients with systemic scleroderma. Diffuse skin involvement, rapid progression of skin thickening, new onset of anemia, duration of scleroderma for less than 4 years, presence of anti-RNA polymerase antibody, a recent cardiovascular event, and use of high-dose glucocorticoids are all associated with a higher risk of scleroderma renal crisis. The poorest prognosis is seen when scleroderma renal crisis is associated with thrombocytopenia, elevated plasma renin levels, and/or hemolytic anemia. Since the typical pathologic progression includes intimal proliferation, medial thinning, and increased collagen deposition in the adventitial layer of the small renal arteries, the clinical result is decreased renal blood flow, hypertension, and progressive renal impairment. Increased plasma levels of renin and angiotensin II contribute further to the worsening hypertension and deteriorating renal function.

DIAGNOSTIC APPROACH

The initial diagnostic and therapeutic approach to a patient with a potential hypertensive crisis involves careful examination of the patient and the urine, an electrocardiogram, and the most recent previous serum creatinine level. If any of these provides evidence of acute, severe TOD, the patient's hypertensive crisis should be classified as an emergency; hospitalization (typically in an ICU) and appropriate parenteral therapy are warranted. Those patients with severely elevated BP and altered mental state, focal neurologic deficit, dissecting aortic aneurysm, or heart failure certainly require the closest monitoring (typically in an ICU). If, on the other hand, there is minimal or mild TOD, and a relatively normal physical examination and laboratory studies, a less-intense effort to lower the BP is appropriate, since the diagnosis is a hypertensive urgency.[20,21]

Hypertensive crises with neurologic manifestations

Table 26.1 summarizes the neurologic manifestations that often present as hypertensive crises. Hypertensive encephalopathy is typically the most difficult diagnosis to establish, as it requires that other causes of the altered mental status be ruled out.[22] In an acute cerebrovascular accident or

Table 26.1   Distinguishing characteristics of neurologic presentations of hypertensive crisis.

	Hypertensive encephalopathy	Acute cerebral infarction	Subarachnoid hemorrhage	Intraparenchymal hemorrhage
History				
Duration of symptoms	Subacute	Acute	Acute	Acute
Headache	Severe	Variable	Severe	Variable
History of hypertension	Nearly universal	Common, but variable	Common, but variable	Common, but variable
Physical examination				
Retinopathy[a]	II–IV (usually III or IV)	Variable: 0–IV	Variable: 0–IV	Variable: 0–IV
Focal neurologic deficits	Unusual; varies with BP level	Characteristic of location of infarction	Variable	Characteristic of location of hemorrhage
Laboratory findings				
Lumbar puncture	Usually normal, except opening pressure	Usually normal, except opening pressure	Xanthochromic or frankly bloody	Xanthochromic or frankly bloody
CT scan	Usually normal	Can show area of infarct	Usually normal	Often shows area of hemorrhage

[a] Graded on the Keith–Wagener–Barker scale. See text for further details.

BP = blood pressure; CT = computed tomography.

subarachnoid hemorrhage, there is usually a sudden deterioration in mental status, as compared to a gradual deterioration that is more common in hypertensive encephalopathy. Patients with encephalopathy often present after a relatively long period of poorly controlled hypertension, with a recent history of very elevated BP, headache, nausea, vomiting, altered mental status, and visual disturbances. If focal neurologic findings are present, serial neurologic examinations should be undertaken, because they often improve dramatically during the initial few minutes of treatment and lowered BP when hypertensive encephalopathy is the correct diagnosis. Grade III or grade IV hypertensive retinopathy is essentially universal in hypertensive encephalopathy; absence of these findings may exclude the diagnosis. When focal neurologic defects are not present, administration of rapidly reversible parenteral therapy to lower the BP into a safer range should be commenced before undertaking other diagnostic procedures. A computed tomography (CT) scan of the head is routinely performed (often with contrast media) when patients present with focal neurologic deficits or altered mental status, to

distinguish between hemorrhagic and thrombic intracranial processes. Intracranial/subarachnoid hemorrhage is a diagnosis that can be easily confused with hypertensive encephalopathy; the CT scan with contrast is a very sensitive and specific test to distinguish between the two. However, it is still sometimes necessary to perform a lumbar puncture to diagnose subarachnoid hemorrhage. This is typically performed after a CT scan shows no intraparenchymal hemorrhage.

Acute cerebrovascular accidents are also frequently accompanied by high BP and can sometimes be confused with hypertensive encephalopathy. The symptoms are usually rapid in onset, and typically manifest as focal neurologic findings that change little during observation. In some severe strokes, the neurologic findings can be so profound acutely that they manifest as mental obtundation. The CT scan of the head is the most helpful diagnostic test, but it may not be abnormal during the very early hours after the acute onset of symptoms. There continues to be major controversy about the wisdom of attempting to lower BP during the first few hours after stroke symptoms begin. Many experts have noted that BP lowering during the hyperacute phase of a stroke may worsen the focal neurologic deficit; others believe that the BP should not be allowed to soar over perhaps 180/110 mmHg during the first few hours of stroke. However, both groups agree that if BP lowering is needed, a short-acting, intravenously administered drug should be used, and the patient examined very frequently in an ICU.[23] The advantage of the intravenously administered antihypertensive drugs is that they can be easily titrated and quickly discontinued if the BP drops unexpectedly.

Hypertensive crises with cardiac manifestations

Pulmonary edema and acute left ventricular failure are the most common varieties of hypertensive crises involving the heart; acute coronary syndromes more commonly manifest with hypotension, but can involve hypertension and be classified as a hypertensive crisis. Therapy for the first two problems is usually directed toward reducing both preload and afterload; this typically also lowers the BP. Most of the drugs used to treat acute pulmonary edema have important antihypertensive actions, including furosemide, nitroglycerin, nitroprusside, and enalaprilat.[24] Most affected patients are treated with a combination of these drugs to acutely reduce both BP and myocardial oxygen demand.

Many patients with unstable angina pectoris or with acute myocardial infarction are anxious and have higher-than-usual BP at presentation. Most emergency rooms now provide intravenous nitroglycerin for these patients, in an effort to dilate the coronary arterial bed. Although nitroglycerin is not a uniformly effective antihypertensive agent in most hypertensives, it is very helpful in relieving symptoms in the clinical setting of ongoing cardiac ischemia. In one of the few comparative trials, nitroglycerin pectoris was not significantly different than nitroprusside in improving long-term prognosis for patients with unstable angina.[25]

Crises with aortic dissection

Since, in aortic dissection, the primary cause of damage to the aorta is the shearing force developed during cardiac contraction, the BP goal for this condition is significantly lower and the rapidity with which that goal should be reached is much greater than with other hypertensive crises.[26]

When aortic dissection is strongly suspected, appropriate BP reduction should be initiated and continued while efforts to confirm the diagnosis, by CT scan, magnetic resonance imaging (MRI), transesophageal echocardiography,[27] or angiography, are in progress.[28] The choice of definitive therapy[29] and the timing and type of surgery, if that option is selected, must be decided upon with dispatch, since aortic dissection still has an extremely poor prognosis if not managed expeditiously.

In contrast to most other hypertensive crises, for which BP reduction should be gradual and accomplished over several hours, in patients with aortic dissection, the systolic BP should be brought to about 120 mmHg within 15–30 minutes. This is necessary to minimize the exposure of the torn aortic intima to excessively high pressures, which could well extend the lesion. Furthermore, the drug used to lower the BP should specifically decrease those shearing forces, usually characterized as the rate of change of pressure with respect to time (or $\delta P / \delta t$). Not all drugs that lower BP also reduce $\delta P / \delta t$; the combination of a beta-blocker and a vasodilator is usually recommended. In the ICU setting, an intravenous beta-blocker, usually esmolol,[30] and either nitroprusside, fenoldopam, or nicardipine is usually used.

Crises related to excess catecholamines

Very elevated blood pressure, diaphoresis, and severe headaches are the typical presenting signs and symptoms of many pheochromocytomas. For a patient in whom this diagnosis is strongly suspected, the collection of a 24-hour urine or venous blood sample for catecholamines and metabolites can be very helpful. Current research suggests that plasma free metanephrines may be the test of choice because of its high sensitivity (99% in a recent series[31]), but the high cost and limited availability are challenges. A finding of normal levels of catecholamines or metabolites during a hypertensive crisis makes the diagnosis of pheochromocytoma very unlikely. It is rarely helpful to perform a Regitine test (measuring BP response to intravenous phentolamine) since both the sensitivity and specificity of the test are low.

Other situations in which hypertensive crises are mediated by excess catecholamines or their metabolites include acute withdrawal from antihypertensive drugs, especially clonidine or beta-blockers. Patients experiencing withdrawal of antihypertensive drug therapy typically need to be given only a single dose of that agent to substantially reduce BP. Patients with other catecholamine excess states can usually be treated with fast-acting alpha-blockers, like prazosin, labetalol, or in difficult or unresponsive cases, intravenous phentolamine.

Crises related to pregnancy

Pre-eclampsia should be treated quickly and intensively because of potential damage to the fetus and the risk to the mother. This form of hypertensive crisis is usually managed in an ICU-like labor and delivery suite. The current definition of pre-eclampsia requires only one BP reading ≥140/90 mmHg in a woman who was normotensive before 20 weeks of pregnancy *and* proteinuria (≥300 mg/24 hours in a full day's collection) or >1+ protein by dipstick without evidence of urinary tract infection.[14] Other features that increase the certainty of the diagnosis include BP ≥160/110 mmHg, proteinuria >2 g/24 hours, new onset of elevated serum creatinine (>1.2 mg/dl), thrombocytopenia (platelets <100 000/mm^3), and/or evidence of microangiopathic hemolytic anemia, or elevated serum concentrations of hepatic enzymes.

An important consideration in the evaluation of pregnant women with hypertension is the special role given to the obstetrician. Although medical treatment for hypertension and pre-eclampsia should not be deferred or delayed, plans for delivery are often hastened when a hypertensive crisis of pregnancy is discovered or suspected.

MANAGEMENT ISSUES IN HYPERTENSIVE EMERGENCIES

Except in aortic dissection, the goal in a hypertensive crisis is to lower the patient's BP gradually to a sufficient degree over an appropriate period of time (typically 6–24 hours) to allow restoration of the autoregulatory capacity of the vasculature. An intravenously administered medication with a short duration of action is almost always used for this purpose, since the hypotensive effect of the drug can be promptly reversed if the response is excessive. With a short-acting, intravenous drug, the clinician has much tighter control over both the rate of BP decline and the ultimate BP target. The intensive monitoring features found in an ICU make this approach very feasible. On the other hand, the onset of action of oral hypotensive medications is almost always too prolonged to avoid significant organ hypofunction, and the hypotensive effects can be unpredictable. These drugs are more appropriate in a nonemergent situation (e.g. hypertensive urgency) on the medical floor or in an Emergency Department.

Unfortunately, it is impossible to know, a priori, the optimal BP goal for each patient, so only general guidelines can be given (Box 26.1). If the patient's clinical condition worsens because the BP has been lowered either too precipitously or to too low a level, a short-acting, intravenously delivered agent can be discontinued and the BP will rise quickly. Most authorities suggest that in most true hypertensive emergencies (with the exception of aortic dissection and some neurologic crises), the mean arterial pressure should be reduced only 10–15% during the first hour. Gradually, thereafter, a diastolic BP target between 100 and 110 mmHg (or a reduction in 25% compared to the initial baseline, whichever is higher) is appropriate. Reduction of BP to less than 90 mmHg diastolic, or even by as little as 35% of the initial mean arterial pressure, has been associated with major organ dysfunction, coma, and death, even in recent years.[32] The greatest risk occurs when BP reduction occurs very quickly: e.g. from using a bolus of diazoxide or a high dose of oral or sublingual nifedipine.[33]

Crises with neurologic signs or symptoms

For patients with hypertensive encephalopathy, it is usually appropriate to reduce mean arterial pressure by 10% during the first hour after presentation. If the patient's state of cognition does not improve during the first few hours, despite proper BP reduction, the physician should reconsider the diagnosis and take steps to exclude other causes of hypertension, headache, and altered mental status (e.g. infection, subarachnoid hemorrhage or stroke, etc.).

Hypertensive crises secondary to intracranial hemorrhage may be treated in a similar fashion, except that there is usually no major and sudden improvement in mental status or neurologic symptoms when the BP is lowered by only 10%. Drugs with a short onset of hypotensive effect are preferred because they can be abruptly discontinued if the patient's neurologic status deteriorates. In these patients, the target BP should be 160–170/95–100 mmHg, although a somewhat more conservative recommendation (180–185/ 105–110 mmHg) is appropriate if the patient has a history of long-standing hypertension.[34]

Box 26.1   Target blood pressures (BPs) for common hypertensive crises

---

Cardiovascular crises

1. **Aortic dissection:** reduce BP to <120/80 mmHg (if no other untoward events occur) within 15–30 minutes.
2. **Left ventricular failure:** reduce BP to a level consistent with improvement in clinical status (typically a BP drop of 10–15% is sufficient, and >25% may be deleterious) within 30–60 minutes.
3. **Angina pectoris/myocardial ischemia:** reduce BP to a level consistent with diminution/cessation of ischemia (typically only 10–15% reduction is sufficient), within 30–60 minutes.

Neurologic crises

1. **Hypertensive encephalopathy:** 10% reduction in mean arterial pressure over the first hour, and up to 25% reduction (typically 160–180/100–110 mmHg) over 2–3 hours.
2. **Intracranial hemorrhage:** 0–25% reduction (controversy exists about the optimal degree of reduction) over 6–12 hours.
3. **Subarachnoid hemorrhage:** up to 25% reduction (typically 170–180/100–110 mmHg for patients with previous chronic hypertension; or 130–160/90–100 mmHg for previously normotensive patients) over 6–12 hours.
4. **Stroke-in-evolution:** no treatment is routinely recommended for BP <180/105 mmHg at presentation. A BP goal of 160–170/95–100 mmHg is recommended for previously normotensive patients or 180–185/105–110 mmHg for patients with previous chronic hypertension.

Other crises

1. A typical goal is reduction of mean arterial pressure by 10% in the first hour, and 25% (to 100–110 mmHg diastolic) within another 1–2 hours.

Pregnancy-related hypertensive crises

1. Eclampsia and pre-eclampsia are special cases, wherein the BP goal is typically much lower, and the patients are much younger.

In an acute ischemic stroke most authorities defer treatment unless the BP is higher than 180/110 mmHg.[23] An intravenously administered agent that can be quickly discontinued is most commonly recommended, along with frequent neurologic examinations in an ICU.

Crises with cardiac signs or symptoms

The target BP for patients with hypertensive crises associated with either cardiac ischemia or left ventricular dysfunction is variable. About 5–10% reduction in BP after the initiation of therapy usually results in a major improvement in coronary ischemia or heart failure. This is probably because the specific agent chosen in these settings is useful in dilating coronary arteries – nitroglycerin for angina – or reducing preload and afterload – diuretic, angiotensin-converting enzyme (ACE) inhibitor, nitrates – and thereby reducing pul-monary congestion, improving cardiac filling, and improving symptoms of heart failure. The situation is completely different in patients with aortic dissection. To minimize the risk of further intimal tearing, both $\delta P/\delta t$ and BP must be reduced, both quickly and effectively to a lower target. The target systolic BP for aortic dissection is typically <120 mmHg, and should be achieved fairly quickly (within 15–30 minutes).

Renal hypertensive crises

For patients who present with very elevated BP and new hematuria or a recent increase in serum creatinine, a reduction in mean arterial pressure of approximately 25% over a 2–3-hour period is most commonly recommended. Patients with only moderately elevated initial serum creatinine concentrations – <5 mg/dl, corresponding to a glomerular filtration rate (GFR) in the 20–

25 ml/min range – seldom require acute dialysis. Unfortunately, patients with presenting serum creatinine concentrations >10 mg/dl, corresponding to GFRs of below 10 ml/min, often require acute dialysis, typically during the same hospitalization.[13] Careful long-term control of BP is very important for patients who present with hypertensive crises and require acute dialysis. A substantial number of these patients recover sufficient renal function to allow discontinuation of chronic dialysis, even after many months, if the BP is well-controlled as the accompanying arteritis heals.[12]

Catecholamine excess hypertensive crises

These patients usually tolerate much lower BPs during treatment than many other patients with hypertensive crises, perhaps because the duration of very high blood pressures is short when blood pressure 'spikes' only briefly. Appropriate treatment with alpha-adrenergic blockade is usually all that is necessary; sometimes vasodilators and/or beta-blockers may be required. Initiating therapy with a beta-blocker in patients with catecholamine excess states may be especially dangerous, since it leads to unopposed alpha-simulation, increased BP, and worsened hypertensive crisis. For patients who are withdrawing from specific antihyperten-sive drugs, a single dose of the missing medication usually restores BP into the nondangerous range.

Pregnancy hypertensive crises

Most obstetricians are very comfortable treating pre-eclamptic patients, using multiple drugs to lower the BP to <140/90 mmHg. Because these patients are generally young, with a short duration of elevated BPs, they also respond very well, with little risk of going beyond the autoregulatory threshold. In some chronically hypertensive pregnant women, a somewhat higher BP can be tolerated, but seldom is it left >160/100 mmHg.

THERAPEUTIC OPTIONS IN THE INTENSIVE CARE UNIT

A list of preferred drugs to treat specific types of hypertensive crises is shown in Table 26.2. There are a broad range of agents that may be selected, depending on the particular type of crisis, and the patient's clinical characteristics.

For many years, *sodium nitroprusside* was the standard intravenously administered drug for all hypertensive crises. Nitroprusside has many desirable attributes. It has a favorable pharmacokinetic profile (with an onset of action within 2–3

Table 26.2 Drugs for hypertensive crises.

Condition	Drug of choice	Contraindicated
Hypertensive encephalopathy	Nitroprusside[a]	Methyldopa
Other CNS catastrophes	Nitroprusside[a]	Methyldopa
Subarachnoid hemorrhage	Nimodipine	
Aortic dissection	Beta-blocker plus nitroprusside[a]	Hydralazine, diazoxide
Eclampsia	Hydralazine	Nitroprusside, trimethaphan
Heart failure	Enalaprilat, nitroglycerin, nitroprusside[a]	Labetalol
Renal impairment/hematuria	Fenoldopam	
Myocardial ischemia/angina pectoris	Nitroglycerin	Hydralazine
Catecholamine-related	Phentolamine	
Clonidine withdrawal	Clonidine	
Postoperative hypertension	Nitroprusside[a]	
Post-CABG hypertension	Nitroglycerin, nicardipine	

[a] Some physicians prefer intravenous nicardipine or fenoldopam (especially in the setting of renal impairment) over nitroprusside, because of the lack of potentially toxic metabolites.

CABG = coronary artery bypass grafting; CNS = central nervous system.

minutes); it is inexpensive; and, perhaps most importantly, it has a long record of effectiveness in treating hypertensive crises of nearly all types.[35] In many ICUs, a patient requiring a nitroprusside infusion is required to have an arterial line, so that BP can be continuously monitored, and the infusion rate can be appropriately adjusted very quickly. This requirement for an intra-arterial line becomes a major limitation for its use, since line placement and calibration takes time and is expensive. Nitroprusside has toxic metabolic products (thiocyanate and cyanide), which is the reason for its absolute contraindication in pregnancy. These metabolites can accumulate when nitroprusside is given either at high doses or during long periods of infusion, and in the setting of significant renal or hepatic impairment. The US Food and Drug Administration (FDA) has recommended that the dose of nitroprusside be kept under 2 µg/kg/min, to avoid these difficulties. Patients with thiocyanate toxicity can appear disoriented and sometimes psychotic, and complain of nausea, fatigue, and muscle spasms. The laboratory signs of toxicity include a widening anion gap and a rising lactate level; serum thiocyanate levels can be measured to confirm toxicity, but the assay takes time and is not routinely available. It is often easier to downtitrate and discontinue nitroprusside, and watch for clinical improvement, than to wait for a serum thiocyanate level. Nitroprusside is typically begun at 0.3 µg/kg/min, and increased by 0.2–1.0 µg/kg/min every 3–5 minutes until the BP reaches the target range.[35] Once the optimal dose of nitroprusside has been found, the process of choosing an oral medication to replace it should begin. In most hospitals, this switch-over must be completed in the ICU, as nitroprusside use is restricted to that setting.

In recent years, two other drugs have begun to displace nitroprusside as the usual drug of first choice; neither has potentially toxic metabolites. *Nicardipine*, a dihydropyridine calcium antagonist, has been available in the USA as an intravenous formulation since 1991. It is an effective antihypertensive agent[36] and may have a special role in patients with coronary disease, or after cardiac surgery.[37] *Fenoldopam mesylate*, a dopamine-1 agonist, was approved in 1998 by the FDA,[38] and has been shown in clinical trials against nitroprusside to have several potentially beneficial renal effects, including increased diuresis, natriuresis, and creatinine clearance.[39] Fenoldopam probably is most useful for BP reduction in the setting of renal impairment or vascular surgery.[40] The acquisition cost of either nicardipine or fenoldopam is higher than nitroprusside, but the total cost of care may be lower, since nitroprusside must be given in an ICU with an arterial line in place, according to nursing policies in most hospitals. Nicardipine is typically begun at 5 mg/h, and increased by 2.5 mg/h every 15 minutes until either the BP goal or a maximum dose of 15 mg/h is reached. This agent has a rather long (~44 minutes) serum half-life,[36] several drug interactions (cyclosporine, cimetidine), and the usual vasodilator side effects (headache, flushing, nausea/vomiting, and reflex tachycardia). Fenoldopam is typically begun at 0.1 µg/kg/min, and increased at 20-minute intervals by 0.1–0.2 µg/kg/min, with a maximum dose of 1.5 µg/kg/min.[38]

There are several other drugs that are being investigated for use in hypertensive crisis, or which are available for this indication in other countries. These include urapidil (an alpha-blocker which also interferes with both central and peripheral uptake of serotonin),[41,42] intravenous felodipine (a dihydropyridine calcium antagonist, similar to nicardipine),[43] and lacidipine (another dihydropyridine calcium antagonist).[44] Whether any of these will have a defined role in treatment in the USA is still unclear.

Other intravenously administered antihypertensive drugs are most useful only in specific clinical situations (see Table 26.2). *Nimodipine* (either oral or intravenous) has a special place in neurologic crises, and has been subjected to clinical trials in acute stroke and subarachnoid hemorrhage. It has both anti-ischemic and antihypertensive effects. Its use has been associated with improved outcomes after subarachnoid hemorrhage,[45] but its use in acute stroke is controversial.[46] Its beneficial effects may be more related to preserving neurons in peril by limiting calcium influx into ischemic cells rather than to its hypotensive effects. The usual oral dose is 60 mg (two 30 mg capsules) every 4 hours for 21 days after the neurologic event. *Nitroglycerin* is useful in the setting of angina pectoris, coronary artery bypass surgery, or neurosurgery, but is now being replaced for these situations in some hospitals by nicardipine. Nitroglycerin has the disadvantages of being unstable in solution, adhering to intravenous lines (leading to variability in the administered dose over time), inducing tolerance during prolonged administration, and causing profound headache. It is typically begun at 5 µg/min, with an increase in dose every 3–5 minutes by 5–10 µg/min, as needed. *Trimethaphan camsylate* is typically used only as a second-line choice in aortic dissection (e.g. in asthmatics who cannot take a beta-blocker), causes profound orthostatic hypotension, and is rarely effective after 24 hours. It is usually given at 0.3 mg/min initially, with a maximum dose of 6 mg/min. *Phentolamine* is a nonselective alpha-antagonist, and is very useful in pheochromocytoma and other catecholamine excess states. It is typically delivered in 2–5 mg 'minibolus' injections, in order to minimize the risk of precipitous falls in BP.

First-choice drug therapy for hypertensive crises during pregnancy is complicated, because there are two patients to be considered, the mother and the baby. Drugs with teratogenic potential (e.g. nitroprusside, ACE inhibitors, and angiotensin II receptor blockers) are contraindicated. Although most obstetricians prefer $MgSO_4$ and *methyldopa* for inpatient and outpatient treatment of gestational hypertension, respectively, parenteral *hydralazine* is the typical drug chosen for initial or parenteral treatment of pre-eclampsia.[47] During a period when it was not available, many studies of *nifedipine* in pregnancy were begun, and there is now a reasonably large literature showing the effectiveness and lack of adverse experiences with this drug in obstetrics.[48–50] Perhaps because most obstetric patients are young, and have only modestly increased BPs with their crises, nifedipine has only rarely been associated with adverse outcomes in this special patient population.[33]

Other agents can be useful in some patients. Labetalol, for example, is easier to use than nitroprusside, since it can be given in multiple miniboluses (25 mg, then 50 mg, then 100 mg, then 200 mg, at 15-minute intervals). But it is not as effective as nitroprusside, since only 80–85% of patients respond, and it may precipitate asthma, systolic dysfunction, or heart failure. Diazoxide was a popular ICU drug in the past, but this drug can cause precipitous hypotension and acute ischemic complications. Its unpredictability in action, striking reflex tachycardia, tendency to exacerbate or cause diabetes mellitus, and retain fluid almost always outweigh its advantages. Diazoxide is now only rarely used for hypertensive emergencies. If needed, however, it should be given as 50-mg miniboluses every 15 minutes or as a continuous infusion. Once the BP of the patient has been adequately controlled with intravenous antihypertensive drugs in the ICU, the infusion rate is reduced and orally acting antihypertensive agents are started. Only after the patient has been weaned off the intravenous infusion and the BP is fairly well controlled on oral antihypertensive drugs is the patient usually transferred out of the ICU for further evaluation and management.

PROGNOSIS

The prognosis for patients with a hypertensive emergency has improved markedly since this clinical syndrome was first recognized. Prior to 1950, no effective antihypertensive drug therapy was available, and few affected patients survived a year. Nearly all reported series since 1990 have reported 1-year survival rates higher than 95%. Now that effective oral antihypertensive drug therapy is available for long-term treatment, the prognosis for patients with a hypertensive crisis depends more on the level of cardiac, renal, and cerebral function at presentation than on the level of blood pressure or the type of therapy chosen.

SUMMARY AND RECOMMENDATIONS

In summary, patients presenting with a true hypertensive emergency should be quickly diagnosed and promptly started on effective parenteral therapy (typically, nitroprusside 0.3 µg/kg/min or fenoldopam 0.1 µg/kg/min) in an intensive care unit. Blood pressure should be reduced about 10% during the first hour and a further 10–15% over the next hour or so. Oral antihypertensive therapy (often with an immediate-release calcium antagonist) may be instituted after 6–12 hours of parenteral therapy, and consideration should be given to secondary causes of hypertension after transfer out of the ICU.

Most patients who present with very elevated BPs without signs or symptoms of acute TOD (i.e. a 'hypertensive urgency') do not require parenteral therapy, and can be managed with any one of a number of oral antihypertensive medications, and long-term follow-up care of their hypertension arranged. During the last 50 years of advances in antihypertensive therapy and management, there has been a progressive improvement in the prognosis of patients with a hypertensive crisis.

REFERENCES

1. Keith NM, Wagener HP, Kernohan JW. The syndrome of malignant hypertension. Arch Intern Med 1928;41:141–53.
2. Gifford RW Jr. Management of hypertensive crises. JAMA 1991;266:829–35.
3. Kaplan NM. Management of hypertensive emergencies. Lancet 1994;344:1335–8.

4. Chobanian AV, Bakris GL, Black HR, et al. Seventh Report of the Joint National Committee on Prevention, Detection, Evaluation, and Treatment of High Blood Pressure (JNC VI). Hypertension 2003;42:1206–52.

5. Burt VL, Whelton PK, Roccella EJ, et al. Prevalence of hypertension in the U.S. adult population: Results from the Third National Health and Nutrition Examination Survey, 1988–91. Hypertension 1995;25:305–13.

6. Sung JF, Harris-Hooker S, Alema-Mensah E, Mayberry R. Is there a difference in hypertensive claim rates among Medicaid recipients? Ethn Dis 1997;7:19–26.

7. Kato J, Kitamura K, Matsui E, et al. Plasma adrenomedullin and natriuretic peptides in patients with essential or malignant hypertension. Hypertension Res 1999;22:61–5.

8. Shea S, Misra D, Francis CK. Predisposing factors for severe, uncontrolled hypertension in an inner-city minority population. N Engl J Med 1992;327:776–81.

9. Davis BA, Crook JE, Vestal RE, Oates JA. Prevalence of renal vascular hypertension in patients with grade III or IV hypertensive retinopathy. N Engl J Med 1979;301:1273–6.

10. Zarifis J, Lip GY, Leatherdale B, Beevers G. Malignant hypertension in association with primary hyperaldosteronism. Blood Press 1996;5:250–4.

11. Oka K, Hayashi K, Nakazato T, et al. Malignant hypertension in a patient with primary hyperaldosteronism with elevated active renin concentration. Intern Med 1997;36:700–4.

12. Bakir AA, Bazilinski N, Dunea G. Transient and sustained recovery from renal shutdown in accelerated hypertension. Am J Med 1986;80:172–6.

13. Jespersen B, Eiskjaer H, Christiansen NO, et al. Malignant arterial hypertension. Relationship between blood pressure control and renal function during long-term observation of patients with malignant nephrosclerosis. J Clin Hypertens 1987;3:409–18.

14. Report of the National High Blood Pressure Education Program Working Group on High Blood Pressure in Pregnancy. Am J Obstet Gynecol 2000;183:S1–22.

15. Lip GY, Beevers M, Beevers DG. Malignant hypertension in young women is related to previous hypertension in pregnancy, not oral contraception. QJM 1997;90:571–5.

16. Petitti DB, Klatsky AL. Malignant hypertension in women 15–44 years, and its relation to cigarette smoking and oral contraceptives. Am J Cardiol 1983;52:297–8.

17. Zahn KA, Li RL, Purssell RA. Cardiovascular toxicity after ingestion of 'herbal ecstacy'. J Emerg Med 1999;17:289–91.

18. Johansson B, Strandgaard S, Lassen NA. The hypertensive 'breakthrough' of autoregulation of cerebral blood flow with forced vasodilation, flow increase, and blood–brain barrier damage. Circ Res 1974;34–35:I167–71.

19. Ahmed MEK, Walker JM, Beevers DG, Beevers M. Lack of difference between malignant and accelerated hypertension. BMJ 1986;292:235–7.

20. Wenzel UO, Stahl RA, Grieshaber M, Schweitzer G. [Diagnostic and therapeutic procedures by doctors for patients in a hypertensive crisis. An inquiry in 56 internal medicine clinics.] Dtsch Med Wochenschr 1998;123:443–7. [in German]

21. Zeller KR, Von Kuhnert L, Matthews C. Rapid reduction of severe asymptomatic hypertension: a prospective controlled trial. Arch Intern Med 1989;149:2186–9.

22. Healton EB, Brust JC, Feinfeld DA, Thomson GE. Hypertensive encephalopathy and the neurological manifestations of malignant hypertension. Neurology 1982;32:127–32.

23. Phillips SJ. Pathophysiology and management of hypertension in acute ischemic stroke. Hypertension 1994;23:131–6.

24. Hirschl MM, Binder M, Bur A, et al. Impact of the renin–angiotensin–aldosterone system on blood pressure response to intravenous enalaprilat in patients with hypertensive crises. J Hum Hypertens 1997;11:177–83.

25. Flaherty JT. Comparison of intravenous nitroglycerin and nitroprusside in acute myocardial infarction. Am J Med 1983;74:53–60.

26. Smith DA, Radvan J. Dissection of the aorta. J Hum Hypertens 1999;13:209–10.

27. Blanchard DG, Kimura BJ, Dittrich HC, DeMaria AN. Transesophageal echocardiography of the aorta. JAMA 1994;272:546–51.

28. Cigarroa JE, Isselbacher EM, DeSanctis RW, Eagle KA. Diagnostic imaging in the evaluation of suspected aortic dissection. Old standards and new directions. N Engl J Med 1993;328:35–43.

29. Miller DC. The continuing dilemma concerning medical versus surgical management of patients with acute type B dissections. Semin Thorac Cardiovasc Surg 1993;5:33–46.

30. O'Connor B, Luntley JB. Acute dissection of the thoracic aorta. Esmolol is safer than and as effective as labetalol. BMJ 1995;310:875.

31. Lenders JW, Pacak K, Walther MM, et al. Biochemical diagnosis of pheochromocytoma: which test is best? JAMA 2002;287:1427–34.

32. Hoshide S, Kario K, Fujikawa H, Ikeda U, Shimada K. Hemodynamic cerebral infarction triggered by excessive blood pressure reduction in hypertensive emergencies. J Am Geriatr Soc 1998;46:1179–80.

33. Grossman E, Messerli FH, Grodzicki T, Kowey P. Should a moratorium be placed on sublingual nifedipine capsules given for hypertensive emergencies and pseudoemergencies? JAMA 1996;276:1328–31.

34. Biller J, Godersky JC, Adams HP. Management of aneurysmal subarachnoid hemorrhage. Stroke 1988;19:1300–5.

35. Cohn JN, Burke LP. Nitroprusside. Ann Intern Med 1979;91:752–7.

36. Wallin JD, Fletcher E, Ram CVS, et al. Intravenous nicardipine for the treatment of severe hypertension. Arch Intern Med 1989;149:2662–9.

37. Vincent JL, Berlot G, Preiser JC, et al. Intravenous nicardipine in the treatment of postoperative arterial hypertension. J Cardiothorac Vasc Anesth 1997;11:160–4.

38. Murphy MB, Murray C, Shorten GD. Fenoldopam: a selective peripheral dopamine-receptor agonist for the treatment of severe hypertension. N Engl J Med 2001;345:1548–57.

39. Shusterman NH, Elliott WJ, White WB. Fenoldopam, but not nitroprusside, improves renal function in severely hypertensive patients with normal or impaired baseline renal function. Am J Med 1993;95:161–8.

40. Oparil S, Aronson S, Deeb GM, et al. Fenoldopam: a new parenteral antihypertensive: consensus roundtable on the management of perioperative hypertension and hypertensive crises. Am J Hypertens 1999;12:653–64.

41. Hirschl MM, Binder M, Bur A, et al. Safety and efficacy of urapidil and sodium nitroprusside in the treatment of hypertensive emergencies. Intensive Care Med 1997;23:885–8.

42. Hirschl MM, Herkner H, Bur A, et al. Course of blood pressure within the first 12 h of hypertensive urgencies. J Hypertens 1998;16:251–5.

43. Risler T, Bohm R, Wetzchewald D, et al. A comparison of the antihypertensive efficacy and safety of felodipine IV and nifedipine IV in patients with hypertensive crisis or emergency not responding to oral nifedipine. Eur J Clin Pharmacol 1998;54:295–8.

44. Sobrino Martinez J, Adrian Martin MJ, Ribera Tello L, Torres Salinas M. [Emergency treatment of hypertension with lacidipine]. Rev Clin Esp 1997;197:211. [in Spanish]

45. Feigin VL, Rinkel GJ, Algra A, Vermeulen M, van Gign J. Calcium antagonists in patients with aneurysmal subarachnoid hemorrhage: a systematic review. Neurology 1998;50:876–83.

46. Gelmers HJ, Gorter K, de Weerdt CJ, Wieser HJA. A controlled trial of nimodipine in acute ischemic stroke. N Engl J Med 1988;318:203–7.

47. Powers DR, Papadakos PJ, Wallin JD. Parenteral hydralazine revisited. J Emer Med 1998;16:191–6.
48. Scardo JA, Vermillion ST, Hogg BB, Newman RB. Hemodynamic effects of oral nifedipine in preeclamptic hypertensive emergencies. Am J Obstet Gynecol 1996;175:336–8.
49. Scardo JA, Vermillion ST, Newman RB, Chauhan SP, Hogg BB. A randomized, double-blind, hemodynamic evaluation of nifedipine and labetalol in preeclamptic hypertensive emergencies. Am J Obstet Gynecol 1999;181:862–6.
50. Vermillion ST, Scardo JA, Newman RB, Chauhan SP. A randomized, double-blind trial of oral nifedipine and intravenous labetalol in hypertensive emergencies of pregnancy. Am J Obstet Gynecol 1999;181:858–61.

27

Pediatric intensive care unit nephrology

Ayesa N Mian and Susan R Mendley

INTRODUCTION

Children in a pediatric intensive care unit (PICU) setting develop a wide range of metabolic disturbances as well as acute renal failure (ARF), and pediatric nephrologists are closely involved in all aspects of diagnosis and management of these patients, beyond merely providing renal replacement therapy (RRT). Despite advances in pediatric critical care, ARF remains a significant source of morbidity for children in the PICU. The causes of ARF in children differ importantly from those in adults.[1,2] Primary renal disease accounts for a larger share of ARF in the PICU than is seen in adults; sepsis and multiorgan failure are proportionally less common in children. The causes of pediatric ARF also differ between industrialized and nonindustrialized countries. Hemolytic uremic syndrome (HUS) and glomerulonephritis (GN) appear to be more common and more severe in developing countries, whereas ARF secondary to other complicated medical illnesses is more likely to occur in industrialized nations which offer more intensive therapies. The clinical picture of ARF may also result from an acute presentation of previously asymptomatic end-stage renal disease or congenital urologic abnormality. Survival of children who require dialysis in the PICU is superior to that of adults and is estimated at approximately 65% in single-center series; in addition, the likelihood of recovery of renal function is high.[3]

EVALUATION OF ACUTE RENAL FAILURE IN CHILDREN

When evaluating children with ARF, the typical paradigm of prerenal, renal, and postrenal causes is still valid, albeit modified in this population. Volume depletion causing prerenal azotemia is well-recognized, particularly in the setting of gastrointestinal losses; however, children usually have robust autoregulatory mechanisms and decreases in glomerular filtration rate (GFR) often respond promptly to volume repletion. A postrenal cause for ARF is common, particularly in infants with congenital urologic malformations. The range of renal parenchymal causes of ARF is extensive, including acute tubular necrosis (ATN), glomerulonephritis, and interstitial nephritis. Box 27.1 summarizes common causes of pediatric ARF. Several renal diseases which are particularly common in children are discussed in greater detail below.

Evaluation of ARF is directed by a history of recent sepsis or hypotension, nephrotoxic medications, abnormal prenatal ultrasound, gross hematuria, or edema. Microscopic examination of the urine may be diagnostic if red blood cell, white blood cell, or tubular cell casts are present. Serologic studies are helpful in patients suspected of having GN (complement components, antinuclear antibody, and antineutrophil cytoplasmic antibodies). Urinary sodium excretion and the fractional excretion of sodium [$FE_{Na} = (U_{Na}/P_{Na}) \times (P_{Cr}/U_{Cr})$] help differentiate prerenal azotemia from intrinsic renal disease in the oliguric patient. The presence of an $FE_{Na} < 1\%$ is generally consistent with a prerenal condition; however, neonates and premature infants may not achieve that level of sodium conservation because of immature tubular function and a level of 2.5% may be considered evidence of a prerenal state.[4]

Renal ultrasonography is indispensable in the evaluation of the pediatric patient with ARF, demonstrating congenital anomalies (e.g. hydronephrosis, cystic disease, hypoplasia/dysplasia, agenesis, etc.)

Box 27.1   Causes of pediatric acute renal failure

Prerenal failure

Hypoxia/ischemia

Gastrointestinal losses (vomiting, diarrhea)

Renal losses (diabetes insipidus, diabetes mellitus)

Third-space losses (post-surgery, nephrosis)

Shock (sepsis, anaphylaxis)

Renovascular disease (stenosis/thrombosis)

Renal vasoconstriction (norepinephrine)

Cardiac failure

Liver failure

Intrinsic renal failure

Glomerulonephritis

Hemolytic uremic syndrome

Systemic vasculitis

Acute tubular necrosis

Pyelonephritis

Interstitial nephritis

Cystic/dysplastic renal disease

Tumor lysis

Nephrotoxins

Postrenal failure

Anatomic obstruction:

- Posterior urethral valves
- Ureteropelvic junction obstruction (bilateral)
- Ureterovesicle junction obstruction (bilateral)
- Urolithiasis
- Blood clot
- Fungal bezoar

---

and obstruction. The presence of small, echogenic kidneys may provide the first clue for previously unrecognized chronic renal failure; these children may also have a history of poor growth. The presence of hydronephrosis suggests the need for further imaging: a voiding cystourethrogram to assess for vesicoureteral reflux and posterior urethral valves, and nuclear renography to detect ureteropelvic or ureterovesicle junction obstruction.

Conservative management

Conservative management of ARF is directed to those correctable causes of azotemia. Worldwide, gastrointestinal disease is the leading cause of pre-renal azotemia in children; prompt and adequate fluid resuscitation is needed to prevent ATN. Initial isotonic crystalloid infusions are scaled to weight or surface area as no standard volume can be assumed. Once circulating volume is restored, intravenous infusion rates are adjusted to accommodate gastrointestinal losses, urine output, and insensible fluid loss. Potassium and bicarbonate supplementation are often needed.

Occasionally, children with volume depletion have preserved, or even massive, urine output as a result of an unrecognized urinary concentrating defect. This may be the result of diabetes insipidus (central or nephrogenic) or polyuric chronic renal failure (often congenital partial obstruction). X-linked nephrogenic diabetes insipidus from a vasopressin-2 receptor mutation is the most dramatic example of polyuric volume depletion, and in this case, male infants present in the first few months of life with failure to thrive, polyuria, and hypernatremic dehydration with urine output which may exceed 10 ml/kg/h.[5,6] Large volumes of hypotonic fluids are used and urine electrolytes may help guide fluid therapy. Dextrose-containing solutions may cause hyperglycemia and an osmotic diuresis, which will complicate therapy. If hypernatremia is severe, serum sodium must be lowered gradually to avoid cerebral edema.

Once oliguric ARF is established, conservative management requires careful balancing of intravenous fluid, nutrition, insensible losses, and urine output. Dietary protein, potassium, and phosphate are restricted and diuretics, sodium polystyrene, sodium bicarbonate, and phosphate binders are used. Precision in measuring intake, output, and body weight is needed as small inaccuracies can dramatically affect fluid balance in small patients. Nutritional needs for infants and young children are large relative to adults and adequate calories and protein are needed to prevent negative nitrogen balance; thus, hyperalimentation solution volumes are proportionally much larger and may cause fluid overload in oliguric patients. However, insensible fluid losses are also larger in small children and, if some urine output remains, it may be possible to provide adequate nutrition. When obligate volume requirements exceed output and insensible losses, RRT is almost always required.

Dose adjustment of medications with renal excretion is critical and pharmacokinetic data in small children are often lacking. Further, one must recognize that a significant loss of GFR may be associated with a serum creatinine value which does not appear abnormal in most hospital laboratory reports, since normal serum creatinine ranges are 0.2–0.4 mg/dl in an infant, 0.4–0.6 mg/dl in a school-age child, and 0.6–0.9 mg/dl in an adolescent.

Hemolytic uremic syndrome

Hemolytic uremic syndrome is the most common cause of ARF requiring dialysis in children.[7,8] This multisystem disease characterized by microangiopathic hemolytic anemia, thrombocytopenia, and ARF has a diarrheal prodrome in over 90% of cases. Shiga toxin-producing *Escherichia coli* (STEC) is the most common pathogen; in the developing world, *Shigella dysenteriae* is also important.[9,10] *E. coli* O157:H7 is the most extensively studied serotype of STEC and has been implicated in many North American outbreaks.[11,12] Nondiarrheal or atypical HUS is much less common, but is important to recognize because of special management issues and overall less-favorable prognosis.

STEC-associated HUS may affect patients of any age, but children under 5 years old are most typical. The gastrointestinal symptoms may include hemorrhagic colitis, but this often resolves before the manifestations of HUS become apparent. Disease models suggest that during the diarrheal phase, Shiga toxin crosses the denuded colon and gains entry to the blood, binding Gb3 (globotriaosylceramide) receptors located on endothelial cells. The toxin undergoes endocytosis and causes protein synthesis inhibition and endothelial cell injury, with subsequent platelet adherence and thrombotic microangiopathy. The mechanism of renal failure is less clearly understood.[7,8] Table 27.1 summarizes reported organ involvement with HUS.[13] Mortality during the acute phase of the illness is estimated at 3–5% in large series.[14] Central nervous system (CNS) involvement, including seizures and coma, is an important prognostic indicator, portending poor outcome.

Antibiotic therapy of STEC-associated HUS is controversial and, when given early in the course of diarrhea, may increase the risk of developing HUS.[15] Antimotility agents appear to increase the risk of HUS.[16] Other therapies, including plasma exchange, glucocorticoids, gamma-globulin, heparin, urokinase, and prostacyclin, have not been proven effective for diarrhea-associated HUS. SYNSORB Pk, an oral silicon dioxide-based resin covalently bound to the trisaccharide moiety of the Gb3 receptor, was recently studied, but found ineffective in reducing mortality, frequency of severe extrarenal complications, and the need for dialysis.[17]

Atypical forms of HUS account for approximately 5% of cases in childhood, consisting of a heterogeneous group of disorders in which endothelial cell injury and platelet activation are prominent.[18] Overall prognosis is poor compared to the favorable outcome expected in diarrheal HUS. Atypical HUS should be distinguished from thrombotic thrombocytopenic purpura (TTP), a condition of impaired proteolytic cleavage of von Willebrand multimers, as therapeutic choices differ. Hereditary forms of HUS may present at any age and family history is illustrative. Repeated plasma exchange is typically required. HUS in children may occur after exposure to cyclosporine or oral contraceptives and after bone marrow transplantation. Withdrawal of offending agents may be sufficient, although plasma exchange is often required. HUS is recognized to occur after *Streptococcus pneumoniae* infection (typically with bacteremia or meningitis).[19] Our current understanding of *S. pneumoniae*-induced HUS assumes that bacterially secreted neuraminidase removes the sialic acid residues which mask the Thomsen–Friedenreich (T-F) antigen on endothelial cells, platelets, and erythrocytes.[20] Human plasma normally contains antibodies against T-F antigen; therefore, once unmasked, the T-F antigen is exposed to these antibodies, which results in hemolysis and endothelial cell injury. Transfusion of even unwashed blood products may, in theory, exacerbate the disease, as they contain small amounts of plasma. Clearly, plasma infusion or plasma exchange is not appropriate.

Sepsis with multiple organ system failure

Septic shock is seen frequently in the PICU in children who are immunocompromised secondary to chemotherapy, HIV (human immunodeficiency virus) infection, or organ transplantation, as well as in normal hosts. ARF in this setting may be the result of ischemia from hypotension or renal vasoconstriction and may be complicated by nephrotoxins. As importantly, the systemic inflammatory response syndrome is well recognized to occur in children, resulting in multiple organ system failure with ARF.[21] The role of endotoxins and cytokines in this process continues to be elucidated; mortality is high, although it appears better than that reported from adult ICU patients. Renal failure is an important feature of the syndrome, and contributes to

Table 27.1 Extrarenal manifestations of diarrhea-associated hemolytic uremic syndrome.

Location	Approximate reported frequency (%)
Gastrointestinal	
Esophagus	<1
Small intestine	4
Large intestine (colitis):	100
• Necrosis/perforation	2
• Intussusception	1
• Prolapse	8
• Stricture	3
• Anal/perianal	10
Pancreas:	
• Pancreatitis	20
• Diabetes mellitus	8
• Exocrine dysfunction	<1
Liver (hepatomegaly/elevated enzymes)	40
Gallbladder (cholelithiasis)	<1
Central nervous system	
Seizures	20
Coma/semicoma/stupor	15
Stroke	4
Cortical blindness	1
Miscellaneous	
Heart (congestive heart failure/ischemia/infarction)	<1
Lung (hemorrhage/edema)	<1
Muscle (rhabdomyolysis)	<1
Skin (necrosis)	<1
Eye (retinal infarction)	<1

Source: adapted from Siegler.[13]

morbidity and mortality. Multiple organ dysfunction is discussed in greater detail in Chapter 3.

Nephrotic syndrome

Nephrotic syndrome in childhood has an estimated prevalence of 5 in 100 000, with steroid responsive minimal change disease as the most common histologic diagnosis, particularly in the toddler and young school-age child. In older children, there is an increased incidence of focal segmental glomerulosclerosis and membrano-proliferative GN. Severe nephrosis with profound hypoalbuminemia can result in intrarenal edema, with decreased GFR or even hemodynamically

mediated ARF.[22,23] Massive ascites, when present, can also contribute to renal hypoperfusion through compression of the renal vessels. ARF in this setting is precipitous and may be prolonged. Management strategies include:

1. The discontinuation of potentially nephrotoxic medications, including cyclosporine and angiotensin-converting enzyme (ACE) inhibitors, which may have been used for disease control.
2. The judicious use of albumin with or without diuretics.
3. Isolated ultrafiltration, with or without albumin infusion to manage hypervolemia and diminish renal edema.

4. Initiation of dialysis, as metabolic disturbances arise.[24,25]

Congenital heart disease

The development of ARF in the postoperative period following repair of congenital heart disease was the most common reason for dialysis in older literature and continues to be an important indication for RRT in neonates and infants. Preoperative risk factors include poor cardiac output and the need for radiocontrast dye during cardiac catheterization. Postoperative risk factors include prolonged time on bypass, hypotension, and poor cardiac function. Hypervolemia occurs commonly, as these children require large fluid volume to accommodate medication and nutrition and may have congestive heart failure immediately after the procedure. Initial management involves diuretics, but RRT is frequently required.[26] Peritoneal dialysis (PD) has traditionally been utilized in this setting, although more recent literature emphasizes continuous renal replacement therapy (CRRT).[27–29]

Tumor lysis

Tumor lysis syndrome occurs in patients with large tumor burdens from hematologic malignancies. Cell death, either spontaneous or chemotherapy-induced, is associated with the release of intracellular contents and results in hyperphosphatemia, secondary hypocalcemia, and hyperkalemia. Calcium phosphate precipitation within renal parenchyma occurs as a result of massive supersaturation of tubular filtrate, and is enhanced by an alkaline urine pH (see below). As the calcium phosphate precipitation proceeds, GFR falls and the phosphate burden overwhelms renal excretion, perpetuating the process. Only vigorous diuresis can ameliorate the supersaturation and diminish the risk of precipitation. However, conservative strategies to increase urine flow rates may be insufficient to permit excretion of the phosphate burden and prevent life-threatening metabolic complications; RRT is often required. Continuous hemofiltration provides more efficient phosphorus removal than intermittent hemodialysis, although both have been used in this clinical setting.[30] Peritoneal dialysis provides somewhat better phosphate clearance than hemodialysis but it is insufficient for the massive phosphate release and is therefore only recommended when no other option exists.

Tumor lysis also results in cellular release of uric acid, with subsequent urinary supersaturation, tubular precipitation, and ARF, so-called acute urate nephropathy. This process is enhanced in acidic urine. Preventive strategies include a forced alkaline diuresis and the use of allopurinol to prevent uric acid formation by xanthine oxidase inhibition. However, allopurinol results in accumulation of the precursor xanthine, which is less water soluble than uric acid and which may itself precipitate, causing acute xanthine nephropathy. Alternatively, recombinant urate oxidase has recently been used successfully to prevent acute urate nephropathy in children with leukemia and lymphoma.[31] Urate oxidase converts uric acid to allantoin, a water-soluble metabolite with renal excretion, and thus directly decreases the uric acid load without the accumulation of toxic precursors. This alternative strategy may make urinary alkalinization less important and may diminish the potential risk of calcium phosphate precipitation and the rate of renal complications.[32]

Acute glomerulonephritis

Acute GN can present floridly with gross hematuria, proteinuria, edema, and ARF. Hypertension is typically present and may be malignant. A variety of immune-mediated conditions may cause this condition and prognosis depends upon the underlying disease. The most common etiology in children is acute post-infectious glomerulonephritis (APIGN) which is most often the result of an antecedent streptococcal infection (pharyngitis or impetigo), although that infection may not have been clinically recognized. A depressed C3 value with antibody evidence of prior streptococcal exposure may be sufficient to make the diagnosis. However, atypical presentations or a confusing serologic picture may mandate renal biopsy to differentiate less common but more aggressive forms of GN. The clinical picture of rapidly progressive glomerulonephritis (RPGN), with loss of renal function over days to months, may be caused by antiglomerular basement membrane antibodies (Goodpasture's disease), pauci-immune GN, membranoproliferative GN, Henoch–Schönlein purpura, immunoglobulin A (IgA) nephropathy, and systemic lupus erythematosus.[33] Management includes control of blood pressure, institution of dialysis, if needed, and immunotherapy, including glucocorticoids, cytotoxic agents, anticoagulants, and plasmapheresis. Prognosis is uncertain despite therapy.[34,35]

RENAL REPLACEMENT THERAPY IN PEDIATRIC ACUTE RENAL FAILURE

Children require RRT in the ICU for many of the same reasons as adult patients, and a few unique ones as well. The most common indication is oligoanuric renal failure requiring fluid or urea removal to optimize nutritional and medical support. Other emergency indications include hypervolemia complicated by congestive heart failure, pulmonary edema, or severe hypertension despite diuretic therapy and fluid restriction; hyperkalemia refractory to medical management or associated with electrocardiogram changes; and metabolic acidosis refractory to medical management with sodium bicarbonate or limited by sodium overload. Chronic renal failure is often silent in children; they may present with advanced, symptomatic uremia, pericarditis, neuropathy, or encephalopathy requiring emergency initiation of dialysis in an ICU setting. Hematologic malignancies resulting in acute tumor lysis syndrome or severe hyperuricemia may require removal of solute and dialysis support. There is an important role for RRT in the management of toxic ingestions, particularly common in children; this is discussed in greater detail in Chapter 18. Lastly, infants with urea cycle defects or other inborn errors of metabolism may require urgent hemodialysis to manage severe, life-threatening hyperammonemia, correct lactic acidosis, and/or remove toxic metabolites.[36,37]

Every treatment modality utilized in adults is available for children; the mechanisms of clearance are the same. However, patient size often affects the choice of modality, and technical challenges are presented by extremely small infants. Small size allows very efficient clearance, which may be lifesaving in hyperammonemia or toxic ingestions, but will need to be tempered in cases of longstanding uremia.

Peritoneal dialysis

Peritoneal dialysis (PD) is most often used in children with ARF. It is a technically simple procedure, not requiring specialized personnel. PICU nurses can be trained to perform the procedure with an acceptably low infection rate. Automated cycler devices permit continuous therapy with frequent dialysis exchanges within a closed circuit, further lowering the infection risk. Vascular access and anticoagulation are avoided. The procedure is well tolerated in the hemodynamically compromised child since fluid and solute removal occur gradually over the course of the day, rather than during a short hemodialysis treatment where the risk of hypotension or dialysis dysequilibrium would be much greater.[38,39]

Solute and fluid removal across the peritoneal membrane are efficient in children; peritoneal membrane surface area correlates with body surface area rather than with body mass, and this ratio is most favorable in infants and young children.[40] Initiating PD in the acute setting can also facilitate the transition to chronic home dialysis should renal recovery be incomplete. Finally, this form of dialysis is somewhat less expensive to perform and requires a smaller initial capital investment than other CRRTs (see below).[41]

There are a few absolute contraindications to PD: abdominal wall defects (e.g. bladder extrophy, omphalocele, and gastroschisis), diaphragmatic lesions (e.g. diaphragmatic hernia and surgical defects), and recent abdominal surgery. A ventriculoperitoneal shunt is a relative contraindication because of the risk of ascending infection should peritonitis develop. Importantly, in those clinical situations where rapid removal of solute (e.g. hyperkalemia), toxin (ingestion), or metabolite (e.g. ammonia) is required, PD is not most appropriate. The gradual nature of the treatment, which is advantageous in uremia, will limit the rapid response those emergencies require. Further, in states of acute volume overload with pulmonary edema or congestive heart failure, the ultrafiltration provided by PD may not be rapid enough to prevent clinical deterioration or the need for intubation.

Technical considerations
PD catheters are available in sizes appropriate for neonates, infants, and children, including acute 'temporary' catheters and chronic catheters for operative placement. Acute catheter placement can be performed percutaneously at the bedside after filling the abdomen with dialysate.[42] However, percutaneous placement can result in injury to or perforation of an abdominal viscus.[43] The catheters are stiff and can cause bowel injury even after successful placement, which necessitates

immobilizing the child. Temporary catheters are also uncuffed and pose a greater risk for dialysate leakage at the exit site and subsequent infection. After 3 days of use, the risk of peritonitis increases significantly; generally, when PD is initiated, it is impossible to predict the time to renal recovery.[44] In most modern PICU settings, the benefits of rapid initiation of PD do not justify the complications associated with acute catheters, and many nephrologists prefer an operatively placed soft silicone catheter.[45]

Commercially available lactate-based dialysis solution is almost always used in pediatric PD. 'Custom-made' bicarbonate-based dialysis solution prepared in the hospital pharmacy has been used in acute dialysis, but it is labor-intensive to produce and carries the very real risk of formulation error.

Acute PD is usually initiated shortly after catheter placement, making dialysate leakage a major concern. Therefore, low fill volumes of approximately 10–15 ml/kg are used initially, although poor drainage, slow clearance, and inadequate ultrafiltration may limit the effectiveness. Fill volumes are gradually increased over several days to a goal of 40–50 ml/kg, as tolerated. Short dwell times (60–90 minutes) may help overcome the limitations of low fill volume and facilitate ultrafiltration by limiting glucose absorption; this is best accomplished with an automated cycler device.[46] Even shorter exchange times are possible but may compromise efficiency, since a larger proportion of time is spent filling and draining, which leaves less time for actual dialysis. Rapid PD exchanges performed in infants and young children can result in unpredictable and sometimes excessive ultrafiltration; careful reassessment of volume status and supplemental fluid, either enteral or parenteral, must be provided to prevent intravascular volume depletion, which, in turn, may impair renal recovery.

The complications of PD, typically catheter malfunction and infection, often dissuade clinicians from undertaking this modality. Catheters may become obstructed by omentum, blood clots, fibrin, or adhesions; omentectomy or the addition of heparin to the dialysate may help avoid these problems. Catheter migration can occur, resulting in painful inflow of dialysate as well as poor outflow. Constipation and intestinal distension often limit outflow and should be managed with stool softeners, enemas, or laxatives (avoiding magnesium and phosphorus).

The catheter may leak externally, around the exit site or the incision, or internally, resulting in a her-

nia. External leaks tend to occur when dialysis is performed with stiff temporary catheters, in malnourished or hypoalbuminemic patients, after repeated catheter manipulation or when large fill volumes are used early after catheter placement.[39,45,47] The use of two purse-string sutures to seal the peritoneum around the catheter and to seal the posterior rectus sheath opening may prevent leakage.[48] Temporary discontinuation of PD and use of smaller fill volumes is the initial approach to catheter leaks, but surgical repair is sometimes required.

Infection may occur at the exit site, within the tunnel, and/or the peritoneum. In the acute setting, an exit site infection is essentially a surgical wound infection and should be managed as such with parenteral antibiotics. It creates a significant risk of dialysate leakage and contamination of the peritoneal space. Peritonitis is a serious complication of acute PD, presenting a tremendous inflammatory burden to an already debilitated, catabolic patient. Skin and genitourinary flora are the most common organisms, but drug-resistant bacteria and fungi are a greater risk in the intensive care setting, where patients are often already receiving antibiotic therapy. Since typical features of peritonitis such as fever, abdominal pain, and cloudy effluent may be difficult to discern in this setting, surveillance cell counts and cultures are advisable.

Metabolic complications can result from acute PD, most often due to glucose absorption. Hyperglycemia may occur and require insulin therapy.[49] Hypertriglyceridemia can result from glucose absorption and be difficult to distinguish from the effects of hyperalimentation. Transperitoneal albumin loss can cause hypoalbuminemia; this loss is dramatically increased with peritonitis. Lactate absorption from the dialysate could cause lactic acidosis, but in fact this is a rare problem; acidosis generally improves with initiation of PD. Hyponatremia is common in very young patients, made worse by the administration of hypotonic fluids; hypernatremia can develop with excessive ultrafiltration and insufficient free water intake.[49]

Hemodialysis

Hemodialysis (HD) can be performed safely and effectively in acutely ill infants and children of all sizes.[50–52] Acute HD is the modality of choice when rapid removal of fluid, solute, or toxins is required, as in hyperammonemic coma or other inborn errors of metabolism, toxic ingestions, or hyper-kalemia.[53] In fact, HD treatments in small children can be extremely efficient as body water space is small relative to the clearance one can provide with standard or high-flux dialyzers and typical blood flows.[54]

Technical considerations

Acute HD in children should only be undertaken by highly trained dialysis nurses, preferably with pediatric experience. Keen observation skills and an awareness of age-dependent norms for vital signs are necessary to assess patients who may not be able to communicate their distress verbally. Agitation or poor perfusion must be recognized quickly as indications of incipient decompensation; hypotension may develop precipitously.

Children have benefited from technological improvements in the design of HD machines, in particular the incorporation of volumetric ultrafil-tration control and blood pumps capable of cali-bration for neonatal, infant, and pediatric blood lines. The blood pump must accurately deliver flow rates within the range 20–300 ml/min, appro-priate for neonates through older adolescents. Accurate volumetric ultrafiltration control is also essential, since errors in ultrafiltration volume of even a few hundred milliliters can cause sympto-matic fluid overload or intravascular volume depletion in a small child.

The extracorporeal circuit volume may represent a significant fraction of total blood volume in an infant or small child and hypotension can occur at initiation of the treatment. The typical blood circuit for adults exceeds 150 ml and neonatal, infant, and pediatric blood lines are available to limit the cir-cuit volume. The blood pump must be recalibrated for the chosen blood line for accurate flow rate. In choosing the smallest available blood lines and dialyzer, one attempts to reduce the extracorporeal volume to less than 10% of the patient's blood vol-ume to avoid hemodynamic decompensation at initiation of treatment. However, in newborns and small infants, it may not be possible to avoid exceeding this circuit volume; if so, the circuit can be primed with blood.[50] Packed red blood cells (RBCs) are diluted with normal saline or 5% albu-min to decrease the hematocrit to approximately 40% and diminish the viscosity and risk of clotting. Blood priming carries its own particular risks: it is a potential infectious exposure and young children may acquire cytomegalovirus infection as a result. Further, even if the primed blood circuit is infused at a low blood flow rate (20–50 ml/min), it repre-sents a very rapid rate of blood transfusion. This may result in a transfusion reaction or hypocal-cemia from citrate infusion. The large potassium load associated with rapid transfusion of packed RBCs may produce sudden hyperkalemia with cardiac arrhythmias, which may not be corrected quickly enough by the HD procedure. This risk is diminished by washing packed RBCs prior to the procedure. Alternatively, one may prime the circuit with saline and transfuse RBCs peripherally at a slower rate. This may prevent instability from rapid transfusion, but the patient develops a dilu-tional anemia and must be closely monitored dur-ing HD. The long-term consequence of transfusion is that of potential antigen exposure, which will complicate future renal transplantation in patients who do not regain renal function. The risk of sen-sitization to antigens is multiplied by the number of HD treatments required, as each will require a separate blood prime.

Dialyzers of all types have been used in children; no pediatric data suggest an advantage of one type of membrane, although studies in adults suggest a benefit of biocompatible membranes on survival and recovery of ARF.[55-57] There are few choices in small dialyzers (surface area less than 0.4 m² and priming volume less than 40 ml) and their availability changes often.

Vascular access remains a challenge in pediatric dialysis; blood vessels in young children only sup-port small-caliber catheters, which may produce suboptimal blood flow rates and are prone to kink-ing. Typically, acute HD is performed with a per-cutaneously placed double-lumen dialysis catheter, ranging from 7F to 12F, although surgical placement is often necessary. Guidelines for catheter size and site are given in Table 27.2.[58] Triple-lumen catheters intended for infusion are not appropriate vascular accesses for hemodialysis because of their flexibility, length, and small lumen size.

Prospective trials to determine the adequacy of acute HD in children with ARF are lacking. Since the causes of ARF are quite different from those in adults, extrapolation from that literature is of lim-ited utility. Thus, the duration, frequency, and effi-ciency of the hemodialysis treatments are a matter of judgment, aided by an understanding of kinetic modeling and of the modifiable variables (blood flow, dialysate flow).[54] Often, a single metabolic derangement (e.g. intoxication, hyperammonemia) defines the length and efficiency of the treatment. Since acute presentations of previously unrecog-nized chronic renal failure often result in PICU

Table 27.2	Vascular access recommendations for the pediatric patient.	
Patient size	**Catheter size**[a]	**Access site**
Neonate	Umbilical artery catheter 3.5–5.0F or Umbilical vein catheter 5.0–8.5F or	Umbilical vessels
	5.0F single-lumen catheter or 7.0F dual-lumen catheter	Femoral vein
5–15 kg	7.0F dual-lumen catheter	Femoral/subclavian vein
16–30 kg	9.0F dual-lumen catheter	Femoral/subclavian/internal jugular vein
>30 kg	11.0F dual-lumen catheter	Femoral/internal jugular/subclavian vein

Source: adapted from Bunchman and Donckerwolcke.[58]

[a]Cather sizes in French (F): 1F = 0.33 mm.

dialysis treatments, it is important to recognize the implications of advanced uremia. Urea clearances in small children may be surprisingly rapid, even when standard dialyzers are used, and true dysequilibrium syndrome or seizures may occur.[59,60] Blood flow rate for the first few treatments may be decreased to target urea clearance of 2–3 ml/kg/min and treatment length will usually be shortened to 1½–2 hours to avoid precipitous falls in blood urea nitrogen.[59,61]

Bicarbonate-based dialysate is the standard for HD in children; during efficient treatments with acetate dialysate, acetate levels rise, resulting in transient acid–base disturbances and potentially less stable treatments.[62] Ultrafiltration must be performed slowly, as it may cause hemodynamic instability in small children.

Most hemodialysis procedures are performed with anticoagulation, particularly since blood flow is often low, increasing the risk of clotting. Systemic heparinization is the most common, with empiric doses scaled to body size (load 10–30 units/kg, maintenance 10–20 units/kg/h) and then adjusted according to activated clotting times (ACT), targeting approximately 150–180% of control for standard heparinization and 125–150% of control for tight heparinization in patients at high risk of bleeding.[63] Alternative strategies for maintaining circuit patency include:

- saline flushes without other anticoagulation
- regional heparinization with protamine reversal
- low-dose heparin
- regional citrate anticoagulation.

Hemodialysis for nonrenal failure indication – inborn errors of metabolism

Hemodialysis prescription considerations are somewhat different when children are dialyzed for nonrenal failure indications such as hyperammonemia, branched-chain amino acids or other inborn errors of metabolism. In this situation, neuronal damage occurs as a result of prolonged exposure to toxic metabolite levels and rapid clearance is of paramount importance to improve neurologic outcome; dialysis therapy must be started without delay. A well-functioning vascular access is essential because blood flow rates as high as 10–15 ml/kg/min may be needed.[37,64] There is no concern for dialysis dysequilibrium to limit therapy; however, such patients are critically ill and often volume depleted if there has been preceding lethargy, poor intake, or vomiting. Hypokalemia and metabolic alkalosis will develop unless dialysate potassium and bicarbonate are adjusted. Phosphorus levels can be expected to fall and supplementation may be required.[53] Metabolite levels are monitored through treatment and dictate the duration, efficiency, and frequency of hemodialysis sessions. Rebound and ongoing production of metabolites following hemodialysis should be anticipated and appropriate conservative therapies should be started immediately. CRRTs have also been used successfully alone and in conjunction with HD to control the rebound metabolite levels.[36,64,65]

Continuous renal replacement therapy

CRRT has certain advantages over other forms of dialysis in children requiring renal replacement therapy. The potential for adsorptive removal of cytokines such as tumor necrosis factor-α (TNF-α) and interleukin-1β (IL-1β) is of theoretical benefit in multiorgan system failure, although that represents only a fraction of children who receive RRT.[66] On a more practical level, CRRT permits gradual, predictable, and efficient correction of hypervolemia and uremia. The predictability of CRRT contrasts with the clearance provided by PD, although there are few direct comparison studies. In one single-center experience of children recovering from repair of congenital heart disease, patients who received CRRT had more successful fluid removal and solute clearance and improved calorie intake compared to those treated with PD.[28] There does not appear to be an absolute lower limit to patient size for CRRT, and it has been performed in neonates and infants at a variety of centers.[36,64-68] In addition to ARF, CRRT has a particular role in the management of tumor lysis syndrome, permitting the correction of hyperphosphatemia without the rebound phenomenon typical of acute hemodialysis, as well as providing ongoing clearance as cell lysis continues.[30,69]

Within the past decade more sophisticated CRRT machines have been developed which are capable of providing precise ultrafiltration control, thermal control, and a variety of blood flow rates appropriate for infants through adolescents. Many machines are now available with pediatric blood lines and hemofilters. These technical advances have contributed to the increasing use of CRRT in the management of childhood ARF. These more sophisticated machines offer a wide range of therapeutic options: slow continuous ultrafiltration (SCUF), continuous venovenous hemofiltration (CVVH), continuous venovenous hemodialysis (CVVHD), or continuous venovenous hemodiafiltration (CVVHDF) with some machines having the added flexibility for use in conventional hemodial-

ysis. A more complete discussion of CRRTs is found in Chapter 14.

SCUF has been used in children after repair of congenital heart disease, where isolated fluid removal is required, and in diuretic-resistant hypervolemia.[70] Since neither dialysate nor replacement fluid is provided, electrolyte disturbances are possible if large ultrafiltration volume is replaced with standard intravenous fluids or parenteral nutrition.[61] Further, hypothermia may occur if warmed dialysate or replacement fluid is not used. In-line blood warmers are usually available, but they add significantly to the volume of the extracorporeal circuit.

Continuous arteriovenous hemofiltration (CAVH) is well tolerated in hemodynamically unstable children and offers the advantages of technical simplicity, low priming volume, and gradual fluid removal.[28,29,67,70,71] However, it requires both arterial and venous vascular access. In the neonate, the umbilical vessels or the femoral vessels may be cannulated; in older children, the choices are much wider. Adequate blood flow rates have been reported, with mean arterial pressures greater than 40 mmHg.[58] Some form of anticoagulation is required to maintain circuit patency. Incorporation of a pump into the circuit to provide more consistent blood flow or ultrafiltration has also been reported.[72,73]

CVVH, CVVHD, and CVVHDF are now the most common of the continuous modalities used in children. It appears safer to avoid arterial catheter placement and its associated risks of bleeding, thrombosis, and limb ischemia with potential impaired future limb growth. Incorporation of a blood pump into the circuit increases the extracorporeal circuit volume and complexity of the procedure but also allows greater consistency in blood flow rate delivery.[74] Modern machines include software interfaces to assist bedside nurses in correcting problems as they arise and maintaining continuous therapy; the procedure can be independent of hemodialysis staff.

Technical considerations

Maintaining vascular access for CRRT raises the same concerns as noted above in hemodialysis and the same lines and sites are used. As in acute hemodialysis, one attempts to limit the total volume of the extracorporeal circuit to 10% of blood volume, or else one primes the circuit with RBCs. When using a blood prime in conjunction with an AN-69 membrane a potentially fatal syndrome of bradykinin release has been reported, with hypotension, tachycardia, vasodilatation, and anaphylaxis within minutes of CRRT initiation.[75]

Strategies for anticoagulation are similar to those used in adults, as detailed in Chapter 12. Many centers have developed a preference for the use of heparin or citrate anticoagulation, although both have been used in children. Heparin anticoagulation is performed, as noted above, with a bolus dose and infusion rate determined by weight, and is monitored by ACT. In one large series, heparin was more commonly used in the smallest children.[68]

The use of regional citrate anticoagulation in pediatrics has been increasing.[76,77] Complications of citrate infusion in children are the result of relatively smaller body mass. In particular, metabolic alkalosis typically arises after 7 days of therapy because the rate of citrate infusion is proportional to the blood flow rate, which is relatively higher in children than in adults.[77] Hypomagnesemia occurs from citrate chelation. Hypernatremia often occurs, particularly when trisodium citrate (4% solution) is used. Anticoagulant citrate dextrose-A (ACD-A: sodium citrate, anhydrous citrate, and dextrose) may be less likely to cause hypernatremia, but the dextrose concentration of 2.45% can cause hyperglycemia in infants and small children. Citrate accumulation (or 'citrate lock') occurs when the infusion rate exceeds hepatic metabolism and clearance and will result in falling ionized calcium despite rising total serum calcium.

A small minority of CRRT procedures can be performed without anticoagulation.[68] There are no published data regarding the use of low molecular weight heparin or hirudin in children on CRRT. Argatroban anticoagulation has been reported in two neonates undergoing extracorporeal membrane oxygenation (ECMO).[78]

Dialysate solutions intended for use with CRRT are available with a choice of lactate or bicarbonate buffer. PD fluid is no longer a standard or desirable choice for dialysate with CRRT; pharmacy-based 'custom-made' dialysate solutions are still used but are less desirable now that industry-manufactured bicarbonate solutions are readily available and not associated with the risk of formulation errors. While a survival advantage of bicarbonate- over lactate-based solutions has not been demonstrated in children with ARF, improved hemodynamic stability and lower lactate levels are seen in CRRT with bicarbonate-based solution.[79]

Guidelines for pediatric CRRT prescription are based upon small published series, extrapolation from adult literature, and individual center experience. Blood flows of 3–21 ml/kg/min in infants and 3–10 ml/kg/min in children have been reported, considerably greater than that used in adults and similar to that used in hemodialysis procedures.[58,68,74] Not surprisingly, once adequate vascular access is achieved, all forms of CRRT are very efficient in small children. Dialysate flow rate generally ranges from 10 to 20 ml/min/m² and is similar to the rate of 2 L/1.73 m²/h used for adults. The rate of fluid removal on CRRT is based upon hemodynamic stability, and there are no firm guidelines; children on multiple vasopressors can receive CRRT.[68] There are no prospective pediatric data indicating that one modality (CVVH vs CVVHD vs CVVHDF) is superior to another. Small molecular weight solutes are removed equally well with continuous hemofiltration and continuous hemodialysis. However, larger molecular weight solutes are cleared better with hemofiltration than hemodialysis; the clinical relevance of this in unclear.[80]

There are a few complications of CRRT which are of particular concern in children. Although the continuous treatment is hemodynamically better tolerated than intermittent hemodialysis, hypotension still occurs particularly at the initiation of therapy when the extracorporeal circuit volume is large relative to the patient's circulating blood volume or when excessive fluid is removed. Unpredictable and excessive fluid removal was a concern in the past when pediatric CRRT was performed using adaptive machinery; the infusion pumps used to measure dialysate and ultrafiltration were often inaccurate, especially at high volumes.[58,74,81] Newer, more sophisticated CRRT machines contain integrated, precise scales or pumps which reduce errors in fluid balance.

Dialysis dysequilibrium, a serious metabolic complication in uremic children beginning intermittent hemodialysis, generally does not occur with continuous therapies because solute removal occurs more slowly; nonetheless, it remains a theoretical risk in a small child with prolonged azotemia treated with high blood and dialysate flow rates. Other metabolic complications can be anticipated with CRRT. Phosphate clearance will result in hypophosphatemia requiring replacement. Glucose-containing replacement fluids may result in hyperglycemia in small children, requiring insulin therapy. In addition, amino acid losses on CRRT may be significant and contribute to negative nitrogen balance.[82] Maintaining positive nitrogen balance may require much higher protein intake (up to 3–4 g/kg/day), although this has not yet been demonstrated to be successful. The potential catabolic complications of pediatric CRRT require further research.

CRRT has been used successfully with extracorporeal membrane oxygenation (ECMO).[83,84] Hypervolemia and ARF are well-recognized complications of ECMO, and CRRT has become an important addition when diuretic therapy alone is insufficient for fluid removal. A hemofilter can be incorporated into the ECMO circuit without the need for additional vascular access or anticoagulation.[83,84] Careful consideration needs to be given to positioning of the hemofilter within the ECMO circuit to minimize blood recirculation and shunting away from the oxygenator.[85] If needed, dialysate can be added to the system to allow continuous hemodialysis and/or hemodiafiltration.

HYPERTENSION IN THE PEDIATRIC INTENSIVE CARE UNIT

Children with hypertensive crisis are usually managed in an ICU setting. Complications such as encephalopathy, seizures, cerebrovascular accidents, and heart failure can occur at blood pressures (BP) much lower than those seen in adults. The likelihood of developing symptomatic hypertension depends on the duration of elevated BP as well as the severity. Normal children with acute disease may manifest malignant hypertension at blood pressures only modestly greater than the 99th percentile (Table 27.3), while those with long-standing unrecognized disease may tolerate extremely elevated BP without symptoms.[86] Recognizing hypertensive infants is a particular challenge because they exhibit nonspecific symptoms: irritability, poor feeding, failure to thrive, emesis, lethargy, seizures, tachypnea, and congestive heart failure.[87] Older children and adolescents may have more classic symptoms such as headaches, visual disturbances, epistaxis, emesis, or chest pain.

Renal parenchymal disease and renovascular disease are the most common causes of hypertensive crisis in children. The former may result from APIGN, HUS, polycystic kidney disease, reflux nephropathy, obstructive uropathy, trauma, or acute or chronic renal failure. Renovascular disease is usually the result of fibromuscular dysplasia, although extrinsic compression from an abdominal mass can occur. Aortic coarctation is usually seen in infants and toddlers. A wide range of other diseases can present in childhood with severe hypertension and are listed in Box 27.2. The etiology of hypertension may be suggested by pertinent aspects of history or physical examination. Blood pressures should be checked in both arms and one leg to screen for aortic coarctation; a discrepancy of 20 mmHg between the right arm and another extremity is highly suggestive. Echocardiography definitively evaluates the thoracic aorta. Renal ultrasonography is done early in the evaluation because of the predominance of renal parenchymal and structural disease. However, if renovascular disease is suspected, angiography remains the gold standard; vascular lesions are

Table 27.3 Severe hypertension in children.		
Age	**Severe HTN systolic BP**	**Severe HTN diastolic BP**
Newborn (<7 days)	≥ 106	
Newborn (8–30 days)	≥ 110	
Infant (<2 years)	≥ 118	≥ 82
Child (3–5 years)	≥ 124	≥ 84
Child (6–9 years)	≥ 130	≥ 86
Child (10–12 years)	≥ 134	≥ 90
Adolescents (13–15 years)	≥ 144	≥ 92
Adolescents (16–18 years)	≥ 150	≥ 98

Source: Values reported correspond to the 99% for age and sex combined and are based on data from the Report of the Second Task Force on Blood Pressure Control in Children.[86]

BP = blood pressure (in mmHg); HTN = hypertension.

<table>
<tr><td colspan="2">

Box 27.2   Etiologies of hypertensive crises in children

</td></tr>
</table>

Renal disease

Glomerulonephritis

Reflux nephropathy

Obstructive uropathy

Hemolytic uremic syndrome

Polycystic kidney disease, autosomal dominant and recessive

Acute renal failure

Liddle syndrome

Renovascular disease

Fibromuscular disease

Systemic vasculitis

Renal trauma (Page kidney)

Neurofibromatosis

Williams syndrome

Renal artery thrombosis

Extrinsic compression by abdominal mass

Cardiovascular disease

Coarctation of the aorta

Mid-aortic syndrome

Endocrine disease

Congenital adrenal hyperplasia

Hyperthyroidism

Cushing's syndrome

Pheochromocytoma

Glucocorticoid therapy

Mineralocorticoid disturbance

• Dexamethasone-suppressible hyperaldosteronism

• Apparent mineralocorticoid excess

Neurologic disease

Elevated intracranial pressure

Tumors

Wilms tumor

Neuroblastoma

Miscellaneous

Drugs – e.g. cocaine, amfetamines

Traction-induced hypertension

Rebound after withdrawal of antihypertensives

often located in intrarenal branch arteries and cannot be adequately detected by Doppler ultrasonography, magnetic resonance angiography, or radionuclide studies.[88] Measures of renin and aldosterone, cortisol, thyroid hormone, plasma and urine catecholamines, and specialized imaging studies are obtained when clinically indicated.

When malignant hypertension is present, immediate lowering of BP is most safely accomplished with a parenteral, titratable agent. Recognizing that long-standing severe hypertension affects cerebral autoregulation in children as well as adults, one avoids precipitous declines in BP with the risk of cerebral ischemia; gradual BP reduction with medications administered by continuous infusion over 3–4 days is less likely to cause neurologic deficits when compared to bolus therapy.[89] An initial decline of systolic BP by 10–20% may be sufficient to control symptoms in chronic hypertension, whereas acute hypertension may require a greater reduction; further gradual decline over the next 12–24 hours can be planned.

Parenteral agents for hypertensive emergencies are the same as those used in adults, including sodium nitroprusside, nicardipine, and labetalol. Published pediatric experience with fenoldopam is limited.[90] Bolus doses of diazoxide have been used frequently in the past; however, it can cause an abrupt, unpredictable drop in BP, which increases the risk for ischemic complications, so other agents are preferred. Medications used to treat hypertensive urgencies and emergencies are given in Table 27.4.[91] Oral nifedipine can cause an unpredictable decline in BP, although the cardiac complications seen in adults have not been reported in children.[92] ACE inhibitors may be particularly effective when renovascular hypertension is present, although patients with bilateral disease may be exquisitely sensitive to ACE inhibition and at increased risk for developing ARF. Neonates are normally hyper-reninemic and renal perfusion may be dependent upon angiotensin II tone, so one starts with low initial doses of ACE inhibitors.

CONCLUSION

A broad array of diseases draw nephrologists into the care of PICU patients. The range of diagnoses is quite distinct from that seen in adults and varies from industrialized to nonindustrialized countries. Pediatric nephrologists must recognize common and rare syndromes in these critically ill children. The full extent of RRT available in adults has been

Table 27.4   Antihypertensive therapy for pediatric hypertensive crisis.

Drug	Route	Dose	Onset of action	Duration
Sodium nitroprusside	IV	0.5–8 µg/kg/min	Within seconds	Seconds to minutes
Nicardipine	IV	1–3 µg/kg/min	Within minutes	~ 10–15 minutes
Labetalol	IV	0.5–3 mg/kg/hour	5–10 minutes	2–3 hours
Hydralazine	IV	0.1–0.5 mg/kg	10–30 minutes	4–12 hours
Esmolol	IV	50–300 µg/kg/min	Within seconds	10–20 minutes
Enalaprilat	IV	0.005–0.01 mg/kg/dose q 8–24 hours	Within 15 minutes	12–24 hours
Nifedipine	PO	0.25–0.5 mg/kg	Within 20–30 minutes	Up to 6 hours

Source: adapted from Adelman et al.[91]

applied in children, although important technical modifications are made to accommodate patients of widely varying size. Certain diseases present unique challenges in providing dialysis clearance, either because of the toxic solute or the coincident medical complications. The field of pediatric ICU nephrology is expanding as technical advances are applied more widely and studied more comprehensively.

REFERENCES

1. Mendley SR, Langman CB. Acute renal failure in the pediatric patient. Adv Ren Replace Ther 1997;4:S93–101.
2. Flynn JT. Causes, management approaches, and outcome of acute renal failure in children. Curr Opin Pediatr 1998;10:184–9.
3. Maxvold NJ, Smoyer WE, Gardner JJ, et al. Management of acute renal failure in the pediatric patient: hemofiltration versus hemodialysis. Am J Kidney Dis Suppl 1997;4:S84–8.
4. Ellis EN, Arnold WC. Use of urinary indexes in renal failure in the newborn. Am J Dis Child 1982;136:615–17.
5. Rosenthal W, Seibold A, Antaramian A, et al. Molecular identification of the gene responsible for congenital nephrogenic diabetes insipidus. Nature 1992;359:233–5.
6. Saborio P, Tipton GA, Chan JC. Diabetes insipidus. Pediatr Rev 2000;21:122–9.
7. Pickering LK, Obrig TG, Stapleton FB. Hemolytic-uremic syndrome and enterohemorrhagic Escherichia coli. Pediatr Infect Dis J 1994;13:459–76.
8. Kaplan BS, Meyers KE, Schulman SL. The pathogenesis and treatment of hemolytic uremic syndrome. J Am Soc Nephrol 1998;9:1126–33.
9. Tarr PI, Neill MA. Perspective: the problem of non-O157:H7 shiga toxin (Verocytotoxin)-producing Escherichia coli. J Infect Dis 1996;174:1136–9.
10. Koster F, Levin J, Walker L, et al. Hemolytic-uremic syndrome after shigellosis. Relation to endotoxemia and circulating immune complexes. N Engl J Med 1978;298:927–33.
11. Bell BP, Goldoft M, Griffin PM, et al. A multistate outbreak of Escherichia coli O157:H7-associated bloody diarrhea and hemolytic uremic syndrome from hamburgers. The Washington experience. JAMA 1994;272:1340–53.
12. Besser RE, Lett SM, Weber JT, et al. An outbreak of diarrhea and hemolytic uremic syndrome from Escherichia coli O157:H7 in fresh-pressed apple cider. JAMA 1993;269:2217–20.
13. Siegler RL. Spectrum of extrarenal involvement in postdiarrheal hemolytic-uremic syndrome. J Pediatr 1994;125:511–18.
14. Repetto HA. Epidemic hemolytic-uremic syndrome in children. Kidney Int 1997;52:1708–19.
15. Wong CS, Jelacic S, Habeeb RL, et al. The risk of hemolytic-uremic syndrome after antibiotic treatment of Escherichia coli O157:H7 infections. N Engl J Med 2000;342:1930–6.
16. Cimolai N, Carter JE, Morrison BJ, et al. Risk factors for the progression of Escherichia coli O157:H7 enteritis to hemolytic-uremic syndrome. J Pediatr 1990;116:589–92.
17. Trachtman H, Cnaan A, Christen E, et al. Effect of an oral Shiga toxin-binding agent on diarrhea-associated hemolytic uremic syndrome in children: a randomized controlled trial. JAMA 2003;290:1337–44.
18. Ruggenenti P, Noris M, Remuzzi G. Thrombotic microangiopathy, hemolytic uremic syndrome, and thrombotic thrombocytopenic purpura. Kidney Int 2001;60:831–46.
19. Cabrera GR, Fortenberry JD, Warshaw BL, et al. Hemolytic uremic syndrome associated with invasive Streptococcus pneumoniae infection. Pediatrics 1998;101:699–703.
20. McGraw ME, Lendon M, Stevens RF, Postlethwaite RJ, Taylor CM. Haemolytic uraemic syndrome and the Thomsen Friedenreich antigen. Pediatr Nephrol 1989;3:135–9 .
21. Proulx F, Fayon M, Farrell CA, et al. Epidemiology of sepsis and multiple organ dysfunction syndrome in children. Chest 1996;109:1033–7.
22. Smith JD, Hayslett JP. Reversible renal failure in the nephrotic syndrome. Am J Kidney Dis 1992;19:201–13.
23. Koomans HA. Pathophysiology of acute renal failure in idiopathic nephrotic syndrome. Nephrol Dial Transplant 2001;16:221–4.
24. Varade WS, McEnery PT, McAdams AJ. Prolonged reversible renal failure with nephrotic syndrome. Pediatr Nephrol 1991;5:685–9.
25. Sakarcan A, Timmons C, Seikaly MG. Reversible idiopathic acute renal failure in children with primary nephrotic syndrome. J Pediatr 1994;125:723–7.
26. Giuffre RM, Tam KH, Williams WW, et al. Acute renal failure complicating pediatric cardiac surgery: a comparison of survivors and nonsurvivors following acute peritoneal dialysis. Pediatr Cardiol 1992;13:208–13.

27. Dittrich S, Dahnert I, Vogel M, et al. Peritoneal dialysis after infant open heart surgery: observations in 27 patients. Ann Thorac Surg 1999;68:160–3.
28. Fleming F, Bohn D, Edwards H, et al. Renal replacement therapy after repair of congenital heart disease in children. A comparison of hemofiltration and peritoneal dialysis. J Thorac Cardiovasc Surg 1995;109:322–31.
29. Paret G, Cohen AJ, Bohn DJ, et al. Continuous arteriovenous hemofiltration after cardiac operations in infants and children. J Thorac Cardiovasc Surg 1992;104:1225–30.
30 Sakarcan A, Quigley R. Hyperphosphatemia in tumor lysis syndrome: the role of hemodialysis and continuous veno-venous hemofiltration. Pediatr Nephro 1994;8:351–3.
31. Pui CH, Jeha S, Irwin D, et al. Recombinant urate oxidase (rasburicase) in the prevention and treatment of malignancy-associated hyperuricemia in pediatric and adult patients: results of a compassionate-use trial. Leukemia 2001;15:1505–9.
32. Wossmann W, Schrappe M, Meyer U, et al. Incidence of tumor lysis syndrome in children with advanced stage Burkitt's lymphoma/leukemia before and after introduction of prophylactic use of urate oxidase. Ann Hematol 2003;82:160–5.
33. A clinico-pathologic study of crescentic glomerulonephritis in 50 children. A report of the Southwest Pediatric Nephrology Study Group. Kidney Int 1985;27:450–8.
34. Roy S 3rd, Murphy WM, Arant BS Jr. Poststreptococcal crescenteric glomerulonephritis in children: comparison of quintuple therapy versus supportive care, J Pediatr 1981;98:403–10.
35. Cunningham RJ 3rd, Gilfoil M, Cavallo T, et al. Rapidly progressive glomerulonephritis in children: a report of thirteen cases and a review of the literature. Pediatr Res 1980;14(2):128–32.
36. Picca S, Dionisi-Vici C, Abeni D, et al. Extracorporeal dialysis in neonatal hyperammonemia: modalities and prognostic indicators. Pediatr Nephrol 2001;16:862–7.
37. Rutledge SL, Havens PL, Haymond MW, et al. Neonatal hemodialysis: effective therapy for the encephalopathy of inborn errors of metabolism. J Pediatr 1990;116:125–8.
38. Reznik VM, Griswold WR, Peterson BM, et al. Peritoneal dialysis for acute renal failure in children. Pediatr Nephrol 1991;5:715–7.
39. Flynn JT, Kershaw DB, Smoyer WE, et al. Peritoneal dialysis for management of pediatric acute renal failure. Perit Dial Int 2001;21:390–4.
40. Esperanca MJ, Collins DL. Peritoneal dialysis efficiency in relation to body weight. J Pediatr Surg 1966;1:162–9.
41. Reznik VM, Randolph G, Collins CM, et al. Cost analysis of dialysis modalities for pediatric acute renal failure. Perit Dial Int 1993;13:311–13.
42. Bunchman TE. Acute peritoneal dialysis access in infant renal failure. Perit Dial Int Suppl 1996;1:S509–11.
43. Day RE, White RH. Peritoneal dialysis in children. Review of 8 years' experience. Arch Dis Child 1977;52:56–61.
44. Stewart JH, Tuckwell LA, Sinnett PF, et al. Peritoneal and haemodialysis: a comparison of their morbidity, and of the mortality suffered by dialysed patients. Q J Med 1966;35:407–20.
45. Wong SN, Geary DF. Comparison of temporary and permanent catheters for acute peritoneal dialysis. Arch Dis Child 1988;63:827–31.
46. Wood EG, Lynch RE, Fleming SS, Bunchman TE. Ultrafiltration using low volume peritoneal dialysis in critically ill infants and children. Adv Perit Dial 1991;7:266–8.
47. Chadha V, Warady BA, Blowey DL, et al. Tenckhoff catheters prove superior to Cook catheters in pediatric acute peritoneal dialysis. Am J Kid Dis 2000;35:1111–16.
48. Alexander SR, Tank ES. Surgical aspects of continuous ambulatory peritoneal dialysis in infants, children, and adolescents. J Urol 1982;127:501–4.
49. Van de Walle J, Raes A, Castillo D, Lutz-Dettinger L, Dejaegher A. New perspectives for PD in acute renal failure related to new catheter techniques and introduction of APD. Adv Perit Dial 1997;13:190–4.
50. Donckerwolcke RA, Bunchman TE. Hemodialysis in infants and small children. Pediatr Nephrol 1994;8:103–6.
51. Sadowski RH, Harmon WE, Jabs K. Acute hemodialysis of infants weighing less than five kilograms. Kidney Int 1994;45:903–6.
52. Bock GH, Campos A, Thompson T, et al. Hemodialysis in the premature infant. Am J Dis Child 1981;135:178–80.
53. Wiegand C, Thompson T, Bock GH, et al. The management of life-threatening hyperammonemia: a comparison of several therapeutic modalities. J Pediatr 1980;96:142–4.
54. Sargent JA, Gotch FA. Mathematic modeling of dialysis therapy. Kidney Int Suppl 1980;10:S2–10.
55. Hakim RM, Wingard RL, Parker RA. Effect of the dialysis membrane in the treatment of patients with acute renal failure. N Engl J Med 1994;331:1338–42.
56. Himmelfarb J, Tolkoff Rubin N, Chandran P, et al. A multicenter comparison of dialysis membranes in the treatment of acute renal failure requiring dialysis. J Am Soc Nephrol 1998;9:257–66.
57. Schiffl H, Lang SM, Konig A, et al. Biocompatible membranes in acute renal failure: prospective case-controlled study. Lancet 1994;344:570–2.
58. Bunchman TE, Donckerwolcke RA. Continuous arterial-venous diahemofiltration and continuous veno-venous diahemofiltration in infants and children. Pediatr Nephrol 1994;8:96–102.
59. Arieff AI. Dialysis disequilibrium syndrome: current concepts on pathogenesis and prevention. Kidney Int 1994;45:629–35.
60. Grushkin CM, Korsch B, Fine RN. Hemodialysis in small children. JAMA 1972;221:869–73.
61. Parekh RS, Bunchman TE. Dialysis support in the pediatric intensive care unit. Adv Ren Replace Ther 1996;3:326–36.
62. Kaiser BA, Potter DE, Bryant RE, et al. Acid–base changes and acetate metabolism during routine and high-efficiency hemodialysis in children. Kidney Int 1981;19:70–9.
63. Geary DF, Gajaria M, Fryer-Keene S, et al. Low-dose and heparin-free hemodialysis in children. Pediatr Nephrol 1991;5:220–4.
64. Schaefer F, Straube E, Oh J, et al. Dialysis in neonates with inborn errors of metabolism. Nephrol Dial Transplant 1999;14:910–18.
65. Falk MC, Knight JF, Roy LP, et al. Continuous venovenous haemofiltration in the acute treatment of inborn errors of metabolism. Pediatr Nephrol 1994;8:330–3.
66. De Vriese AS, Colardyn FA, Philippe JJ, et al. Cytokine removal during continuous hemofiltration in septic patients. J Am Soc Nephrol 1999;10:846–53.
67. Zobel G, Rodl S, Urlesberger B, et al. Continuous renal replacement therapy in critically ill neonates. Kidney Int Suppl 1998;66:S169–73.
68. Symons JM, Brophy PD, Gregory MJ, et al. Continuous renal replacement therapy in children up to 10 kg. Am J Kidney Dis 2003;41:984–9.
69. Saccente SL, Kohaut EC, Berkow RL. Prevention of tumor lysis syndrome using continuous veno-venous hemofiltration. Pediatr Nephrol 1995;9:569–73.
70. Zobel G, Stein JI, Kuttnig M, et al. Continuous extracorporeal fluid removal in children with low cardiac output after cardiac operations. J Thorac Cardiovasc Surg 1991;101:593–7.
71. Ronco C, Parenzan L. Acute renal failure in infancy: treatment by continuous renal replacement therapy. Intensive Care Med 1995;21:490–9.
72. Ellis EN, Pearson D, Belsha CW, et al. Use of pump-assisted hemofiltration in children with acute renal failure. Pediatr Nephrol 1997;11:196–200.
73. Chanard J, Milcent T, Toupance O, et al. Ultrafiltration-pump assisted continuous arteriovenous hemofiltration (CAVH). Kidney Int Suppl 1988;24:S157–8.

74. Bunchman TE, Maxvold NJ, Kershaw DB, et al. Continuous venovenous hemodiafiltration in infants and children. Am J Kidney Dis 1995;25:17–21.

75. Brophy PD, Mottes TA, Kudelka TL, et al. AN-69 membrane reactions are pH-dependent and preventable. Am J Kidney Dis 2001;38:173–8.

76. Mehta RL, McDonald BR, Aguilar MM, et al. Regional citrate anticoagulation for continuous arteriovenous hemodialysis in critically ill patients. Kidney Int 1990;38:976–81.

77. Bunchman TE, Maxvold NJ, Barnett J, Hutchings A, Benfield MR. Pediatric hemofiltration: Normocarb dialysate solution with citrate anticoagulation. Pediatr Nephrol 2002;17:150–4.

78. Kawada T, Kitagawa H, Hoson M, Okada Y, Shiomura J. Clinical application of Argatroban as an alternative anticoagulant for extracorporeal circulation. Hematol Oncol Clin North Am 2000;14:445–57.

79. Maxvold NJ, Flynn JT, Smoyer WE, et al. Prospective, crossover comparison of bicarbonate versus lactate-based dialysate for pediatric CVVHD. Blood Purif 1999;17:27.

80. Jeffrey RF, Khan AA, Prabhu P, et al. A comparison of molecular clearance rates during continuous hemofiltration and hemodialysis with a novel volumetric continuous renal replacement system. Artif Organs 1994;18:425–8.

81. Jenkins R, Harrison H, Chen B, et al. Accuracy of intravenous infusion pumps in continuous renal replacement therapies. ASAIO J 1992;38:808–10.

82. Maxvold NJ, Smoyer WE, Custer JR, et al. Amino acid loss and nitrogen balance in critically ill children with acute renal failure: a prospective comparison between classic hemofiltration and hemofiltration with dialysis. Crit Care Med 2000;28:1161–5.

83. Sell LL, Cullen ML, Whittlesey GC, et al. Experience with renal failure during extracorporeal membrane oxygenation: treatment with continuous hemofiltration. J Pediatr Surg 1987;22:600–2.

84. Heiss KF, Pettit B, Hirschl RB, et al. Renal insufficiency and volume overload in neonatal ECMO managed by continuous ultrafiltration. ASAIO Trans 1987;33:557–60.

85. Yorgin PD, Kirpekar R, Rhine WD. Where should the hemofiltration circuit be placed in relation to the extracorporeal membrane oxygenation circuit? ASAIO J 1992;38:801–3.

86. Report of the Second Task Force on Blood Pressure Control in Children – 1987. Task Force on Blood Pressure Control in Children. National Heart, Lung, and Blood Institute, Bethesda, Maryland. Pediatrics 1987;79:1–25.

87. Adelman RD. The hypertensive neonate. Clin Perinatol 1988;15:567–85.

88. Deal JE, Snell MF, Barratt TM, et al. Renovascular disease in childhood. J Pediatr 1992;121:378–84.

89. Deal JE, Barratt TM, Dillon MJ. Management of hypertensive emergencies. Arch Dis Child 1992;67:1089–92.

90. Strauser LM, Pruitt RD, Tobias JD. Initial experience with fenoldopam in children. Am J Ther 1999;6(5):283–8.

91. Adelman RD, Coppo R, Dillon MJ. The emergency management of severe hypertension. Pediatr Nephrol 2000;14:422–7.

92. Blaszak RT, Savage JA, Ellis EN. The use of short-acting nifedipine in pediatric patients with hypertension. J Pediatr 2001;139:34–7.

Index

Note: Page references in *italics* refer to tables or boxes, where these do not occur within page ranges; those in **bold** refer to figures